DSM-IV Sourcebook

Volume 1

DSM-IV Sourcebook

Volume 1

Edited by

Thomas A. Widiger, Ph.D.
Allen J. Frances, M.D.
Harold Alan Pincus, M.D.
Michael B. First, M.D.
Ruth Ross, M.A.
Wendy Davis, Ed.M.

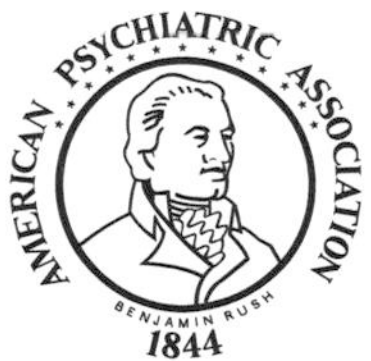

Published by the American Psychiatric Association
Washington, DC

Note: The authors have worked to ensure that all information in this book concerning drug dosages, schedules, and routes of administration is accurate as of the time of publication and consistent with standards set by the U.S. Food and Drug Administration and the general medical community. As medical research and practice advance, however, therapeutic standards may change. For this reason and because human and mechanical errors sometimes occur, we recommend that readers follow the advice of a physician who is directly involved in their care or the care of a member of their family.

The findings, opinions, and conclusions of this report do not necessarily represent the views of the officers, trustees, all members of the task force, or all members of the American Psychiatric Association. The views expressed are those of the authors of the individual chapters. Task force reports are considered a substantive contribution of the ongoing analysis and evaluation of problems, programs, issues, and practices in a given area of concern.

Manufactured in the United States of America on acid-free paper
First Edition
97 96 95 94 4 3 2 1
American Psychiatric Association
1400 K Street, N.W., Washington, DC 20005

Library of Congress Cataloging-in-Publication Data
DSM-IV sourcebook. — 1st ed.
p. cm.
Developed by the DSM-IV Task Force of American Psychiatric Association.
Includes bibliographic references and index.
ISBN 0-89042-065-3
1. Diagnostic and statistical manual of mental disorders.
2. Mental illness—Classification. 3. Mental illness—Diagnosis.
I. American Psychiatric Association. Task Force on DSM-IV.
II. Title: DSM-IV sourcebook.
[DNLM: 1. Mental Disorders—classification. 2. Psychiatry—nomenclature. WM 15 D277 1994]
RC455.2.C4D754 1994
616.89′075—dc20
DNLM/DLC
for Library of Congress 93-48304
CIP

British Library Cataloguing in Publication Data
A CIP record is available from the British Library.

Contents

SECTION II

DELIRIUM, DEMENTIA, AND AMNESTIC AND OTHER COGNITIVE DISORDERS

SECTION III

SCHIZOPHRENIA AND OTHER PSYCHOTIC DISORDERS

Section IV
Medication-Induced Movement Disorders

Section V
Sleep Disorders

Contributors

Gerard Addonizio, M.D. Associate Professor of Clinical Psychiatry, The New York Hospital–Cornell Medical Center, White Plains, New York

Lenard A. Adler, M.D. Associate Professor of Clinical Psychiatry, New York University School of Medicine, and Staff Psychiatrist, New York Veterans Affairs Medical Center, New York, New York

Nancy Andreasen, M.D., Ph.D. Andrew H. Woods Professor, Department of Psychiatry, College of Medicine; Director, Mental Health Clinical Research Center, The University of Iowa Hospitals and Clinics, Iowa City, Iowa

Burt Angrist, M.D. Professor of Psychiatry, New York University School of Medicine, and Staff Psychiatrist, New York Veterans Affairs Medical Center, New York, New York

J. Hampton Atkinson, M.D. Adjunct Professor, Department of Psychiatry, University of California, San Diego, California

Stephen Brown, M.D. Assistant Clinical Professor, University of California, San Diego, HIV Neurobehavioral Research Center, San Diego, California

Daniel J. Buysse, M.D. Assistant Professor of Psychiatry, University of Pittsburgh Medical Center, Sleep and Chronobiology Center, Pittsburgh, Pennsylvania

John Cacciola, Ph.D. Research Assistant Professor of Psychology and Psychiatry, University of Pennsylvania, Philadelphia VA Medical Center, Philadelphia, Pennsylvania

Eric D. Caine, M.D. Professor of Psychiatry and Neurology and Associate Chairman for Academic Affairs, University of Rochester Medical Center, Rochester, New York

Daniel E. Casey, M.D. Chief, Psychiatry Research and Psychopharmacology, Veterans Affairs Medical Center; Professor of Psychiatry and Associate Professor of Neurology, Oregon Health Sciences University, Portland; Collaborative Scientist, Oregon Regional Primate Research Center, Beaverton, Oregon

Patricia A. Coble, R.N. Assistant Professor of Psychiatry, Co-Director of Sleep Evaluation Center, University of Pittsburgh, Western Psychiatric Institute, Pittsburgh, Pennsylvania

Thomas J. Crowley, M.D. Professor of Psychiatry, University of Colorado Medical School, Denver, Colorado

Wendy Davis, Ed.M. Editorial Coordinator, DSM-IV

Amy Fasiczka, B.A. Research Associate, University of Pittsburgh, Western Psychiatric Institute and Clinic, Pittsburgh, Pennsylvania

Wayne S. Fenton, M.D. Director of Research, Chestnut Lodge Research Institute, Rockville, Maryland

Michael B. First, M.D. Assistant Professor of Clinical Psychiatry, Columbia University, New York, New York

Marian W. Fischman, Ph.D. Professor of Behavioral Biology, Department of Psychiatry, College of Physicians and Surgeons, Columbia University, New York, New York

Michael Flaum, M.D. Assistant Professor, Department of Psychiatry, The University of Iowa, and Co-Director, Mental Health Research Center, Iowa City, Iowa

Marshal F. Folstein, M.D. Chairman, Department of Psychiatry, New England Medical Center Hospital, Boston, Massachusetts

Allen J. Frances, M.D. Chairman, Department of Psychiatry, Duke University Medical Center, Durham, North Carolina; Chair, Task Force on DSM-IV, American Psychiatric Association, Washington, DC

Alan J. Gelenberg, M.D. Professor and Head, Department of Psychiatry, University of Arizona Health Sciences Center, Tucson, Arizona

Gary L. Gottlieb, M.D., M.B.A. Executive Vice Chairman, Department of Psychiatry, Associate Dean for Managed Care, University of Pennsylvania Medical Center, Philadelphia, Pennsylvania

Igor Grant, M.D. Professor and Vice Chairman, Department of Psychiatry, San Diego School of Medicine, University of California, San Diego, California

Rosben Gutierrez, M.D. Psychiatrist, Private Practice, Poway, California

John E. Helzer, M.D. Professor and Chairman, Department of Psychiatry, University of Vermont College of Medicine, Burlington, Vermont

John R. Hughes, M.D. Professor, Department of Psychiatry, University of Vermont College of Medicine, Burlington, Vermont

Michael R. Irwin, M.D. Associate Professor, Department of Psychiatry, Veterans Affairs Medical Center, University of California, San Diego, San Diego, California

James W. Jefferson, M.D. Distinguished Senior Scientist, Dean Foundation, and Clinical Professor of Psychiatry, University of Wisconsin Medical School, Madison, Wisconsin

Dilip V. Jeste, M.D. Professor of Psychiatry and Neurosciences, University of California, San Diego; Director, Geriatric Psychiatry Clinical Research Center, Veterans Affairs Medical Center, San Diego, California

Jerry C. Johnson, M.D. Associate Professor of Medicine, and Director, Geriatric Medicine Fellowship Program, University of Pennsylvania, Philadelphia, Pennsylvania

John Kane, M.D. Chairperson, Department of Psychiatry, Hillside Hospital, Long Island Jewish Medical Center, Glen Oaks, New York

Samuel J. Keith, M.D. Professor and Chairman, Department of Psychiatry, University of New Mexico, Albuquerque, New Mexico

Kenneth H. Kendler, M.D. Rachel Brown Banks Distinguished Professor of Psychiatry, Department of Psychiatry, and Professor, Department of Human Genetics, Medical College of Virginia, Richmond, Virginia

Thomas Kosten, M.D. Associate Professor, Department of Psychiatry, Yale University School of Medicine, New Haven, Connecticut

David J. Kupfer, M.D. Professor and Chairman, Department of Psychiatry, Western Psychiatric Institute, University of Pittsburgh, Pittsburgh, Pennsylvania

Sue E. Levkoff, Sc.D. Director, Harvard Geriatric Education Center, Harvard Medical School, Boston, Massachusetts

Jeffrey Lieberman, M.D. Director of Research, Hillside Hospital, Long Island Jewish Medical Center, Glen Oaks, New York

Benjamin Liptzin, M.D. Chairman, Department of Psychiatry, Baystate Medical Center, Springfield, Massachusetts

Susan M. Matthews, M.D. Assistant Director for Research Activities, Division of Clinical and Treatment Research, National Institute of Mental Health, Rockville, Maryland

Thomas H. McGlashan, M.D. Psychiatrist-in-Chief, Yale Psychiatric Institute, New Haven, Connecticut

Peter E. Nathan, Ph.D. Vice President for Academic Affairs, Dean of the Faculties, and University of Iowa Distinguished Professor of Psychology, The University of Iowa, Iowa City, Iowa

Eric A. Nofzinger, M.D. Assistant Professor of Psychiatry, University of Pittsburgh Medical Center, Sleep and Chronobiology Center, Pittsburgh, Pennsylvania

Harold Alan Pincus, M.D. Deputy Medical Director and Director, Office of Research, American Psychiatric Association, Washington, DC

Michael K. Popkin, M.D. Professor of Psychiatry and Medicine, University of Minnesota Medical School; Chief, Psychiatry, Hennepin County Medical Center, Minneapolis, Minnesota

George W. Rebok, Ph.D. Associate Professor, Department of Mental Hygiene, School of Hygiene and Public Health, Johns Hopkins University, Baltimore, Maryland

Quentin R. Regestein, M.D. Professor, Division of Psychiatry, Department of Medicine, Brigham and Women's Hospital, Boston, Massachusetts

Charles F. Reynolds III, M.D. Professor of Psychiatry and Neurology, and Director of Sleep and Chronobiology Center, Department of Psychiatry, Western Psychiatric Institute, University of Pittsburgh, Pittsburgh, Pennsylvania

Ruth Ross, M.A. Science Writer, DSM-IV, American Psychiatric Association, Washington, DC

Michael J. Sateia, M.D. Director, Sleep Disorders Center, Dartmouth-Hitchcock Medical Center, Lebanon, New Hampshire

Marc A. Schuckit, M.D. Professor, Department of Psychiatry, Veterans Affairs Medical Center, University of California, San Diego, San Diego, California

Samuel G. Siris, M.D. Director, Adult Psychiatric Day Programs, Hillside Hospital, Long Island Jewish Medical Center, Glen Oaks; Professor of Psychiatry, Albert Einstein College of Medicine, Bronx, New York

Virginia L. Susman, M.D. Associate Professor of Clinical Psychiatry, The New York Hospital–Cornell Medical Center, White Plains, New York

Sally Szymanski, D.O. Research Psychiatrist, Psychiatry Research Department, Hillside Hospital, Long Island Jewish Medical Center, Glen Oaks, New York

Michael J. Thorpy, M.D. Director, Sleep-Wake Disorders Center, Montefiore Medical Center; Associate Professor, Department of Neurology, Albert Einstein College of Medicine, Bronx, New York

John W. Tsuang, M.D. Substance Abuse Fellow, Department of Psychiatry, Veterans Affairs Medical Center, University of California, San Diego, San Diego, California

Gary J. Tucker, M.D. Professor and Chairman, Department of Psychiatry and Behavioral Sciences, University of Washington, Seattle, Washington

Harold C. Urschel III, M.D. Associate Medical Director and Director, Chemical Dependency Treatment Program, Southwestern Psychiatric Services, Dallas, Texas

Peter J. Weiden, M.D. Director, Schizophrenia Program, Department of Psychiatry, St. Luke's–Roosevelt Hospital Center, New York, New York

Thomas A. Widiger, Ph.D Professor, Department of Psychology, University of Kentucky, Lexington, Kentucky

George E. Woody, M.D. Chief, Substance Abuse Treatment Unit, Philadelphia VA Medical Center, and Clinical Professor of Psychiatry, Department of Psychiatry, University of Pennsylvania, Philadelphia, Pennsylvania

Ramzy Yassa, M.D. Professor of Psychiatry, McGill University; Psychiatrist, Douglas Hospital Center, Verdun, Quebec, Canada

Preface

DSM-IV Sourcebook: Volumes 1–3—Literature Reviews

For more than 5 years the Task Force on DSM-IV and members of the DSM-IV Work Groups participated in a comprehensive effort of empirical review leading to the publication of the fourth edition of the American Psychiatric Association's *Diagnostic and Statistical Manual of Mental Disorders* (DSM-IV). The *DSM-IV Sourcebook* chronicles these efforts and their results, documenting the rationale and empirical support for the text and criteria sets presented in DSM-IV. The major emphasis in the DSM-IV process has been on empirical review and documentation, and the Sourcebook, published in five volumes, is an important means of presenting that documentation. The first three volumes contain the DSM-IV literature reviews and summarize the DSM-IV Work Groups' efforts that led to the publication of the *DSM-IV Options Book* in 1991. The fourth volume contains the results of the DSM-IV data reanalyses, and the fifth volume contains the results of the DSM-IV field trials.

The *DSM-IV Sourcebook* is the culmination of a process that began in September 1987, when the American Psychiatric Association (APA) Committee on Psychiatric Diagnosis and Assessment met to explore possible timetables for the publication of DSM-IV. Because of the work already proceeding on the 10th edition of the International Classification of Diseases (ICD-10) by the World Health Organization (1992), the Committee concluded that work should also begin on DSM-IV to allow for mutual influence and convergence of the two systems (Frances et al. 1989). From the outset, the Committee recommended that review of the empirical evidence on diagnostic issues—often stimulated by the publication of DSM-III (American Psychiatric Association 1980) and DSM-III-R (American Psychiatric Association 1987)—be the centerpiece for the development of DSM-IV.

In May of 1988, the Board of Trustees of the APA appointed a Task Force to undertake the preparation of DSM-IV. Thirteen Work Groups were formed, each chaired by a member of the Task Force. These Work Groups covered the Anxiety Disorders; Child and Adolescent Disorders; Eating Disorders; Late Luteal Phase Dysphoric Disorder; Mood Disorders; the Multiaxial system; Delirium, Dementia, and Amnestic and Other Cognitive ("Organic") Disorders; Personality Disorders;

Psychiatric System Interface Disorders (consisting of Somatoform, Factitious, Dissociative, Impulse Control, and Adjustment Disorders); Psychotic Disorders; Sexual Disorders; Sleep Disorders; and Substance-Related Disorders.

Two conferences were held to develop the process by which DSM-IV would be constructed. These conferences were attended by representatives of the DSM-IV Task Force; the various Work Groups; and expert consultants on the design, analysis, and review of empirical research. The first Methods Conference was held in August 1988 to discuss procedures for gathering and analyzing data from different studies to achieve a comprehensive and objective consideration of the empirical literature. The second Methods and Applications Conference was held in November 1988 to discuss in more detail procedures for reviewing research, for selecting validators for existing and proposed items, for conducting field trials, and for resolving the various issues that would be addressed by the respective Work Groups. It was decided that the development of DSM-IV should proceed through three interactive stages of empirical review and documentation: 1) literature reviews, 2) reanalyses of existing data sets, and 3) focused field trials (Widiger et al. 1991). The goal of this process was to maximize the impact of empirical research on the deliberations and decisions of the DSM-IV Work Groups and Task Force and to document the empirical support for the resulting recommendations and proposals (Frances et al. 1990).

For any substantial revision of, addition to, or deletion from DSM-III-R to be considered for DSM-IV, it had to be accompanied by a review of the empirical and clinical literature (Widiger et al. 1990). Those conducting the reviews were to function as if they were consensus scholars (persons with no preconceptions who are fully aware of the clinical and research literature) (Cooper 1984). The reviews were not to be position papers arguing for particular proposals, but rather systematic, comprehensive, and objective overviews of the most relevant empirical research. These literature reviews are presented in the first three volumes of the *DSM-IV Sourcebook.*

The literature reviews also served to identify gaps and inadequacies within the literature on questions of crucial importance to the DSM-IV Work Groups. Fortunately, in many such instances, relevant existing data sets were available that had not yet been analyzed in a fashion that would provide useful answers. Therefore, the second stage of the DSM-IV development process was to obtain and reanalyze multiple data sets to address questions not answered in the published literature. This also allowed us to generate and pilot new proposals for criteria sets for DSM-IV (Widiger et al. 1991). These efforts were funded in part by the John D. and Catherine T. MacArthur Foundation, and the results will be presented in Volume 4 of the *DSM-IV Sourcebook.*

The culmination of the literature review and data reanalysis process was the publication of the *DSM-IV Options Book* (American Psychiatric Association 1991). The purpose of the *Options Book* was both to present the major diagnostic issues, and options for dealing with them, that had been identified by the Task Force on DSM-IV and to encourage review, comments, and the contribution of additional available data. Summaries describing how the information from the literature reviews and data reanalyses aided the Task Force and Work Groups in developing these options are presented in the Sourcebook. It is hoped that the publication of this information will provide an explanation and documentation for the decisions made in DSM-IV.

The third stage of the DSM-IV development process was to perform focused field trials to assess the extent to which proposed revisions would actually improve the reliability and/or validity of criteria sets and to address the issues identified by the literature reviews. The field trials allowed the DSM-IV Work Groups to compare alternative options (usually DSM-III, DSM-III-R, ICD-10 research criteria, and the various proposals for DSM-IV that had been generated during the first two steps) and to study the possible impact of any suggested changes. Funding for the field trials was obtained from the National Institute of Mental Health in collaboration with the National Institute on Drug Abuse and the National Institute on Alcohol Abuse and Alcoholism. The results of the focused field trials and the rationale for the final decisions of the Work Groups and Task Force will be presented in Volume 5 of the *DSM-IV Sourcebook*.

The culmination of this final stage in the DSM-IV development process was the publication of the *DSM-IV Draft Criteria* (American Psychiatric Association 1993). The purpose of this document was to invite review and comment on the proposed criteria before they appeared in DSM-IV. Readers were asked to help identify any mistakes, inconsistencies, oversights, unforeseen problems, potential for misuse, or boundary confusions.

In the rest of this Preface, we deal in more detail with the organization and format of the literature reviews presented in the first three volumes of the *DSM-IV Sourcebook*. Separate introductions to Volume 4 and Volume 5 will deal with issues specific to the data reanalyses and field trials, respectively.

The DSM-IV literature reviews are divided into three volumes, organized with respect to shared concerns and issues. Volume 1 presents the reviews for Substance-Related Disorders; Delirium, Dementia, and Amnestic and Other Cognitive Disorders (including a review on Mental Disorders Due to a General Medical Condition); Schizophrenia and Other Psychotic Disorders; Medication-Induced Movement Disorders; and Sleep Disorders. Volume 2 presents the reviews for the Mood Disorders, Late Luteal Phase Dysphoric Disorder, Anxiety Disorders, Personality Disorders, Psychiatric System Interface Disorders (consisting of Somatoform, Factitious, Dissociative, Impulse Control, and Adjustment Disorders), and

Sexual Disorders. Volume 3 presents the reviews for Childhood Disorders, Eating Disorders, Family-Relational Issues, Multiaxial Issues, and Cultural Issues. The section for each group of disorders begins with an introductory chapter that provides an executive summary of the material contained within that section as well as an overview of the activities and procedures of the Work Group. This is followed by the individual literature reviews dealing with the specific questions addressed by the Work Group.

Experts on the methodology of literature review provided guidelines for performing systematic, objective, and comprehensive evaluation of the available clinical research literature (Cooper 1984). The authors of the reviews were encouraged to follow an explicit format for conducting the review and presenting its findings. Successive drafts of each review were distributed widely to the advisers to each Work Group, who were specifically chosen to include individuals who represented a wide range of viewpoints on any given issue. Many of the reviews have also been published in revised form in professional and scientific journals and presented at conferences and meetings. We have encouraged the authors to publish and present their findings and interpretation to receive as much peer review and critical commentary as possible. This iterative process and the explicit format have been very helpful in identifying the various inadequacies, gaps, and biases that occurred in earlier drafts (e.g., failure to cover an important issue, a bias in the selection of studies, gaps in the coverage or presentation of the literature, disagreements concerning the interpretation of empirical findings, and failure to consider alternative options).

Each review contains the following sections: Statement of the Issues, Significance of the Issues, Methods, Results, Discussion, and Recommendations (Widiger et al. 1990). The purpose of the "Statement of the Issues" section is to outline explicitly the issues being addressed in the review and to keep the review focused on the pertinent nosological questions. This section informs the reader of the focus and scope of the review.

The purpose of the "Significance of the Issues" section is to frame the importance of the issue and discuss its clinical and/or empirical significance.

The purpose of the "Methods" section is to ensure replicability of the review and to document the extent to which the reviews were systematic and comprehensive in their coverage of the literature. This section indicates the types of studies that were considered and the ways they were identified with any explicit inclusion or exclusion criteria (e.g., requirements with respect to the populations sampled, the criteria sets used, how recently the study was conducted, and other methodological features). Authors were instructed to conduct computerized literature searches, to review specified journals systematically, and to solicit input from all the leading researchers in the field to minimize bias in the identification and consideration of studies that might result from the authors' own perspective on the literature.

The purpose of the "Results" section is to provide an objective and thorough, yet succinct, summary of the findings most relevant to the issues. To facilitate a balanced presentation of the findings, the authors were discouraged from presenting their own conclusions or recommendations in this section.

The purpose of the "Discussion" section is to address the implications of the clinical research findings for DSM-IV. Authors were encouraged to delineate and discuss all meaningful options for resolving the issues (including those they might not favor) and to outline the advantages and disadvantages of each option.

In the "Recommendations" section, the authors were encouraged to present their own recommendations for DSM-IV based on their review of the literature. In a few instances, these recommendations were not shared by the respective Work Group. In such cases, the recommendations were revised or the authors were requested to be explicit regarding their disagreements and to indicate the advantages and disadvantages of the various options. Authors were also encouraged to make suggestions for future research that would be helpful to the authors of DSM-V.

It is unlikely that readers will agree with all the recommendations presented in these reviews. Many of the issues do not have clear or obvious solutions, and more or less plausible arguments can often be made for a variety of alternative viewpoints. Our efforts have been directed toward achieving solutions that provide an optimal balance between false positives and false negatives in the diagnostic process. The advance of fundamental understanding of mental disorders will undoubtedly provide much clearer (and probably often very different) answers to the questions raised here.

In preparing the first three volumes of the *DSM-IV Sourcebook*, we have kept in mind that not all readers will be interested in all the fine points concerning every issue. For this reason, the chair of each Work Group prepared an introductory section for each group of disorders, including an executive summary of the important points in each review. For those interested in pursuing a subject in more detail, the individual reviews discuss the questions at hand in much greater depth and provide extensive reference sections.

Thomas A. Widiger, Ph.D.
Allen J. Frances, M.D.
Harold Alan Pincus, M.D.
Michael B. First, M.D.
Ruth Ross, M.A.
Wendy Davis, Ed.M.

References

American Psychiatric Association: Diagnostic and Statistical Manual of Mental Disorders, 3rd Edition. Washington, DC, American Psychiatric Association, 1980

American Psychiatric Association: Diagnostic and Statistical Manual of Mental Disorders, 3rd Edition, Revised. Washington, DC, American Psychiatric Association, 1987

American Psychiatric Association: DSM-IV Options Book: Work in Progress 9/9/91. Washington, DC, American Psychiatric Association, 1991

American Psychiatric Association, Task Force on DSM-IV: DSM-IV Draft Criteria 3/1/93. Washington, DC, American Psychiatric Association, 1993

Cooper HM: The Integrative Research Review: A Systematic Approach, Vol 2. Beverly Hills, CA, Sage, 1984

Frances AJ, Widiger TA, Pincus HA: The development of DSM-IV. Arch Gen Psychiatry 46:373–375, 1989

Frances AJ, Pincus HA, Widiger TA, et al: DSM-IV: work in progress. Am J Psychiatry 147:1439–1448, 1990

Widiger TA, Frances AJ, Pincus HA, et al: DSM-IV literature reviews: rationale, process, and limitations. Journal of Psychopathology and Behavioral Assessment 12:189–202, 1990

Widiger TA, Frances AJ, Pincus HA, et al: Toward an empirical classification for the DSM-IV. J Abnorm Psychol 100:280–288, 1991

World Health Organization: The ICD-10 Classification of Mental and Behavioral Disorders: Clinical Descriptions and Diagnostic Guidelines. Geneva, World Health Organization, 1992

Acknowledgments

DSM-IV has been a team effort with more than 1,000 people (and numerous professional organizations) helping us in its preparation. The Task Force on DSM-IV and Work Group members have worked hard and cheerfully through the demanding process of developing DSM-IV. Without their energy and expertise, this project would not have been possible.

Bob Spitzer has our thanks for his untiring efforts and unique perspective. Norman Sartorius, Michael Rutter, Darrel Regier, Lewis Judd, Fred Goodwin, and Chuck Kaelber were instrumental in facilitating a mutually productive interchange between the American Psychiatric Association (APA) and the World Health Organization. Dennis Prager, Peter Nathan, and David Kupfer helped us in developing a novel data reanalysis strategy that has been supported with funding from the John D. and Catherine T. MacArthur Foundation.

There are several individuals within the APA who deserve special recognition. Mel Sabshin's special wisdom and grace made even the most tedious tasks seem worth doing. The APA Committee on Diagnosis and Assessment (chaired by Layton McCurdy) provided valuable direction and counsel. We would also like to thank the APA Presidents (Drs. Fink, Pardes, Benedek, Hartmann, English, and McIntyre) and Assembly Speakers (Drs. Cohen, Flamm, Hanin, Pfaehler, and Shellow), who helped with the planning of our work. Carolyn Robinowitz and her staff in the APA Medical Director's office provided valuable assistance in the organization of the project.

The energy, intelligence, and scholarship of the authors of the DSM-IV literature reviews have surpassed our highest demands and expectations. Each review was read and commented on by many authorities in the field. Reviews often went through as many as half a dozen revisions. We would like to thank all those who contributed to this tremendous effort (in particular the Work Group chairs, literature review authors, and commentators) for their unflagging efforts and good nature throughout this effort.

Excellent administrative and editorial support was provided by Myriam Kline, Gloria Miele, Sarah Tilly, Willa Hall, Kelly MacKinney, Helen Stayna, Nina Rosenthal, Susan Mann, Joanne Mas, Nancy Vettorello, Nancy Sydnor-Greenberg,

Cindy Jones, Rebekah Brown, and Stacey Tipp, without whose help these volumes would have been impossible. Finally, we thank Ron McMillen, Claire Reinburg, Pam Harley, and Karen Sardinas-Wyssling for their expert production and editorial assistance.

We thank our patient readers. We hope that our efforts are useful to you.

Allen J. Frances, M.D.
Chair, Task Force on DSM-IV

Harold Alan Pincus, M.D.
APA Deputy Medical Director

Michael B. First, M.D.
Editor, DSM-IV Text and Criteria

Thomas A. Widiger, Ph.D.
Research Coordinator

Wendy Davis, Ed.M.
Editorial Coordinator

Ruth Ross, M.A.
Science Writer

Section I

Substance-Related Disorders

Contents

Section I
Substance-Related Disorders

Introduction to Section I

Substance-Related Disorders

Marc A. Schuckit, M.D.

The Substance Use Disorders Work Group was formed in 1988 with the goal of using the best data possible to formulate diagnostic criteria for DSM-IV. A small working group of six individuals was constituted to carry out the majority of the day-to-day work. The membership of this core committee included individuals with expertise with alcohol, opiates, stimulants, and polysubstances, and spanned a variety of clinical and research interests in psychiatry and psychology. Conference calls of this working group have been carried out every 2 weeks since the inception of the process; members meet face-to-face three to five times per year; and the core group is also responsible for presentations and major meetings that have included the American Psychiatric Association, the American College of Neuropsychopharmacology, the Committee for Problems in Drug Dependence, the American Psychological Association, the Research Society on Alcoholism, and others.

Detailed minutes of all interactions of the core working group are shared twice a month with a series of 12 close consultants. These include individuals who were very active in DSM-III-R (American Psychiatric Association 1987), representatives of both the National Institute on Alcohol Abuse and Alcoholism and the National Institute on Drug Abuse, as well as other leaders in the substance use disorders field.

All major reports and drafts of criteria and text are then shared with a cadre of more than 50 advisers. This is a heterogeneous group representing both clinical and research arenas, basic and applied sciences, and a host of groups with special interests. The latter include individuals actively carrying out care in geriatrics, adolescent and child psychiatry, women's groups, and ethnic populations.

This work was supported by the Veterans Affairs Research Service and National Institute on Alcohol Abuse and Alcoholism Grants 05226, 08401, and 08403.

The Decision-Making Process

The first step in establishing a working relationship among members of the core Work Group was to discuss a philosophy for approaching the task. All members agreed that they would enter the process with no preconceived notions regarding final decisions about changes from DSM-III-R. In addition, we accepted the premise that because such major changes had been made in 1980 for DSM-III (American Psychiatric Association 1980) and in 1987 for DSM-III-R, further alterations in the diagnostic criteria in the early 1990s would be made only if there appeared to be a solid basis for the alterations. Stability in diagnostic criteria is an important component of both treatment and research endeavors. Also, there was general concurrence that those changes that are instituted as part of DSM-IV must be based as much as possible on the best data available. Additional guidelines for the Work Group were the requirements of drafting criteria that were broad enough to be relevant to all of the classes of substances of abuse, formulating an approach that would apply at least in general to various ethnic and the gender groups, and developing a rubric that adequately translates to the International Classification of Diseases, 10th Revision (ICD-10) (World Health Organization 1992), because government and insurance agencies use this international numbering system. Finally, we concurred that when a problem in criteria appears to be present but data are inadequate to indicate an obvious solution, the committee would highlight these areas for future research in an attempt to optimize the decision-making process for DSM-V.

These biases, especially the heavy reliance on data, had some important practical implications. The first was the need to utilize input from close consultants and advisers to generate a long list of potential areas of focus for the group over the subsequent 5 years. This "wish list" was evaluated, and items were highlighted based on their clinical and research impact, as well as the practical issue of whether it seemed likely that an informed decision could be made through either existing reports by extracting information from existing data sets or from a planned field trial. The need to reanalyze existing data resulted in funding from the John D. and Catherine T. MacArthur Foundation; the field trial was financed by the Alcohol, Drug, and Mental Health Administration. The field work has generated data from more than 1,200 men and women in six centers in the United States and at least three groups in Europe. The results of the MacArthur analyses and field trial will be reported in greater detail in subsequent volumes.

In the sections that follow, the authors outline in some detail the deliberations that surrounded the major issues considered by the Work Group. Few other topics were considered to have the appropriate combination of clinical and/or research impact along with appropriate data to allow for informed decisions. An example of a topic not evaluated in detail is the potential relevance of the diagnostic term of *codependency,* an interesting and potentially important area that, unfortunately, suffers from a large diversity of definitions and a paucity of robust research. The only topic covered in great depth but not represented in this Sourcebook is the issue of the potential meaning of alcoholic dementia. Although a report was developed by Maristella Monteiro and subsequently published (Monteiro 1990), the decision by the DSM-IV Task Force to revise thoroughly the organization of the "organic" disorders for DSM-IV made it difficult to place that fine review into a perspective relevant to the revised format of the diagnostic manual.

In the remainder of this chapter, I offer an executive summary of the reports relevant to the substance use disorders that are incorporated in this volume of the Sourcebook. For ease of reference, the reports are somewhat arbitrarily divided into those missives that were associated with potentially important alterations in the new diagnostic manual, and those that resulted in no changes from DSM-III-R to DSM-IV. When perusing these reports, readers should be aware that as this volume goes to press the deliberations and accumulation of information are continuing; thus, the *recommendations* presented in these reports may change somewhat as the decision-making process moves into its final stages.

Reports Associated With Potentially Important Changes From DSM-III-R to DSM-IV

Eight full reports in the Sourcebook that deal with key issues related to DSM-IV are highlighted. For each topic, the Work Group felt that the extensive literature review generated enough data to warrant alterations that impacted on the text and/or the criteria in the new diagnostic manual. Although each report stands on its own in describing the rationale, methodologies, and discussions that support the *recommendations,* they are briefly highlighted here.

The Optimal Criteria for Abuse

The change between DSM-III and DSM-III-R represented an entire reorientation in the concept of abuse and dependence. As is described in more detail below, the term *dependence* was broadened considerably. As a consequence, the framers of DSM-III-R originally proposed to delete the concept of abuse, feeling that the entire spectrum of substance-related problems was now incorporated into the broad concept of dependence. At the last minute, however, pressure from the field required that the term *abuse* be reinserted into the manual. However, abuse was now viewed as a residual diagnosis that was to be applied only to individuals who still had some substance-related difficulties but who did not fit into even a broad approach to dependence.

As documented in Chapter 1 by Dr. John E. Helzer, the residual label of abuse posed several problems. First, because the criteria required that only one item be met, it was difficult to conceive of abuse as a true syndrome. Second, the two items chosen for the definition of abuse were selected from among the list of nine items for dependence, with no clear rationale about why these specific issues were more relevant to the concept of abuse than the others. Reflecting the large change in the structure of both diagnoses, the relationship between the diagnostic categories of abuse and dependence could not be fully understood.

The results of the literature review, substantiated by the MacArthur analyses and the field trial, supported the advisability of continuing to incorporate the concept of abuse into DSM-IV. This would enable the newer manual to relate appropriately to ICD-10, a rubric that also has two major entities subsumed under substance use disorders. The literature review further supported the appropriateness of focusing on social manifestations of problems in the concept of abuse, and demonstrated how these, in general, crosswalk favorably across different cultures. The review documented that a considerable number of individuals will meet criteria only for abuse and not go on to dependence, thereby demonstrating the potential clinical relevance of maintaining abuse as a diagnostic entity. At the same time, the search of the existing literature and additional data analyses revealed a disturbing lack of reliability for the existing diagnostic criteria for abuse, as well as problems in translation between abuse as diagnosed in the DSM system and its partner labeled "harmful use" in ICD.

These considerations resulted in a series of *recommendations*. Thus, the material presented in Chapter 1 suggests that the term *abuse* be retained in DSM-IV and that the emphasis remain on social difficulties. However, it also suggests that the number of items used to arrive at a diagnosis be expanded, and that the wording of the criteria, as well as the examples given within the diagnostic set, be honed down for improved clarity and clinical relevance. Readers may notice that in Chapter 1, Dr. Helzer lists five criteria for Abuse, whereas four criteria are listed in the *DSM-IV Options Book* (American Psychiatric Association 1991). The criterion added by Dr. Helzer is the first given in Table 1–1 in Chapter 1 (i.e., "Continued substance use despite knowledge of persistent or recurrent social, psychological, or physical problem(s) caused or exacerbated by the use of the substance"). At the time that Dr. Helzer originally developed his chapter, the Work Group was of the opinion that this symptom was a manifestation of a *social problem* and therefore an appropriate criterion for Abuse. However, by the time the *Options Book* was published, the consensus of the Work Group was that this symptom was rather a manifestation of *compulsive behavior* and thus appropriate for inclusion in the criteria for Dependence but not Abuse. This symptom was therefore deleted from the criteria for Abuse listed in the *Options Book*. Since publication of the *Options*

Book, as more information has become available, the Work Group has come to favor a third option: that is, that this criterion contains elements of both Abuse and Dependence and should therefore be divided between these two diagnoses.

Modifications for the Criteria for Dependence

In DSM-III, dependence incorporated a concept of repeated problems related to substances, requiring that at least one of those difficulties include the demonstration of tolerance and/or the signs and symptoms of a physical abstinence or withdrawal syndrome when substance intake was stopped. In stark contrast to this view of dependence, the framers of DSM-III-R turned to the idea of a broad concept of dependence developed by Griffith Edwards and Milton Gross (Edwards 1986; Edwards and Gross 1976). This was viewed as a multidimensional syndrome with social, behavioral, and biological components that signaled evidence of impaired control over substance use. This DSM-III-R approach, which was subsequently echoed in ICD-10, was felt to have the strengths of integrating a single theoretical concept, diminishing what was felt to be an inappropriate emphasis on tolerance and withdrawal, and allowing for the incorporation of a broader array of problems into a single diagnostic approach.

However, Dr. Peter E. Nathan, in his literature review in Chapter 2, bolstered by data analyses, reveals a number of potentially serious problems with the DSM-III-R approach to dependence. First, a large change in the concept of the diagnosis of dependence was instituted without adequate data to demonstrate the potential impact of these alterations on the prognostic and treatment requirements of individuals who are assigned the new label. Second, the marked shift away from the centrality of the concept of tolerance and withdrawal was contrary to a large literature and a long tradition in psychiatry. Third, the DSM-III-R criteria paid less attention to social consequences and other concepts related to substance use problems that had been a relatively central feature of prior diagnoses. Finally, there are dangers in assuming that one theoretical approach to dependence, to the exclusion of all others, is an appropriate basis for a new diagnostic scheme.

These considerations resulted in several *recommendations.* The Work Group recognized that large changes in the concept of dependence occurred in 1980 with DSM-III, and even larger alterations were incorporated into DSM-III-R in 1987. Thus, in the absence of compelling data indicating that yet another large change will be justified, the committee agreed to try to remain within the broadened concept of dependence. Once that general decision was reached, two relevant modifications were developed and tested as part of the MacArthur analyses and the field trial. Both options incorporated relatively minor rewording of the original nine criteria items for DSM-III-R, while offering more clinically relevant examples.

Option Two would have called for the same polythetic approach, but would require that one or more of the three items indicating evidence of either tolerance or withdrawal must be present to establish a diagnosis of substance dependence. This change would have meant a compromise midway between DSM-III and DSM-III-R and would have allowed the field another decade or so to gather additional data in preparation for a more definitive decision in DSM-V. However, the field trial data indicated that the less severe changes proposed in Option One would accomplish the same benefits but with less need for adjustment by clinicians and researchers. In this approach, the one most likely to be incorporated into DSM-IV, the same basic nine items (with rewording and additional examples) that were used in DSM-III-R, are maintained, but the clinician is requested to take two steps. The first step is to establish a diagnosis of dependence (the major diagnostic numbering to be used), after which the clinician should subtype dependence as existing with or without evidence of tolerance or physical withdrawal. This final compromise would mean no major change for the field, but will help ensure that both clinical and research data sets will allow administrators and researchers to use information garnered over the next decade to determine what relevance, if any, tolerance and withdrawal have for prognosis and treatment across the various substances.

Diagnostic Guidelines for Dealing With Psychiatric Syndromes in Individuals With Substance Use Disorders

Consistent with prior diagnostic approaches dating back to Kraepelin and before, DSM-III-R recognized the problems involved in attempting to diagnose major psychiatric disorders during the course of an organic mental condition. Implicit in this approach is the recognition, for example, that depressions developing during hypothyroidism are not likely to have the same prognostic and treatment implications as similar conditions that develop outside the context of a preexisting major disorder. Similarly, hallucinations documented after head trauma are not likely to imply a future clinical course of schizophrenia.

Consistent with prior diagnostic approaches, DSM-III-R recognized the problems with arriving at psychiatric diagnoses based on signs and symptoms that developed during substance intoxication or withdrawal. Although this general caveat was offered within DSM-III-R, only 17 of the possible 292 diagnoses made specific mention of the need to rule out intoxication and withdrawal from drugs before the psychiatric label could be applied, although an additional 13 labels warned clinicians that these diagnoses could not be established if there was evidence that an organic factor initiated and maintained the disturbance. Finally, an additional 19 labels reminded clinicians of the general caveat of not assigning a diagnosis if the symptoms were part of any other established Axis I disorder.

Although these diagnostic rules were relatively straightforward, Dr. Marc A. Schuckit, in his literature review in Chapter 3, revealed a number of problems. It appears as if many clinicians may have ignored the warnings and assigned multiple diagnostic labels, even in the face of obvious intoxication or withdrawal syndromes. An additional complicating factor was the apparent lack of realization on the part of many clinicians that severe depressive, anxiety, and psychotic symptoms not only develop during intoxication and active withdrawal, but frequently linger at clinically relevant levels of symptomatology for 2 or 3 weeks, and sometimes for as long as 5 or 6 weeks. An additional difficulty is that even some of those clinicians who recognized these potential problems appeared to need frequent reminders throughout the text in a consistent approach applied to each relevant psychiatric diagnosis, rather than a piecemeal set of reminders presented "here or there" within the text.

As a result of this review, several *recommendations* were set forth. First, DSM-IV should maintain the general approach of DSM-III-R and prior diagnostic manuals of reminding clinicians that psychiatric symptoms occurring in the context of an organic mental condition do not carry the same prognostic and treatment implications as independent psychiatric disorders. Second, a consistent guideline regarding the application of this concept to substance intoxication and withdrawal should be presented clearly within the Introduction to DSM-IV, should be mentioned within each of the major sections of the text, and should be incorporated into the actual diagnostic criteria themselves. Third, when one considers the different types of drugs, the huge range in half-lives of these substances of abuse, and the variability in substance-related clinical syndromes, it was felt appropriate to advise clinicians not to diagnose major psychiatric disorders definitively based on symptoms that occur during intoxication or within 6 weeks of abstinence. Fourth, at the same time, the manual emphasizes that individuals with substance use disorders are at least as likely as the general population to have any other major psychiatric syndrome, and that for at least two Axis I disorders (mania and schizophrenia) as well as one Axis II disorder (the antisocial personality disorder), significantly elevated rates of substance use disorders can be expected in the course of the major psychiatric syndrome.

Thus, the diagnostic manual emphasizes the need for clinicians to attempt to establish whether psychiatric syndromes began before the onset of an actual substance use disorder, or were observed during periods of abstinence that exceeded 6 weeks, or, in the present clinical condition, if the psychiatric symptomatology is intense and long-lasting enough to justify an independent psychiatric disorder following 6 weeks of abstinence.

The Diagnostic Criteria for Remission Deserved Further Scrutiny

DSM-III-R provides two categories for remission among patients formerly dependent on a psychoactive substance: partial and full. The diagnosis of partial remission is made when, during the past 6 months, there has been some use of the substance and some symptoms of dependence. A diagnosis of full remission indicates that during the past 6 months there has either been no use of the substance or use of the substance and no symptoms of dependence. However, as Dr. George E. Woody and Dr. John Cacciola indicate in their literature review in Chapter 4, the guidelines for appropriate use of these criteria give little information on how to label temporary "slips," offer little advice about the potential relevance of substitution therapies (e.g., methadone), and might not have paid appropriate attention to the periods of time when relapse is most likely to occur. Nor is significant information offered about how to deal with individuals who are continuing sporadically to use their major problematical drug, similar substances, or other drugs of abuse.

The literature review, supplemented by data analyses, resulted in a number of *recommendations*. It was felt that remission should include a subtype of early remission, indicating the time of greatest danger of relapse: the first 6 months following termination of use. This concept of early remission would then be further subdivided into clearly stating whether an individual 1) has any continued use of the substance, 2) is participating in a substitution or agonist therapy but has no illegal use of the substance, or 3) is not participating in a substitution therapy and there is no use of the major problematical substance or any closely related drug. After 6 months, it is suggested that an individual be labeled as having entered sustained remission, which is further subtyped as with or without substitution or agonist therapies, with the latter further subdivided into full abstinence, non-problematical use, or partial remission. Finally, clinicians are advised to use their own clinical judgment regarding the potential for dropping any notation of a current substance-dependent problem, even in remission, after 3 or more years of continued abstinence.

Since Dr. Woody and Dr. Cacciola originally developed their chapter (and since publication of the *Options Book*), there have been many discussions with advisers and members of ICD-10 on the subject of the remission criteria. These meetings have resulted in a number of suggested changes that are somewhat different from those presented by Dr. Woody and Dr. Cacciola, although the main concepts are retained. The new categories are believed to reflect the available data accurately and in general to provide an improved level of compatibility with ICD-10. Specifically, the changes that are recommended include removing agonist treatment from the remission category (and placing it in a separate category), providing only one category for early remission, and extending the "preremission" category from 6 to 12 months.

The Need to Define Severity More Clearly

DSM-III-R provides vague guidelines to allow clinicians to divide individuals with substance dependence into those with a few problems (mild dependence), those with many symptoms (severe dependence), and those whose substance-related problems fall between the two extremes (moderate dependence). However, as explained in Chapter 5 by Dr. George E. Woody and Dr. John Cacciola, there are few instructions about how to distinguish between the three subgroups; the validity and reliability of the subtyping have not been established; treatment and prognostic implications of the subdivisions have not been thoroughly studied; and few data exist on even the most tentative application of the severity criteria to drugs other than alcohol.

As a result of these considerations, several *recommendations* were set forth. First, if the same vague descriptors are used, at the very least it is important to remind clinicians that there are few data to validate these criteria. Second, efforts should be made to encourage the field to study the existing criteria more thoroughly and to attempt to develop more precise severity ratings for which validity and reliability can be established. Third, the results of the literature review and the field trial considered the possibility of more precisely defining mild dependence as three or four of the nine potential symptoms, moderate dependence as five or six of the nine symptoms, and severe dependence as seven or more. Unfortunately, probably as a consequence of the need for more sophisticated weighting of each of the items, this approach at present does not appear to have great prognostic implications and, thus, even this mild modification was not recommended for incorporation into DSM-IV.

A Reorganization of the "Organic" Sections Resulted in Changes in Notation of Some Substance Use Disorders

As is described in Section II, Chapter 19, considering some psychiatric syndromes as "organic" and others as "not organic" raised some serious potential problems. The general reorganization of the concept of organic (now called cognitive) disorders justified several changes that affected the substance use disorders. These included the appropriateness of moving discussions of substance-related anxiety, depressive, and psychotic states to the anxiety, depressive, and psychotic disorders sections of the manual. In addition, a decision was made to incorporate the discussion of "intoxication" and "withdrawal" into the same section with the presentation of information on abuse and dependence.

As a consequence of Dr. Thomas J. Crowley's literature review in Chapter 6, which supported the optimal manner of conforming with the overall changes within the new diagnostic manual as they relate to the old "organic" disorders, several other problems emerged. The literature review and data analyses revealed marked inconsistencies in how depressive, anxiety, psychotic, and personality alterations were used within the manual as they related to a variety of substances and alcohol- or drug-related states. Regarding the latter, there was a lack of clear guidelines on how appropriately to label a clinical condition such as an anxiety state if it developed during intoxication or withdrawal or appeared to be a more persisting condition.

As a result of these considerations, several *recommendations* were set forth. The most significant of these alterations is the development of guidelines to help the clinician to indicate consistently for each relevant condition the substance involved (e.g., alcohol, hallucinogens), the clinical state during which the condition developed (e.g., intoxication, withdrawal, or persisting conditions), and the symptom pattern being described (e.g., anxiety, mood disorder, psychosis, or personality alterations). For example, the condition that had previously been labeled as an "organic mood disorder" in the context of alcoholism, would in DSM-IV be likely to be labeled alcohol intoxication mood disorder. This concept, originally alluded to in the *Options Book,* has been developed in a more definitive manner in Chapter 6.

Since publication of the *Options Book,* one additional issue related to cognitive problems has been discussed. Thus, Dr. Crowley explains in his chapter the need to define more fully the concept of "maladaptive behavior," especially as it might impact on medical as opposed to legal problems.

The Appropriate Handling of Nicotine Withdrawal in DSM-IV

In his careful review of the literature, Dr. John R. Hughes reveals in Chapter 7 a number of potential problems with the DSM-III-R concept of nicotine withdrawal. These included the recognition that this clinical condition was one of the few withdrawal states where "craving" was a specific diagnostic item, whereas the remainder of the withdrawal conditions assumed that craving was prominent and that there was no need to list that difficulty specifically. The literature review further documented the potential importance of some symptoms not previously listed within DSM-III-R, including the relevance of dysphoric or depressed mood, insomnia, impatience, and increased consumption of sweets during nicotine withdrawal. Finally, the literature review was used to consider whether it was appropriate that nicotine remain the only substance for which dependence but not abuse criteria were set forth.

These considerations resulted in a number of *recommendations.* First, for the sake of consistency, craving will be considered as an implicit part of the syndrome and will be highlighted in the text describing nicotine withdrawal, but will not be listed as a specific item. Second, the data from the literature are adequate to support the addition of several new items to the criteria set, including dysphoric or depressed mood and evidence of insomnia. Third, the literature review supports the relevance of using "impatience" as an alternate criterion for "restlessness," but, fourth, does not offer enough new data to support the inclusion of a new diagnostic category of nicotine abuse. The first and third of these issues (i.e., deletion of craving and using impatience as an alternative to restlessness) developed through questions raised since publication of the *Options Book.*

Should Alcohol Idiosyncratic Intoxication Be Deleted From DSM-IV?

A review was carried out by Dr. Harold C. Urschel III and Dr. George E. Woody in Chapter 8 to question whether the English language literature offers enough convincing data to support the existence of a syndrome characterized by severe violence occurring within a short time of the consumption of relatively small amounts of alcohol (e.g., one or two drinks) as a separate entity. Although studies published to date confirmed the likelihood of a high sensitivity to alcohol among some individuals with brain damage, the psychiatric, medical, and neurological publications gave little support to a unique syndrome in other individuals that would conform to the criteria outlined in the earlier diagnostic manuals.

It was the *recommendation* of this report that, reflecting the paucity of appropriate data, this diagnostic entity be deleted from DSM-IV.

Reports Resulting in No Major Significant Alterations in DSM-IV

A number of additional issues raised in the early months of discussions of the Work Group were also closely scrutinized through literature reviews and related data analyses. In contrast to the questions highlighted earlier, the reviews related to these questions led to the conclusion that no changes in the diagnostic approach are justified. Reflecting that negative response, the executive-type summary of those considerations is relatively brief.

Should Caffeine Abuse and Dependence Be Added to the Diagnostic Manual?

The last decade has witnessed an expansion of scientific understanding of the clinical relevance of this very common drug, caffeine. During the last several years, an increasing number of case reports have appeared describing levels of discomfort among heavy coffee drinkers when they cease caffeine intake. This raises the question of whether there are sufficient data to support diagnoses of caffeine withdrawal, dependence, and abuse in the new diagnostic manual. Although Dr. John R. Hughes supported the potential usefulness of these concepts in his detailed literature review in Chapter 9, their inclusion in DSM-IV was jeopardized by several issues. These included the observations that only three symptoms of withdrawal have been validated (headache, fatigue, and drowsiness), and that two of these symptoms (fatigue and drowsiness) basically represent the same concept. In addition, all three of these symptoms have a high prevalence in the general population unrelated to caffeine intake and can be mimicked by many noncaffeine-related conditions.

It is the *recommendation* of this report that the concepts of withdrawal, abuse, and dependence on caffeine are worthy of further evaluation, with a hope for their inclusion in DSM-V. On the other hand, the low number of symptoms and their lack of specificity do not justify their inclusion in DSM-IV.

The Potential Importance of Highlighting Anabolic Steroid Dependence

This group of body-building hormones has been used since the 1950s by athletes to enhance body mass, strength, and endurance. In recent years, an increasing proportion of young people have sought out these drugs for similar reasons or to enhance personal appearance. In his literature review in Chapter 10, Dr. John W. Tsuang documented an increasing number of convincing clinical descriptions of what would appear to be patterns of uncontrolled use that might approach the threshold for criteria for abuse and dependence. On the other hand, there are only limited animal data and no large-scale epidemiological or clinical studies. Consequently, only limited data are available to date on the validity and reliability of applying the general criteria for abuse or dependence to individuals with intake of these steroids. In addition, there are only limited data regarding the prognostic and treatment implications of these diagnoses if they were applied.

It is the *recommendation* of the literature review that anabolic steroid withdrawal, abuse, and dependence are potentially relevant clinical syndromes. All possible efforts should be made to encourage more vigorous studies of these phenomena over the next decade in the hopes that an increased volume of investigations might justify the development of specific criteria that would relate to an itemized and individually numbered diagnostic approach to these substances. Until that time, it is recommended that the text of DSM-IV note the potential importance of these substances, highlight them under the "Other (or Unknown) Substance Use

Disorders" category, and encourage greater research on this potentially important topic.

The Potential Relevance of Protracted Abstinence (Withdrawal) Syndromes

There are three categories of drugs known to produce physical withdrawal syndromes: opiates, stimulants (including amphetamines and cocaine), and depressants (including alcohol). For each of these substances, both animal and human data document a continuation of some level of symptomatology beyond the initial acute withdrawal syndrome. As documented in the literature review by Dr. Marc A. Schuckit, Dr. Thomas Kosten, and Dr. Marian W. Fischman in Chapter 11, it appears clear that uncomfortable and even at times distressing physiological and psychological symptoms, often less intense remnants of conditions observed during acute withdrawal, often persist for months following the immediate postwithdrawal period. These longer-term or protracted symptoms appear to be observed in a substantial proportion of individuals recovering from substance use disorders and are hypothesized to contribute to relapse. Despite these data, however, the level of documentation at present does little to highlight specific criteria that might be incorporated into a new diagnostic entity. Nor are the data on the usual clinical course or treatments of these protracted symptoms adequate.

It is the *recommendation* of this literature review that the current paucity of vigorous, large-scale studies outlining the specific parameters of a syndrome precludes the development of valid and reliable criteria for DSM-IV. At the same time, it is hoped that aspects of this potential syndrome will be outlined within the text of DSM-IV, that protracted abstinence conditions will be highlighted for potential consideration for DSM-V, and that all possible steps will be taken to encourage research in this important clinical area.

The Potential Relevance of a New Subtype of Dependence Based on the Familial Pattern of the Disorder

As described in Chapter 12 by Dr. Marc A. Schuckit, the research literature has long documented that, at least for alcoholism, dependent individuals with alcoholic close family members are likely to have some predictable characteristics. These include an earlier onset of drinking, more alcohol-related life problems, and a younger age at admission for their first inpatient rehabilitation. At the same time, alcohol-dependent individuals with or without histories of alcoholism in close family members tend be relatively similar on cognitive functioning, health problems, drug use patterns, education, and occupation. However, although the literature review documented some interesting clinical correlates of the presence of alcoholism in close family members, the clinical utility of this potential subtype of dependence was undermined by a number of issues. These included difficulties in extracting consistent data from the literature because of divergent approaches to defining a positive family history, the possibility that it is not alcohol dependence but the presence of *any* major psychiatric disorder in the family that correlated with outcome, and a confounding variable where most studies did not appropriately control for the impact of the antisocial personality disorder.

Considering all of these data, it was the *recommendation* of the Work Group that, despite the limited amount of useful information offered by this subtyping, once additional factors are controlled, it does not appear as if there is sufficient reason to incorporate a new diagnostic entity into the manual. On the other hand, the text will encourage clinicians to pay close attention to family history information, and it is hoped that further and better-controlled studies will be carried out in preparation for DSM-V.

Should Amphetamines and Cocaine Be Combined Into One Large Category Labeled Stimulants?

As described in Chapter 13 by Dr. Michael R. Irwin, the animal and human literature clearly indicate many similarities in the central nervous system effects, behavioral correlates, and clinical syndromes associated with amphetamines and the various forms of cocaine. Consistent with this conclusion, most diagnostic manuals over the years have used similar, and sometimes identical, criteria for withdrawal, abuse, dependence, and substance-related "organic" conditions when describing amphetamines and cocaine. Thus, the literature review clearly documented the potential scientific and clinical appropriateness of combining the two types of drugs into one large category.

Reflecting these factors, it was the *recommendation* of this report that the diagnostic manual be simplified by combining all information on amphetamines and cocaine into a single section on stimulants. However, although this recommendation made great clinical and scientific sense, there were a number of extraneous factors that convinced the Work Group to allow the two types of substances to remain as independent categories in DSM-IV. Most compelling was the need for DSM-IV to remain compatible, at least on diagnostic numbering, with ICD-10. That international manual has maintained a distinction between amphetamines and cocaine. In addition, even though it would be more scientifically correct to combine the two categories of drugs, little harm would be likely to result from allowing for separate diagnostic numbering for the two types of stimulants. Thus, the Work Group decided to remain consistent with the prior DSMs and with the ICD and allow for separate diagnostic assignments for amphetamines and cocaine.

Some Conclusions

The DSM-IV working groups are the first given the opportunity to document all stages of deliberations carefully and to make decisions based on carefully constructed criteria. The 5-year process encouraged the use of detailed literature reviews and allowed members of the working groups to generate data from both MacArthur analyses and field trials to make the most appropriate decisions possible.

The Substance Use Disorders Work Group was faced with a potentially infinite number of questions that could be asked. The guidelines presented at the beginning of this introduction, especially the focus on areas where data are already available or might potentially be generated from a field trial, allowed our Work Group to focus on a limited number of questions. With rare exceptions, each of these areas was evaluated by the thorough literature reviews that have resulted in the series of chapters that make up this section of the Sourcebook.

Our goals are relatively straightforward. It is important that clinicians, researchers, administrators, and those men and women who will work in the DSM-V process have full access to the state of the literature that existed in the late 1980s and early 1990s, and the decision-making process that was used to address the issues that impacted on DSM-IV. It is hoped that the following pages will not only help readers to understand both how and why the DSM-IV Substance Use Disorders Work Group made the relevant decisions, but will also encourage active research to answer more fully the potentially important questions raised in these reviews.

References

American Psychiatric Association: Diagnostic and Statistical Manual of Mental Disorders, 3rd Edition. Washington, DC, American Psychiatric Association, 1980

American Psychiatric Association: Diagnostic and Statistical Manual of Mental Disorders, 3rd Edition, Revised. Washington, DC, American Psychiatric Association, 1987

American Psychiatric Association: DSM-IV Options Book: Work in Progress 9/9/91. Washington, DC, American Psychiatric Association, 1991

Edwards G: The alcohol dependence syndrome: a concept as stimulus to enquiry. Br J Addict 81:171–183, 1986

Edwards G, Gross MM: Alcohol dependence: provisional description of a clinical syndrome. BMJ 1:1058–1061, 1976

Monteiro MG: DSM-III-R diagnostic criteria for dementia associated with alcoholism: a critical review. Annals of Clinical Psychiatry 2:263–275, 1990

World Health Organization: The ICD-10 Classification of Mental and Behavioural Disorders: Clinical Descriptions and Diagnostic Guidelines. Geneva, World Health Organization, 1992

Chapter 1

Psychoactive Substance Abuse and Its Relation to Dependence

John E. Helzer, M.D.

Statement of the Issues

In this report, I examine the appropriateness of a diagnostic label of substance "abuse," the definition of abuse, and the relationship between abuse and dependence. On the basis of an extensive review of the existing literature, I then make recommendations for the DSM-IV treatment of these issues.

Although substance abuse has long been used as a diagnostic label, and was so used in both DSM-III (American Psychiatric Association 1980) and DSM-III-R (American Psychiatric Association 1987), to some it is a pejorative term with no place in a diagnostic nomenclature. Furthermore, the definition of abuse has varied. In DSM-III, the definition was relatively clear conceptually, requiring some evidence of both a pattern of pathological use of a substance and of impairment in social or occupational functioning. By definition, abuse was closely related to dependence. In DSM-III-R, abuse essentially became a residual of dependence. The definition of dependence was based on the alcohol dependence syndrome of Griffith Edwards and colleagues (Edwards and Gross 1976). Without a clear theoretical rationale or data base, two of the dependence symptoms were used to define abuse.

There are a number of possibilities regarding the definition of substance abuse and its relationship to dependence:

1. Provide a specified definition for dependence but view abuse as a less specifically defined, residual category for those who manifest involvement with psychoactive substances that is not sufficient to meet criteria for dependence.
2. View abuse and dependence as a continuum of drug involvement, with abuse having a lower threshold. Thus, one who met criteria for dependence would also meet criteria for abuse. Abuse would have a specific definition (i.e., a

specific threshold on the continuum) and would not constitute a "residual" category as in the first conceptualization.

3. Provide specific definitions for both abuse and dependence but view them as orthogonal concepts rather than a single continuum. That is, the universe of symptoms utilized for abuse would differ from that of dependence, and each category would have a specific definition based on its own set of symptoms.
4. Eliminate the concept of abuse altogether and make substance dependence the only diagnosis available in the substance use disorders category. An elaboration of this possibility is to identify risky behaviors as they relate to substance abuse, such as harmful and/or hazardous use, but not give these diagnostic status.

Significance of the Issues

There is evidence from the Epidemiologic Catchment Area (ECA) survey (Regier et al. 1984) that the substance use disorders are the most prevalent forms of psychopathology in the general population. It is also well known from the study of multiple clinical populations that the treatment of these disorders often has a low success rate. Furthermore, the public health implications of these disorders are great. To the degree that distinct diagnostic entities can be identified within the broader category of the substance use disorders, the opportunity for progress in understanding their etiology and for finding effective treatments is improved. In addition, to the degree that abuse is a distinct entity, separate from substance dependence, recognition of this fact is important for etiological, natural history, and treatment studies. Finally, to the degree that substance abuse is a prodrome of dependence, recognition of this fact is important for the prevention of the latter.

Methods

This review began with an automated literature search, conducted by the American Psychiatric Association, for publications relevant to the definition of, and longitudinal studies examining, substance abuse. Bibliographies from articles found in the automated review led to additional relevant papers, and investigators and clinicians interested in this area were invited to give their own ideas and to contribute other relevant literature.

Early drafts of this report were circulated to consultants and advisers to the Substance Use Disorders Work Group and to other interested experts. Most of the literature relevant to the topics covered in this report relates to alcohol, because the pertinent literature relating to illicit drugs is rather meager.

Results

I now briefly review the data concerning the dimensions of substance use, the relationship between substance abuse and dependence, objections to the term *abuse*, and arguments in favor of the term *abuse* as a construct and as a label.

Dimensions of Substance Use

In a study of the dimensions of problem drinking and their stability across time in adolescents, White (1987) found that traditional measures of problem drinking represent at least two distinct dimensions: intensity of use (based on measures of alcohol consumption) and use-related problems. Using confirmatory factor analytic techniques, White found that a two-dimensional model fit the data on the adolescents much better than a unidimensional model. Considerable dimensional stability through adolescence and up to age 24 years was also found. In other words, both intensity of use and alcohol-related problems tended to remain stable over this period of time.

Perceptions of the dimensions of substance involvement are encompassed in the definitions of substance use that have evolved over time. For both drugs and alcohol, the definitions of dependence have been more numerous and seemingly of greater interest to the field than definitions of abuse. The substance definitions that have captured the bulk of most recent attention have been those relating to the "dependence syndrome" concept as enunciated by Edwards and Gross (1976). Much of the existing work has been carried out conceptualizing the alcohol dependence syndrome as a dimensional model rather than a categorical one, and Skinner and Allen (1982) did an early review of research examining the scalar properties of measures of the alcohol dependence syndrome.

Babor and colleagues (1987) assessed the predictive validity of the dependence syndrome by examining how well severity of dependence correlated with reinstatement of substance use after a period of abstinence. They found that severity of alcohol dependence was a good predictor of reinstatement among those who used alcohol, but severity of drug dependence did not predict reinstatement as consistently in those who used opiates. Among female alcoholic patients, "recent dependence was only a modest predictor, and lifetime dependence did not significantly predict reinstatement" (p. 402). Work by Kosten and colleagues (1987) and Hasin and colleagues (1988) examined the applicability of the dependence syndrome concept across many substance categories. Results showed high clustering of dependence symptoms with each other and with health, social, and emotional problems attributed to drug use.

In sum, there is evidence that alcoholism, and perhaps other substance involvement, is multidimensional and that dimensions may be differentially predictive.

Relationship of Substance Abuse to Dependence

In a detailed analysis of the DSM-III criteria, Rounsaville (1987) indicated that the relationship between substance abuse and dependence as defined in DSM-III can be considered inconsistent and illogical in several of the substance categories. For example, although iatrogenically addicted persons often do not exhibit social consequences of addiction or a pathological pattern of use, self-induced addicted persons typically exhibit both social consequences and evidence of dependence.

Using a Delphi technique and a panel of 99 substance abuse experts, Rinaldi and colleagues (1988) evolved a definition of (drug) dependence as "a generic term that relates to physical or psychological dependence, or both. It is characteristic for each pharmacological class of psychoactive drugs. Impaired control over drug-taking behavior is implied" (p. 557). The definition they evolved for drug abuse is "any use of drugs that causes physical, psychological, economic, legal, or social harm to the individual user or to others affected by the drug user's behavior" (p. 557). This is consistent with the idea that abuse and dependence are seen by many in the field as orthogonal constructs.

There are only a few studies that have examined the relationship of components of a dependence syndrome to consequences of substance use. Skinner and Goldberg (1986) found that three dependence items clustered together in a factor distinct from social and health problems. Skinner and Allen (1982) found that high levels of alcohol dependence are associated with social consequences from drinking. However, these studies do not address the obverse: that is, the prevalence of dependence symptoms among those selected on the basis of having social consequences. Such information would be very helpful in the development of definitions for abuse and dependence and the relationship of abuse to dependence.

Hasin and colleagues (1990) examined the longitudinal course of alcohol problems over a 4-year period in a group of men selected from the general population by the Alcohol Research Group. At follow-up, 70% of the subjects who were initially classified as abusing alcohol were still either classifiable as abusing alcohol or were remitted. Only 30% reported indicators of dependence. Among those initially classified as dependent, 46% still had current symptoms of dependence, and 39% had remitted. Overall, the difference in outcome between those with abuse only and dependence at index was statistically significant ($P < .05$).

In a personal communication to the Substance Use Disorders Work Group, Dr. Hasin also reviewed unpublished work in progress from three other data sets that provide additional evidence of longitudinal distinctions between alcohol abuse and dependence. These data are reviewed in detail in a previous committee report (J. E. Helzer, unpublished manuscript, September 1989), but are consistent with Dr. Hasin's work in suggesting that social problems due to alcohol are not necessarily more likely to remit, but rather often remain consistent over time, showing neither escalation (either in terms of numbers of social problems or type) nor diminution. Hasin's findings are also consistent with earlier work by Cahalan and colleagues (1969) and Bejerot (1972).

In summary, these data are suggestive of at least two diagnostic dimensions, at least for alcoholism: one (the dependence dimension) involving physiological factors and perhaps signs of compulsive use and the other (the abuse dimension) relating more to personal, social, or legal consequences of substance use. Although the two are often aggregated in the same individual, abuse may occur without dependence and is not necessarily just a prodrome of dependence.

Objections to the Term *Abuse*

At this point, it is important to review objections to *abuse* as a diagnostic term. First, although *abuse* is defined in DSM-III and DSM-III-R in a relatively specific way, the term is often also used as a more generic descriptive one implying misuse of substances. Many consider *abuse* to be a pejorative term that should be avoided in a scientific nomenclature (Blackwell 1987; Peyser and Gitlow 1988), and some prefer to reserve the term for heavy drinking that is induced by a social context.

Miller and Gold (1989) pointed out that confusion is sometimes created because abuse is a concept that depends on the standard of use for a particular societal context. However, it is sometimes used interchangeably with other terms implying abnormal use of a drug, such as *addiction*. They also feel that the way abuse is defined in DSM-III-R, it is a subcategory of addiction rather than a deviance from social norms. They suggested that *abuse* be retained only as a descriptive term and not as a diagnostic category.

In a personal communication to the Substance Use Disorders Committee, Richard Frances recalled that there was an attempt to drop the term *abuse* in the DSM-III-R criteria, but that it was reinstituted at the time of the field trials by the popular demand of those attempting to use the new DSM-III-R criteria. He also suggested that one desirable feature of the dependence criteria is they are probably less culturally influenced than are the adverse social consequences that might go into an abuse definition.

Skodol (1989) noted that there were criticisms of the division of substance use disorders into abuse and dependence syndromes on the basis that the "distinctions were arbitrary, inconsistently applied, and gave inadequate coverage in the classification itself to the psychopathology encountered in clinical practice" (p. 123). He suggested that clinicians typically think of abuse as synonymous with psychological addiction, and dependence as corresponding to physiological addiction.

There is presumably considerable overlap between cases identified as substance abuse and those as dependent, at least for alcoholic inpatients. For instance,

Schuckit and colleagues (1985) found that the index clinical characteristics and clinical course over 1 year failed to differentiate those who met criteria for DSM-III alcohol abuse versus DSM-III dependence.

Hasin and Grant (1987) compared the Schedule for Affective Disorders and Schizophrenia (Endicott and Spitzer 1978) and Research Diagnostic Criteria (Spitzer et al. 1978) system of diagnosing substance involvement with diagnoses obtained in the same sample by the Diagnostic Interview Schedule (Robins et al. 1981) and DSM-III. They found the procedures agreed fairly well on global assessment of substance problems, but that distinctions between abuse and dependence were not reliable within the separate drug classes.

Arguments Favoring *Abuse* as a Construct and as a Label

Setting aside for a moment the desirability of *abuse* as a term, there are some points that can be raised in defense of substance abuse as a construct. It seems not inappropriate that social manifestations be considered a legitimate part of a substance involvement diagnosis, as they are for other psychiatric disorders. Antisocial personality disorder is an obvious example of a diagnosis that is partially defined by social consequences; indeed, social consequences are implied in the diagnostic label itself. Social consequences are also included in the DSM-III-R definitions of some of the major "endogenous" disorders, as illustrated by the B criterion for schizophrenia and the C criterion for mania. Furthermore, social manifestations of substance use are both consistent across cases and highly predictive of outcome.

Regarding the label itself, use of the term *abuse* acknowledges that the problems encompassed are not at the same level as those encompassed in a stronger term like *dependence.* The term *abuse* also implies that the symptoms encompassed do not constitute essential aspects of an underlying disease process in the same way that symptoms of a dependence syndrome likely do. If a syndromal definition is based exclusively on social consequences, the use of a term like *abuse* to identify this syndrome does not seem inappropriate; the label actually implies use to the extent that social consequences result. The charge that this is a pejorative term carries more weight when *abuse* is applied more generically to cases such as those with iatrogenic use. This argues in favor of specific criteria for an operational definition of *abuse,* rather than using it as a residual term, since the latter approach tends to promote both pejorative and inconsistent application.

At least for alcohol, a syndrome based on adverse social consequences in the absence of dependence symptoms does appear qualitatively different from dependence and not simply a prodrome of dependence (see work by Hasin and others, cited above). Thus, dropping the abuse category would leave a group of people with clear alcohol problems uncovered by a diagnostic category, whereas lowering the threshold of dependence to include those who meet criteria for abuse would increase the heterogeneity of a category that is probably quite heterogeneous already.

Regarding the cultural relativity of social criteria, Helzer and Canino (1989) have shown that social consequences of alcoholism are applicable in widely diverse cultures in North America, Europe, and Asia, and that the vast majority of clinicians in these cultures consider the DSM-III social criteria to be highly appropriate in their own cultures. Helzer and colleagues (1990) have shown cross-cultural rank order frequency correlations ranging from .66 to .94 for social consequences related to drinking behavior. That is, the frequency of specific consequences in the general population was highly consistent across widely diverse cultures. Furthermore, even within the United States, there are regional differences in the acceptability of substance use. However, by definition, the occurrence of social "consequences" indicates that behavior has exceeded acceptable norms in the region. Even if those norms change (e.g., if driving-while-intoxicated laws are tightened), it is the individual's responsibility to conform to a new set of standards. It seems appropriate to label significant failures to do so as substance abuse.

In their analysis of DSM-III-R field trial data, Rounsaville and colleagues (1987) found that discrepant diagnoses of substance abuse between DSM-III and DSM-III-R related in part to removal of social consequences as a requirement for the DSM-III-R diagnoses. They also suggested that substance abuse as defined in DSM-III-R will be uncommon and that the large majority of those who would meet DSM-III criteria for abuse or dependence would also meet DSM-III-R criteria for dependence. However, there is evidence from the ECA survey that the distinction between alcohol abuse and dependence, at least as it appears in DSM-III, is worth preserving (Helzer et al. 1991). In their analysis of approximately 20,000 general population respondents, Helzer and colleagues found that about 10% of men and 2% of women met criteria for alcohol abuse but not dependence, and approximately 3% of men and 1% of women met criteria for dependence without also having abuse. Those with dependence had roughly twice as many lifetime alcohol symptoms as those who abused alcohol, and the distribution of symptoms between the two groups was distinctly different. In addition, heavy drinking was significantly more common in those meeting dependence criteria. In her analysis of ECA respondents age 65 or older, Bucholz (1988) also found fewer alcohol symptoms in those with a current or past history of abuse as compared with dependence. Therefore, it is apparent that these distinctions persist into later life and are not simply a matter of the persons abusing alcohol being identified at an early stage of an invariably progressive illness.

Finally, there is a potential difficulty in applying the DSM-III-R criteria in family history studies. Because the criteria exclude social consequences of substance involvement from the diagnostic definitions, it is difficult to make a substance-related diagnosis on the basis of family history information. A family member is less likely to have information about the behaviors encompassed in the dependence syndrome concept than about more externally visible social consequences that made up a good part of the DSM-III definitions.

Discussion

A disadvantage in deleting social consequences from the taxonomy and diagnosing only a dependence syndrome, as it is conceptualized in DSM-III-R, is that the latter lacks the necessary follow-up and other data to establish predictive validity, particularly for substances other than alcohol (Rounsaville 1987). Substance use taxonomies based on social consequences of use have been used for many years, and thus more validity data are available.

For a variety of reasons, it seems appropriate to base an abuse diagnosis on the occurrence of substance-related adverse social consequences (Table 1–1). Specifically, the benefits of such a definition include

1. It would provide a definition for substance abuse that is consistent with DSM-III, the Feighner criteria (Feighner et al. 1972), and the Research Diagnostic Criteria.

Table 1–1. Diagnostic criteria items for abuse

1. Continued substance use despite knowledge of persistent or recurrent social, psychological, or physical problem(s) caused or exacerbated by the use of the substance (e.g., daily cigarette smoking despite a known diagnosis of emphysema or chronic bronchitis, cocaine use despite cocaine-induced depression, or continued drinking despite an ulcer made worse by alcohol consumption).
2. Recurrent substance use resulting in inability to fulfill major role obligations at work, school, or home (e.g., repeated absences or poor work performance related to substance use; substance-related absences, suspensions, or expulsions from school; or neglect of children or household).
3. Recurrent substance use in situations in which it is physically hazardous (e.g., driving an automobile or operating a machine when impaired by substance use).
4. Important social, occupational, or recreational activities given up or reduced because of substance use.
5. Recurrent substance-related legal or interpersonal problems (e.g., substance-related arrests and traffic accidents, or physical fights related to substance use).

Note. Field trials will be used to determine whether abuse can be diagnosed with only one item, or if two or more items are required.

2. It retains elements from previous criteria (adverse consequences) that have proven to be highly reliable and consistent over time.
3. There is evidence that cases defined in this way may have a different natural history than those having evidence of tolerance, withdrawal, and compulsive use.
4. It broadens one's repertoire of constructs for those few substances that have been hard to fit into previous diagnostic systems (e.g., tobacco dependence is often hard to diagnose because many smokers never quit for a long enough period to know if they would develop withdrawal symptoms).
5. Given the current state of knowledge about the predictive validity of the dependence syndrome, it seems premature to eliminate adverse social consequences from the DSM-IV taxonomy. Inclusion of adverse consequences in some form in the new criteria encourages comparative research between consequences of substance use and the elements of dependence.
6. It provides a definition of abuse that is conceptually clearly separable from dependence, rather than a definition that is a residual of dependence or shares most of the same elements.

Such a definition of *abuse* would provide a contrast with a diagnosis of substance dependence based on the recognized physiological and behavioral elements such as tolerance, withdrawal, and compulsive use. A definition of *dependence* that is orthogonal to the social consequences of substance use is useful in that the latter may have an inconsistent relationship to the core psychopathology because of social mores and other factors external to the individual. On the other hand, retention of social consequences as a separate dimension is also useful since its predictive validity has been more thoroughly examined and since these criteria may be more objective and utilitarian in certain contexts, such as family history studies of substance use. Orthogonal dimensions of social consequences and a dependence syndrome, each identified with its own label, also have the advantage of a taxonomy based on two definitionally independent (although obviously related) constructs rather than a single more complex construct.

The stability of criteria, with minor modification, is another advantage of this proposal. In their comparison of DSM-III and DSM-III-R criteria for schizophrenia, Fenton and colleagues (1988) advised against changing diagnostic criteria too frequently and were in favor of maintaining links between a particular taxonomy and its predecessors. In his related editorial, Gift (1988) suggested that the "issue might be stated in terms of locating a middle ground between unwarranted flux and undesirable stasis" (p. 1414).

Skodol (1989) pointed out that a dependence syndrome may establish itself before social consequences are evident, or even in some cases in the absence of social consequences. Therefore, for some persons, a dependence definition that is conceptualized independently from use-related social consequences may lead to earlier identification of a dependent state. However, Skodol goes on to say that

> research in substance dependence has yet to face adequately the need for external validation of alternative concepts of dependence. Shifts in concept like the one introduced in DSM-III-R need to be shown to define a population that has a maximally positive family history or maximal evidence of other known risk factors, suggests a particular treatment approach, or has a more uniform prognosis or short- or long-term outcome. Until such time as that is achieved, the concepts remain the products of strong opinions of certain professionals, but are of unknown scientific significance. (p. 139)

One obvious implication of orthogonal concepts for abuse and dependence is that a given subject can meet criteria for one but not the other, or for both simultaneously. Some decisions need to be made about how to deal diagnostically with the various possible combinations. First, abuse without dependence will likely be found to occur not infrequently (see ECA data) but is not a diagnostic problem. Second, the question arises whether one should give diagnoses of both abuse and dependence to those who meet criteria for both. This seems unnecessarily complicated. Many if not most of those with substance dependence will either currently or in the past have also had sufficient social and/or other external consequences from their substance involvement that they will have met criteria for abuse. To acknowledge this fact formally with an additional diagnosis of abuse is not entirely redundant, but is probably largely so, and there would seem to be little gain in diagnostic clarity. It seems reasonable, therefore, that one of the criteria for substance abuse is that the respondent has never met criteria for dependence for the same substance. However, a specific designation of dependence without abuse, when applicable, would appear to be a more meaningful diagnostic possibility. This latter category might be particularly appropriate for 1) iatrogenic cases of dependence (as in the use of narcotics for pain relief), 2) those who are dependent on atypical substances (such as anabolic steroids) but have not had adverse social consequences from their use, or 3) physicians and other medical personnel who are dependent on drugs without manifesting adverse social consequences because they have a more available source of supply.

Recommendations

In conclusion, on the basis of this review of the literature, it is recommended that DSM-IV develop orthogonal concepts for substance abuse and dependence. That is, the universe of symptoms utilized for abuse would differ from that of dependence, and each category would have a specific definition based on its own set of symptoms. The abuse diagnosis, based on the occurrence of substance-related adverse social consequences, would thus be conceptually clearly separable from dependence, rather than a residual of dependence as was essentially the case in DSM-III-R.

References

American Psychiatric Association: Diagnostic and Statistical Manual of Mental Disorders, 3rd Edition. Washington, DC, American Psychiatric Association, 1980

American Psychiatric Association: Diagnostic and Statistical Manual of Mental Disorders, 3rd Edition, Revised. Washington, DC, American Psychiatric Association, 1987

Babor TF, Cooney NL, Lauerman RJ: The dependence syndrome concept as a psychological theory of relapse behaviour: an empirical evaluation of alcoholic and opiate addicts. Br J Addict 82:393–405, 1987

Bejerot N: A theory of addiction as an artificially induced drive. Am J Psychiatry 128:842–846, 1972

Blackwell J: Proposed changes in DSM-III substance dependence criteria (letter). Am J Psychiatry 144:258, 1987

Bucholz K: Alcohol abuse versus alcohol dependence in community-dwelling elders. Paper presented at the Midwest Sociological Society, March 24, 1988

Cahalan D, Cisin III, Crossley HM: American Drinking Practices: A National Study of Drinking Behavior and Attitudes. New Brunswick, NJ, Rutgers Center of Alcohol Studies, 1969

Edwards G, Gross MM: Alcohol dependence: provisional description of a clinical syndrome. BMJ 1:1058–1061, 1976

Endicott J, Spitzer RL: A diagnostic interview: the Schedule for Affective Disorders and Schizophrenia. Arch Gen Psychiatry 35:837–844, 1978

Feighner JP, Robins E, Guze SB, et al: Diagnostic criteria for use in psychiatric research. Arch Gen Psychiatry 26:57–63, 1972

Fenton WS, McGlashan TH, Heinssen RK: A comparison of DSM-III and DSM-III-R schizophrenia. Am J Psychiatry 145:1446–1449, 1988

Gift TE: Changing diagnostic criteria (editorial). Am J Psychiatry 145:1414–1415, 1988

Hasin DS, Grant BF: Assessment of specific drug disorders in a sample of substance abuse patients: a comparison of the DIS and the SADS-L procedures. Drug Alcohol Depend 19:165–176, 1987

Hasin DS, Grant BF, Harford TC, et al: The drug dependence syndrome and related disabilities. Br J Addict 83:45–55, 1988

Hasin DS, Grant B, Endicott J: The natural history of alcohol abuse: implications for definitions of alcohol use disorders. Am J Psychiatry 147:1537–1541, 1990

Helzer JE: Working paper on the relationship of psychoactive substance abuse to substance dependence. Prepared for the DSM-IV Substance Use Committee, September 25, 1989

Helzer JE, Canino GJ: The implications of cross-national research for diagnostic validity, in The Validity of Psychiatric Diagnosis. Edited by Robins LN, Barrett JE. New York, Raven, 1989

Helzer JE, Canino GJ, Yeh EK, et al: Alcoholism: North America and Asia: a comparison of population surveys with the Diagnostic Interview Schedule. Arch Gen Psychiatry 47:313–319, 1990

Helzer JE, Burnam A, McEvoy LT: Alcohol abuse and dependence, in Psychiatric Disorders in America. Edited by Robins LN, Regier DA. New York, Free Press, 1991

Kosten TR, Rounsaville BJ, Babor TF, et al: Substance-use disorders in DSM-III-R: evidence for the dependence syndrome across different psychoactive substances. Br J Psychiatry 151:834–843, 1987

Miller NS, Gold MS: Suggestions for changes in DSM-III-R criteria for substance use disorders. Am J Drug Alcohol Abuse 15:223–230, 1989

Peyser HS, Gitlow SE: Substance abuse category in DSM-III-R (letter). Am J Psychiatry 145:279–280, 1988

Regier DA, Myers JK, Kramer M, et al: The NIMH Epidemiologic Catchment Area program: historical context, major objectives, and study populations characteristics. Arch Gen Psychiatry 41:934–941, 1984

Rinaldi RC, Steindler EM, Wilford BB, et al: Clarification and standardization of substance abuse terminology. JAMA 259:555–557, 1988

Robins LN, Helzer JE, Croughan J, et al: National Institute of Mental Health Diagnostic Interview Schedule: its history, characteristics, and validity. Arch Gen Psychiatry 38:381–389, 1981

Rounsaville BJ: An evaluation of the DSM-III substance-use disorders, in Diagnosis and Classification in Psychiatry: A Critical Appraisal of DSM-III. Edited by Tischler GL. Cambridge, NY, Cambridge University Press, 1987

Rounsaville BJ, Kosten TR, Williams JB, et al: A field trial of DSM-III-R psychoactive substance dependence disorders. Am J Psychiatry 144:351–355, 1987

Schuckit MA, Zisook S, Mortola J: Clinical implications of DSM-III diagnoses of alcohol abuse and alcohol dependence. Am J Psychiatry 142:1403–1408, 1985

Skinner HA, Allen BA: Alcohol dependence syndrome: measurement and validation. J Abnorm Psychol 91:199–209, 1982

Skinner HA, Goldberg AE: Evidence for a drug dependence syndrome among narcotics users. Br J Addict 81:479–484, 1986

Skodol AE: Problems in Differential Diagnosis: From DSM-III to DSM-III-R in Clinical Practice. Washington, DC, American Psychiatric Press, 1989

Spitzer RL, Endicott J, Robins E: Research Diagnostic Criteria: rationale and reliability. Arch Gen Psychiatry 35:773–782, 1978

White HR: Longitudinal stability and dimensional structure of problem drinking in adolescence. J Stud Alcohol 48:541–550, 1987

Chapter 2

Psychoactive Substance Dependence

Peter E. Nathan, Ph.D.

Statement of the Issues

The diagnostic criteria for Psychoactive Substance Dependence in DSM-III (American Psychiatric Association 1980) and DSM-III-R (American Psychiatric Association 1987) have generated both admirers and critics. Both sets of criteria have been lauded because they provide operational criteria that enhance diagnostic reliability and permit diagnostic distinctions between abuse and dependence that have demonstrable diagnostic validity and utility.

The DSM-III approach to the diagnosis of the Psychoactive Substance Use Disorders has been criticized 1) because it lacks an underlying theoretical rationale; 2) because only modest empirical data informed its development; 3) because it does not make clear the conceptual basis on which it distinguishes between abuse and dependence; and 4) because that distinction is only moderately valid and useful (Rounsaville 1987; Rounsaville et al. 1986; Schuckit et al. 1985). The DSM-III-R approach has been questioned 1) because it seems to rely on a single conceptual view of dependence, Edwards' (1986) alcohol dependence syndrome, with insufficient empirical support; 2) because it appears to have broadened the scope of dependence at the expense of abuse; and 3) because, like DSM-III, it has proven to be only moderately useful and valid (Hasin et al. 1989; T. A. Kosten and T. R. Kosten: The dependence syndrome concept as applied to alcohol and other substances of abuse, Yale University, unpublished manuscript 1989; Rounsaville et al. 1987).

In this review, I evaluate the strengths and weaknesses of the conceptual and empirical bases for the DSM-III and DSM-III-R criteria for Psychoactive Substance Dependence, as well as the empirical data on the utility and validity of those criteria. The central issue for the review is whether the DSM-III criteria for dependence, the DSM-III-R criteria, or criteria representing some combination of the two yield diagnostic distinctions that differ in conceptual soundness, reliability, usefulness, and validity.

Significance of the Issues

The issue of the reliability, utility, and validity of the diagnosis of Psychoactive Substance Dependence is most significant. In essence, the issue affects the relative proportions of persons using psychoactive substances who are considered to be either abusing them or dependent on them. An ideal distinction between abuse and dependence would yield quite separate groups of persons differing in symptomatology, predicted course of illness, and likely response to treatment. Maximizing the predictive significance of the distinction between abuse and dependence would almost certainly enhance the ability of clinicians to provide more effective prevention and treatment for the victims of these disorders.

Methods

This review included a computer-based search for both conceptual and empirical studies of definitions, correlates, and predictors of substance (alcohol and drug) dependence according to DSM-III, DSM-III-R, and ICD-9 (World Health Organization 1977) criteria. Most of the literature reviewed related to alcohol dependence since relatively few studies on dependence on other drugs have been reported. More than 125 citations, dating to 1981, were generated. Drafts of this review were shared with members of the Substance Use Disorders Work Group, as well as with consultants and advisers to the Work Group.

Results and Discussion

The Evolution of Diagnostic Conceptions of Dependence

Alcoholism and drug dependence appeared in DSM-I (American Psychiatric Association 1952), the first broadly conceived American nomenclature, as subsets of "Sociopathic Personality Disturbance," a catchall diagnostic category that also included antisocial behavior and the sexual deviations, including homosexuality. DSM-II (American Psychiatric Association 1968) categorized all four patterns of behavior essentially the same way. In both these editions of DSM, the implication of the placement of these conditions was that all constituted behaviors of which society strongly disapproved (Nathan and Harris 1975).

DSM-III moved away from the implicit moralizing burdening those portions of DSM-I and DSM-II devoted to substance abuse and dependence, the sexual deviations, and antisocial behavior. It did so, in part, by allocating a separate category to the substance use disorders, thereby avoiding the guilt by association implicit in their 1952 and 1968 placement. In addition, the text of the 1980 manual highlighted research findings implicating sociocultural and genetic factors in the etiology of these disorders, thereby emphasizing the role that scientists and clinicians had begun to play in their study and treatment.

The DSM-III Conception of Abuse and Dependence

DSM-III divided the substance use disorders into two major categories—abuse and dependence—even though until very recently clinical data, but no empirical research, justified the definition of an abuse category. However, Hasin and colleagues (1990), investigating the natural history of abuse and dependence, found a significant number of persons with a history of abuse who never progressed to dependence, thereby justifying a category of abuse separate from dependence.

Spitzer and colleagues (1980) defined the DSM-III conception of substance dependence as follows:

> The presence of either tolerance or withdrawal. For Alcohol and Cannabis Dependence, impairment in social or occupational functioning is also required. In the case of tobacco, the presence of a serious physical disorder that the individual knows is exacerbated by tobacco use is also considered evidence of Dependence. (p. 157)

The empirical data accumulated over the years in support of the validity of the DSM criteria for (largely) alcohol abuse and dependence have, with some exceptions (e.g., Schuckit et al. 1986), found the distinction between abuse and dependence predictive of disorder severity and treatment outcome to a moderate degree (e.g., Hermos et al. 1988; Kosten and Kosten, unpublished manuscript 1989; Rounsaville et al. 1987). Other predictors, however, including age at onset and intensity of alcohol or drug use (e.g., Schuckit 1985), family history of substance abuse and/or dependence (e.g., Buydens-Branchey et al. 1989), and number and severity of comorbid conditions, especially antisocial personality (e.g., Hesselbrock et al. 1985a, 1985b; Rounsaville et al. 1986, 1987; Stabenau 1984), have predicted both severity and outcomes at least as robustly.

Critiques of the DSM-III Criteria for Abuse and Dependence

Although widely hailed as less stigmatizing and more reliable than its predecessors, DSM-I and DSM-II, and despite the empirical data in support of its concurrent and predictive validity cited above, the DSM-III concept of abuse and dependence was widely criticized (e.g., Rounsaville 1987; Rounsaville et al. 1986; Schuckit et al. 1985). Most authors based their critiques on the voluminous literature on the sensitivity, specificity, and utility of the DSM-III criteria.

For example, Rounsaville (1987) identified four key problems with DSM-III.

1. The Substance Use Disorder section of DSM-III does not adequately conceptualize or denote the coexistent features of these disorders. Most clinicians and researchers agree that there is much more to substance use and abuse than simply the use of psychoactive drugs. The criteria for abuse and dependence in DSM-III do not reflect this clinical diversity.
2. The DSM-III conceptualization of the substance use disorders is unhelpfully atheoretical. By contrast, the consensus statement of the World Health Organization Working Group 4 (Edwards et al. 1981) represents a cogent and convincing statement of the need for a theory-driven conceptualization of the substance use disorders. The World Health Organization model proposal in that statement, influenced by Edwards and Gross' (1976) alcohol dependence syndrome (described below), is a complex, dynamic scheme based on behavioral principles that puts forward a "system of reinforcement which initiates and perpetuates substance taking and dependence" (Rounsaville 1987, p. 183).
3. Tolerance is a poor criterion for determining dependence. Tolerance in DSM-III is not specified in a complex manner, even though clinical tolerance phenomena are complex and varied. In addition, wide individual differences in initial levels of tolerance to drugs are the rule rather than the exception. Accordingly, it is easy for nontolerant persons to meet the tolerance criterion the way it is written in DSM-III.
4. The relationship between substance abuse and substance dependence is inconsistent and illogical in several substance categories in DSM-III. As they are written, the dependence criteria include, and sometimes mix, two different concepts: "psychological" dependence characterized by a pathological pattern of use, and "physiological" dependence demonstrated by a substance-specific withdrawal syndrome.

The DSM-III-R Conception of Dependence

The DSM-III-R conception of dependence owes a heavy debt to the alcohol dependence syndrome, described by Edwards and Gross in 1976, and elaborated by Edwards and colleagues in 1981 and Edwards in 1986. As described by Rounsaville and Kranzler (1989) in a review of the theoretical basis and empirical grounding for DSM-III-R, the alcohol dependence syndrome develops

> . . . in accordance with behavioral principles via a system of reinforcement that initiates and perpetuates substance taking and dependence. The positive and negative reinforcement contingencies involved in heavy alcohol use lead to the development of a core set of symptoms designated as the *dependence syndrome*; it is seen as multidimensional with *biologic, social, and behavioral components.* The cardinal feature of this syndrome is impaired control over alcohol use. The syndrome elements, most of which are incorporated into DSM-III-R criteria, are as follows: 1) narrowing of the substance use repertoire such that substance use becomes stereotyped around a regular schedule of almost continuous or daily consumption; 2) salience of substance-taking behavior such that, despite negative consequences, substance use is given higher priority than are other activities that previously had been important; 3) increased tolerance; 4) withdrawal symptoms; 5) substance use to avoid withdrawal; 6) subjectively experienced compulsion to use the substance; and 7) readdiction liability. (pp. 324–326)

The substance dependence syndrome concept appears to address most of the concerns about the four key problems with the DSM III approach to the substance use disorders identified by Rounsaville (1987). Thus, the substance dependence syndrome constitutes: 1) a theoretical, integrating statement about substance dependence that 2) clarifies the relationship between abuse and dependence, 3) diminishes the importance of both tolerance and withdrawal in the diagnosis of dependence, and 4) permits the incorporation of coexisting features of the substance use disorders in the diagnosis.

The substance dependence syndrome seems to be valid for drugs other than alcohol, the drug from which it was originally developed (e.g., Phillips et al. 1987; Stripp et al. 1990; Sutherland et al. 1986), and the syndrome has also been independently validated for alcohol by research workers other than Edwards and his colleagues (e.g., Babor et al. 1987a; Drummond 1990).

Concerns About the DSM-III-R Conception of Dependence

Despite the hypothetical advantages of conceptual reliance on the substance dependence syndrome in DSM-III-R, the dependence criteria that resulted from that reliance have in turn produced problems for diagnosticians and clinicians.

Moving away from the greater emphasis in DSM-III on the physical aspects of dependence (exemplified by tolerance and withdrawal symptoms) has appeared to some to dispute both widespread clinical conviction and empirical data attesting to the predictive validity of these symptoms (e.g., Hasin et al. 1989; Kosten and Kosten, unpublished manuscript 1989; Rounsaville et al. 1987). Shifting the criteria away from social consequences of alcohol abuse and dependence has also seemed to some to be a movement away from a central feature of the syndrome. Others have also noted that the concept of dependence in the DSM-III-R criteria is so broad that it has increased the heterogeneity of labeled patients and obscured traditional concepts of the substance use disorders so that clinicians are tempted to arrive at unsubstantiated syndromes such as shopping and sexual dependencies. The changes in criteria have also reduced the meaning of the concept of abuse to a "residual" label lacking documented prognostic and treatment implications, despite some empirical evidence to the contrary reported by Hasin et al. (1990). Despite encouraging empirical and conceptual reports on the advantages of the substance dependence syndrome (e.g., Babor et al. 1987a, 1987b; Skinner and Goldberg 1986), a direct comparison of the DSM-III and DSM-III-R criteria with a range of patients in a variety of clinical settings would appear requisite to a fully informed decision on the differential predictive validity of the two sets of criteria.

Recommendations

In each of two alternative sets of proposed DSM-IV criteria (Tables 2–1 and 2–2), dependence incorporates the DSM-III-R emphasis on an expanded concept of dependence (including compulsive use), as well as the DSM-III reliance on impairment in social and occupational functioning and pathological use.

By using the first proposed set of criteria (Table 2–1), which represents an effort to resolve the continuing question of the proper diagnostic emphasis placed on tolerance and withdrawal, the diagnostic utility of subtyping dependence into Physiological Dependence and Behavioral Dependence can be explored. Diagnosis of either of the two would require that a specified number of criteria for dependence be met; the exact number of criteria will be determined by field trial. Patients who met criteria for dependence that included tolerance, withdrawal, or both would merit the diagnosis Physiological Dependence; those who met criteria for dependence that did not include tolerance or withdrawal would receive the diagnosis Behavioral Dependence (i.e., substance dependence without physiological dependence).

In the second of the proposed sets of criteria (Table 2–2), satisfying a specified number of criteria (to be determined by field trial) describing compulsive use, impairment in social and occupational functioning, or pathological use without demonstrating tolerance or withdrawal would yield the diagnosis of substance abuse. An additional demonstration of tolerance or withdrawal would result in the diagnosis of substance dependence.

A principal source of data to evaluate DSM-III-R and any possible changes for DSM-IV will be a field trial with at least six data collection sites within the United States and five outside the United States. Together, they will survey more than 1,500 patients diverse in age, ethnicity, gender, and treatment status. These men and

Table 2–1. Proposed DSM-IV diagnostic criteria set 1: Psychoactive Substance Dependence

A. A maladaptive pattern of substance use, leading to clinically significant impairment or distress, as manifested by ? of the following [items and thresholds to be determined by field trial]:

(1) tolerance, as defined by any of the following:

(a) need for markedly increased amounts of the substance to achieve intoxication or desired effect

(b) markedly diminished effect with continued use of the same amount of the substance

(c) has functioned adequately at doses or blood levels of the substance that would produce significant impairment in a casual user

(2) the characteristic withdrawal syndrome for the substance

(3) the same substance is often taken to relieve or avoid withdrawal symptoms

(4) the substance is often taken in larger amounts or over a longer period than intended

(5) any unsuccessful effort or persistent desire to cut down or control substance use

(6) a great deal of time is spent in activities necessary to obtain the substance (e.g., visiting multiple doctors or driving long distances), take the substance (e.g., chain-smoking), or recover from its effects

(7) recurrent substance use resulting in inability to fulfill major role obligations at work, school, or home (e.g., repeated absences or poor work performance related to substance use; substance-related absences, suspensions, or expulsions from school; neglect of children or household)

(8) recurrent substance use in situations in which it is physically hazardous (e.g., driving an automobile or operating a machine when impaired by substance use)

(9) important social, occupational, or recreational activities given up or reduced because of substance use

(10) recurrent substance-related legal or interpersonal problems (e.g., substance-related arrests and traffic accidents, physical fights related to substance use)

(11) continued substance use despite knowledge of a persistent or recurrent problem(s) caused or exacerbated by the use of the substance (e.g., keeps using heroin despite family arguments about it, cocaine use despite recognition of cocaine-induced depression, or continued drinking despite recognition that an ulcer was made worse by alcohol consumption)

Options for Criterion B: (duration of symptoms):

Option B1:

B. Some symptoms of the disturbance have occurred most days for at least 1 month, or have occurred repeatedly over a longer period of time.

Option B2: no duration specified (i.e., omit criterion B)

Specify if:

With Physiological Dependence: Evidence of tolerance or withdrawal (i.e., any of items A(1), A(2), or A(3) are present).

Without Physiological Dependence: No evidence of tolerance or withdrawal (i.e., none of items A(1), A(2), and A(3) is present).

Table 2–2. Proposed DSM-IV diagnostic criteria set 2: Psychoactive Substance Dependence

A. Any of the following:
   (1) tolerance, as defined by any of the following:
      (a) need for markedly increased amounts of the substance to achieve intoxication or desired effect
      (b) markedly diminished effect with continued use of the same amount of the substance
      (c) has functioned adequately at doses or blood levels of the substance that would produce significant impairment in a casual user
   (2) the characteristic withdrawal syndrome for the substance
   (3) the same substance is often taken to relieve or avoid withdrawal symptoms

B. A pattern of repeated problems with the substance as indicated by at least ? of the following [items and thresholds to be determined by field trial]:
   (1) the substance is often taken in larger amounts or over a longer period than intended
   (2) any unsuccessful effort or persistent desire to cut down or control substance use
   (3) a great deal of time is spent in activities necessary to obtain the substance (e.g., visiting multiple doctors or driving long distances), take the substance (e.g., chain-smoking), or recover from its effects
   (4) recurrent substance use resulting in inability to fulfill major role obligations at work, school, or home (e.g., repeated absences or poor work performance related to substance use; substance-related absences, suspensions, or expulsions from school; neglect of children or household)
   (5) recurrent substance use in situations in which it is physically hazardous (e.g., driving an automobile or operating a machine when impaired by substance use)
   (6) important social, occupational, or recreational activities given up or reduced because of substance use
   (7) recurrent substance-related legal or interpersonal problems (e.g., substance-related arrests and traffic accidents, and physical fights related to substance use)
   (8) continued substance use despite knowledge of a persistent or recurrent problem(s) caused or exacerbated by the use of the substance (e.g., keeps using heroin despite family arguments about it, cocaine use despite recognition of cocaine-induced depression, or continued drinking despite recognition that an ulcer was made worse by alcohol consumption)

Options for Criterion C: (duration of symptoms)

Option C1:

C: Some symptoms of the disturbance have occurred most days for at least 1 month, or have occurred repeatedly over a longer period of time.

Option C2: no duration specified (i.e., omit criterion C)

women will be drawn from the general population as well as from treatment samples suffering from a range of substance use disorders. The patients' abuse and/or dependence will be diagnosed according to DSM-III, ICD-10 (World Health Organization 1992), and DSM-III-R criteria, as well as the two sets of criteria proposed for DSM-IV pending the evaluation of their reliability and validity.

In addition, several existing sets of previously unanalyzed clinical data are being analyzed under a grant from the John D. and Catherine T. MacArthur Foundation. These data were gathered from general population samples, such as the Epidemiologic Catchment Area projects (Regier et al. 1984), as well as from groups of individuals using cocaine, heroin, and alcohol. The diagnosis of abuse or dependence of these individuals will be established according to the proposed DSM-IV criteria, as well as by those from the three other diagnostic systems.

The saliency of the groups of patients diagnosed by the four criteria sets will be judged on multiple levels. These include the relative homogeneity, clinical characteristics, and "coverage" of relevant clinical cases labeled by the different diagnostic schemes. In addition, some samples will be followed over 3 or more months to determine the course of the substance use disorder. Outcomes will include such indices as whether or not drinking or drug use resumes, the pattern and malignancy of resultant alcohol- or drug-related problems, presence and severity of alcohol or drug withdrawal symptoms, occurrence and nature of co-morbidity, and, when relevant, the nature of subsequent alcohol- or drug-related diagnoses.

Following the analysis of unanalyzed data sets and data from the field trial, the differential predictive and concurrent validity of the four sets of diagnostic criteria will be examined. Although the ultimate validator of criteria defining abuse or dependence will be how well abuse and dependence independently predict course of illness, other relevant predictors will include number and malignancy of substance-related signs and symptoms; associated physical, psychological, psychiatric, social, familial, and vocational status; and response to treatment and other measures of involvement in treatment.

References

American Psychiatric Association: Diagnostic and Statistical Manual: Mental Disorders. Washington, DC, American Psychiatric Association, 1952

American Psychiatric Association: Diagnostic and Statistical Manual of Mental Disorders, 2nd Edition. Washington, DC, American Psychiatric Association, 1968

American Psychiatric Association: Diagnostic and Statistical Manual of Mental Disorders, 3rd Edition. Washington, DC, American Psychiatric Association, 1980

American Psychiatric Association: Diagnostic and Statistical Manual of Mental Disorders, 3rd Edition, Revised. Washington, DC, American Psychiatric Association, 1987

Babor TF, Cooney NL, Lauerman RJ: The drug dependence syndrome concept as a psychological theory of relapse behavior: an empirical evaluation. Br J Addict 82:393–405, 1987a

Babor TF, Lauerman RJ, Cooney NL: In search of the alcohol dependence syndrome: a cross-national study of its structure and validity, in Cultural Studies on Drinking and Drinking Practices. Edited by Paakkanen P, Sulkunen P. Helsinki, Social Research Institute on Alcohol Studies, 1987b

Buydens-Branchey L, Branchey MH, Noumair D: Age of alcoholism onset: relationship to susceptibility. Arch Gen Psychiatry 46:225–230, 1989

Drummond DC: The relationship between alcohol dependence and alcohol-related problems in a clinical population. Br J Addict 85:357–366, 1990

Edwards G: The alcohol dependence syndrome: a concept as stimulus to enquiry. Br J Addict 81:171–183, 1986

Edwards G, Gross MM: Alcohol dependence: provisional description of a clinical syndrome. BMJ 1:1058–1061, 1976

Edwards G, Arif A, Hodgson R: Nomenclature and classification of drug- and alcohol-related problems: a WHO memorandum. Bull WORLD Health Organ 59:225–242, 1981

Hasin DS, Endicott J, Keller MB: RDC alcoholism in patients with major affective syndromes: two-year course. Am J Psychiatry 146:318–323, 1989

Hasin DS, Grant B, Endicott J: The natural history of alcohol abuse: implications for definitions of alcohol use disorders. Am J Psychiatry 147:1537–1541, 1990

Hermos JA, Locastro JS, Glynn RJ, et al: Predictors of reduction and cessation of drinking in community-dwelling men: results from the normative aging study. J Stud Alcohol 49:363–368, 1988

Hesselbrock MN, Weidenman MA, Reed HBC: Effect of age, sex, drinking history and antisocial personality on neuropsychology of alcoholism. J Stud Alcohol 46:313–319, 1985a

Hesselbrock MN, Meyer RE, Keener JJ: Psychopathology in hospitalized alcoholics. Arch Gen Psychiatry 42:1050–1055, 1985b

Nathan PE, Harris SL: Psychopathology and Society. New York, McGraw-Hill, 1975

Phillips GT, Gossop MR, Edwards G, et al: The application of the SODQ to the measurement of the severity of opiate dependence in a British sample. Br J Addict 82:691–699, 1987

Regier DA, Myers JK, Kramer M, et al: The NIMH Epidemiologic Catchment Area program: historical context, major objectives, and study populations characteristics. Arch Gen Psychiatry 41:934–941, 1984

Rounsaville BJ: An evaluation of the DSM-III substance-use disorders, in Diagnosis and Classification in Psychiatry: A Critical Appraisal of DSM-III. Edited by Tischler GL. New York, Cambridge University Press, 1987

Rounsaville BJ, Kranzler HR: The DSM-III-R diagnosis of alcoholism, in American Psychiatric Press Review of Psychiatry, Vol 8. Edited by Tasman A, Hales RE, Frances AJ. Washington, DC, American Psychiatric Press, 1989

Rounsaville BJ, Spitzer RL, Williams JBW: Proposed changes in DSM-III substance use disorders: description and rationale. Am J Psychiatry 143:463–468, 1986

Rounsaville BJ, Dolinsky ZS, Babor TF, et al: Psychopathology as a predictor of treatment outcome in alcoholics. Arch Gen Psychiatry 44:505–513, 1987

Schuckit MA: The clinical implications of primary diagnostic groups among alcoholics. Arch Gen Psychiatry 42:1043–1049, 1985

Schuckit MA, Zisook S, Mortola J: Clinical implications of DSM-III diagnoses about alcohol abuse and alcohol dependence. Am J Psychiatry 142:1403–1408, 1985

Schuckit MA, Schwei MG, Gold E: Prediction of outcomes in inpatient alcoholics. J Stud Alcohol 47:151–155, 1986

Skinner HA, Goldberg AE: Evidence for a drug dependence syndrome among narcotics users. Br J Addict 81:479–484, 1986

Spitzer RL, Williams JB, Skodol AE: DSM-III: The major achievements and an overview. Am J Psychiatry 137:151–164, 1980

Stabenau JR: Implications of family history of alcoholism, antisocial personality, and sex differences in alcohol dependence. Am J Psychiatry 141:1178–1182, 1984

Stripp AW, Burgess PM, Pattison PE, et al: An evaluation of the psychoactive substance dependence syndrome in its application to opiate users. Br J Addict 85:621–627, 1990

Sutherland G, Edwards G, Taylor C, et al: The measurement of opiate dependence. Br J Addict 81:485–494, 1986

World Health Organization: International Classification of Diseases, 9th Revision. Geneva, World Health Organization, 1977

World Health Organization: The ICD-10 Classification of Mental and Behavioural Disorders: Clinical Descriptions and Diagnostic Guidelines. Geneva, World Health Organization, 1992

Chapter 3

The Relationship Between Alcohol Problems, Substance Abuse, and Psychiatric Syndromes

Marc A. Schuckit, M.D.

Statement of the Issues

1. Should DSM-IV include more specific exclusion criteria for the diagnosis of mental disorders in the presence of alcohol or drug abuse/dependence?
2. If so, how should these exclusion criteria be framed?

Significance of the Issues

The crossover between substance intake and symptoms of psychopathology is important to DSM-IV for a number of reasons. For example, the interactions must be considered in the process of developing appropriate exclusion criteria for psychiatric disorders. The topic has a potential impact on prognostic factors associated with both substance-related and major psychiatric problems. The interrelationship among these problems affects notations of severity of psychopathology. Several potential subtypings of diagnostic categories change dramatically in light of different ways of viewing the interactions. In this chapter, I attempt to outline the wide-ranging implications of these interactions for both the structure and content of DSM-IV. (Note: In this chapter, I use the term *substance abuse* to

---

This chapter is an abridged version of a report in the author's file.

include alcohol and to relate to both abuse and dependence; alcoholism is used as a shorthand for alcohol abuse or dependence.)

Factors Contributing to the High Rate of Comorbidity

One reason the relationship between substance abuse and psychiatric problems, especially depression and anxiety, is so visible is because both types of disorders are very common. Thus, by chance alone, psychiatric symptomatology and substance abuse problems should be expected to occur concomitantly in many individuals (Helzer et al. 1988; Robins et al. 1984; Schuckit 1985b). Related to the high prevalence, there is consistent evidence that when an individual demonstrates symptoms in two or more areas, he or she is more likely to come in for treatment than the average individual and thus is more likely to be identified as a potential case (Weissman 1980).

A second major reason why problems of substance abuse often co-occur with other psychiatric symptoms has a more direct relationship to potential causes. There is evidence that intake of many of the drugs of abuse, including alcohol, can produce psychiatric symptoms that mimic major psychiatric disorders. This might be true of any type of drug of abuse, but most data have been generated regarding the brain stimulants (e.g., cocaine, amphetamine) and brain depressant drugs (e.g., alcohol, benzodiazepines, barbiturates) (Schuckit 1989). In short, intoxication with *brain stimulants* can cause many symptoms of *anxiety,* with intake of larger doses even producing syndromes that can look similar to obsessive-compulsive disorder, panic disorder, and generalized anxiety disorder. Withdrawal from brain stimulants as well as repeated and prolonged intoxication with *brain depressants* can cause sadness that might even produce severe and incapacitating *depression* that resembles a major depressive episode. Withdrawal from brain depressant drugs is likely to produce intense and acute anxiety, with the probability of prolonged, but less severe, anxiety during what might be considered a protracted abstinence syndrome. Repeated stimulant intoxication, especially with amphetamines and cocaine, is likely to produce a syndrome of auditory hallucinations along with paranoid delusions that can temporarily resemble *schizophrenia.*

The Approach Used by DSM-III-R

DSM-III-R (American Psychiatric Association 1987) combines elements of several schemes that are used for dealing with multiple diagnoses (Skodol 1989). If a patient fulfills criteria for both a psychiatric syndrome and a drug-related difficulty, the case usually falls into one of four conditions. First, the criteria for some psychiatric disorders note that alcohol- and drug-related problems are *specific exclusions* for the label, a case that applies to 17 of the DSM-III-R labels as shown in Table 3–1. Second, some psychiatric syndromes mention substance- or alcohol-related diffi-

Table 3–1. DSM-III-R diagnoses with specific substance-related exclusions

Diagnosis number	Diagnosis	Comment noted in criteria
295.6X	Schizophrenia, Residual Phase	Not due to a Psychoactive Substance Use Disorder
301.13	Cyclothymia	It cannot be established that an organic factor initiated and maintained the disturbance (e.g., repeated intoxication from drugs or alcohol)
300.21, .01, .22	Panic Disorder	It cannot be . . . (e.g., amphetamine or caffeine intoxication, hyperthyroidism)
300.02	Generalized Anxiety Disorder	It cannot be . . . (e.g., hyperthyroidism, caffeine intoxication)
300.30	Obsessive Compulsive Disorder	. . . the content of the obsession is not . . . about drugs in the presence of a Psychoactive Substance Use Disorder
300.81	Somatization Disorder	No organic pathology or pathophysiologic mechanism (e.g., a physical disorder or the effects of injury, medication, drugs, or alcohol) to account for the symptom
300.70	Undifferentiated Somatoform Disorder	Appropriate evaluation uncovers no organic pathology or pathophysiologic mechanism (e.g., a physical disorder or the effects of injury, medication, drugs, or alcohol) to account for the physical complaints
300.12	Psychogenic Amnesia	The disturbance is not due to Multiple Personality Disorder or to an Organic Mental Disorder (e.g., blackouts during alcohol intoxication)
307.42	Insomnia Related to Another Mental Disorder (Nonorganic)	This category is not used if the Insomnia Disorder is related to an Axis I Disorder involving a known organic factor such as Psychoactive Substance Use Disorder (e.g., Amphetamine Dependence)
780.50	Insomnia Related to a Known Organic Disorder	The known organic disorder . . . Axis I (if Psychoactive Substance Use Disorder)
307.42	Primary Insomnia	. . . that apparently is not maintained by . . . Psychoactive Substance Use Disorder
780.50	Hypersomnia Related to a Known Organic Factor	. . . is related to a known organic, such as . . . Psychoactive Substance Use Disorder (e.g., Cannabis Dependence)
780.54	Primary Hypersomnia	. . . is apparently not maintained by another mental disorder or any known organic factor such as . . . a Psychoactive Substance Use Disorder

(continued)

Table 3–1. DSM-III-R diagnoses with specific substance-related exclusions *(continued)*

Diagnosis number	Diagnosis	Comment noted in criteria
312.34	Intermittent Explosive Disorder	The . . . loss of control does not occur during . . . intoxication with a Psychoactive Substance
307.23	Tourette's Disorder	Occurrence not exclusively during Psychoactive Substance Intoxication
307.22	Chronic Motor or Vocal Tic Disorder	Same as above
307.21	Transient Tic Disorder	Same as above

culties indirectly, noting the need to exclude cases related to organic disorders. These syndromes include schizophrenia; delusional (paranoid) disorder; brief reactive psychosis, schizophreniform disorder, schizoaffective disorder, and psychotic disorder not otherwise specified (NOS) (atypical psychoses); manic episode, major depressive episode, and dysthymia; psychogenic fugue; and dream anxiety disorder, sleep terror disorder, and sleepwalking disorder. Third, some labels call for the exclusion of individuals with any Axis I label. They include the sexual desire disorders, the sexual arousal disorders, inhibited female and male orgasm, and vaginismus, together with hypersomnia related to another mental disorder (nonorganic), factitious disorders with physical and psychological symptoms, and all adjustment disorders. Fourth, the majority of psychiatric labels make no mention of substance-related difficulties as potential exclusionary criteria. (Note: the unabridged version of this report in the author's files includes tables that further detail each of these four conditions.)

The present state of affairs in DSM-III-R raises several questions. Are the exclusionary criteria consistent with the data generated in the literature? Are clinicians appropriately considering the exclusionary criteria? If diagnoses are established for their prognostic and treatment implications, do more specific exclusion rules need to be developed? If more specific or extensive exclusion criteria are justified for the diagnosis of mental disorders in the presence of alcohol or drug abuse or dependence, are these most appropriately incorporated into the diagnostic criteria themselves, should they be placed in the background paragraphs for diagnostic sections, or is it appropriate to place them only within the Sourcebook? After DSM-IV is finalized, what additional data need to be gathered so that DSM-V can subsequently represent a step forward in the clear utilization of data to justify diagnostic schemes with the maximal impact on prognosis and treatment? This daunting list of questions underscores the significance of these issues and more than justifies the time and effort expended on the data evaluation.

Methods

In preparing this overview, it became apparent that to answer and document these general issues adequately, enough material would be generated to fill several full-length texts. Therefore, I have opted to place a major emphasis on the *global scheme,* focusing on specific items only when such expansions are useful in helping our committee to develop a more global approach. It is assumed that once an overall paradigm is adopted, it may be necessary to go back to the literature to expand the information as it relates to more specific queries.

In light of these considerations, I present in the results section a more global overview of the relationship between psychiatric syndromes and substances of abuse. To make the task "doable," I focus primarily on two categories of drugs likely to be involved with psychiatric syndromes: the brain stimulants and the brain depressants. At the same time, recognizing the impossibility of paying adequate homage to all psychiatric syndromes, I focus specifically on anxiety disorders, psychoses, and depressive syndromes. However, the selection of depressants and stimulants as the examples of drug classes and the focus on anxiety, psychotic, and depressive states is not meant to imply that other drugs and diagnoses are less relevant. The unabridged version of this report outlined some of those relationships.

A computerized literature search was carried out utilizing Medline. The specific descriptors used included drug abuse and alcohol interacting with anxiety, depression, and psychoses. The search generated 200 citations that were briefly reviewed, with special care devoted to references listed in the diagnostic categories as they interact predominantly with the two categories of substances involved. Of these references, 120 are listed in the unabridged report.

Results

Anxiety Disorders and Substance Abuse

The data that support the contention that substances of abuse can cause anxiety syndromes, the data indicating that abuse of substances can exacerbate preexisting anxiety disorders, and the subsequent high rate of co-occurrence of anxiety and substance-related problems are briefly reviewed. Some tentative conclusions are also drawn.

Intoxication with stimulant drugs has been documented to produce many symptoms of anxiety. Animals administered a diverse range of stimulants (usually amphetamines or cocaine) demonstrate evidence of increased motor activity. Humans frequently show signs of anxiety or nervousness and can also develop cardiac arrhythmias and full-blown panic attacks with resulting groups of symptoms that can resemble generalized anxiety disorder or panic disorder (Anthony et al. 1989; Gawin and Ellinwood 1988; Lowenstein et al. 1987). These data are corroborated by the high rate of panic and anxiety symptoms among those who abuse stimulants and those who indulge in large amounts of coffee (Anthony et al. 1989). The most potent stimulants, such as amphetamines and cocaine, can also produce striking obsessive-compulsive behavior (Segal and Schuckit 1983). However, as described below, if the anxiety developed in the context of drugs, the symptoms are likely to improve rapidly with abstinence.

The repeated intake of higher doses of the more powerful stimulants is likely to induce tolerance and evidence of physical dependence. The subsequent stimulant withdrawal or abstinence syndrome is likely to include numerous symptoms of anxiety such as insomnia and subjective complaints of nervousness (Wood and Lal 1987). Once again, unlike symptoms observed in the context of major anxiety syndromes, problems related to stimulant withdrawal are likely to decrease over time, although a period of several months might be involved (Gawin and Ellinwood 1988).

Brain depressant drugs (e.g., alcohol, the benzodiazepines, the barbiturates) are also likely to produce anxiety syndromes in the context of withdrawal. The acute abstinence syndrome associated with brain depressants almost invariably includes symptoms of anxiety and insomnia, along with evidence of autonomic nervous system overactivity (e.g., increased pulse, respiratory rates, and blood pressure) (Schuckit 1989; Sellers 1988). Problems with anxiety in this context can also include panic attacks and phobic syndromes. Although these symptoms are likely to decrease rapidly within the first 4–10 days of abstinence, many autonomic and electrophysiological changes persist with decreasing levels of intensity over a much more extended period of time, often several months (De Soto et al. 1985; Roelofs and Dikkenberg 1987). There is also evidence that acute intoxication with higher doses of alcohol or benzodiazepines can actually increase anxiety feelings, especially if people are asked to perform tasks while intoxicated (Monteiro et al. 1990).

Consumption of stimulants or withdrawal from depressants can intensify preexisting major psychiatric disorders. For example, individuals with panic disorder are likely to report an intensification of their symptoms after consuming caffeine (Bruce and Lader 1989; Gawin and Ellinwood 1988; Schuckit 1985a). Similar reactions have also been documented after the abuse of cocaine (Aronson and Craig 1986). Thus, it may be difficult to establish the severity of even a preexisting anxiety syndrome in the context of use or abuse of stimulants. According to anecdotal reports, many patients with anxiety syndromes refrain from drinking or drug use because they recognize that these substances worsen their condition (Tilley 1987).

There are consistent data documenting the high prevalence of anxiety symptoms among those who abuse alcohol and drugs (Kushner et al. 1990; Ross et al. 1988). The greatest likelihood of symptoms of anxiety is during acute withdrawal from brain depressants or intoxication with stimulants, conditions for which the anxiety is likely to disappear with time alone. Unfortunately, many of the studies in the literature report the presence of anxiety symptoms during periods contiguous with substance intake, making it difficult to determine what proportion of patients have independent disorders. For example, after a brief period of abstinence, of 84 male and 18 female alcoholic inpatients, 13% of the men and 33% of the women showed clinical pictures similar to agoraphobia; 25% and 17%, respectively, demonstrated evidence of social phobias (Mullaney and Trippett 1979). Invoking similar cross-sectional descriptions of alcoholic or other drug-abusing persons soon after abstinence from drugs (frequently within 2 weeks), similar high rates of symptoms of phobias, panic attacks, and general anxiety have frequently been documented (George et al. 1988; Hesselbrock et al. 1985; Smail et al. 1984; Stockwell and Bolderston 1987). On the other hand, studies using more restrictive criteria have reported lower levels of severe states of anxiety (Rounsaville et al. 1980), and others question such high rates of anxiety disorders among substance-abusing persons overall (Christie et al. 1988; Powell et al. 1982; Stravynski et al. 1986). Other studies have corroborated the high level of anxiety syndromes observed in the context of drug intoxication or withdrawal, but offer little evidence of elevated rates of major anxiety syndromes before the onset of severe alcohol or drug problems or persisting beyond the abstinence syndrome (Brown et al. 1991; Schuckit 1985a).

The co-occurrence of anxiety syndromes and actual abuse of substances is less impressive when the population under study is from psychiatric samples. Considering the high prevalence of alcohol abuse or dependence, as well as the enhanced likelihood that the co-occurrence of symptoms will bring an individual into treatment, the finding that between 10% and perhaps 20% of patients with a variety of anxiety disorders might also fulfill criteria for alcoholism or drug abuse is not very impressive (Bibb and Chambless 1986; Breier et al. 1986; Cloninger et al. 1981; Samarasinghe et al. 1984). One additional study of a diverse sample of 42 patients with anxiety disorders or depression reported that more than 40% were alcoholic, but considering the sample selection procedures, many subjects may have had primary alcoholism to begin with (Van Valkenburg et al. 1984). This is not to say that the literature documents that the two types of disorders are totally independent, but only that it highlights the lack of evidence for a remarkably enhanced rate of alcoholism or substance abuse in anxious patients.

There are a number of lines of evidence consistent with the probability that anxiety disorders and substance abuse disorders are usually discrete diagnoses. It may be that in most patients the two syndromes do *not* have a unique and close relationship, but rather that there is a temporary crossover of symptoms. First, as briefly alluded to above, when anxiety occurs in the context of abuse or dependence on drugs or alcohol, the symptoms tend to be temporary and, in distinction to what would be observed with the major anxiety disorders themselves, tend to disappear fairly rapidly over time. Brown and colleagues (1991) used the State-Trait Anxiety Inventory (Spielberger et al. 1968) with 171 alcoholic men who were followed over a 3-month period. Although on admission (after about 1 week of abstinence) 40% of these individuals scored in the 75th percentile or higher on anxiety symptoms, the levels of anxiety returned to normal within 2–4 weeks. On follow-up, it was only the alcoholic men who had gone back to drinking who were likely to demonstrate any significant increase in anxiety scores at 3 months. Similarly, Roelofs and Dikkenberg (1987) reported that the level of anxiety decreases with the length of abstinence.

Another line of reasoning supporting the relative independence of substance-related and anxiety syndromes comes from family and genetic studies. Schuckit (1987) compared anxiety scores and diagnoses of anxiety disorders from 237 sons of an alcoholic parent, ages between 18 and 25 years, with the scores from 237 control subjects. No increased prevalence of either anxiety symptoms or disorders was found in the group at high future alcoholism risk (i.e., sons of an alcoholic parent). Similarly, all known adoption studies of children of an alcoholic parent have failed to demonstrate an increased risk for major anxiety disorders in these children, even when they were followed into their mid-30s (Goodwin et al. 1973; Schuckit 1990; Schuckit and Winokur 1972). Also consistent with these conclusions is the study demonstrating that when alcoholic twin pairs are followed over time, it is only the heavy drinking member of the pair who is also likely to show anxiety (Mullan et al. 1986). Additionally, prospective studies of teenagers who were identified and followed up over a long period have also not demonstrated any close association between preexisting anxiety syndromes and the later development of alcohol or drug abuse (Vaillant 1983). Personality evaluations of individuals who eventually became alcoholic have also failed to show a close association between anxiety pictures and alcoholism or drug abuse at a later date (Kammeier et al. 1973).

Other studies have evaluated the rate of alcoholism among close relatives of individuals with panic disorder, although these investigations are hampered by the possibility that some of the original subjects were actually alcoholic or abusing drugs and had secondary anxiety syndromes. Only modest levels of increased rates of alcohol-related problems have been documented within those family groups in most studies (Crow et al. 1983; Harris et al. 1983; Munjack and Moss 1981). Although some investigations did report a markedly increased rate of alcohol problems, these were data gathered only from the subject and at times using only telephone interviews without any personal contact with close family members (Harris et al. 1983; Munjack and Moss 1981). Finally, several long-term studies of general population groups revealed no increased rate of anxiety syndromes among those who later went on to develop severe abstinence problems (Kammeier et al. 1973; Vaillant 1983).

In conclusion, the data do show a high level of co-occurrence of anxiety and substance-related problems. However, they also indicate that when anxiety syndromes occur in the context of alcohol or drug abuse, the prognostic and treatment implications may be different than when anxiety occurs in the absence of substance problems. The prognostic and treatment implications of even severe anxiety syndromes in the context of substance abuse are diverse and do not necessarily indicate syndromes that are identical to independent anxiety disorders. It may make more sense to consider these as potentially different from major anxiety disorders. Placing anxiety states related to substance abuse into a separate category avoids the danger of indicating they have the same prognostic and treatment needs as primary anxiety states.

Psychotic Syndromes and Substance Abuse

Here I review the evidence that drugs of abuse can cause psychoses, document the relatively high prevalence of co-occurrence of psychotic and drug-related syndromes, and draw some related conclusions.

The most compelling evidence that drugs can cause and exacerbate psychoses are the data (from both animal and human studies) that document the likelihood of developing psychotic symptoms or their animal equivalents following the administration of a diverse range of stimulant drugs (Janowsky and Risch 1979; Segal and Schuckit 1983). These appear to include all stimulants, but with a greater likelihood of symptoms and an enhanced severity of the symptomology when more potent drugs are used (e.g., amphetamines and cocaine), especially in higher and/or repeated doses. Human studies have documented perseveration and picking behaviors along with paranoid feelings, actual paranoid delusions, and auditory hallucinations occurring in a clear sensorium without insight in research subjects (Griffith 1977). Similarly, there is evidence from several investigations that stimulant drugs, including amphetamine and methylphenidate (Ritalin), are likely to increase psychotic symptoms among individuals with preexisting schizophrenia

(Janowsky and Risch 1979; Negrete 1989; Segal and Schuckit 1983). In addition, animal studies have demonstrated a broad range of psychostimulant effects in a number of species (Segal and Schuckit 1983). These usually include perseverative behaviors such as searching patterns and motor stereotypies, including picking of the skin (at modest doses) and inhibited behaviors (at higher doses).

The data suggest there is a high prevalence of co-occurrence of drug and psychotic problems. Many persons who abuse drugs report histories of psychotic symptoms in the recent past. This includes 50%–90% of stimulant-abusing hospitalized inpatients who reported past paranoid delusions (Gawin and Ellinwood 1988; Segal and Schuckit 1983), and up to 90% who related a history of hallucinations (Segal and Schuckit 1983). For phencyclidine (PCP), such symptoms usually occur during a state of confusion, where 90% have reported feelings of unreality, 75% paranoia, and 60% hallucinations (Schuckit 1989). A minority of alcoholic persons (perhaps about 3%) may also develop paranoid delusions and auditory hallucinations that can resemble schizophrenia (Glass 1989; Schuckit 1989).

Similarly, there are numerous anecdotal reports and some systematic surveys indicating elevated rates of intemperance among schizophrenic patients and others with psychotic disorders (Alterman et al. 1984; Barbee et al. 1989; Drake et al. 1989). Unfortunately, many of these studies involve individual case reports or descriptions of a limited number of research subjects. In addition, several studies disagree with the assumption that actual diagnosable substance abuse or dependence is more common among schizophrenic patients than among psychiatric patients in general. For instance, one such study reported a 9% rate of substance abuse in a carefully described group meeting criteria for schizophrenia according to Research Diagnostic Criteria (Spitzer et al. 1978) in a Maudsley Hospital sample (Schneier and Siris 1987), and others that 23% of schizophrenic patients had alcohol problems (not necessarily alcohol dependence). These rates are not higher than those reported in other patients (Schneier and Siris 1987).

In conclusion, many drugs of abuse, especially stimulants, are capable of producing temporary psychotic pictures that closely resemble clinical syndromes observed in the course of schizophrenia. This finding, along with the likelihood that the co-occurrence of psychoses and substance abuse increases the chance that an individual will seek out help or be diagnosed as a case, help contribute to the probable higher rate of combined abuse of substances and psychotic syndromes than might be expected from chance alone.

The joint occurrence of these syndromes has several potential prognostic and treatment implications. Based on clinical reports as well as investigations carried out with humans, when psychoses develop only in the context of substance abuse, they are likely to disappear spontaneously and not require long-term treatment with antipsychotic drugs. Therefore, the recognition of the occurrence of psychoses during the abuse of stimulants or other drugs helps to identify a group whose prognoses and treatment needs are distinct from those who might otherwise fulfill criteria for schizophrenia. However, when a psychotic picture develops in the course of abuse of drugs such as stimulants and persists for 6 or more months consecutively, the prognosis may be more severe and more likely to indicate an independent psychotic disorder.

Depressive Symptoms and Substance Abuse

Here I describe how the co-occurrence of syndromes of sadness and abuse of substances occurs for a number of reasons, document the high rate of comorbidity, and draw some tentative conclusions.

Most studies evaluating the development of depressive symptoms in the context of substance intoxication have focused on brain depressants, especially alcohol. Administration of low to modest doses of ethanol in a research protocol is likely to result in minor symptoms of irritability and sadness, even when subjects are healthy individuals and the doses of alcohol are limited to between three and five drinks (Schuckit 1987). Similar alcohol challenges with healthy women subjects have reportedly produced modest mood disruptions that can still be measured the day after the experiment (Birnbaum et al. 1983).

Other studies and clinical observations have focused on higher levels of alcohol intake over longer periods of time. These investigations have demonstrated alcohol's potential for producing severe states of sadness, often accompanied by significant elevations in depression rating scale scores, and at times clinical pictures that resemble major depressive episodes (Gibson and Becker 1973; Schuckit 1986). It is thus not surprising that alcohol has also been reported to increase preexisting feelings of depression (Aneshensel and Huba 1983).

The literature supports similar findings regarding depressed feelings expressed by subjects following the acute elation caused by stimulants, as well as more intense sadness in those abusing substances during stimulant withdrawal. Thus, as described below, sadness, irritability, and sleep disturbances are common among those who abuse stimulant drugs (Gawin and Ellinwood 1988). Although less data are available, mood disturbances are also reported to be common during more intense intoxication with cannabinols and with most other categories of drugs (Schuckit 1989).

Repeated intoxication with depressants and withdrawal from stimulants can produce serious states of depression, but there is consistent evidence that these affective disturbances are likely to improve markedly and fairly rapidly with abstinence. Thus, alcoholic inpatients often present with severe depressions, but these are likely to decrease in intensity over the subsequent 2–4 weeks (Brown and

Schuckit 1988; Gawin and Ellinwood 1988; Jaffe and Ciraulo 1985; Willenbring 1986). A study of 191 carefully diagnosed alcoholic men demonstrated that after approximately 1 week of abstinence, 42% had Hamilton Rating Scale for Depression (Hamilton 1960) scores of at least 20 (Brown and Schuckit 1988). However, after 2 additional weeks, only 12% of this population had similar levels of depression, and only 6% had elevated depression scores by the fourth week. This clinical recovery occurred without the use of antidepressant medications. Other studies are consistent with a high rate of depressive symptoms among alcoholic patients entering treatment and a rapid clearing of this clinical picture (Brown and Schuckit 1988; Liskow et al. 1982; Nakamura et al. 1983; Schuckit 1985a, 1986; Willenbring 1986). A subsequent follow-up of the 191 subjects demonstrated no increased rate of reoccurrence of depressive symptoms *except* among those individuals who returned to the abuse of drugs or alcohol (Brown and Schuckit 1988).

Clinical evaluations of those who abuse alcohol and those who abuse depressant drugs reveal a high rate of depressive symptoms (Brown and Schuckit 1988; Helzer and Pryzbeck 1988; Penick et al. 1988; Schuckit 1986). The specific figures vary according to 1) the type of sample selected (with higher rates among individuals who come to mental health centers than those who appear at substance abuse treatment programs); 2) the criteria used (the more demanding criteria for major depressive disorder the less the prevalence reported); 3) the research invoked (with descriptive instruments such as the Minnesota Multiphasic Personality Inventory (MMPI) (Hathaway and McKinley 1970) reporting much higher rates of problems than the more demanding Schedule for Affective Disorders and Schizophrenia (Endicott and Spitzer 1978)); and 4) the emphasis on recent or lifetime histories (with the latter obviously reporting higher rates).

Although depressive symptoms are very common (up to 98%) at some time in the life histories of alcoholic persons, only about one-third meet the more stringent criteria that demand persistent depressions interfering with functioning over a period of 2 or more weeks (Schuckit 1985a, 1986). However, after 2–4 weeks of abstinence, only perhaps 5%–10% of alcoholic men and perhaps 15% of alcoholic women are likely still to evidence severe depressions (Brown and Schuckit 1988; Keeler et al. 1979; Overall et al. 1985; Schuckit 1986; Weissman and Myers 1980). Thus, although many alcoholic persons report severe symptoms of depression, and a significant minority (perhaps up to one-third) have had depressions lasting 2 or more weeks that interfered with functioning (usually while intoxicated or going through withdrawal), a much lower percentage of alcoholic persons appear to have depressions that last for extended periods of time after abstinence or that develop independently of heavy drinking episodes. There are also data that adequately document the high rate of co-occurrence of depressive symptoms among individuals on methadone maintenance, those with repeated opiate intoxication, and those undergoing withdrawal from stimulants (Gawin and Ellinwood 1988; Rounsaville et al. 1986; Weiss et al. 1989).

There are, of course, reasons to note the secondary affective disturbances when they appear. Being severely depressed probably increases the risk for suicide in the near future; concomitant depression might impact on the decision to seek treatment (Brown and Schuckit 1988; Howes and Hokanson 1979); and the syndromes might relate to outcome (Hasin et al. 1989; Penick et al. 1984). Some studies report a poorer course over time, and others a better course for alcohol problems occurring in individuals who also exhibit depressive symptoms (Hatsukami and Pickens 1982; Pettinati et al. 1982; Rounsaville et al. 1987). Studies of those abusing opiates have indicated that depression may have a relationship to a poorer 2.5-year outcome, even after one controls for the possible effects of general levels of psychopathology (Rounsaville et al. 1986).

There are indications that substance-related depression may be a separate phenomenon from major depression. Investigations suggest that for the average alcoholic person it is not likely that the severe depressive symptoms antedated the alcohol or drug abuse or dependence. A study by Schuckit (1986) of sons of an alcoholic parent and control subjects revealed no differences in clinical pictures or scores on personality measures that would indicate higher levels of affective disturbances among individuals at high future risk for alcoholism. In addition, Goodwin and colleagues (1973, 1977) demonstrated no marked increase for depressive syndromes in adopted-out sons of an alcoholic parent (daughters of an alcoholic parent did show an increased rate of depressive symptoms *but only when raised by the alcoholic parent*). Knop and colleagues (1985) reported similar negative findings, as did Cadoret (1978), and Valliant (1983) reported no increased rate of depressive disorders among adolescents and young adults who later went on to develop alcoholism. Finally, an evaluation of scores on the MMPI carried out in individuals who subsequently developed alcoholism revealed no evidence of significant elevations in clinically relevant symptoms of depression at the earlier testing time (Kammeier et al. 1973).

There are a number of additional lines of evidence supporting the conclusion that abuse of alcohol or drugs and major affective disturbances are often (but not always) independent disorders. Although both alcoholism and depressive disorders appear to be familial and genetically influenced (Schuckit 1987), family studies have indicated that they often appear to be genetically distinct (Cloninger et al. 1979; Merikangas et al. 1985a, 1985b; Reich 1990). In addition, once one controls for the effects of assortative mating, patients with bona fide major depressive disorders are not likely to have markedly elevated rates of alcoholism among their close family members (Zisook and Schuckit 1987). In one study, evaluations of 377 primary alcoholic persons (based on interviews with the individual and at least two resource persons) indicated that only 10% of the subjects had a relative who demonstrated a clear affective disorder in the absence of abuse of drugs or alcohol (Zisook and Schuckit 1987). Also, an 18-year follow-up of 80 persons who demonstrated severe depressive episodes in childhood or adolescence revealed no increased risk for the future development of alcoholism (Harrington et al. 1990).

Of course, the possible independence of substance abuse and primary depressive disorder is far from certain. Winokur and colleagues (1975) and Liskow and colleagues (1982) commented on the higher prevalence of alcoholism in men and affective disorder in women and noted the possibility of an increased risk for the second disorder in relatives of individuals with the first. Although this observation is important, other studies have not demonstrated an increased crossover for depressive disorder and alcoholism within families when clearly defined diagnostic groups are studied (James and Chapman 1975; Robins et al. 1977; Schuckit 1985a, 1986; Zisook and Schuckit 1987). Thus, although it is possible that future research might indicate that some forms of alcoholism and some affective disorders are genetically related, the present evidence does not strongly support such a conclusion.

In summary, the data reviewed here support a number of possible conclusions. First, intoxication or withdrawal from a variety of substances can cause severe and at times even suicidal depressive disturbances. Second, as distinct from independent major depressive disorders, when these symptoms develop in the context of abuse of drugs or alcohol, they are likely to improve markedly with abstinence. Third, related to a variety of complex issues, there is a high level of co-occurrence of sadness, intense short-lived depressive episodes, as well as disturbances of affect that meet DSM-III-R criteria for major depressive disorders among those who abuse alcohol and other drugs.

Even though alcoholic persons with depressions occurring in the context of their heavy drinking or withdrawal have many symptoms similar to those seen in individuals with major depressive disorders, the "sociodemography," family histories, and early life course of problems in the alcoholic persons tend to be more similar to those observed for alcoholic individuals than for individuals with major depression (Merikangas et al. 1985b; Schuckit 1983, 1986). As discussed above, consistent with the independence of the alcoholism and affective disorders, children of an alcoholic parent do not appear to have a significant increase in depressive disease. Finally, an evaluation of 864 university students who responded to a questionnaire revealed no correlation between the number of alcoholic relatives and the incidence of depressive episodes in either the students themselves or their other relatives (Schuckit and Sweeney 1987).

Thus, in the final analysis, a high rate of co-occurrence for depressive symptoms and alcoholism or drug abuse has been documented. However, the causal nature of their relationship has not been definitively established. Most importantly, there is consistent evidence that depressions occurring in the context of abuse of alcohol or drugs are likely to improve rapidly with abstinence and are not likely to run the clinical course typical of independent major depressions.

The Importance of Recognizing Independent Psychiatric Disorders in the Context of Substance Problems

Because this document was prepared for its relevance to a psychiatric diagnostic and statistical manual, the major emphasis has been on a clinically relevant series of problems for which general psychiatrists would benefit from a literature review. Of equal importance are patients who clearly have an independent major psychiatric disorder but also demonstrate problems associated with substance abuse and dependence. However, the discussion of this aspect of the interaction between substances of abuse and psychiatric labels was brief because much of the relevant background material is described in the sections dealing with the specific disorders, and additional important items regarding optimal diagnostic criteria for major psychiatric disorders are covered in reports generated by other Work Groups. These issues are described in detail in the unabridged version of this report; they are briefly alluded to below.

1. It is important to note that there are a number of psychiatric syndromes for which secondary alcohol and drug problems are prominent, including schizophrenia, mania, and the antisocial personality disorder (Drake et al. 1989; Gorelick et al. 1990). The literature regarding the prevalence of preexisting major anxiety disorders among alcoholic and drug-abusing persons is somewhat less clear (Brown et al. 1991; Kushner et al. 1990; Schneier and Siris 1987; Schuckit 1985a; Schuckit et al. 1990). Of course, when phobic symptoms or syndromes exist in the context of substance abuse, they can adversely impact on treatment and must be clinically addressed and labeled (e.g., organic anxiety syndrome), but these do not necessarily indicate that an anxiety disorder predated and "caused" the substance problems.
2. Regardless of the causative nature of the interactions, it is probable that the combination of severe psychiatric syndromes and substance-related problems identifies men and women who may have poorer prognoses and additional treatment needs (Woody et al. 1984).
3. It is possible that drug use might contribute to the precipitation of psychiatric syndromes of a more severe nature or with an earlier onset among individuals who are predisposed to the disorders (Andreasson et al. 1989; Bowers 1987; Manschreck et al. 1988).

There are numerous additional potential relationships that are not covered within this report but that have a great deal of clinical relevance. For example, the clinical impact, etiology, and optimal treatment for relatively mild but persistent depressions in the context of methadone maintenance deserve mention. Such a clinical picture could be the result of hormonal changes in the context of methadone treatment; the result of more direct changes in opiate receptors in the context of therapy; or a reaction to changes in the life situation, including giving up a life-style that many addicted persons find exciting. Although this report cannot comment extensively on this and other related problems, it is important to note the need for generation of additional data that might help with the reformulation of interactions for DSM-V.

Discussion

In this review, I have documented the clinical relevance of the relationship between psychiatric disorders and abuse of substances. Recognizing the great complexity inherent in the questions being raised, I opted to offer a more global overview emphasizing two groups of drugs (brain stimulants and depressants) and three categories of psychiatric pathology (anxiety, psychoses, and depression).

In my opinion, because the interrelationship between substance-related and more typical psychiatric disorders is so complex, there are not enough clear data to justify major changes in the diagnostic manual. As previously discussed, DSM-III-R *did,* at least indirectly, recognize the possibility that abuse of some substances can cause temporary psychiatric pictures that resemble major psychiatric disorders. Thus, clinicians are directly warned not to diagnose residual phase of schizophrenia in the presence of substance disorder, with similar caveats regarding cyclothymia, panic disorder, generalized anxiety disorder, obsessive-compulsive disorder, somatization disorder, and so on. A conservative approach to DSM-IV is to continue to recognize the possible uniqueness of clinical syndromes that occur in the context of active abuse or withdrawal from substances by presenting those drug and alcohol conditions as prominent exclusion criteria. This *warns the diagnostician that such complex pictures might not run the predicted course and that optimal treatments may be different* from those appropriate for independent depressions, anxiety disorders, and so on.

In a review, Skodol (1989) presented a decision tree. It is basically these rules that, depending on the specific diagnosis being considered, are already implied or directly stated by DSM-III-R and that I propose be used in DSM-IV. Of course, as is true of any diagnostic scheme, this approach is not without its liabilities. Some relevant *potential* caveats may be extracted from the discourse on the primary versus secondary approach presented by Rounsaville and Kranzler (1989). These potential problems and relevant responses are discussed in the unabridged version of this report.

In summary, there are many reasons for considering the continuation of the use of careful exclusionary criteria in evaluating patients with multiple psychiatric syndromes in the context of abuse or dependence on alcohol or other drugs. First, this approach is consistent with what has been carefully outlined in DSM-III-R. Second, it appears as if independent psychiatric disorders can be recognized in the context of substance problems. Third, there are data that suggest that even intense psychiatric symptoms occurring in the context of stimulant or depressant intoxication or withdrawal are likely to improve markedly within a fairly short period of time. Thus, they carry prognoses different from those likely to be observed in psychiatric syndromes that developed in the absence of substance intoxication or withdrawal.

Recommendations

In conclusion, DSM-III (American Psychiatric Association 1980) and DSM-III-R present us with some guidelines regarding what a diagnosis should accomplish, and we have been given criteria of what should be required for major modifications in a diagnostic scheme. As is outlined earlier in this chapter, there is no simple and perfect way to use multiple diagnoses in the context of substance use and abuse to indicate prognosis and treatment. Even with the amount of data that have accrued on the high prevalence of multiple labels among patients meeting criteria for alcohol- or drug-related problems, no single theoretical approach discussed earlier in this report appears to accomplish the goals clearly. In light of these results, the Work Group more clearly highlights the need not to diagnose psychiatric syndromes based on symptoms observed only during intoxication or withdrawal from substances. These issues are highlighted in the introduction to DSM-IV, in each relevant section of the manual, and within relevant criteria sets.

References

Alterman AI, Ayre FR, Williford WO: Diagnostic validation of conjoint schizophrenia and alcoholism. J Clin Psychiatry 45:300–303, 1984

American Psychiatric Association: Diagnostic and Statistical Manual of Mental Disorders, 3rd Edition. Washington, DC, American Psychiatric Association, 1980

American Psychiatric Association: Diagnostic and Statistical Manual of Mental Disorders, 3rd Edition, Revised. Washington, DC, American Psychiatric Association, 1987

Andreasson S, Allebeck P, Rydberg U: Schizophrenia in users and nonusers of cannabis. Acta Psychiatr Scand 79:505–510, 1989

Aneshensel C, Huba G: Depression, alcohol use and smoking. J Abnorm Psychol 92:134–150, 1983

Anthony JC, Tien AY, Petronis KR: Epidemiologic evidence on cocaine use and panic attacks. Am J Epidemiol 129:543–549, 1989

Aronson TA, Craig TJ: Cocaine precipitation of panic disorder. Am J Psychiatry 143:643–645, 1986

Barbee JG, Clark PD, Crapanzano BS, et al: Alcohol and substance abuse among schizophrenic patients presenting to an emergency psychiatric service. J Nerv Ment Dis 177:400–407, 1989

Bibb JL, Chambless DL: Alcohol use and abuse among diagnosed agoraphobics. Behav Res Ther 24:49–58, 1986

Birnbaum I, Taylor T, Parker E: Alcohol and sober mood state in female social drinkers. Alcoholism: Clinical and Experimental Research 7:362–368, 1983

Bowers MB Jr: The role of drugs in the production of schizophreniform psychoses and related disorders, in Psychopharmacology: The Third Generation of Progress. Edited by Meltzer HY. New York, Raven, 1987

Breier A, Charney DS, Heninger GR: Agoraphobia with panic attacks: development, diagnostic stability, and course of illness. Arch Gen Psychiatry 43:1029–1036, 1986

Brown SA, Schuckit MA: Changes in depression among abstinent alcoholics. J Stud Alcohol 49:412–417, 1988

Brown SA, Irwin M, Schuckit MA: Changes in anxiety among abstinent male alcoholics. J Stud Alcohol 52:55–61, 1991

Bruce MS, Lader M: Caffeine abstention in the management of anxiety disorders. Psychol Med 19:211–214, 1989

Cadoret RJ: Psychopathology in adopted-away offspring of biologic parents with antisocial behavior. Arch Gen Psychiatry 35:176–184, 1978

Christie KA, Burke JD Jr, Regier DA, et al: Epidemiologic evidence for early onset of mental disorders and higher risk of drug abuse in young adults. Am J Psychiatry 145:971–975, 1988

Cloninger CR, Reich T, Wetzel R: Alcoholism and affective disorders: familial associations and genetic models, in Alcoholism and Affective Disorders: Clinical, Genetic, and Biochemical Studies. Edited by Goodwin DW, Erickson DK. New York, SP Medical & Scientific Books, 1979

Cloninger CR, Martin RL, Clayton P, et al: A blind follow-up and family study of anxiety neurosis: preliminary analysis of the St. Louis 500, in Anxiety: New Research and Changing Concepts. Edited by Klein DF, Rabkin J. New York, Raven, 1981

Crow RR, Noyes R, Pauls DL, et al: A family study of panic disorder. Arch Gen Psychiatry 40:1065–1069, 1983

De Soto CB, O'Donnell WE, Allred LJ, et al: Symptomatology in alcoholics at various stages of abstinence. Alcoholism: Clinical and Experimental Research 9:505–512, 1985

Drake RE, Osher FC, Wallach MA: Alcohol use and abuse in schizophrenia: a prospective community study. J Nerv Ment Dis 177:408–414, 1989

Endicott J, Spitzer RL: A diagnostic interview: the Schedule for Affective Disorders and Schizophrenia. Arch Gen Psychiatry 35:837–844, 1978

Gawin FH, Ellinwood EH: Cocaine and other stimulants: actions, abuse, and treatment. N Engl J Med 318:1173–1182, 1988

George DT, Zerby A, Noble S, et al: Panic attacks and alcohol withdrawal: can subjects differentiate the symptoms? Biol Psychiatry 24:240–243, 1988

Gibson S, Becker J: Changes in alcoholics' self-reported depression. Quarterly Journal of Studies on Alcohol 34:829–836, 1973

Glass IB: Alcoholic hallucinosis: a psychiatric enigma-1: the development of an idea. Br J Addict 84:29–41, 1989

Goodwin DW, Schulsinger F, Hermansen L, et al: Alcohol problems in adoptees raised apart from alcoholic biological parents. Arch Gen Psychiatry 28:238–243, 1973

Goodwin D, Schulsinger F, Knop J: Psychopathology in adopted and non-adopted daughters of alcoholics. Arch Gen Psychiatry 34:1005–1009, 1977

Gorelick DA, Irwin MR, Schmidt-Lackner S: Alcoholism among male schizophrenic inpatients. Annals of Clinical Psychiatry 2:19–22, 1990

Griffith JD: Amphetamine dependence: clinical features, in Drug Addiction, II. Edited by Martin JR. New York, Springer-Verlag, 1977

Hamilton M: A rating scale for depression. J Neurol Neurosurg Psychiatry 23:56–62, 1960

Harrington R, Fudge H, Rutter M, et al: Adult-outcome of childhood and adolescent depressions. Arch Gen Psychiatry 47:465–473, 1990

Harris EL, Noyes R, Crowe RR, et al: Family study of agoraphobia. Arch Gen Psychiatry 40:1061–1064, 1983

Hasin DS, Endicott J, Keller MB: RDC alcoholism in patients with major affective syndromes: two-year course. Am J Psychiatry 146:318–323, 1989

Hathaway SR, McKinley JC: Minnesota Multiphasic Personality Inventory, Revised. Minneapolis, MN, University of Minnesota, 1970

Hatsukami D, Pickens RW: Posttreatment depression in an alcohol and drug abuse population. Am J Psychiatry 139:1563–1566, 1982

Helzer JE, Pryzbeck TR: The co-occurrence of alcoholism with other psychiatric disorders in the general population and its impact on treatment. J Stud Alcohol 49:219–224, 1988

Helzer JE, Canino GJ, Hwu HG, et al: Alcoholism: a cross-national comparison of population surveys with the diagnostic interview schedule, in Alcoholism: Origins and Outcome. Edited by Rose RM, Barrett J. New York, Raven, 1988

Hesselbrock MN, Meyer RE, Keener JJ: Psychopathology in hospitalized alcoholics. Arch Gen Psychiatry 42:1050–1055, 1985

Howes MJ, Hokanson JE: Conversational and social responses to depressive interpersonal behavior. J Abnorm Psychol 88:625–634, 1979

Jaffe JH, Ciraulo DA: Drugs used in the treatment of alcoholism, in The Diagnosis and Treatment of Alcoholism. Edited by Mendelson JH, Mello NK. New York, McGraw-Hill, 1985

James J, Chapman C: A genetic study of bipolar affective disorder. Br J Psychiatry 126:449–456, 1975

Janowsky DS, Risch C: Amphetamine psychosis and psychotic symptoms. Psychopharmacology (Berlin) 65:73–77, 1979

Kammeier ML, Hoffmann H, Loper RG: Personality characteristics of alcoholics as college freshmen and at time of treatment. Quarterly Journal of Studies on Alcohol 34:390–399, 1973

Keeler MH, Taylor CI, Miller WC: Are all recently detoxified alcoholics depressed? Am J Psychiatry 136:586–588, 1979

Knop J, Teasdale TW, Schulsinger F, et al: A prospective study of young men at high risk for alcoholism: school behavior and achievement. J Stud Alcohol 46:273–278, 1985

Kushner M, Sher K, Beitman B: The relationship between alcohol problems and anxiety disorders. Am J Psychiatry 147:685–695, 1990

Liskow B, Mayfield D, Thiele J: Alcohol and affective disorder: assessment and treatment. J Clin Psychiatry 43:144–147, 1982

Lowenstein DJ, Massa SM, Rowbotham MC, et al: Acute neurologic and psychiatric complications associated with cocaine abuse. Am J Med 83:841–846, 1987

Manschreck TC, Laughery JA, Weisstein CC, et al: Characteristics of freebase cocaine psychosis. Yale J Biol Med 61:115–122, 1988

Merikangas DR, Weissman MM, Prusoff BS: Depressives with secondary alcoholism: psychiatric disorders in offspring. J Stud Alcohol 46:199–204, 1985a

Merikangas DR, Leckman JF, Prusoff BA, et al: Familial transmission of depression and alcoholism. Arch Gen Psychiatry 42:367–372, 1985b

Monteiro M, Schuckit MA, Irwin M: Subjective feelings of anxiety in young men after ethanol and diazepam infusions. J Clin Psychiatry 51:12–16, 1990

Mullan MJ, Gurling HM, Oppenheim BE, et al: The relationship between alcoholism and neurosis: evidence from a twin study. Br J Psychiatry 148:435–441, 1986

Mullaney JA, Trippett CJ: Alcohol dependence and phobias: clinical description and relevance. Br J Psychiatry 135:565–573, 1979

Munjack DJ, Moss GB: Affective disorder and alcoholism in families of agoraphobics. Arch Gen Psychiatry 38:869–871, 1981

Nakamura MM, Overall JL, Kelley JT, et al: Persistence of depression in detoxified alcoholics. Alcoholism: Clinical and Experimental Research 7:188–193, 1983

Negrete JC: Cannabis and schizophrenia. Br J Addict 84:349–351, 1989

Overall JE, Reilly EL, Kelley JT, et al: Persistence of depression in detoxified alcoholics. Alcoholism: Clinical and Experimental Research 9:331–333, 1985

Penick EC, Powell BJ, Othmer E: Subtyping alcoholics by co-existing psychiatric syndromes: course, family history, outcome, in Longitudinal Research in Alcoholism. Edited by Goodwin DW, Van Dusen RT, Mendick SA, et al. Boston, MA, Kluwer-Nijhoff Publishing, 1984

Penick EC, Powell BJ, Liskow BI, et al: The stability of coexisting psychiatric syndromes in alcoholic men after one year. J Stud Alcohol 49:395–405, 1988

Pettinati HM, Sugerman AA, Maurer HS: Four year MMPI changes in abstinent and drinking alcoholics. Alcoholism: Clinical and Experimental Research 6:487–494, 1982

Powell BJ, Penick EC, Othmer E, et al: Prevalence of additional psychiatric syndromes among male alcoholics. J Clin Psychiatry 43:404–407, 1982

Reich T: The familial transmission of alcoholism and related disorders, in Genetics and Biology of Alcoholism. Edited by Cloninger CR, Begleiter H. Plainview, NY, Cold Spring Harbor, 1990

Robins E, Gentry KA, Munoz RA: A contrast of the three more common illnesses with the ten less common in a study and 18-month follow-up of 14 psychiatric emergency room patients, II: characteristics of patients with the three more common illnesses. Arch Gen Psychiatry 34:269–281, 1977

Robins LN, Helzer JE, Weissman MM, et al: Lifetime prevalence of specific psychiatric disorders in three sites. Arch Gen Psychiatry 41:949–958, 1984

Roelofs SM, Dikkenberg GM: Hyperventilation and anxiety: alcohol withdrawal symptoms decreasing with prolonged abstinence. Alcohol 4:215–220, 1987

Ross HE, Glaser FB, Germanson T: The prevalence of psychiatric disorders in patients with alcohol and other drug problems. Arch Gen Psychiatry 45:1023–1031, 1988

Rounsaville BJ, Kranzler HR: The DSM-III-R diagnosis of alcoholism, in American Psychiatric Press Review of Psychiatry, Vol 8. Edited by Tasman A, Hales RE, Frances AJ. Washington, DC, American Psychiatric Press, 1989

Rounsaville BJ, Rosenberger P, Wilber C, et al: A comparison of the SADS/RDC and the DSM-III. J Nerv Ment Dis 168:90–97, 1980

Rounsaville BJ, Kosten TR, Weissman MM, et al: Prognostic significance of psychopathology in treated opiate addicts. Arch Gen Psychiatry 43:739–745, 1986

Rounsaville BJ, Dolinsky ZS, Babor TF, et al: Psychopathology as a predictor of treatment outcome in alcoholics. Arch Gen Psychiatry 44:505–513, 1987

Samarasinghe DS, Tilley S, Marks IM: Alcohol and sedative drug use in neurotic outpatients. Br J Psychiatry 145:45–58, 1984

Schneier FR, Siris SG: A review of psychoactive substance use and abuse in schizophrenia: patterns of drug choice. J Nerv Ment Dis 175:641–652, 1987

Schuckit MA: Alcoholic patients with secondary depression. Am J Psychiatry 140:711–714, 1983

Schuckit MA: The clinical implications of primary diagnostic groups among alcoholics. Arch Gen Psychiatry 42:1043–1049, 1985a

Schuckit MA: Overview: epidemiology of alcoholism, in Alcohol Patterns and Problems. Edited by Schuckit MA. New Brunswick, NJ, Rutgers Center of Alcohol Studies, 1985b

Schuckit MA: Genetic and clinical implications of alcoholism and affective disorder. Am J Psychiatry 143:140–147, 1986

Schuckit MA: Biological vulnerability to alcoholism. J Consult Clin Psychol 55:301–309, 1987

Schuckit MA: Drug and Alcohol Abuse: A Clinical Guide to Diagnosis and Treatment, 3rd Edition. New York, Plenum, 1989

Schuckit MA: Treatment of anxiety in patients who abuse alcohol and drugs, in Handbook of Anxiety, Vol 4. Edited by Noyes R, Roth M, Burrows GD. Amsterdam, Elsevier Science Publishers, 1990

Schuckit MA, Sweeney S: Substance use and mental health problems among sons of alcoholics and controls. J Stud Alcohol 48:528–534, 1987

Schuckit MA, Winokur G: A short term follow up of women alcoholics. Diseases of the Nervous System 33:672–678, 1972

Schuckit MA, Irwin M, Brown S: The history of anxiety symptoms among 171 primary alcoholics. J Stud Alcohol 51:34–41, 1990

Segal DS, Schuckit MA: Animal models of stimulant-induced psychosis, in Stimulants: Neurochemical, Behavioral and Clinical Perspectives. Edited by Creese I. New York, Raven, 1983

Sellers EM: Alcohol, barbiturate and benzodiazepine withdrawal syndromes: clinical management. Can Med Assoc J 139:113–123, 1988

Skodol AE: Problems in Differential Diagnosis: From DSM-III to DSM-III-R in Clinical Practice. Washington, DC, American Psychiatric Press, 1989

Smail P, Stockwell T, Canter S, et al: Alcohol dependence and phobic anxiety states, I: a prevalence study. Br J Psychiatry 144:53–57, 1984

Spielberger CD, Gorsuch RL, Lushene R: State-Trait Anxiety Inventory. Palo Alto, CA, Consulting Psychologists Press, 1968

Spitzer RL, Endicott J, Robins E: Research Diagnostic Criteria: rationale and reliability. Arch Gen Psychiatry 35:773–782, 1978

Stockwell T, Bolderston H: Alcohol and phobias. Br J Addict 82:971–979, 1987

Stravynski A, Lamontagne Y, Lavallee Y: Clinical phobias and avoidant personality disorder among alcoholics admitted to an alcoholism rehabilitation setting. Can J Psychiatry 31:714–719, 1986

Tilley S: Alcohol, other drugs and tobacco use and anxiolytic effectiveness: a comparison of anxious patients and psychiatric nurses. Br J Psychiatry 151:389–392, 1987

Vaillant GE (ed): The Natural History of Alcoholism. Cambridge, MA, Harvard University Press, 1983

Van Valkenburg C, Akiskal HS, Puzantian V, et al: Anxious depressions: clinical, family history, and naturalistic outcome: comparisons with panic and major depressive disorders. J Affective Disord 6:67–82, 1984

Weiss RD, Griffin ML, Mirin SM: Diagnosing major depression in cocaine abusers: the use of depression rating scales. Psychiatry Res 28:335–343, 1989

Weissman MM: Alcoholism and depression: separate entities? Paper presented at the Cambridge Hospital 7th Annual Alcoholism Symposium, Boston, MA, 1980

Weissman MM, Myers JK: Clinical depression in alcoholism. Am J Psychiatry 137:372–373, 1980

Willenbring ML: Measurement of depression in alcoholics. J Stud Alcohol 47:367–372, 1986

Winokur G, Cadoret R, Baker M: Depression spectrum disease versus pure depressive disease: some further data. Br J Psychiatry 127:75–77, 1975

Wood DM, Lal H: Anxiogenic properties of cocaine withdrawal. Life Sci 41:1431–1436, 1987

Woody GE, McLellan AT, Luborsky L, et al: Psychiatric severity as a predictor of benefits from psychotherapy: the Penn-VA Study. Am J Psychiatry 141:1172–1177, 1984

Zisook S, Schuckit MA: Male primary alcoholics with and without family histories of affective disorder. J Stud Alcohol 48:337–344, 1987

Chapter 4

Review of Remission Criteria

George E. Woody, M.D.
John Cacciola, Ph.D.

Statement of the Issues

DSM-III-R (American Psychiatric Association 1987) provides two categories for remission among individuals who were formerly dependent on a psychoactive substance: partial and full. *Partial* is applied to those who, during the last 6 months, have experienced some use of the substance and some symptoms of dependence. *Full* remission is applied when, during the past 6 months, there has been either no use of the substance or use with no symptoms of dependence. Thus, level of remission is determined by taking into account use and associated symptoms, as well as time since last use. However, there are some potential problems with the existing criteria. Should the criteria for relapse 1) address differences in risk that may occur as a function of time since last use, 2) distinguish between different patterns in drug use that may occur following abstinence, or 3) provide different remission criteria for drug abuse than for dependence?

Significance of the Issues

Although the categories for remission in DSM-III-R adequately describe two common adjustment patterns that follow detoxification and rehabilitation, their specificity could be improved. A review of the literature on remission indicates that there is a strong relationship between risk for relapse and time of last drug use. Essentially, risk for relapse diminishes as a function of time spent abstinent. The literature also indicates that there is a wide range of outcomes following abstinence. People often move from abstinence to sporadic use, relapse to dependence, and then resume abstinence.

A. Thomas McLellan, Ph.D., and Arthur A. Alterman, Ph.D., both provided valuable assistance in preparing this report.

The existing criteria for remission do not address the issues of differences in risk for relapse as a function of time since last use, nor do they provide many options for coding the wide range of drug use patterns that occur following abstinence. Remission criteria could be strengthened by addressing this relationship between time of last use and probability of relapse. They could also be improved by a modest expansion of the number of possible outcome categories so as to describe better the range of clinical situations that occur following discontinuation or reduction of drug use.

Furthermore, the existing categories for remission apply only to dependence. The addition of remission criteria for abuse may be appropriate, especially in view of the proposal to make abuse a more definitive diagnosis in DSM-IV.

These issues are considered significant for the following reasons:

1. The literature indicates that the likelihood of relapse is extremely high during the first 3–6 months following discontinuation of dependence, and that it becomes substantially lower after 3 years of abstinence. Modifying current remission criteria to reflect these data could be helpful to clinicians and researchers.
2. The literature review indicates that nonabstinent use patterns following detoxification and rehabilitation are common. Patients commonly move from abstinence, to "slips," to abuse or dependence, and back to abstinence. Current remission criteria lack guidelines for when an individual should be moved from partial to full remission, or vice versa, and provide a very limited menu that can be used to describe these varying outcomes. Criteria could be improved by a modest expansion of the outcome categories.
3. Substitution therapy is widely used for opiate dependence and is beginning to be used for nicotine dependence. Some patients treated with substitution therapy discontinue use of all unprescribed medications. Current remission criteria have no category for substitution therapy.
4. Although current criteria for dependence require 1 month of problematic use to make the diagnosis of dependence, the literature on remission indicates that relapse to dependence usually occurs within days. DSM-IV criteria could be improved by shortening the time for diagnosing relapse to dependence.

These issues are discussed in turn in the results section of this chapter.

Methods

In this review, we focus on published studies pertaining to remission and relapse to psychoactive substance dependence. The studies were located by consulting with other professionals so as to identify the major studies that should be included in this review, by a recent Medline search, and by general readings in the major psychiatric and drug dependence journals.

Especially important to the literature review was the *National Institute on Drug Abuse Research Monograph 72: Relapse and Recovery in Drug Abuse* (Tims and Leukefeld 1986). Also useful are the findings from a study of treatment outcome and relapse by Pettinati (1991). This study is especially important as it includes weekly, detailed follow-up interviews with 150 patients who were treated at the Carrier Foundation, Belle Mead, New Jersey, for problems with cocaine, alcohol, or both.

Efforts were made to include literature that deals with remission from a wide range of substances. The largest number of studies addressed remission from dependence on alcohol and opiates, although studies on nicotine and stimulants are also available. Approximately 125 studies were scanned. Of these studies, 50–60 were subject to more detailed examination.

RESULTS

Relationship Between Time Since Last Use and Chances for Relapse

Time since last use has historically been considered an important variable in determining remission. The Hunt curves (Hunt et al. 1971) clearly displayed the rapid relapse to dependence on heroin, tobacco, and alcohol as a function of time since last use. This downward sloping and negatively accelerated curve showed a consistency among relapse rates to these three substances, with 60% relapsing within the first 3 months following treatment, and another 10%–15% relapsing during the next 3 months. Relapse continued after the 6-month point but at a much slower rate, and flattened considerably by 3 years.

Although others have criticized the specific percentages cited by Hunt and colleagues (1971), especially as they pertain to individual drugs of abuse (Litman et al. 1977), the "curve" indicating that risk of relapse is greatest in the first few months following a period of abstinence has also been observed in other studies (Hubbard and Marsden 1986; Pettinati 1991; Tønnesen et al. 1991).

The literature that examines the timing of relapse to different drugs of abuse is variable. Although a number of studies have examined relapse to opiates, alcohol, and nicotine, much less has been written about cocaine, marijuana, sedatives, and amphetamines. The literature that is available, however, supports the conclusion that a very high risk for relapse occurs following abstinence from dependence on any drug of abuse. The timing of relapse to these various drugs is examined below.

Opiates. Several follow-up studies of patients with opiate dependence indicate that relapse is particularly common and that it usually occurs within hours to a few months after the end of treatment.

Hunt and Odoroff (1962) followed up a large sample of opiate-dependent patients after treatment at the Public Service Hospital in Lexington, Kentucky, and found that 83% were readdicted within 6 months. Maddux and Desmond (1981) found that 70% of a large sample of opiate-dependent subjects relapsed within 1 month following treatment or release from incarceration. Simpson and Sells (1982) found that 56%–77% of opiate-dependent patients used opiates within the first year following treatment. The range varied according to treatment program, and the studies implied that use of opiates in formerly dependent addicted persons was almost synonymous with relapse to dependence, although this distinction was not always clearly made. Hubbard and Marsden (1986) found that approximately 60% of opiate-addicted persons used opiates within the first year following treatment. Among those who used and ultimately relapsed to daily use in the first year, approximately 80% did so within the first 3 months after treatment.

Although these studies often differ in the criteria used to define *relapse*, their findings are remarkably consistent given the different patient cohorts and types of programs. Reinstitution of opiate use occurs in the majority of treated patients within the first year after treatment, and use usually results in relapse to dependence. Those studies that specifically measure time to daily use (Hubbard and Marsden 1986) find that the first 3 months is a time of particularly great risk, although relapse continues to occur throughout the follow-up period, even up to 12 years (Simpson and Marsh 1986; Vaillant 1966).

Alcohol. Representative studies of patients with alcohol dependence following treatment exhibit relapse curves similar to Hunt's (Hunt et al. 1971), although the percentage of relapse is somewhat more variable at the different time frames. Pettinati and colleagues (1982) found that 28% of 225 alcoholic patients maintained complete abstinence during a 1-year follow-up for alcoholism treatment. An additional 12% were abstinent, with only occasional "slips" and good overall adjustment. Almost all of the remaining sample returned to problem drinking. Schuckit and colleagues (1986) followed up 464 alcoholic men from treatment at a Veterans Administration program and found at 1-year follow-up that only one-third had remained abstinent for 300 or more days.

In a Veterans Administration cooperative study (Dorus et al. 1989), 457 men hospitalized for treatment of alcohol dependence were followed in a double-blind, placebo-controlled study to assess the efficacy of lithium carbonate in the treatment of depressed and nondepressed alcoholic patients. Relapse rates were similar for depressed and nondepressed patients whether treated with lithium or placebo.

Approximately 40% had drunk alcohol at 3-month follow-up, 50% at 6 months, and two-thirds by 1 year. It is not clear how many of those who drank relapsed to alcohol dependence, but one-quarter of the sample had been hospitalized for treatment of alcohol problems by the 1-year follow-up. In a sample of stable alcoholic patients treated at a private center, Wallace and colleagues (1988) reported 66% continuously abstinent at 6-month follow-up. Nevertheless, even in this group, which might be considered to have a better-than-average prognosis, one-third consumed alcohol within the first 6 months following treatment.

In a study of 95 alcoholic men, Orford and colleagues (1976) revealed that at 3-month follow-up from outpatient treatment, approximately 85% had at least one drink, and approximately 50% had returned to problem drinking. At 6 months, 90% had drunk alcohol, and 65% had returned to problem drinking.

The Hunt curves (Hunt et al. 1971) and an article by DeSoto and colleagues (1989) indicate that the risk for relapse is substantially lower after 3 or more years of abstinence.

Nicotine. Cohen and colleagues (1989) reported data from 10 long-term prospective studies that examined rates of self-quitting by cigarette smokers. Approximately 5,000 subjects were involved. Reports of abstinence were verified either through contacting informants or with biochemical procedures. Almost all of those who resumed use relapsed to dependence, a finding consistent with other studies, which show that intermittent use of cigarettes, especially among formerly dependent subjects, is rare (Brandon et al. 1986). Continuous abstinence at 6-month follow-up ranged from 4.6% to 16.3% (median 6.0%), and 3.9% to 10.6% (median 4.3%) at 1 year. The median point prevalence rates of abstinence at 6 months and 1 year were 13.2% and 13.9%, respectively. These data indicate that the overwhelming majority relapsed to dependence within 6 months. This figure is somewhat lower than that obtained by a variety of smoking cessation programs, which report a 1-year point prevalence rate of abstinence of approximately 20% (e.g., Schwartz 1987).

Other treatment programs have reported higher success rates. For example, Hall and Kilen (1985) reported abstinence rates approaching 50% at 1 year. Nevertheless, even among those programs reporting more successful interventions, the majority relapsed to dependence within the first year. Brandon and colleagues (1986) reported on the process of smoking relapse in a more detailed manner for 82 subjects participating in a 2-week smoking cessation program. Of the 82 subjects, 72 achieved abstinence. During the 2-year follow-up period, 54 subjects smoked, and 49 returned to daily smoking. The time between treatment termination and first cigarette averaged 58 days, although daily smoking did not begin until 41 days on average after the first cigarette. This also supports a 3-month point of highest risk for relapse to dependence, although relapse continued well beyond that point, as seen with other drugs. Similar high relapse rates in the first 3–6 months were reported by Tønnesen and colleagues (1991).

Cocaine. Relapse to cocaine dependence has not been studied as extensively as heroin, alcohol, or tobacco, but literature continues to accumulate. Hubbard and Marsden (1986) found that 65% of those reporting weekly or more frequent cocaine use at treatment intake ($N > 1{,}000$) relapsed to some cocaine use by the first year. Three-quarters of those who relapsed to daily use did so within the first 3 months.

In evaluating early abstinence from cocaine, Gawin and Kleber (1986) presented clinical evidence for a model in which vulnerability to relapse is especially high during the first 3 months. These data are similar to those reported by Pettinati (1991), where the greatest proportion of subjects who relapsed to cocaine dependence did so within the first month, with another, but lower, peak in relapse rates occurring at 3–4 months.

Other drugs. Hubbard and Marsden (1986), in the Treatment Outcome Prospective Study (TOPS), evaluated outcome according to four drug classes: heroin, other narcotics, cocaine, and "other nonnarcotics." This latter category included marijuana, sedatives, alcohol, and amphetamines. Relapse to daily use was greater for those using narcotics than for the other drug classes. Use of other nonnarcotics was reported by approximately 80% of all subjects within the first year of follow-up. Some subjects who reported other drug use at follow-up had not reported such use at intake.

These data suggest that there was often continued abuse or dependence but that the use patterns had shifted to less addicting drugs. Approximately 80% of those who used other nonnarcotics on a daily basis within the first year did so within the first 3 months. It is unclear what proportion of subjects met full dependence criteria, although some most probably did meet the criteria since they used daily. Again, these data indicate that the first 90 days following treatment is a period of special vulnerability to relapse, even among this mixed category of drugs.

Nonabstinent Use Patterns: The Primary Drug

Alcohol. Although occasional use of alcohol by alcoholic persons—for example, "normal drinking" (Davies 1962) or "controlled drinking" (Orford et al. 1976)—remains a controversial issue, several studies (Davies 1962; Helzer et al. 1985; Orford et al. 1976) indicate that some individuals who were formerly dependent can sometimes resume social drinking. The study by Orford and colleagues (1976) indicated that almost all dependent individuals who become "controlled" drinkers have mild forms of dependence.

A study by Helzer and colleagues (1985) specifically addressed the issue of controlled drinking as a long-term outcome among alcoholic persons. They examined the 5- to 7-year outcome for 1,289 alcoholic subjects from a variety of programs. They found that 15% were totally abstinent; 6.2% were controlled drinkers; 12.2% were heavy nonproblem drinkers; and 66.5% continued to be alcohol dependent. The predictors of controlled drinking were being female and having less severe alcoholism. This 6.2% rate is quite similar to Davies' (1962) controversial report that normal drinking was achieved several years after treatment in 7 of 93 (7.5%) alcoholic persons. Severity of dependence was not assessed, and thus conclusions cannot be made about the relationship between severity and outcome.

Heroin. Similar data also indicate that some former heroin-addicted persons can engage in sporadic opiate use without relapse to dependence. An example is the study of opiate-addicted persons by Hunt and Odoroff (1962), who reported an 83% relapse rate within 6 months following hospitalization (relapse in this study was defined as at least 2 weeks of daily opiate use) and 87.3% by 1 year. By the end of the follow-up, which ranged from 12 to 54 months, 90.1% were readdicted, 6.6% were abstinent, and 3.3% had irregular or undetermined use. This study indicates that with opiates, as with alcohol but probably more so, use is extremely likely to result in readdiction, but that irregular use can occur. Vaillant (1966) followed up a smaller but similar sample of opiate-addicted persons treated at the U.S. Public Health Service Hospital in Lexington, Kentucky, and found a similar outcome. That is, within 2 years after treatment, 90.9% became readdicted at some time during the follow-up period, 3% had a single 1-day slip, and 1% used opiates on an irregular basis. The other 5.1% remained continuously abstinent.

Simpson and Marsh (1986) reported on the outcome of 405 opiate-dependent male patients at various Drug Abuse Reporting Programs (i.e., methadone maintenance, therapeutic community, outpatient drug free, outpatient detoxification, and intake only). At 1-year follow-up, 63% had used opiates, and 47% of the overall sample had relapsed to daily use. Thus, 75% of those who had used any opiates relapsed to daily use within the first year. Throughout a 12-year follow-up, the rates of daily use fell to 24%, and rates for any use fell to 39%. Consistently throughout each year assessed, approximately 60% of the patients with any opiate use returned to daily use. Although any use usually led to relapse, a small proportion of patients engaged in nonabstinent use patterns without relapse.

Hubbard and Marsden (1986) reported similar findings in the TOPS study. They found that among 720 patients who used any heroin within the year following treatment, 54% relapsed to daily use. Interestingly, of the 626 patients who used any opiates other than heroin during the 1-year follow-up, only 25% relapsed to daily use. These differences could be due to differences in route of administration—intravenous for heroin versus oral for Percodan (oxycodone and aspirin) or codeine.

Findings significantly different from these treatment follow-up studies were reported by Robins and colleagues (1980) in their epidemiological study of Vietnam-era veterans. In this study, approximately half of the soldiers who had been addicted to heroin in Vietnam reported ever having used opiates after their return to the United States. Among these formerly dependent persons who had ever used opiates, only about one-eighth had become readdicted at the time of the follow-up. Among a subgroup of those who had used heroin often, including some who used weekly or more often, only about one-half had become readdicted. These findings differ from those typically reported from treatment follow-up studies and may relate to differences in subject characteristics of treated versus epidemiological samples. Alternatively, the lower relapse rates may be due to differences in cues that were associated with drug taking in Vietnam, but that were no longer present on return to the United States.

Tobacco. For tobacco-dependent individuals, any use seems to be particularly dangerous. For instance, Brandon and colleagues (1986) found that 91% of the subjects who "tasted" a cigarette returned to regular daily smoking. However, relapse to daily smoking occurred on average 41.3 days following the first cigarette. Similarly, Cohen and colleagues (1989) found that rates of those who had "not a puff" throughout a 1-year period were comparable to abstinence rates as defined by engaging in no smoking during the week prior to evaluation. These data indicate that nonabstinent use patterns occur in tobacco dependence, but that this outcome is rare.

Nonabstinent Use Patterns: Other Drugs

An important point to consider in assessing relapse is that focusing only on use of the primary pretreatment drug may underestimate overall drug use due to the high prevalence of polydrug abuse (Ball et al. 1988). Many studies show that patients may shift drug-taking patterns from one substance to another. This can occur when the primary drug is not available, when rewarding effects of the primary drug are diminished by treatment with pharmacological agents such as methadone or naltrexone, or when there are other circumstances.

For example, in Hubbard and Marsden's (1986) sample of 1,163 opiate patients, 13% engaged in frequent use of non-opiate drugs. A special situation occurs among methadone maintenance patients. Research (e.g., Ball et al. 1988) indicates that with adequate methadone doses and appropriate levels of psychosocial services, more than 90% of patients in methadone treatment are abstinent from heroin in the month preceding evaluation. However, the work of Ball and colleagues and that of others also shows that use of other abusable substances such as cocaine and unprescribed benzodiazepines is common among methadone patients (Iguchi et al. 1990). Wolf and colleagues (1990) have also documented problematic use of benzodiazepines and sedative-hypnotics among alcoholic persons in outpatient treatment. Additionally, occasional use of opiates within the context of treatment in a methadone program may be a reasonably stable outcome, whereas use outside of methadone treatment is extremely likely to result in relapse to uncontrolled use.

Since dependence is defined in terms of the primary drug, these patterns involving other drugs are probably best avoided in establishing criteria for remission. If use of other drugs becomes more intense or problematic, it may require an additional diagnosis.

Substitution Therapy and Prescribed Medication

During the last 20 years, an increasing number of studies have documented the usefulness of pharmacotherapies for drug dependence. Three of these are agonists that have effects that are very similar to the original drug of dependence. These agonists are methadone and *levo*-alpha-acetylmethadol for opiate dependence, and nicotine polacrilex gum (Nicorette) for cigarette smoking. Many subjects treated in programs using substitution therapy discontinue use of all unprescribed drugs. Such patients can be stably maintained on methadone for years and show no signs or symptoms of dependence other than tolerance or withdrawal.

Remission criteria could probably be improved by adding a category for patients who are treated with psychotropic agents for dependence that have agonist properties that are similar to the original drug. This is especially true for methadone, which as of this writing is being used in the treatment of approximately 115,000 patients in the United States alone.

Time Required to Make the Diagnosis of Relapse to Dependence

Criteria for a diagnosis of dependence or abuse require that the behavior be present for 1 month or longer. This originally seemed to be a reasonable time for making the diagnosis, but several studies indicated that relapse to dependence usually occurs more rapidly. For example, Pettinati (1991) used 1 week of regular cocaine use to rediagnose dependence, Hunt and Odoroff (1962) used 2 weeks for opiates, and Brandon and colleagues (1986) used 3 days of consecutive smoking to diagnose relapse to nicotine dependence. Thus, it may be appropriate to rediagnose dependence if problematic and/or regular use occurs over a period shorter than 1 month.

Although data are sparse on this point, 1 week of regular use is probably appropriate for rediagnosing dependence.

One month may be appropriate for abuse since, by definition, abuse consists of less regular consumption than dependence and the pattern should be observed over a longer period of time. However, one could argue that one or a few episodes of high-dose use occurring over a period of days is sufficient to diagnose relapse to abuse.

Parallel Criteria for Abuse

Abuse is a residual category in DSM-III-R. Perhaps because it was classified as such, criteria for remission and relapse focus only on dependence. As of this writing, there has been no research on whether the remission issues that apply to dependence also apply to abuse.

Dropping the Dependence Diagnosis

DSM-III-R text does not address the question of when, if ever, the clinician may drop the dependence diagnosis. Follow-up studies of Vietnam veterans indicate that relapse is not an inevitable consequence for opiate dependence (Robins et al. 1975). Other studies mentioned in this review indicate that some formerly dependent individuals have very extended (or even permanent) periods of abstinence (Vaillant 1973, 1988). The question then arises: Should there be a time after which the clinician may have the option of dropping the diagnosis of dependence in remission? Data reviewed here indicate that the risk for relapse drops considerably after 3 or more years of successful abstinence.

Discussion

Although it is difficult to characterize the long-term course of substance dependence, the literature points to several generalities that can be stated with a fair degree of confidence. These generalizations form the basis for our recommendations for DSM-IV regarding these issues (see below), and include

1. A consistent and continuous pattern of nonuse (or use) is the exception rather than the rule. Most patients manifest a shifting longitudinal pattern in which they are remitting and relapsing from use, abuse, and dependence.
2. The first 3–6 months following treatment stands out as a time during which the risk for relapse to all drugs of abuse/dependence is greatest.
3. Relapse to dependence usually involves daily use of the substance and occurs

over a much shorter time than it originally takes to become dependent. There is very little written about time for relapse to abuse.

4. Some data support 1–2 years of abstinence or nonproblematic use as a good predictor of future outcome. However, 3 or more years seems to improve predictability of future good outcome status even more.
5. Longer periods of abstinence predict the likelihood of continued abstinence or good outcome. However, relapse to dependence has been reported even after many years of abstinence or irregular use. Risk for relapse appears to drop considerably after 3 or more years of successful abstinence.
6. Drugs with agonist properties that are similar to the drug of dependence are prescribed for treatment of dependence on opiates and nicotine. Patients treated with substitution therapy have variable patterns of drug use, as do those in abstinence treatment. Some are stably maintained with no signs or symptoms of dependence other than tolerance and withdrawal.
7. Remission criteria for abuse are not mentioned in DSM-III-R, and there is little or no literature on remission and relapse following a diagnosis of abuse.

Recommendations

At this point in our thinking we recommend the following scheme for DSM-IV, a scheme in which there are two types of remission from dependence: early and sustained.

Early Remission

Early remission will be used during the first 6 months following the termination of drug use and/or acute withdrawal symptoms. Generally, acute withdrawal symptoms end within 1 week after the substance is discontinued.

Early remission has the following three subcategories:

- *With Use:* With use of this (or a closely related) substance.
- *Without Use:* No use of this (or a closely related) substance and not on agonist treatment.
- *With Agonist Treatment:* No use of this (or a closely related) substance other than prescribed agonist treatment.

If 6 months or more have passed without relapse to dependence, the person then moves from early to sustained remission.

Sustained Remission

Sustained remission has four subcategories, depending on the use pattern during the previous 6 months:

- *Partial:* During the past 6 months, some use of the substance and some symptoms of dependence.
- *Full With Nonproblematic Use:* During the past 6 months, some use of this (or a closely related) substance but no symptoms of dependence.
- *Full With Abstinence:* During the past 6 months, no use of this (or a closely related) substance.
- *Full With Agonist Treatment:* During the past 6 months, no use of this (or a closely related) substance and taking prescribed agonist.

If a person relapses to dependence while in sustained remission, he or she must recycle to early remission and remain there for 6 months before again being eligible for sustained remission.

Additions to the existing criteria or text that are recommended are

1. A statement that the clinician has the option of dropping the "remission" diagnosis if the patient has been in sustained remission with abstinence for 3 or more years. If the clinician chooses to drop the diagnosis, it becomes a lifetime part of the medical history, but not a current problem that is always coded as "in remission."
2. A statement that relapse to dependence is diagnosed if dependence criteria are met for 1 week.
3. A statement that remission from abuse should be determined by clinical judgment. There are no data available that can be used to develop specific criteria for remission from abuse at this time.

References

American Psychiatric Association: Diagnostic and Statistical Manual of Mental Disorders, 3rd Edition, Revised. Washington, DC, American Psychiatric Association, 1987

Ball JC, Lange WR, Myers CP, et al: Reducing the risk of AIDS through methadone maintenance treatment. J Health Soc Behav 29:214–226, 1988

Brandon TH, Tiffany ST, Baker TB: The process of smoking relapse, in RAUS: Relapse and Recovery in Drug Abuse (NIDA Research Monograph No 72). Edited by Tims FM, Leukefeld CG. Washington, DC, U.S. Government Printing Office, 1986

Cohen S, Lichtenstein E, Prochaska JO, et al: Debunking myths about self-quitting: evidence from 10 prospective studies of persons who attempt to quit smoking by themselves. Am Psychol 44:1355–1365, 1989

Davies DL: Normal drinking in recovered alcohol addicts. Quarterly Journal of Studies on Alcohol 23:94–104, 1962

DeSoto CB, O'Donnell WE, DeSoto JL: Long-term recovery in alcoholics. Alcoholism: Clinical and Experimental Research 13:693–697, 1989

Dorus W, Ostrow DG, Anton R, et al: Lithium treatment of depressed and nondepressed alcoholics. JAMA 262:1646–1652, 1989

Gawin FH, Kleber HD: Abstinence symptomatology and psychiatric diagnosis in cocaine abusers. Arch Gen Psychiatry 43:107–113, 1986

Hall S, Kilen JD: Psychological and pharmacological approaches to smoking relapse prevention, in Pharmacological Adjuncts in Smoking Cessation (NIDA Research Monograph No 53). Edited by Grabowski J, Hall S. Washington, DC, U.S. Public Health Service, 1985

Helzer JE, Robins LN, Taylor JR, et al: The extent of long-term moderate drinking among alcoholics discharged from medical and psychiatric treatment facilities. N Engl J Med 312:1678–1682, 1985

Hubbard RL, Marsden ME: Relapse to use of heroin, cocaine and other drugs in the first year after treatment, in RAUS: Relapse and Recovery in Drug Abuse (NIDA Research Monograph No 72). Edited by Tims FM, Leukefeld CG. Washington, DC, U.S. Government Printing Office, 1986

Hunt GH, Odoroff ME: Followup study of narcotic drug addicts after hospitalization. Public Health Rep 77:41–54, 1962

Hunt WA, Barnett LW, Branch LG: Relapse rates in addiction programs. J Clin Psychol 27:455–456, 1971

Iguchi M, Griffiths R, Bashel W, et al: Relative abuse liability of benzodiazepines in methadone maintained populations in three cities, in Problems of Drug Dependence 1989 (NIDA Research Monograph No 95). Edited by Harris LS. Washington, DC, U.S. Government Printing Office, 1990

Litman GK, Eiser JR, Rawson NSB, et al: Towards a typology of relapse: a preliminary report. Drug Alcohol Depend 2:157–162, 1977

Maddux JF, Desmond DP: Careers of Opioid Users. New York, Praeger, 1981

Orford J, Oppenheimer E, Edwards G: Abstinence or control: the outcome for excessive drinkers two years after consultation. Behav Res Ther 14:409–418, 1976

Pettinati HM: The use of patient matching in a private psychiatric setting to evaluate treatment outcome for addiction, in Models and Methods for Patient Matching (McLellan AT, Chair). Workshop conducted at the NIDA National Conference on Drug Abuse Research & Practice, Washington, DC, January 1991

Pettinati HM, Sugerman AA, DiDonato N, et al: The natural history of alcoholism over four years after treatment. J Stud Alcohol 43:201–215, 1982

Robins LH, Helzer JE, Davis DH: Narcotic use in southeast Asia and afterward: an interview study of 898 Vietnam returnees. Arch Gen Psychiatry 32:955–961, 1975

Robins LH, Helzer JE, Hesselbrock M, et al: Vietnam veterans three years after Vietnam: how our study changed our view of heroin, in Yearbook of Substance Use and Abuse, Vol 2. Edited by Brill I, Winick C. New York, Human Sciences Press, 1980, pp 213–230

Schuckit MA, Schwei MG, Gold E: Prediction of outcome in inpatient alcoholics. J Stud Alcohol 47:151–155, 1986

Schwartz JL: Review and evaluation of smoking cessation methods: the United States and Canada (NIH Publ No 87-2940). Washington, DC, U.S. Department of Health and Human Services, 1987

Simpson DD, Marsh KL: Relapse and recovery among opioid addicts 12 years after treatment, in RAUS: Relapse and Recovery in Drug Abuse (NIDA Research Monograph No 72). Edited by Tims FM, Leukefeld CG. Washington, DC, U.S. Government Printing Office, 1986

Simpson DD, Sells S: Effectiveness of treatment for drug abuse: an overview of the DARP research program. Adv Alcohol Subst Abuse 2:7–29, 1982

Tims FM, Leukefeld CG (eds): RAUS: Relapse and Recovery in Drug Abuse (NIDA Research Monograph No 72). Washington, DC, U.S. Government Printing Office, 1986

Tønnesen P, Nørregaard J, Simonsen K, et al: A double-blind trial of a 16-hour transdermal nicotine patch in smoking cessation. N Engl J Med 325:311–315, 1991

Vaillant GE: Twelve year follow-up of New York narcotic addicts, II: the natural history of a chronic disease. N Engl J Med 275:1282–1288, 1966

Vaillant GE: A 20-year follow-up of New York narcotic addicts. Arch Gen Psychiatry 29:237–241, 1973

Vaillant GE: What can long-term follow-up teach us about relapse and prevention of relapse in addiction? Br J Addict 83:1147–1157, 1988

Wallace J, McNeill D, Gilfillan D, et al: I. Six-month treatment outcomes in socially stable alcoholics: abstinence rates. J Subst Abuse Treat 5:247–252, 1988

Wolf B, Iguchi M, Griffiths R: Sedative/tranquilizer use and abuse in alcoholics currently in outpatient treatment: incidence, pattern and preference, in Problems of Drug Dependence 1989 (NIDA Research Monograph No 95). Edited by Harris LS. Washington, DC, U.S. Government Printing Office, 1990

Chapter 5

Severity of Dependence

George E. Woody, M.D.
John Cacciola, Ph.D.

Statement and Significance of the Issues

DSM-III-R (American Psychiatric Association 1987) provides three criteria for severity of psychoactive substance dependence: mild, moderate, and severe. *Mild* dependence is defined as having "few, if any, symptoms in excess of those required to make the diagnosis, and the symptoms result in no more than mild impairment in occupational functioning or in usual social activities or relationships with others" (p. 168). *Moderate* is defined as "symptoms or functional impairment between 'mild' and 'severe'" (p. 168). *Severe* is having "many symptoms in excess of those required to make the diagnosis, and the symptoms markedly interfere with occupational functioning or with usual social activities or relationships with others" (p. 168). These three criteria are intended to be used by clinicians in making a global assessment of the severity of dependence. Implicit in these criteria is the concept that dependence is a syndrome of graded severity rather than a unitary categorical state, as was the case in DSM-III (American Psychiatric Association 1980). Four issues are being considered in this literature review on severity of dependence.

First, the concept of dependence as dimensional rather than categorical and of having graded levels of severity originates in the work of Edwards and Gross (1976) on the alcohol dependence syndrome. Perhaps as a consequence of the strength of the data supporting the alcohol dependence syndrome (reviewed below), the framers of DSM-III-R applied the ideas of Edwards and Gross not only to alcohol, but to *all other substances of abuse* as well. This extension of the ideas of Edwards and Gross to other substances was done in the relative absence of data supporting the validity of their concept for other types of substance use disorders. Thus, there

Arthur A. Alterman, Ph.D., Jack Blaine, M.D., and A. Thomas McLellan, Ph.D., provided valuable assistance in preparing this chapter.

is a need for data indicating whether or not the dependence syndrome, with its varying levels of severity, does in fact apply to substances other than alcohol.

A second issue emerges when one compares the way the alcohol dependence syndrome is used in studies of severity with the way the term *dependence* is used in the DSM-III-R and ICD-10 (World Health Organization 1992). For example, in DSM-III-R the "residual" abuse category is applied to individuals who have a maladaptive pattern of use as indicated by either "continued use despite knowledge of having a persistent or recurrent social, occupational, psychological, or physical problem that is caused or exacerbated by use of the psychoactive substance" (p. 169), or "recurrent use in situations in which use is physically hazardous" (p. 169). These symptoms must have persisted for at least 1 month, and the individual must never have met criteria for dependence for that substance. In ICD-10, the term *harmful use* is similar to abuse insofar as it represents a pattern of nondependent but problematic use. It differs, however, in that it is restricted to use that results *only* in *actual* psychological or physical harm. As in DSM-III-R, ICD-10 requires three or more symptoms to meet criteria for dependence.

The criteria used to diagnose abuse or harmful use are also present as single items in the list of criteria used to make DSM-III-R or ICD-10 diagnoses of dependence. However, the categories of abuse or harmful use are generally not mentioned in the papers that examine severity of alcohol dependence. This is best seen in studies that describe the instruments that have been designed to measure the alcohol dependence syndrome, such as the Severity of Alcohol Dependence Questionnaire (SADQ) (Stockwell et al. 1979). Rather than identify those individuals with only abuse or harmful use and exclude them from the analyses, it appears that severity of dependence is usually determined by administering the SADQ (or another related instrument) to all individuals who present for treatment and have *either alcohol problems or alcohol dependence.* The category of mild dependence is applied to those having low scores on the SADQ, and moderate or severe dependence is applied to those with higher scores. By using the SADQ in this way, it appears that mild dependence may be applied to persons who would be classified as having abuse or harmful use according to DSM-III-R or ICD-10. Thus, even in the relatively extensive literature on severity of alcohol dependence, we require further data that examine the significance of severity *after* those subjects with abuse or harmful use have been excluded from the analyses.

Third, there is a growing literature on the prognostic significance of associated problems as determinants of outcome (e.g., Glassman et al. 1990; McLellan et al. 1983). Especially important appear to be psychiatric symptoms or diagnoses that are found in the context of substance use disorders. Specifically, diagnoses of depression and antisocial personality disorder (ASPD) have been found to have a negative influence on prognosis in most subjects with alcohol and drug use disorders (e.g., Breslau et al. 1991; Kosten et al. 1986; Rounsaville et al. 1986, 1987; Schuckit et al. 1986; Woody et al. 1985). Ratings of "psychiatric severity," which are essentially global measures of the intensity and frequency of psychiatric symptoms, have also been found to be associated with a negative outcome (McLellan et al. 1983). The interface between these associated problems and substance use disorders is examined in detail by Marc A. Schuckit in Chapter 3 of this volume. However, for our purposes, it suffices to note that the inclusion of severity ratings for dependence implies that severity has clinical meaning, such as being prognostic of outcome. The studies that suggest that associated problems may be significant predictors of outcome, even more than severity, suggest that severity may be only one of several clinically important aspects of dependence. Furthermore, its significance may differ according to the drug(s) of dependence.

In fact, even more areas have been identified as influencing outcome. Among these are social adjustment and stability (Nordström and Berglund 1987) and beliefs and preferences (Miller et al. 1992; Orford and Keddie 1986). Some studies have found that severity does not predict outcome at all, but this finding occurs less often than one showing that severity is a significant predictor (Miller et al. 1992; Nordström and Berglund 1987).

Finally, the criteria for severity in DSM-III-R are perhaps too general and might be difficult to use in clinical practice or research. Because they lack precision, severity ratings can easily be applied differently in various settings. Assuming severity is a valid and clinically meaningful concept that applies to all or most abusable substances, it might be helpful to define it more precisely. One way to do so might be to specify exactly how many symptoms are necessary for the groupings of mild, moderate, and severe. Another approach might be to determine whether only a few of the dependence criteria are associated with tolerance or withdrawal and thus might be associated with more "severe" symptoms, as in a study by Cottler and colleagues (1991). For example, in DSM-III-R, the nine criteria for dependence are weighted equally in one sense because a symptom count is required to determine severity. But in another sense, there is an implicit assumption that "impairment in occupational functioning or in usual social activities or relationships with others" (p. 168) is weighted in determining the level of severity. Severity might be rated in an easier and more valid manner if it is found that only a few criteria carry the "weight" for determining levels of severity, and these criteria were clearly tied to each severity level.

Methods

We reviewed mainly published studies that pertain to dependence, abuse, and severity. These studies were located 1) by scanning the literature that was circulated to the Substance Use Disorders Work Group; 2) through discussions with advisers and consultants; 3) by examining general psychiatric and substance abuse journals; and 4) by a recent Medline search. Other useful sources include the unpublished findings from a study of treatment outcome conducted by Pettinati (1991) at the Carrier Foundation, Belle Mead, New Jersey, and a secondary analysis supported by funds from the John D. and Catherine T. MacArthur Foundation on treatment outcome for persons with cocaine and alcohol use disorders from studies done at the University of Pennsylvania, Philadelphia VA Substance Abuse Treatment and Research Center (Alterman et al., in press; Arndt et al. 1992).

Although efforts were made to include literature that deals with severity of dependence on a wide range of substances, most studies that were found dealt with alcohol dependence. Approximately 200 studies were scanned. Of these studies, 60–70 papers were subject to more detailed examination.

Results

Severity of Dependence for Alcohol Use Disorders

The concept of a dependence syndrome of graded severity originates in the work of Edwards and Gross (Edwards 1986; Edwards and Gross 1976; Edwards et al. 1981). The great bulk of the work supporting the validity of severity of dependence has been done with individuals presenting for treatment of alcohol problems. In these studies, the dependence syndrome has been found to have both internal consistency and external validity.

Instruments have been developed to measure the individual elements of the alcohol dependence syndrome (Cottler et al. 1989; Davidson et al. 1989; Robins et al. 1983; Skinner 1981; Skinner and Allen 1982; Stockwell et al. 1979; Vaillant 1983). Among these instruments, the most commonly used is the SADQ. As summarized by Rounsaville and Kranzler (1989), measures of severity using the SADQ or other similar instruments predict the following: attendance at a treatment clinic and severity of associated problems (Skinner and Allen 1982); craving after a priming dose of alcohol (Hodgson et al. 1979); relapse after a "slip" (Orford et al. 1976; Polich et al. 1981); and poorer posttreatment outcome (Babor et al. 1987b; Rounsaville et al. 1987).

Few, if any, of these studies appear to have excluded subjects who met DSM-III-R criteria for abuse or ICD-10 criteria for harmful use before examining severity of dependence. Thus, it is difficult to ascertain whether subjects classified as having mild dependence were, in fact, those with DSM-III-R abuse or ICD-10 harmful use, rather than dependence. This methodological problem could be important, as suggested in studies by Hasin and colleagues (1990), and Pickens and colleagues

(1991). The study by Hasin and colleagues implied that subjects classified as having alcohol abuse according to DSM-III-R had a significantly better long-term prognosis than those classified as being dependent. The study by Pickens and colleagues found evidence of genetic transmission for subjects with a DSM-III diagnosis of dependence, but not abuse. Thus, studies that exclude subjects with abuse, and examine only those meeting DSM-III-R criteria for dependence, may find less prognostic significance accorded to severity than has been found in studies that have included these subjects.

With few exceptions (Cottler et al. 1991; Doherty and Webb 1989), studies have not specifically examined the three DSM-III-R categories of severity (mild, moderate, and severe) and their relationship to outcome, but rather have looked at the extremes of severe versus mild/moderate dependence. In fact, in a study that measured speed of drinking, Hodgson and colleagues (1979) described only two types of alcohol dependence: mild/moderate and severe. Those with severe dependence developed craving for alcohol after a priming dose, but this outcome was not seen in subjects with mild/moderate dependence. Most studies that have examined clinical correlates of severity find that patients with severe dependence have a history that is consistent with very significant physiological dependence on alcohol, as indicated by withdrawal symptoms such as seizures, a history of delirium tremens, or withdrawal signs and symptoms indicating the need for pharmacotherapy (Skinner 1981).

Few studies have examined the relationship between functional impairment, severity, and outcome. Those that have, find a correlation between severity of dependence and social, legal, medical, and psychiatric problems (Drummond 1990). Generally, this relationship is significant only at the extremes, where severe dependence is associated with repeated detoxification, compulsive drinking style, social deterioration, and increased psychopathology (Skinner 1981). Hasin and colleagues (1988) found a series of complex relationships between severity, age, and antisocial behaviors. This study gave support for a series of characteristics that fall into two types of alcohol dependence, much like that described by Cloninger and colleagues (1988).

Severity of Dependence for Substance Use Disorders Other Than Alcohol

Although developed from work with alcoholic persons, Edwards and Gross' (1976) concept of dependence was applied to other drugs as well in DSM-III-R. At the time the DSM-III-R criteria were developed, very little work had been done to examine how well these criteria applied to dependence on substances other than alcohol. In a study carried out after DSM-III-R was written, Phillips and colleagues (1987) described the development and pilot testing of the Severity of Opiate Dependence

Questionnaire, which was modeled after the SADQ but developed for application to patients with opiate dependence. The results of preliminary field trials indicated that all of the items in the Severity of Opiate Dependence Questionnaire loaded on two factors: withdrawal symptoms (both physical and affective) and withdrawal-relief drug taking. Thus, the data suggested that the items that are used in the SADQ for diagnosing dependence (and are derived from Edwards and Gross) may have different internal relationships in opiate-addicted subjects than among subjects with alcohol dependence, according to DSM-III-R criteria. This finding may be a consequence of the fact that most individuals with opiate dependence are at the high end of the severity scale. Thus, the opiate-dependent population has less "spread" on the severity dimension than is found in those with alcohol dependence.

Babor and colleagues (1987a) measured severity of dependence in alcoholic and opiate-addicted patients undergoing treatment. They found that the severity of dependence predicted outcome consistently in the alcoholic patients, but not in the opiate-addicted patients. Although this study had methodological limitations, it suggested that severity may be a better predictor of outcome for alcohol than for opiate dependence. The data suggested that severity, as defined in DSM-III-R, may not be as clinically meaningful when used for patients with opiate dependence, and perhaps also for dependence on other substances, than when applied to alcohol dependence. Again, this finding may be a function of differences in distribution along the severity continuum among the different groups; the opiate-addicted patients are all more severe.

Kosten and colleagues (1987) published one of the few reports that examined the application of Edwards and Gross' (1976) concepts to *several* other drugs of dependence. Their study found that Edwards and Gross' definition of the dependence syndrome, with graded levels of severity, applied to opiates, cocaine, and alcohol but not to hallucinogens, sedatives, marijuana, or stimulants other than cocaine. This work must be viewed as preliminary since it was a retrospective analysis of data from other studies and was not designed specifically to explore Edwards and Gross' ideas. Furthermore, the number of subjects in some of the groups studied was very small. A second study by Kosten and colleagues (1989) found that the severity of opioid withdrawal after a naloxone challenge test was positively correlated with a score of severity of dependence as determined by a symptom count of DSM-III-R criteria. In addition, opiate withdrawal was not correlated with a global measure of social problems or the frequency or length of drug use. These findings were interpreted as supporting the applicability of the dependence syndrome to opiate-addicted persons because severity was correlated with the number of dependence symptoms, but was not related to associated social problems.

Bryant and colleagues (1991) examined the applicability of the dependence syndrome in cocaine-abusing patients. They found that the nine DSM-III-R items formed a single factor, thus supporting the validity of the dependence syndrome among a sample of 399 treatment-seeking cocaine-abusing patients. More than 60% of the sample met seven to nine of the DSM-III-R dependence criteria, and 19% reported having all nine. Preoccupation with cocaine was found to be the most central criterion in defining cocaine dependence. Avoiding withdrawal by using other drugs was associated with the highest level of severity. In this study, as with those examining opiate-addicted persons, there was a constricted range of severity groupings, with most subjects scoring on the high side of the continuum. This finding could serve to weaken the influence of severity on outcome in this treatment-seeking population.

In fact, a secondary analysis of data on outcome in patients seeking treatment for cocaine problems suggested that the DSM-III-R severity criteria may be less meaningful descriptors of prognosis for patients seeking treatment for cocaine use disorders than is found in the literature on severity and alcohol dependence (Cacciola and Woody, in press). In this study, three groupings of severity were made by counting the number of dependence symptoms rated as being present on the Diagnostic Interview Schedule (Robins et al. 1981). These were related to other measures of clinical status such as amount and frequency of drug use and associated problems. The differences between the severity ratings were strongest at the extremes, similar to the findings of Hodgson and colleagues (1979) with alcohol dependence. However, unlike most of the alcohol studies, severity of dependence did not predict outcome among this group of patients. In fact, there was some evidence that patients with severe dependence had better outcomes than those with mild or moderate dependence.

There was, however, an interesting finding that suggested that a comorbid condition, ASPD, interacts with severity to influence outcome negatively. This is not unexpected because other studies have shown that ASPD generally has a negative influence on outcome (Schuckit et al. 1986; Woody et al. 1985). The effect of ASPD on outcome was tested by dividing the subjects into those with ASPD and those without ASPD and repeating the analyses. Generally, the results were similar to those obtained when all subjects were grouped together, but there were two noteworthy exceptions. The first was that ASPD subjects in the severe dependence group were using more cocaine at 3-month follow-up than ASPD subjects in the moderate and (particularly) the mild groups. Thus, *severity did predict outcome among those with ASPD.* For the non-ASPD subjects, severity groupings did not predict outcome, at least as judged by drug use at 3-month follow-up. The second interesting finding was that ASPD and non-ASPD were equally distributed among the moderately dependent patients. In contrast, more ASPD patients had severe dependence, and more non-ASPD patients had mild dependence.

Other data indicate that the dependence syndrome applies to nicotine, and that severity in persons with nicotine dependence may be related to outcome, as well as to comorbid disorders such as major depression and anxiety disorders (Breslau et al. 1991; Glassman et al. 1990). In the study by Breslau and colleagues, which examined subjects drawn at random from the rolls of a health maintenance organization, only two levels of severity were found according to symptom counts using DSM-III-R items: mild and moderate. Persons with moderate dependence smoked significantly more cigarettes and were much less likely to be in remission in the last year than were those with mild dependence (24% versus 14%). In this study, like those of Babor and colleagues (1987a) with opiate-addicted persons and J. Langenbucher (Supplement to DAO5699, the "Multisite study of substance use disorders," unpublished report, 1991) with alcoholic persons, there was a constricted range of severity ratings. However, unlike these other two studies, where severity ratings using DSM-III-R items were grouped at the high end of the scale, there were no subjects who met criteria for severe dependence in the study by Breslau and colleagues. This may reflect the fact that the sample was drawn from the community and the persons were not seeking treatment.

Prognostic Significance of Associated Problems

Data from patients with cocaine and nicotine dependence relate to a body of evidence suggesting that associated problems, especially comorbid psychiatric symptoms and/or diagnoses, are good predictors of outcome in many patients with substance use disorders. The evidence for the predictive power of comorbid psychopathology is strongest in the literature on drug and nicotine dependence, but there are also examples from studies on alcohol.

One example is the study by McLellan and colleagues (1983), who found that the best predictor of outcome for treatment-seeking opiate and alcohol-dependent persons was a psychiatric severity scale obtained by the Addiction Severity Index. Other studies have found that depression (Kosten et al. 1986; Loosen et al. 1990; Rounsaville et al. 1986) and ASPD (Rounsaville et al. 1987; Schuckit et al. 1986; Woody et al. 1985) are significant predictors of outcome for substance use disorders, including nicotine dependence (Anda et al. 1990; Breslau et al. 1991; Glassman et al. 1990).

The strength of the relationship between severity of dependence, its associated problems, and outcome may differ according to drug class. This could be true simply as a consequence of the different behavioral and pharmacological toxicities of the various drugs of abuse. For example, alcoholic persons are more likely to have cognitive impairment than opiate-addicted persons; cocaine-addicted persons are more likely to have symptoms of paranoia and anxiety than opiate-addicted persons; opiate-addicted persons are more likely to have legal problems than alcoholic persons; and persons with nicotine dependence often have few associated problems unless they have been smoking for such a long time that they develop medical problems. It may also be a function of the range of dependence symptoms that are found among various populations (e.g., treatment-seeking versus community samples) with dependencies on different drug classes, as discussed earlier. Thus, the relationship between severity of dependence, outcome, and associated problems may depend on the primary drug of abuse or dependence, the length of the dependence, the nature of the associated problems, the area of impairment that is being assessed, the population from which the sample is drawn, or the posttreatment environment. Thus, severity may be only one of many factors that can influence outcome.

Discussion

Studies that examine the relationship between severity and outcome for a range of drug dependencies are in a relatively early stage of development. Most of the work has been done with alcohol dependence, and this work indicates that severity of dependence is probably a clinically meaningful predictor of outcome. However, more work needs to be done (even with alcohol dependence) in examining the three DSM-III-R severity ratings (mild, moderate, and severe) after having removed subjects with abuse or harmful use from the analyses. A related issue is determining the point at which abuse ends and dependence begins. Perhaps examining an entire data set, without first attempting to remove subjects with abuse, is the best way to define both abuse *and* severity.

A review of the studies that are available for other drug dependencies indicates that the relationship between severity and outcome that has been found in persons with alcohol dependence is applicable to nicotine and may also apply to cocaine and other drug dependencies. However, it is important to keep in mind the fact that associated problems and other subject characteristics may be even stronger predictors of outcome. Much more work needs to be done in this area, especially with drugs other than alcohol. If associated problems are found to predict outcome better than severity, at least for some substances, it might be helpful to add text in DSM-IV to indicate the additional importance of concurrent psychiatric symptoms or disorders, both Axis I and II, or the limited prognostic significance of severity.

Because severity criteria are very general in DSM-III-R, it might be helpful to clinicians and researchers if more precision could be added to the terms *mild, moderate,* and *severe* in DSM-IV. This could be done by identifying a few factors that are major determinants of levels of severity across drug classes, perhaps by using data from the DSM-IV field trials. For example, Bryant and colleagues (1991) found that taking drugs to avoid withdrawal was associated with the most severe levels of cocaine dependence. The current DSM-IV field trials are obtaining data that can be used in similar analyses with other drug classes. Another approach might be to specify the exact number of positive dependence criteria that must be met for each level of severity.

There is no literature that examines severity of abuse and outcome. In fact, DSM-III-R does not specify any criteria for severity of abuse. Due to the difficulties in determining the significance of severity for dependence, it may be premature to attempt to define and evaluate the significance of severity of abuse, if indeed this task can be accomplished.

Recommendations

Our recommendations are either to make no changes in severity ratings or to define severity more precisely by having a specific symptom count or symptom weighting for the categories of mild, moderate, and severe (e.g., mild = 3–4 symptoms of dependence, moderate = 5–6 symptoms, and severe = 7 or more symptoms of dependence).

However, this latter recommendation will be strongly influenced by the results of analyses from the field trials and from any additional studies that may emerge before the publication of DSM-IV. An important focus of the field trials will be an attempt to identify specific items or combinations of items that are correlated with severity groupings across all substances. Validation of these groupings could be attempted by comparing them with measures of amount and frequency of use or with outcome if additional data are available. If successful, this effort could provide a better foundation for a current definition, and for future studies of severity, especially as it relates to outcome for a range of substances.

References

Alterman AA, McLellan AT, O'Brien CP: Comparative effectiveness and costs of inpatient vs day hospital treatment for cocaine dependence. J Nerv Ment Dis (in press)

American Psychiatric Association: Diagnostic and Statistical Manual of Mental Disorders, 3rd Edition. Washington, DC, American Psychiatric Association, 1980

American Psychiatric Association: Diagnostic and Statistical Manual of Mental Disorders, 3rd Edition, Revised. Washington, DC, American Psychiatric Association, 1987

Anda RF, Williamson DF, Escobedo LG, et al: Depression and the dynamics of smoking. JAMA 264:1541–1545, 1990

Arndt IA, Dorozynsky L, McLellan AT, et al: Desipramine treatment of cocaine dependence in methadone maintained patients. Arch Gen Psychiatry 49:888–893, 1992

Babor TF, Cooney NL, Lauerman RJ: The dependence syndrome as a psychological theory of relapse behavior: an empirical evaluation of alcoholic and opiate addicts. Br J Addict 82:393–405, 1987a

Babor TF, Lauerman R, Cooney N: In search of the alcohol dependence syndrome: a cross-national study of its structure and validity, in Cultural Studies on Drinking and Drinking Practices. Edited by Paakkanen P, Sulkunen P. Helsinki, Social Research Institute of Alcohol Studies, 1987b

Breslau N, Kilbey M, Andreski P: Nicotine dependence, major depression, and anxiety in young adults. Arch Gen Psychiatry 48:1069–1074, 1991

Bryant KJ, Rounsaville BJ, Babor TF: Coherence of the dependence syndrome in cocaine users. Br J Addict 86:1299–1310, 1991

Cacciola J, Woody GE: Cocaine abuse vs dependence and levels of severity: a secondary analysis for DSM-IV, in DSM-IV Sourcebook, Vol 4. Washington, DC, American Psychiatric Association (in press)

Cloninger CR, Sigvardsson S, Bohman M: Childhood personality predicts alcohol abuse in young adults. Alcoholism: Clinical and Experimental Research 12:494–505, 1988

Cottler LB, Robins LN, Helzer JE. The reliability of the Composite International Diagnostic Interview Substance Abuse Module (CIDI-SAM): a comprehensive substance abuse interview. Br J Addict 84:801–814, 1989

Cottler LB, Helzer JE, Mager D, et al: Agreement between DSM-III-R Substance Use Disorders. Drug Alcohol Depend 29:17–25, 1991

Davidson R, Bunting B, Raistrick D: The homogeneity of the alcohol dependence syndrome: a factorial analysis of the SADQ questionnaire. Br J Addict 84:907–914, 1989

Doherty B, Webb M: The distribution of alcohol dependence severity among inpatient problem drinkers. Br J Addict 84:917–922, 1989

Drummond DC: The relationship between alcohol dependence and alcohol-related problems in a clinical population. Br J Addict 85:357–366, 1990

Edwards G: The alcohol dependence syndrome: a concept as stimulus to enquiry. Br J Addict 81:171–183, 1986

Edwards G, Gross MM: Alcohol dependence: provisional description of a clinical syndrome. BMJ 1:1058–1061, 1976

Edwards G, Arif A, Hodgson R: Nomenclature and classification of drug- and alcohol-related problems. Bull WORLD Health Organ 59:225–242, 1981

Glassman AH, Helzer JE, Covey LS, et al: Smoking cessation and major depression. JAMA 264:1546–1549, 1990

Hasin DS, Grant BF, Endicott J: Severity of alcohol dependence and social/occupational problems: relationship to clinical and familial history. Alcoholism: Clinical and Experimental Research 12:660–664, 1988

Hasin DS, Grant B, Endicott J: The natural history of alcohol abuse: implications for definitions of alcohol use disorders. Am J Psychiatry 147:1537–1541, 1990

Hodgson R, Rankin H, Stockwell T: Alcohol dependence and the priming effect. Behav Res Ther 17:379–387, 1979

Kosten TR, Rounsaville BJ, Kleber HD: A 2.5 year follow-up of depression, life crises, and treatment effects on abstinence among opioid addicts. Arch Gen Psychiatry 43:733–738, 1986

Kosten TR, Rounsaville BJ, Babor TF, et al: Substance-use disorders in DSM-III-R: evidence for the dependence syndrome across different psychoactive substances. Br J Psychiatry 151:834–843, 1987

Kosten TR, Jacobsen LK, Kosten T: Severity of precipitated opiate withdrawal predicts drug dependence by DSM-III-R criteria. Am J Drug Alcohol Abuse 15:237–250, 1989

Loosen PT, Dew BW, Prange AW: Long-term predictors of outcome in abstinent alcoholic men. Am J Psychiatry 147:1662–1666, 1990

McLellan AT, Luborsky L, Woody GE, et al: Predicting response to alcohol and drug abuse treatments: role of psychiatric severity. Arch Gen Psychiatry 40:620–625, 1983

Miller WR, Lechman AL, Delaney HD, et al: Long-term follow-up of behavioral self-control training. J Stud Alcohol 53:242–261, 1992

Nordström G, Berglund M: A prospective study of successful long-term adjustment in alcohol dependence: social drinking versus abstinence. J Stud Alcohol 48:95–103, 1987

Orford J, Keddie A: Abstinence or controlled drinking in clinical practice: a test of the dependence and persuasion hypotheses. Br J Addict 81:495–504, 1986

Orford J, Oppenheimer E, Edwards G: Abstinence or control: the outcome for excessive drinkers two years after consultation. Behav Res Ther 14:409–418, 1976

Pettinati HM: The use of patient matching in a private psychiatric setting to evaluate treatment outcome for addiction, in Models and Methods for Patient Matching (McLellan AT, Chair). Workshop conducted at the NIDA National Conference on Drug Abuse Research & Practice, Washington, DC, January 1991

Phillips GT, Gossop MR, Edwards G, et al: The application of the SODQ to the measurement of the severity of opiate dependence in a British sample. Br J Addict 82:691–699, 1987

Pickens RW, Svikis DS, McGue M, et al: Heterogeneity in the inheritance of alcoholism. Arch Gen Psychiatry 48:19–28, 1991

Polich JM, Armor DJ, Braiker HB: The Course of Alcoholism: Four Years After Treatment. New York, Wiley, 1981

Robins LN, Helzer JE, Croughan J, et al: National Institute of Mental Health Diagnostic Interview Schedule: its history, characteristics, and validity. Arch Gen Psychiatry 38:381–389, 1981

Robins LN, Cottler LB, Babor T: WHO/ADAMHA Composite International Diagnostic Interview—Substance Abuse Module (SAM). St. Louis, MO, 1983

Rounsaville BJ, Kranzler HR: The DSM-III-R diagnosis of alcoholism, in American Psychiatric Press Review of Psychiatry, Vol 8. Edited by Tasman A, Hale RE, Frances AJ. Washington, DC, American Psychiatric Press, 1989

Rounsaville BJ, Kosten TR, Weissman MM, et al: Prognostic significance of psychopathology in treated opiate addicts. Arch Gen Psychiatry 43:739–745, 1986

Rounsaville BJ, Dolinsky ZS, Babor TF, et al: Psychopathology as a predictor of treatment outcome in alcoholics. Arch Gen Psychiatry 44:505–513, 1987

Schuckit MA, Schwei MG, Gold E: Prediction of outcome in inpatient alcoholics. J Stud Alcohol 47:151–155, 1986

Skinner HA: Primary syndromes of alcohol abuse: their measurement and correlates. Br J Addict 76:63–76, 1981

Skinner HA, Allen BA: Alcohol dependence syndrome: measurement and validation. J Abnorm Psychol 91:199–209, 1982

Stockwell T, Hodgson R, Edwards G, et al: The development of a questionnaire to measure alcohol dependence. Br J Addict 74:79–87, 1979

Vaillant GE: The Natural History of Alcoholism. Cambridge, MA, Harvard University Press, 1983

Woody GE, McLellan AT, Luborsky L, et al: Sociopathy and psychotherapy outcome. Arch Gen Psychiatry 42:1081–1086, 1985

World Health Organization: The ICD-10 Classification of Mental and Behavioural Disorders: Clinical Descriptions and Diagnostic Guidelines. Geneva, World Health Organization, 1992

Chapter 6

The Organization of Intoxication and Withdrawal Disorders

Thomas J. Crowley, M.D.

Statement and Significance of the Issues

DSM-III-R (American Psychiatric Association 1987) provides the following categories of Organic Mental Syndromes: Delirium, Dementia, Amnestic Syndrome, Organic Hallucinosis, Organic Delusional Syndrome, Organic Mood Syndrome, Organic Anxiety Syndrome, Organic Personality Syndrome, Intoxication, Withdrawal, and Organic Mental Syndrome Not Otherwise Specified (NOS). Intoxication and Withdrawal are *residual diagnoses*; that is, they are to be made only after the other Organic Mental Syndromes have been ruled out. For example, if a person is delirious from an intoxication, the diagnosis is Delirium rather than Intoxication. Moreover, the table of Organic Mental Syndromes Associated With Psychoactive Substances in DSM-III-R (p. 124) provides 19 additional drug-related diagnoses[1]

[1] 1) Amphetamine or Similarly Acting Sympathomimetic Delirium; 2) Cocaine Delirium; 3) Phencyclidine (PCP) or Similarly Acting Arylcyclohexylamine Delirium; 4) Alcohol Withdrawal Delirium; 5) Sedative, Hypnotic, or Anxiolytic Withdrawal Delirium; 6) Amphetamine or Similarly Acting Sympathomimetic Delusional Disorder; 7) Cannabis Delusional Disorder; 8) Cocaine Delusional Disorder; 9) Hallucinogen Delusional Disorder; 10) PCP or Similarly Acting Arylcyclohexylamine Delusional Disorder; 11) Hallucinogen Mood Disorder; 12) PCP or Similarly Acting Arylcyclohexylamine Mood Disorder; 13) Alcohol Idiosyncratic Intoxication; 14) Alcohol Hallucinosis; 15) Alcohol Amnestic Disorder; 16) Dementia Associated With Alcoholism; 17) Posthallucinogen Perception Disorder; 18) PCP or Similarly Acting Arylcyclohexylamine Organic Mental Disorder NOS; and 19) Sedative, Hypnotic, or Anxiolytic Amnestic Disorder.

that are to be ruled out before a residual diagnosis of Intoxication or Withdrawal may be made.

Not stated, but implicit in DSM-III-R is the following diagnostic algorithm:

- Render one or more of the other 19 tabulated diagnoses (instead of Intoxication or Withdrawal) if the patient qualifies for one or more of those 19. Otherwise . . .
- Render a diagnosis of one or more of the other Organic Mental Syndromes (listed in the first sentence of this chapter) if the patient qualifies. For example, diagnose Inhalant Delirium if a patient is intoxicated with an inhalant and meets criteria for Delirium. Otherwise . . .
- Make the residual diagnosis of either Intoxication or Withdrawal for the appropriate substance (e.g., Inhalant Intoxication).

The DSM-III-R treatment of these diagnoses raises many significant issues and questions as regards the potential organization of intoxication and withdrawal disorders in DSM-IV:

Issue 1

States of intoxication and withdrawal are highly variable, depending on doses consumed, time since last dose, chronicity of dosing, the environmental setting for the dosing, and individual biological and psychological factors. It is possible that the 19 tabulated diagnoses may be an incomplete listing of the varied states that may occur in intoxication or withdrawal.

Issue 2

Few of the 19 tabulated diagnoses, and none of the other 7 relevant organic mental syndromes (Delirium, Amnestic Syndrome, Organic Hallucinosis, Organic Delusional Syndrome, Organic Mood Syndrome, Organic Anxiety Syndrome, and Organic Mental Syndrome NOS), are named for intoxication versus withdrawal states. For example, "Barbiturate Mood Disorder" does not convey the basic information of whether the patient is experiencing intoxication or withdrawal. However, intoxication states differ from withdrawal states in both course and treatment. Moreover, evidence presented below suggests that a Delusional Disorder may occur either during chronic intoxication with alcohol or during withdrawal from alcohol. Although these two Delusional Disorders would have different courses and treatments, DSM-III-R does not distinguish between them by providing different diagnoses for Alcohol Intoxication Delusional Disorder and Alcohol Withdrawal Delusional Disorder.

Issue 3

Although the algorithm given earlier seems implicit in DSM-III-R, it is not explicitly stated, and the manual does not provide specific rules for applying it. For example, chronic, prolonged intoxication with alcohol may produce profound, clinically dangerous depression. Depression is cited as one feature of Alcohol Intoxication. But the severely depressed, chronically intoxicated alcoholic patient also appears to qualify for a diagnosis of Organic Mood Syndrome, and Alcohol Intoxication is a residual diagnosis for patients who do not qualify for other Organic Mental diagnoses (such as Organic Mood Syndrome). Is the proper diagnosis here Alcohol Intoxication or Organic Mood Syndrome? Are both diagnoses made? Must the mood disorder predominate for the mood diagnosis, or must it exist alone without other signs of intoxication?

Issue 4

DSM-III-R states that "the essential features of Intoxication are maladaptive behavior and a substance-specific syndrome that are due to the recent ingestion of a psychoactive substance" (p. 116). The term *maladaptive behavior* is the key to this definition, and that term is not defined. A drug-related behavioral change may be adaptive or maladaptive, depending on the social setting. For example, DSM-III-R states that "social drinking frequently causes loquacity, euphoria, and slurred speech; but this should not be considered Intoxication unless maladaptive behavior, such as fighting, impaired judgment, or impaired social or occupational functioning, results" (p. 116). Although loquacity, euphoria, and slurred speech would be maladaptive in a roadside sobriety test or a job interview, the same behaviors might be considered adaptive at a fraternity party. Fighting with a police officer would be maladaptive, but fighting might be adaptive for a person attacked by a mugger; alcohol-induced *impairment* in fighting ability might then be dangerous.

Issue 5

DSM-III-R intermingles descriptions of intoxications and withdrawals with descriptions of disorders that persist long after actual intoxication or withdrawal. These include Amphetamine (and Related) Delusional Disorder; Cocaine (and Related) Delusional Disorder; Alcohol Amnestic Disorder; Dementia Associated With Alcoholism; Posthallucinogen Perception Disorder; and Sedative, Hypnotic, or Anxiolytic Amnestic Disorder. Perhaps this section should distinguish these more persistent disorders from briefer intoxications and withdrawals. Also, questions arise about definition and substantiation for some of these disorders.

Methods

For this report I reviewed published descriptions of states of intoxication and withdrawal for alcohol, sedative-hypnotics and anxiolytics, phencyclidine and related compounds, cocaine, amphetamine and related compounds, cannabis, hallucinogens, inhalants (as described in DSM-III-R), opioids, nicotine, and caffeine. I utilized the *cocaine* listings on Medline from 1988 to August 1989, since studies of cocaine intoxication are relatively new. For the other drugs, systematic studies of intoxication and withdrawal began almost 40 years ago, and I used hand and computer searches of my own files of about 5,300 reprints. Since I study behavioral intoxication in animals, these files are a reasonably rich source for descriptions of intoxications and withdrawals. I also obtained some articles cited in bibliographies of papers found in the above ways. Further, I reference a paper prepared by a consultant to our Work Group.

I examined about 150–200 papers and cite about 50. They are of decidedly mixed quality. Some are prospective laboratory studies of induced chronic intoxications and withdrawals; others are case reports, and a few are reviews. One citation to *Physicians' Desk Reference* (Medical Economics Co 1989) accesses case reports available to the manufacturer of meperidine.

Papers were selected because they described the development during intoxication or withdrawal of the signs and symptoms needed to diagnose one of the following Organic Mental Syndromes: Delirium, Delusional Disorder, Mood Disorder, Anxiety Disorder, Amnestic Disorder, Hallucinosis, and residual Intoxication and Withdrawal. I have ignored Dementia and Organic Personality Disorder since both appear more persistent than the briefer syndromes of Intoxication and Withdrawal.

Caution is warranted in interpreting these papers. Many are quite old and did not contemplate the diagnostic niceties of DSM-III-R, DSM-III (American Psychiatric Association 1980), or even of DSM-II (American Psychiatric Association 1968). They also tend to focus more on withdrawal than intoxication. Another difficulty is that DSM-III-R bans most other organic diagnoses in the presence of Delirium. The cited articles seldom indicated whether anxiety, for example, did or did not coexist with delirium, although I considered the presence of anxiety as probable evidence that the drug would produce an Organic Anxiety Syndrome.

Results

Issue 1

The DSM-III-R table of Organic Mental Syndromes Associated With Psychoactive Substances (p. 124) may be an incomplete listing of the Organic Mental Disorders that may develop during substance intoxication and withdrawal. The 19 DSM-III-R diagnoses for Organic Mental Syndromes associated with psychoactive substances as well as the 16 residual Intoxication and Withdrawal diagnoses (see American Psychiatric Association 1987, p. 124) are shown in bold type in Table 6–1. However, the text of DSM-III-R suggests that substance Intoxication or Withdrawal may also be associated with other types of syndromes. For example, the text for Amphetamine Organic Mental Disorder mentions "anxiety" and "apprehension" (p. 135) as possible associated features, although Amphetamine Anxiety Disorder is not listed as a separate diagnosis on page 124 of DSM-III-R. Those diagnoses that were suggested by the text of DSM-III-R are indicated by the notation 3R in Table 6–1. Finally, many references supporting the existence of more diagnoses than the 19 included in DSM-III-R were identified by the literature review. Each reference is listed in Table 6–1 under the specific diagnosis it supports.

It should be noted that DSM-III-R awkwardly names the residual Withdrawal state from alcohol and sedative-hypnotics and anxiolytics as Uncomplicated Alcohol Withdrawal and Uncomplicated Sedative, Hypnotic, or Anxiolytic Withdrawal. Major motor seizures are listed as complications for both. It seems illogical to list such major complications as part of a condition that is labeled "Uncomplicated." It should also be noted that the Delirium and Hallucinosis reference under opioids in the table refers to conditions developing during high-dose meperidine intoxications.

In general, the multiple additional diagnoses suggested in Table 6–1 are not proposals for new diagnoses; they result from applying the rules that appear to be implicit in DSM-III-R. However, DSM-III-R very pointedly does not provide a diagnosis for Cannabis Withdrawal. The literature cited in Table 6–1 appears to make a compelling case for this rare but real diagnosis.

Issue 2

DSM-III-R does not separate Intoxication diagnoses from Withdrawal diagnoses. Table 6–1 suggests that a single drug may produce the same Organic Mental Syndrome during intoxication, and separately, during withdrawal. For example, depression (Mood Syndrome) occurs during chronic intoxication from alcohol and is also observed during withdrawal from alcohol. Because of its importance in predicting course and determining treatment, the name of the drug state (Intoxication or Withdrawal) should perhaps be included in the name of the diagnosis. Few of the 19 tabulated diagnoses and none of the other drug-related Organic Mental Syndrome diagnoses (e.g., Barbiturate Delusional Syndrome) are designated as specifically related to intoxication or withdrawal, although that designation is important in considerations of course and treatment.

Table 6–1. DSM-III-R review table

Organic Mental Syndrome	Alcohol	Sedative-hypnotics/ anxiolytics	Phencyclidine related	Cocaine	Amphetamine related
Drug state: Intoxication					
Delirium	3R Charness et al. 1989 Mendelson & LaDou 1964 Tamerin & Mendelson 1969	Khantzian & McKenna 1979 Isbell et al. 1950 Essig 1968	**PCP-Related Delirium**	**Cocaine Delirium**	**Amphetamine-Related Delirium**
Delusional Syndrome	3R Nathan et al. 1970 Mendelson & LaDou 1964	Khantzian & McKenna 1979	**PCP-Related Delusional Disorder**	**Cocaine Delusional Disorder** (Brief): Sherer et al. 1988 Manschreck 1987 Siegel 1979, 1982 Elpern 1988 Lesko et al. 1982	**Amphetamine-Related Delusional Disorder** (Brief): Angrist & Gershon 1970 Griffith et al. et al. 1970 Bell 1973
Mood Syndrome	McNamee et al. 1968 Nathan & O'Brien 1971 Nathan et al. 1970 Mendelson & LaDou 1964 Tamerin & Mendelson 1969	Isbell et al. 1950	**PCP-Related Mood Disorder**	3R Lowenstein et al. 1987 Manschreck et al. 1987 Siegel 1979, 1982	3R Griffith et al. 1970 Smith 1969
Anxiety Syndrome	McNamee et al. 1968 Nathan & O'Brien 1971 Nathan et al. 1970 Mendelson & LaDou 1964		3R Burns et al. 1975	3R Anthony et al. 1989 Louie et al. 1989 Pohl et al. 1987 Lowenstein et al. 1987 Post & Weiss 1988 Siegel 1982	3R Ellinwood 1967
Amnestic Syndrome	Mello 1972 Charness et al. 1989 Mendelson & LaDou 1964 Goodwin et al. 1969				

Cannabis	Hallucinogens	Inhalants	Opioids	Nicotine	Caffeine
Talbott & Teague 1969 Baker & Lucas 1969	Nicholi 1984	Schuckit 1989 Glaser & Massengale 1962	3R Medical Economics Co 1989		
Cannabis Delusional Disorder	**Hallucinogen Delusional Disorder**	Schuckit 1989			
	Hallucinogen Mood Disorder	Schuckit 1989 Glaser & Massengale 1962	Meyer & Mirin 1979		
3R Kaplan 1971	Nicholi 1984 Frosch et al. 1965 Freedman 1969	Schuckit 1989			3R

(continued)

Table 6–1. DSM-III-R review table *(continued)*

Organic Mental Syndrome	Alcohol	Sedative-hypnotics/ anxiolytics	Phencyclidine related	Cocaine	Amphetamine related
Hallucinosis			3R Burns et al. 1975	3R Lowenstein et al. 1987 Manschreck et al. 1987 Lesko et al. 1982 Siegel 1982	3R Sato et al. 1983 Ellinwood 1967 Angrist & Gershon 1970 Griffith et al. 1970 Bell 1973 Smith 1969
Residual Intoxication	Alcohol Intoxication Alcohol Idiosyncratic Intoxication	SHA Intoxication	PCP-Related Intoxication	Cocaine Intoxication	Amphetamine-Related Intoxication
Drug state: Withdrawal					
Delirium	Alcohol Withdrawal Delirium	SHA Withdrawal Delirium			
Delusional Syndrome		3R Wikler 1968			
Mood Syndrome	3R Nathan et al. 1970	Wikler 1968		3R Gawin & Kleber 1986	3R Ellinwood 1967 Beamish & Kiloh 1960 Smith 1969
Anxiety Syndrome	3R Nathan et al. 1970	3R Isbell et al. 1950 Essig 1968		Gawin & Kleber 1986	
Amnestic Syndrome					
Hallucinosis	Alcohol Hallucinosis	3R Khantzian & McKenna 1979 Wikler 1968 Allgulander 1978			
Residual Withdrawal	Uncomplicated Alcohol Withdrawal	Uncomplicated SHA Withdrawal		Cocaine Withdrawal	Amphetamine-Related Withdrawal
Drug State: Other or Persisting					
	Alcohol Amnestic Disorder Dementia Associated With Alcoholism	SHA Amnestic Disorder	PCP-Related Organic Mental Disorder NOS		

Cannabis	Hallucinogens	Inhalants	Opioids	Nicotine	Caffeine
3R Kaplan 1971	Hallucinogen Hallucinosis		Medical Economics Co 1989		
Cannabis Intoxication	3R Freedman 1969	Inhalant Intoxication	Opioid Intoxication		Caffeine Intoxication
Jones 1971, 1978 Mendelson et al. 1984			Opioid Withdrawal	Nicotine Withdrawal	Hughes 1989
	Posthallucinogenic Perception Disorder				

Note. Diagnoses in bold type indicate the 19 DSM-III-R diagnoses for Organic Mental Syndromes associated with psychoactive substances and the 16 residual Intoxication and Withdrawal diagnoses. 3R = those diagnoses suggested by the text of DSM-III-R. PCP = phencyclidine. SHA = sedative-hypnotic/anxiolytic. NOS = not otherwise specified.

Issue 3

Although the residual nature of Intoxication and Withdrawal in DSM-III-R implies an algorithm (outlined above) of alternative diagnoses that take precedence over Intoxication and Withdrawal, specific rules for proceeding through that algorithm are not provided. Although Table 6–1 illustrates the many diagnoses that might be rendered under the DSM-III-R system, the rules for an explicitly stated algorithm would be quite cumbersome. Alternatives should be considered.

Issue 4

Maladaptive behavior is an essential feature of the diagnosis of Intoxication, but maladaptive behavior is not clearly defined. Many questions arise from leaving the term *maladaptive* undefined. Is drunk driving maladaptive behavior? Is it maladaptive behavior only if the intoxicated person is arrested or injured in an accident? Are slurred speech, loquacity, and euphoria during a job interview maladaptive? Whether a particular behavior is maladaptive may depend as much on the setting as on the pharmacology of the occurrence. Leaving the term undefined permitted DSM-III-R to steer a course between those who did not want all voluntary intoxications labeled as mental disorders and those who felt that any impairment of mental functioning is a mental disorder even if it results from voluntary intoxication. Unfortunately, diagnostic precision probably suffers from this lack of definition.

Issue 5

DSM-III-R provides several drug-related diagnoses that describe conditions persisting long after intoxication or withdrawal, and the organization and content of those descriptions deserve consideration. The persisting Psychoactive Substance-Induced Organic Mental Disorders tabulated in DSM-III-R (p. 124) include the following: Alcohol Amnestic Disorder; Dementia Associated with Alcoholism; Sedative, Hypnotic, or Anxiolytic Amnestic Disorder; Posthallucinogen Perception Disorder; and the Delusional Disorders associated with amphetamine, cocaine, cannabis, and hallucinogens. For Cocaine Delusional Disorder, DSM-III-R states that "delusions can linger for a week or more, but occasionally last for over a year" (p. 144). DSM-IV may avoid confusion among clinicians by more clearly differentiating in text the very persistent drug-related disorders from those observed during intoxications and withdrawals.

In addition, a question arises about the validity of Delusional Disorders triggered by substances that persist long after the direct substance effect ends. Many people do develop long-lasting delusions, and some of them may have been using amphetamines, cocaine, or hallucinogens at the time that their disorder began. However, a term such as *Cocaine Delusional Disorder* clearly implies causation by cocaine. The literature cited in Table 6–1 for Delusional Syndromes (brief) for cocaine and amphetamines clearly supports the development of brief delusional disorders from these drugs, but support for the persisting delusional disorders is less clear.

Discussion and Recommendations

Issues 1, 2, and 3

DSM-IV could maintain the present organization, making the algorithm explicit. But the rules of the algorithm would be cumbersome, and the names would not distinguish intoxication from withdrawal. Another possibility would be to cite the phenomenologic name of the condition along with the name of the drug and the drug state. Examples would be Organic Mood Disorder due to Alcohol Intoxication, Organic Delusional Disorder due to Cocaine Intoxication, and Delirium due to Phenobarbital Withdrawal.

An alternative three-part naming system would first list the drug, then the drug state (Intoxication, Withdrawal, Persisting), and then any associated mental syndrome. Examples would be Alcohol Intoxication Mood Disorder, Pentobarbital Withdrawal Delirium, Cocaine Intoxication Delusional Disorder, and Alcohol Persisting Amnestic Disorder. The residual category, in which the maladaptive behavior does not meet criteria for one of the other Organic Mental Syndromes, is indicated by simply not adding a third-part modifier; examples would be Cocaine Intoxication, Alcohol Withdrawal, or Cannabis Intoxication. The latter approach requires the use of the terms *Intoxication* or *Withdrawal* in all mental disorders resulting from physiologic intoxication or withdrawal, whereas DSM-III-R permits the use of those terms only in the limited residual cases. This change seems valuable since clinicians must recognize and treat intoxication and withdrawal as separate disorders. This change is recommended strongly.

Issue 4

One option is to leave the term *maladaptive behavior* undefined. Much political and social criticism could result if millions of annual episodes of simple intoxication were to be defined as "mental disorders." Leaving the term vague might help to avoid that possibility.

A second option would be to define the term, perhaps as follows:

> The essential features of Intoxication are maladaptive behavior and a substance-specific syndrome that are due to the recent ingestion of a psychoactive substance. The essential features of Withdrawal are the development of maladaptive behavior and a substance-specific syndrome that follows the cessation of, or reduction in, intake of a psychoactive substance that the person previously used regularly. In this context, drug-induced "maladaptive behavior" is behavior developing during drug intoxication or withdrawal that places the drug-using person at significant risk of adverse effects in four life areas: medical, social and family relationships, vocational and financial matters, or legal problems. Drug-induced changes in behavior are, or are not, maladaptive, depending on social or environmental circumstances. For example, occasional moderate alcohol intoxication with slurring, loquacity, euphoria, and some motor impairment may not be maladaptive at a college fraternity party, but becomes highly maladaptive if the student attempts to drive home. Some drug-induced changes in mental state, such as delusions, severe depression, or elation, are so likely to result in maladaptive behavior that the mental states themselves are always viewed as maladaptive. In diagnosing intoxication or withdrawal states as mental disorders, the clinician must ascertain that the person experienced those mental states or behaved in a way that was maladaptive in that person's environment as a result of drug intoxication or withdrawal.
>
> The use of an illegal drug may be a crime, but is not in itself a mental disorder. Only when use of the drug results in intoxication or withdrawal with maladaptive behavior as described above is that state of intoxication or withdrawal a mental disorder.
>
> Intoxication and Withdrawal resulting in maladaptive behavior are mental disorders. But that medical definition does not influence considerations of criminal culpability for drug-influenced behavior. Culpability is a legal concept determined on legal, rather than medical, grounds.

This detailed definition of *maladaptive behavior* may increase diagnostic reliability in this area and is recommended.

Issue 5

DSM-IV could maintain the organization of DSM-III-R; alternatively, it could separately label Persisting Disorders. These would include Alcohol Persisting Amnestic Disorder, Alcohol Persisting Dementia, Cocaine Persisting Delusional Disorder, Amphetamine Persisting Delusional Disorder, Posthallucinogen Persisting Perception Disorder, and Hallucinogen Persisting Delusional Disorder. Since the course and treatment of intoxications, withdrawals, and persisting disorders are clearly different, those differences should be emphasized in the naming of the syndromes and in the organization of the text. Therefore, this reorganization is recommended.

The literature review leaves questions about the authenticity of Persisting Delusional Disorders associated with cocaine, amphetamine, and hallucinogens, and about Persisting Amnestic Disorders associated with sedative-hypnotics and anxiolytics.

References

Allgulander C: Dependence on sedative and hypnotic drugs: a comparative clinical and social study. Acta Psychiatr Scand Suppl 270:1–102, 1978

American Psychiatric Association: Diagnostic and Statistical Manual of Mental Disorders, 2nd Edition. Washington, DC, American Psychiatric Association, 1968

American Psychiatric Association: Diagnostic and Statistical Manual of Mental Disorders, 3rd Edition. Washington, DC, American Psychiatric Association, 1980

American Psychiatric Association: Diagnostic and Statistical Manual of Mental Disorders, 3rd Edition, Revised. Washington, DC, American Psychiatric Association, 1987

Angrist BM, Gershon S: The phenomenology of experimentally induced amphetamine psychosis: preliminary observations. Biol Psychiatry 2:95–107, 1970

Anthony JC, Tien AY, Petronis KR: Epidemiologic evidence on cocaine use and panic attacks. Am J Epidemiol 129:543–549, 1989

Baker AA, Lucas EG: Some hospital admissions associated with cannabis. Lancet 1:148, 1969

Beamish P, Kiloh LG: Psychoses due to amphetamine consumption. Journal of Mental Sciences 106:337–343, 1960

Bell DS: The experimental reproduction of amphetamine psychosis. Arch Gen Psychiatry 29:35–40, 1973

Burns RS, Lerner SE, Corrado R, et al: Phencyclidine: states of acute intoxication and fatalities. West J Med 123:345–349, 1975

Charness ME, Simon RP, Greenberg DA: Ethanol and the nervous system. N Engl J Med 321:442–454, 1989

Ellinwood EH Jr: Amphetamine psychosis, I: description of the individuals and process. J Nerv Ment Dis 144:273–283, 1967

Elpern DJ: Cocaine abuse and delusions of parasitosis. Cutis 42:273–274, 1988

Essig CF: Addiction to barbiturate and nonbarbiturate sedative drugs, in Association for Research in Nervous and Mental Disease, The Addictive States: Proceedings of the Association, December 2 and 3, 1966, New York, N.Y. Baltimore, MD, Williams & Wilkins, 1968

Freedman DX: The psychopharmacology of hallucinogenic agents. Annu Rev Med 20:409–418, 1969

Frosch WA, Robbins ES, Stern M: Untoward reactions to lysergic acid diethylamide (LSD) resulting in hospitalization. N Engl J Med 273:1235–1239, 1965

Gawin FH, Kleber HD: Abstinence symptomatology and psychiatric diagnosis in cocaine abusers: clinical observations. Arch Gen Psychiatry 43:107–113, 1986

Glaser HH, Massengale ON: Glue-sniffing in children: deliberate inhalation of vaporized plastic cements. JAMA 181:300–303, 1962

Goodwin DW, Crane JB, Guze SB: Alcoholic "blackouts": a review and clinical study of 100 alcoholics. Am J Psychiatry 126:191–198, 1969

Griffith JD, Cavanaugh JH, Held J, et al: Experimental psychosis induced by the administration of D-amphetamine, in Amphetamines and Related Compounds: Proceedings of the Mario Negri Institute for Pharmacological Research, Milan, Italy. Edited by Costa E, Garattini S. New York, Raven, 1970

Hughes JR: Review paper on whether caffeine withdrawal should be added to DSM-IV: a report for the Alcohol and Substance Abuse Work Group on DSM-IV. Washington, DC, American Psychiatric Association, 1989

Isbell H, Altschul S, Kornetsky CH, et al: Chronic barbiturate intoxication: an experimental study. Arch Neurol 64:1–28, 1950

Jones RT: Tetrahydrocannabinol and the marijuana-induced social "high," or the effects of the mind on marijuana. Ann N Y Acad Sci 191:155–165, 1971

Jones RT: Marihuana: human effects, in Handbook of Psychopharmacology, Vol 12: Drugs of Abuse. Edited by Iversen LL, Iversen SD, Snyder SH. New York, Plenum, 1978

Kaplan HS: Psychosis associated with marijuana. N Y State J Med 71:433–435, 1971

Khantzian EJ, McKenna GJ: Acute toxic and withdrawal reactions associated with drug use and abuse. Ann Intern Med 90:361–372, 1979

Lesko LM, Fischman MW, Javaid JI, et al: Iatrogenous cocaine psychosis (letter). N Engl J Med 307:1153, 1982

Louie AK, Lannon RA, Ketter TA: Treatment of cocaine-induced panic disorder. Am J Psychiatry 146:40–44, 1989

Lowenstein DH, Massa SM, Rowbotham MC, et al: Acute neurologic and psychiatric complications associated with cocaine abuse. Am J Med 83:841–846, 1987

Manschreck TC, Allen DF, Neville M: Freebase psychosis: cases from a Bahamian epidemic of cocaine abuse. Compr Psychiatry 28:555–564, 1987

McNamee HB, Mello NK, Mendelson JH: Experimental analysis of drinking patterns of alcoholics: concurrent psychiatric observations. Am J Psychiatry 124:1063–1069, 1968

Medical Economics Co: Physicians' Desk Reference, 43rd Edition. Oradell, NJ, Medical Economics Co, 1989

Mello NK: Behavioral studies of alcoholism, in The Biology of Alcoholism, Vol 2: Physiology and Behavior. Edited by Kissin B, Begleiter H. New York, Plenum, 1972

Mendelson JH, LaDou J: Experimentally induced chronic intoxication and withdrawal in alcoholics, Part I: background and experimental design. Quarterly Journal of Studies on Alcohol (Suppl) 2:53–73, 1964

Mendelson JH, Mello NK, Lex BW, et al: Marijuana withdrawal syndrome in a woman. Am J Psychiatry 141:1289–1290, 1984

Meyer RE, Mirin SM: The Heroin Stimulus: Implications for a Theory of Addiction. New York, Plenum Medical, 1979

Nathan PE, O'Brien JS: An experimental analysis of the behavior of alcoholics and nonalcoholics during prolonged experimental drinking: a necessary precursor of behavior therapy? Behavior Therapy 2:455–476, 1971

Nathan PE, Titler NA, Lowenstein LM, et al: Behavioral analysis of chronic alcoholism: interaction of alcohol and human contact. Arch Gen Psychiatry 22:419–430, 1970

Nicholi AM Jr: Phencyclidine hydrochloride (PCP) use among college students: subjective and clinical effects, toxicity, diagnosis, and treatment. J Am Coll Health 32:197–200, 1984

Pohl R, Balon R, Yeragani VK: More on cocaine and panic disorder (letter). Am J Psychiatry 144:1363, 1987

Post RM, Weiss SRB: Psychomotor stimulant vs local anesthetic effects of cocaine: role of behavioral sensitization and kindling, in Mechanisms of Cocaine Abuse and Toxicity (NIDA Research Monograph No 88) (DHHS Publ No ADM-88-1588). Edited by Clouet D, Asghar K, Brown R. Washington, DC, U.S. Department of Health and Human Services, 1988

Sato M, Chen CC, Akiyama K, et al: Acute exacerbation of paranoid psychotic state after long-term abstinence in patients with previous methamphetamine psychosis. Biol Psychiatry 18:429–440, 1983

Schuckit MA: Glues, solvents, and aerosols. Drug Abuse and Alcoholism Newsletter 18, 1989

Sherer MA, Kumor KM, Cone EJ, et al: Suspiciousness induced by four-hour intravenous infusions of cocaine: preliminary findings. Arch Gen Psychiatry 45:673–677, 1988

Siegel RK: Cocaine smoking (letter). N Engl J Med 300:373, 1979

Siegel RK: Cocaine smoking. J Psychoactive Drugs 14:271–359, 1982

Smith DE: The characteristics of dependence in high-dose methamphetamine abuse. Int J Addict 4:453–459, 1969

Talbott JA, Teague JW: Marihuana psychosis: acute toxic psychosis associated with the use of cannabis derivatives. JAMA 210:299–302, 1969

Tamerin JS, Mendelson JH: The psychodynamics of chronic inebriation: observations of alcoholics during the process of drinking in an experimental group setting. Am J Psychiatry 125:886–899, 1969

Wikler A: Diagnosis and treatment of drug dependence of the barbiturate type. Am J Psychiatry 125:758–765, 1968

Chapter 7

Nicotine Withdrawal, Dependence, and Abuse

John R. Hughes, M.D.

Statement of the Issues

This report was commissioned to examine the data on nicotine withdrawal, dependence, and abuse, and to use this information to assess the adequacy and appropriateness of the existing diagnostic criteria for these disorders. In particular, the goals of the report are to determine whether sufficient data exist to 1) add four new withdrawal symptoms to the nicotine withdrawal criteria and 2) add a diagnosis of nicotine abuse.

Significance of the Issues

After caffeine, nicotine is the most widely used psychoactive drug and causes more morbidity and mortality than all other forms of drug abuse combined (U.S. Department of Health and Human Services 1988). Nicotine dependence is especially prevalent in psychiatric patients (Hughes et al. 1986) and in those who abuse alcohol and drugs (DiFranza and Guerrera 1990). Unlike alcohol and opiate withdrawal and dependence, rigorous studies of nicotine withdrawal and dependence have only recently been undertaken (U.S. Department of Health and Human Services 1988).

Methods

The review was based on 1) computerized searches of *Index Medicus* and *Psychological Abstracts* using the term *nicotine* crossed with *drug dependence, drug abuse,* and *withdrawal* for the period 1980–1990 (more than 200 articles were generated); 2) references found in the bibliographies of scientific papers (e.g., Hughes et al. 1990); 3) press articles and papers presented at recent conventions; and 4) material supplied by consultants. A more detailed report including more references is available from the author on request.

Results

Nicotine Withdrawal

Craving as a criterion for nicotine withdrawal. Several reviews concluded that with one exception most of the existing DSM-III-R (American Psychiatric Association 1987) symptoms of nicotine withdrawal are valid (Hughes et al. 1990; U.S. Department of Health and Human Services 1988, 1990). The problem item is "craving," a criterion in nicotine withdrawal but not in most other withdrawal syndromes in DSM-III-R (Hughes et al. 1990; U.S. Department of Health and Human Services 1990). This could imply that craving is more prominent or more closely tied to withdrawal from nicotine than other withdrawal syndromes. However, there are no data to support this notion (Kozlowski and Wilkinson 1987; Kozlowski et al. 1989; West 1987; West and Kranzler 1992). For example, craving is rated high even while smokers are smoking and clearly not in withdrawal (Hughes et al. 1991). Second, it is debatable whether craving during cigarette cessation is actually influenced by nicotine administration (Hughes and Hatsukami 1985; West 1984; West and Schneider 1987). Third, craving appears to be controlled by nonpharmacological factors such as environmental setting (Kozlowski and Wilkinson 1987; West and Kranzler 1992; West and Schneider 1987).

Although these data suggest that craving should be dropped as a criterion—an option not included in the *DSM-IV Options Book* (American Psychiatric Association 1991)—other data suggest the opposite. First, craving is one of the more common and reliable effects of tobacco abstinence (Hughes and Hatsukami 1986; Hughes et al. 1990; Kozlowski and Wilkinson 1987; West and Schneider 1987). Second, if phrased correctly, craving-like constructs (e.g., thinking about smoking) can be shown to be relieved by nicotine (Hughes et al. 1991; Schneider and Jarvik 1985; West and Schneider 1987). Third, several papers indicate that craving prospectively predicts relapse (Covey et al. 1990; Gritz et al. 1991; West et al. 1989a). Finally, because of the ubiquity of environmental cues for smoking compared with cues for other substances of abuse (e.g., opioids, alcohol), craving for tobacco may be more pervasive than for alcohol and other substances of abuse.

Possible new items. Four additional symptoms not presently included in the DSM-III-R criteria for nicotine withdrawal may actually deserve inclusion. These symptoms are depressed mood, disrupted sleep, impatience, and desire for sweets.

Although early evidence about depressed mood as a withdrawal syndrome was mixed (Hughes et al. 1990; U.S. Department of Health and Human Services 1990), more recent data from a number of studies indicate that dysphoria 1) occurs on cessation of smoking in both clinic attendees (Covey et al. 1990; West 1984; West et al. 1989a) and in self-quitters (Hughes et al. 1991); 2) has a time-limited course (Hughes et al. 1990; West et al. 1987, 1989b); 3) is decreased by nicotine administration (West 1984); and 4) is precipitated by cessation of nicotine alone (Hughes et al. 1986). Depression during abstinence is more likely to occur in subjects with a past history of depression (Covey et al. 1990; Hall et al. 1990), and withdrawal-induced depressed mood prospectively predicted relapse in two studies (Covey et al. 1990; West et al. 1989a). Finally, although case reports suggest that abstinence from smoking can induce clinical depressions (Flanagan and Maany 1982; Glassman et al. 1989), true empirical evidence of this phenomenon is not available.

The evidence tends to suggest that disrupted sleep is a symptom of nicotine withdrawal (Hughes et al. 1990; U.S. Department of Health and Human Services 1990). Self-reports of increased numbers of awakenings and intense dreams are common in nicotine withdrawal (Hughes et al. 1990). Cessation of smoking increases the intensity and duration of rapid-eye-movement sleep (Kales et al. 1970), which may account for the increased awakening and intense dreaming. On the other hand, these sleep changes have not been shown to be reversed with nicotine (Hughes et al. 1990).

Another possible addition, not mentioned in the *DSM-IV Options Book,* is impatience. Impatience is often described on smoking cessation, is relieved by nicotine administration, and is precipitated by cessation of nicotine alone (Hughes et al. 1990). Impatience has been operationalized as false positive responding on a computer task and shown to be worsened by smoking cessation (Hughes et al. 1989). Although impatience might be expected to be highly related to the existing criterion of restlessness, in some studies, impatience and restlessness are only modestly correlated ($r = .42–.52$) (Hughes and Hatsukami 1986; Hughes et al. 1991).

In nonhumans, nicotine deprivation increases consumption of sweet foods more than bland or salty foods (Grunberg 1990; U.S. Department of Health and Human Services 1990). Clinicians and ex-smokers often anecdotally report increased desire for sweets after cessation of smoking. However, contrary to these clinical reports, several studies have failed to demonstrate that smoking cessation increased sweet consumption (Gritz et al. 1989; Klesges et al. 1990).

Changes in the description of nicotine withdrawal. First, several studies concur that most withdrawal symptoms peak at 1–2 weeks and decline to baseline levels around 1 month (Gritz et al. 1991; Gross and Stitzer 1989; Hughes et al. 1991; U.S.

Department of Health and Human Services 1990; West et al. 1987, 1989b). Hunger and craving appear to be the exceptions in that these persist for longer than 1 month. Second, four recent prospective studies have tested whether more severe withdrawal predicts relapse. One found withdrawal immediately after cessation predicted short-term (less than 1 month) but not long-term (6 and 12 month) outcome (Gritz et al. 1989). Two studies found certain symptoms predicted short-term (less than 1 month) abstinence at certain follow-ups (Covey et al. 1990; West et al. 1989b). On the other hand, a fourth study reported that none of the withdrawal symptoms predicted short-term or long-term outcome (Hughes et al. 1991). The reason for the discrepancy across these studies is not clear. Third, research has consistently failed to find that headaches and gastrointestinal complaints are associated symptoms of nicotine withdrawal (Hughes et al. 1990).

Changes in Nicotine Dependence

The following findings may prompt changes in the DSM-III-R description of nicotine dependence. First, smokeless tobacco use has become a more common cause of nicotine dependence (Connolly et al. 1986). Second, abstinence rates based on true self-quitters (Cohen et al. 1989) differ from those cited in DSM-III-R, which were based on smokers seen in specialized cessation programs. Third, increased evidence of genetic effects in smoking initiation and cessation has been reported (Carmelli et al. 1990; Hughes 1986). The concordance of DSM-IV and ICD-10 (World Health Organization 1992) will need to be examined. ICD-9 (World Health Organization 1977) lists no diagnosis of tobacco or nicotine dependence under "Drug Dependence (304)." The diagnosis "Tobacco Use Disorder (305.1)" is included under the heading "Drug Abuse (305)" with a descriptor of "tobacco dependence."

Nicotine Abuse

At present, nicotine is the only drug in DSM-III-R to have a dependence but not an abuse disorder. The rationale for this exclusion stated in DSM-III-R is that "although Nicotine Abuse is logically possible . . . virtually no one who has not previously been dependent on nicotine uses nicotine-containing substances in a maladaptive way, e.g., episodic use of cigarettes that exacerbates a physical disorder" (pp. 169–170).

One criterion for Psychoactive Substance Abuse is "continued use despite knowledge of having a persistent or recurrent social, occupational, psychological, or physical problem that is caused or exacerbated by use of the psychoactive substance" (p. 169). Although social, occupational, and psychological problems may be caused by smoking (e.g., in restricted areas), there is no evidence that these are due to an intoxicated state or reach clinical significance. In terms of physical problems, the percentage of smokers who know that they have a specific smoking-induced illness has not been studied in larger surveys.

A second criterion for Psychoactive Substance Abuse is "recurrent use in situations in which use is physically hazardous" (p. 169). There are empirical data that demonstrate that smokers have a higher risk for many types of accidents (e.g., fires, motor vehicle accidents) (U.S. Department of Health and Human Services 1988). Cases in which one can directly attribute a fire or motor vehicle accident to smoking do occur; however, these appear to be due not to nicotine intoxication, but rather to the mechanical act of smoking.

A third criterion for Psychoactive Substance Abuse is "never met the criteria for Psychoactive Substance Dependence for this substance" (p. 169). The percentage of smokers who would fulfill nicotine abuse but do not have a present or past history of nicotine dependence is unknown.

Discussion

The work reviewed suggests three major questions: 1) whether to delete craving as a criterion for nicotine withdrawal; 2) whether to add depression, disrupted sleep, impatience, and increased consumption of sweets as criteria for nicotine withdrawal; and 3) whether to add a category of nicotine abuse.

The generic problems with use of the term *craving* in drug abuse research have been discussed (Kozlowski and Wilkinson 1987). In defining the withdrawal syndromes of alcohol, amphetamine, cocaine, and sedative-hypnotics, DSM-III-R has not included craving. This does not imply that craving is not a reliable and common outcome of cessation of these drugs. Rather, it probably implies that inclusion of the term does not add substantially to the understanding of these syndromes. Thus, the question arises whether there is a sufficient amount of scientific information that indicates craving is more important in nicotine withdrawal than in other drug withdrawal syndromes. Data on this question are not available.

The evidence for adding depression and disrupted sleep to nicotine withdrawal appears straightforward. Although the evidence for impatience is also strong, one could question whether this symptom adds anything to a description already including irritability, anger, frustration, and restlessness. One alternative proposal would be to add impatience as an alternative to restlessness since the two are correlated. The nonhuman data and clinical observations would argue for the inclusion of increased consumption of sweets as a withdrawal criterion; however, the presence of several failures to verify this effect in humans argues against its inclusion.

With increased social pressure against smoking, increased interpersonal, occupational, and social problems may occur in the future (Coombs et al. 1989). However, these problems will not be due to nicotine intoxication. In addition, whether they will reach a magnitude requiring clinical treatment remains to be seen.

Recommendations

1. Delete craving as a criterion for nicotine withdrawal.
2. Add dysphoric or depressed mood and insomnia as criteria for nicotine withdrawal.
3. Add impatience as an alternate criterion for restlessness.
4. Do not add a category of nicotine abuse.

References

American Psychiatric Association: Diagnostic and Statistical Manual of Mental Disorders, 3rd Edition, Revised. Washington, DC, American Psychiatric Association, 1987

American Psychiatric Association: DSM-IV Options Book: Work in Progress 9/9/91. Washington, DC, American Psychiatric Association, 1991

Carmelli D, Swan GE, Robinette D, et al: Heritability of substance use in the NAS-NRC twin registry. Acta Genet Med Gemellol (Roma) 39:91–98, 1990

Cohen S, Lichtenstein E, Prochaska JO, et al: Debunking myths about self-quitting. Am Psychol 44:1355–1365, 1989

Connolly GN, Winn DM, Hecht SS, et al: The reemergence of smokeless tobacco. N Engl J Med 314:1020–1027, 1986

Coombs RB, Kozlowski LT, Ferrence RG: The future of tobacco use and smoking research, in Smoking and Human Behavior. Edited by Ney T, Gale A. New York, Wiley, 1989

Covey LS, Glassman AH, Stetner F: Depression and depressive symptoms in smoking cessation. Compr Psychiatry 31:350–354, 1990

DiFranza JR, Guerrera MP: Alcoholism and smoking. J Stud Alcohol 51:130–135, 1990

Flanagan J, Maany I: Smoking and depression. Am J Psychiatry 139:541, 1982

Glassman AH, Covey LS, Stetner F: Smoking cessation, depression and antidepressants. Abstract presented at the 142nd Annual Meeting of the American Psychiatric Association, May 1989

Gritz ER, Klesges RC, Meyers AW: The smoking and body weight relationship: implications for intervention and post-cessation weight control. Annals of Behavioral Medicine 11:144–153, 1989

Gritz ER, Carr CR, Marcus AC: The tobacco withdrawal syndrome in unaided quitters. Br J Addict 86:57–69, 1991

Gross J, Stitzer ML: Nicotine replacement: ten-week effects on tobacco withdrawal symptoms. Psychopharmacology (Berlin) 98:334–341, 1989

Grunberg NE: The inverse relationship between tobacco use and body weight, in Research Advances in Alcohol and Drug Problems, Vol 10. Edited by Kozlowski LT, Annis H, Cappell HD, et al. New York, Plenum, 1990

Hall SM, Munoz R, Reus V: Smoking cessation, depression and dysphoria, in Problems of Drug Dependence, 1990 (NIDA Research Monograph No 105). Edited by Harris LS. Washington, DC, U.S. Government Printing Office, 1990

Hughes JR: Genetics of smoking: a brief review. Behavior Therapy 17:335–345, 1986

Hughes JR, Hatsukami DK: Short-term effects of nicotine gum, in Pharmacological Adjuncts in Smoking Cessation (NIDA Research Monograph No 53) (DHHS Publ No ADM-85-1333). Edited by Grabowski J, Hall S. Washington, DC, U.S. Government Printing Office, 1985

Hughes JR, Hatsukami DK: Signs and symptoms of tobacco withdrawal. Arch Gen Psychiatry 43:289–294, 1986

Hughes JR, Hatsukami DK, Skoog K: Physical dependence on nicotine gum: a placebo-substitution trial. JAMA 255:3277–3279, 1986

Hughes JR, Keenan R, Yellin A: Effect of tobacco withdrawal on sustained attention. Addict Behav 14:577–580, 1989

Hughes JR, Higgins ST, Hatsukami DK: Effects of abstinence from tobacco: a critical review, in Research Advances in Alcohol and Drug Problems, Vol 10. Edited by Kozlowski LT, Annis H, Cappell HD, et al. New York, Plenum, 1990

Hughes JR, Gust SW, Skoog K, et al: Symptoms of tobacco withdrawal: a replication and extension. Arch Gen Psychiatry 48:52–59, 1991

Kales J, Allen C, Preston T, et al: Changes in REM sleep and dreaming with cigarette smoking and following withdrawal. Psychophysiology 7:347–348, 1970

Klesges RC, Meyers AW, Winders SE, et al: Determining the reasons for weight gain following smoking cessation: current findings, methodological issues, and future directions for research. Annals of Behavioral Medicine 11:134–143, 1990

Kozlowski LT, Wilkinson DA: Use and misuse of the concept of craving by alcohol, tobacco and drug researchers. Br J Addict 82:31–45, 1987

Kozlowski LT, Wilkinson DA, Skinner W, et al: Comparing tobacco cigarette dependence with other drug dependencies. JAMA 261:898–901, 1989

Schneider NG, Jarvik ME: Nicotine gum vs placebo gum: comparisons of withdrawal symptoms and success rates, in Pharmacological Adjuncts in Smoking Cessation (NIDA Research Monograph No 53) (DHHS Publ No ADM-85-1333). Edited by Grabowski J, Hall SM. Washington, DC, U.S. Government Printing Office, 1985

U.S. Department of Health and Human Services: The Health Consequences of Smoking: Nicotine Addiction. Washington, DC, U.S. Government Printing Office, 1988

U.S. Department of Health and Human Services: Health Consequences of Smoking Cessation: A Report of the US Surgeon General. Washington, DC, U.S. Government Printing Office, 1990

West RJ: Psychology and pharmacology in cigarette withdrawal. J Psychosom Res 28:379–386, 1984

West RJ: Use and misuse of craving. Br J Addict 82:39–40, 1987

West RJ, Kranzler HR: Craving for cigarettes and psychoactive drugs, in Addiction Controversies. Edited by Warburton D. New York, Harwood Academic Publishers, 1992

West RJ, Schneider N: Craving for cigarettes. Br J Addict 82:407–415, 1987

West RJ, Hajek P, Belcher M: Time course of cigarette withdrawal symptoms during four weeks of treatment with nicotine gum. Addict Behav 12:1–5, 1987

West RJ, Hajek P, Belcher M: Severity of withdrawal symptoms as a predictor of outcome of an attempt to quit smoking. Psychol Med 19:981–985, 1989a

West RJ, Hajek P, Belcher M: Time course of cigarette withdrawal symptoms while using nicotine gum. Psychopharmacology (Berlin) 99:143–145, 1989b

World Health Organization: International Classification of Diseases, 9th Revision. Geneva, World Health Organization, 1977

World Health Organization: The ICD-10 Classification of Mental and Behavioural Disorders: Clinical Descriptions and Diagnostic Guidelines. Geneva, World Health Organization, 1992

Chapter 8

Alcohol Idiosyncratic Intoxication

A Review of the Data Supporting Its Existence

Harold C. Urschel III, M.D.
George E. Woody, M.D.

Statement of the Issues

DSM-III-R (American Psychiatric Association 1987) diagnostic criteria for Alcohol Idiosyncratic Intoxication (AII)—a diagnosis that has also been called Pathological Intoxication (PI)—is provided in Table 8–1.

DSM-III-R discusses the essential features of AII as consisting of a spectrum of behaviors that might reasonably be anticipated from an individual while he or she is intoxicated. Additional significant features that are associated with the syndrome include

1. The abnormal behavior in response to the alcohol ingestion usually begins while the person is drinking or shortly thereafter within minutes. The duration is usually brief, and the symptoms will usually cease within a few hours of onset (Jacoby and Galanter 1986).
2. Classically, psychotic and/or violent symptoms have been associated with the syndrome, including hallucinations and/or paranoid or persecutory delusions (Hollender 1979).
3. After the symptoms resolve, the patient usually experiences a prolonged period of undisturbed sleep (Coid 1979).
4. On awakening, the patient usually has complete amnesia for the period of intoxication (Coid 1979).
5. Brain injury, most commonly from trauma and encephalitis, may predispose

a patient to this syndrome. Individuals who are extremely fatigued, or who have debilitating physical illnesses, may similarly be predisposed to AII.

Like many other DSM-III-R diagnoses, the criteria for AII have continued to be refined with each successive revision (Perr 1986). However, this syndrome may rest on a somewhat weak data base. Furthermore, although the criteria and associated symptoms for AII appear very straightforward, there are significant problems that may compromise the validity of this diagnosis. These problems include the following:

1. The concept of an amount of alcohol insufficient to induce intoxication in most people is a critical factor in the definition of AII, yet no study has shown through reliable eyewitness accounts or experimental evidence that small quantities of alcohol have ever induced the condition. Although most clinicians or researchers would agree that one or two drinks is a "small amount of alcohol," most articles never attempt to define the amount necessary to produce AII (Coid 1979; Hollender 1979) and often include people who have taken large quantities of alcohol. In fact, every paper on AII but one reports cases and/or experiments in which the patients were subjected to intoxicating levels of alcohol before the symptoms of AII were elicited.
2. The preponderance of the literature on AII indicates that most people with this syndrome have a history of head trauma, an abnormal electroencephalogram (EEG), or symptoms of other psychiatric illnesses (Maletzky 1976). These associated factors could be intimately related to the symptoms of AII and are in direct conflict with criterion C of the DSM-III-R definition, which states that AII is not due to any physical or other mental disorder.
3. The characteristics of the period of amnesia reported to be associated with AII are vague and confusing (Jacoby and Galanter 1986). They do not clearly differentiate this syndrome from other psychiatric disorders, such as an alcoholic blackout, in which a patient may experience any of the behavioral or psychiatric symptoms found in AII (e.g., rage reaction, episodes of violence or destruction, paranoid delusions).

Table 8–1. DSM-III-R diagnostic criteria for Alcohol Idiosyncratic Intoxication

A. Maladaptive behavioral changes, e.g., aggressive or assaultive behavior, occurring within minutes of ingesting an amount of alcohol insufficient to induce intoxication in most people.

B. The behavior is atypical of the person when not drinking.

C. Not due to any physical or other mental disorder.

The purpose of this review is to assess the literature regarding the existence of AII and the problems associated with its diagnosis to determine whether DSM-IV should retain or delete AII.

Significance of the Issues

A diagnostic entity in DSM-IV implies that a specific condition has been clearly identified and that useful information is available on the prognosis and treatment of the disorder. Also, AII has significant forensic implications. For instance, in some court cases the accused may claim AII as a defense to avoid punishment for a crime committed when he or she was drunk. If a careful literature review reveals insufficient data to support the usefulness of a diagnosis, continuing the entity can mislead clinicians and impact on important clinical conditions. On the other hand, if there are sufficient clinical data, the diagnostic entity should be continued into DSM-IV.

Methods

In this review, we focus on studies pertaining to AII and PI published over the last 150 years. These studies were located by using several major computer-assisted Medline and other psychiatric/medical data base literature searches, which included both international and American sources. Several key articles were identified through these searches, and references within those articles served as guides to other articles published on the subject. Approximately 34 studies from both peer-reviewed journals and books were evaluated. Especially important to this literature review were articles by Perr (1986), Jacoby and Galanter (1986), and Coid (1979).

Results

The Evolution of the Diagnosis of AII

Krafft-Ebing first described the condition of "pathological intoxication," the old terminology for AII, in 1869. The initial reports described AII episodes as an acute delirium with hallucinations and delusions of a depressive and persecutory nature. The early investigators also noted that during the AII episode, the individual frequently displayed an irresistible desire for destruction. These reports also noted the occurrence of seizures. For approximately the next 80 years, other writers contributed alternative descriptive criteria as well as psychodynamic formulations for AII. A thorough review of these early investigations can be found in Banay (1944).

It is important to remember that the formulation of AII as a specific disease entity was developed during a less critical era of psychiatry. At that time, the diagnosis of a disorder usually had no specific guidelines, and operational definitions of the major psychiatric disorders were poorly standardized. These difficulties are further compounded by the fact that such a small number of case reports exist that a meaningful analysis of the data is difficult to develop. In fact, a majority of the more recent authors in this area have not personally seen a case of AII (Jacoby and Galanter 1986).

In the first DSM (American Psychiatric Association 1952), PI was described under the category of acute brain syndrome. PI was defined as a marked behavioral or psychotic reaction after minimal alcohol intake, and where there was no other preexisting mental disorder. When the symptoms of another disorder were exaggerated with the use of alcohol, the case would be classified under the diagnosis of the underlying condition. DSM-II (American Psychiatric Association 1968) defined PI as an acute brain syndrome manifested by psychosis after minimal alcohol intake. Finally, in the DSM-III (American Psychiatric Association 1980) definition, the name of the disorder was changed to AII. In addition, the previous criteria were altered by focusing on behavioral changes with aggressivity, and they did not specify that psychosis or an acute brain syndrome must be present (Perr 1986). The DSM-III criteria for AII are very similar to those found in DSM-III-R.

The Controversy Over the Existence of AII

Despite the continuing evolution of the diagnosis of AII, several reports over the last 50 years have strongly disputed its existence. For example, May and Ebaugh (1953) stated that

> There is no justification for continuing to believe in the existence of pathological intoxication as a special diagnostic category. It is a diagnostic catch-all, and difference of opinion, as to its symptomatology may be attributed to failure to distinguish between the various reaction types. (p. 205)

More recent reviews (Coid 1979; Hollender 1979; Jacoby and Galanter 1986) also appear to express skepticism as to the authenticity of AII. Many of these authors make reference to the similarity of AII to other states of acute behavioral disinhibition, such as "Negi Negi," which appears in the Bena Bena tribe of New Guinea. Also called "hysterical psychosis" (Langness 1965), Negi Negi appears with the same symptoms as those of AII, except for the fact that no alcohol is ingested prior to the episode. In addition, Jacoby and Galanter (1986) reviewed many other examples of cultures in which the symptoms of AII occur without the complicating issue of concomitant alcohol ingestion. They imply that AII symptoms may be unrelated to the amount of alcohol ingested because these "aberrant states" also occur in patients in the absence of alcohol. This view is expressed by Redlich and Freedman (1966) who commented that "the existence of the syndrome is not universally recognized" (p. 755). Maletzky (1976) also questioned the existence of AII when he discussed the confusing reports on PI and its lack of empirical support in the literature. In addition, Hollender (1979) emphasized that PI symptoms represent dissociative reactions; the fact that each patient may have consumed a small amount of alcohol is purely incidental. He stated that "it is high time that we ask ourselves, if a notion without substance is being perpetuated. Are we attributing a disturbed state to pathological intoxication when alcohol is incidental rather than causal—merely a culturally-fostered rationalization?" (p. 426).

Similarly, Coid (1979) noted that the majority of experimental studies failed to find an underlying etiological explanation for AII. He hypothesized that the early German writers, in describing PI, looked at a highly heterogeneous group of patients. He then suggested that the many states that may occur during alcohol intoxication, and which may be diagnosed as AII, would be better served if they were transferred to more appropriate categories. Coid also noted the trend in psychiatric diagnosis to split up multiple concepts into individual component parts. He also discussed the fact that no etiological factors for AII have been established, other than suggestions of EEG abnormalities or brain injury such as head trauma or encephalitis. Coid also noted that the theory of an epileptic component has not been able to bear up under double-blind conditions or replications (Bach-y-Rita et al. 1970; Maletzky 1976).

Finally, Cohen (1981, 1985), in discussing PI, emphasized the rareness of the actual entity. He created six specific criteria that are similar to those found in DSM-III but are based on a more scientific approach. These include rechallenging a patient with the same amount of alcohol to reproduce the explosive behavior. Cohen (1985) noted that patients with organic disorders may lose tolerance to alcohol and suggested that, "in order to make a secure diagnosis of Pathological Intoxication, a blood alcohol concentration of less than 0.1% would seem necessary. Otherwise Pathological Intoxication could not be differentiated from alcohol intoxication with an associated rage reaction" (p. 107). In summary, Cohen (1981) stated that "a wide variety of bellicose disturbances that happen to occur in connection with drinking are randomly grouped together by some clinicians as pathological intoxication. Unfortunately, no reliable objective tests are available to support the diagnosis" (p. 3).

The Controversy Over the Amount of Alcohol Involved in the Diagnosis of AII

Many authors question the merits of AII/PI as a type of disinhibition that results from an amount of minimal alcohol intake that never seems to be measured accurately. In reviewing several reasons for the confusing nature of AII, Coid (1979) focused on the concept of a "small amount" of alcohol as being a crucial factor in making the diagnosis. He emphasized that it is impossible to define a relatively small amount of alcohol, because it is a substance having a variety of dose-related effects for individuals who use it in diverse amounts.

May and Ebaugh (1953) discussed the inconsistencies and variations in clinical descriptions of AII, as well as the difficulties involved in verifying the accuracy or reliability of informants in the specific cases that have been reported in the literature. These complexities are very important, especially in light of the fact that many alcoholic persons and those who abuse alcohol have been shown to be unreliable reporters of their alcohol intake. Also, many of the cases in the literature utilize reports from nonprofessionals and others who may be less than impartial witnesses. May and Ebaugh concluded that there is a great lack of reliable evidence for PI, and that in none of the reported cases had symptoms arisen after the ingestion of such a small amount of alcohol that it would have been without an effect on the average individual.

Another important factor in this controversy over the amount of alcohol needed to produce AII is that in DSM-III-R there is little difference between the definition of alcohol intoxication and that of AII. The criteria for Alcohol Intoxication are provide in Table 8–2.

The primary difference between alcohol intoxication and AII is the amount of alcohol ingested, plus the existence of one of the physical symptoms of intoxication. The importance of this difference is magnified when the literature consistently does not support the ability of a "small amount" of alcohol to elicit the AII symptoms and when no studies using double-blind administration of alcohol that result in the symptoms of AII have been reported.

Table 8–2. DSM-III-R diagnostic criteria for Alcohol Intoxication

A. Recent ingestion of alcohol (with no evidence suggesting that the amount was insufficient to cause intoxication in most people).

B. Maladaptive behavioral changes, e.g., disinhibition of sexual or aggressive impulses, mood lability, impaired judgment, impaired social or occupational functioning.

C. At least one of the following signs:
   (1) slurred speech
   (2) incoordination
   (3) unsteady gait
   (4) nystagmus
   (5) flushed face

D. Not due to any physical or other mental disorder.

In reviewing the literature on AII and PI, only two papers attempt to characterize the quantity of alcohol ingested. Kosbab and Kuhnley (1978) and Skelton (1970) both presented single cases that they felt represented AII. However, on closer examination, Skelton's patient had consumed significant amounts of alcohol (wine and beer) earlier in the day, which, by definition, is not consistent with "minimal" alcohol intake. Kosbab and Kuhnley described the patient who ingested the smallest amount of alcohol reported in any of the AII literature's case reports reviewed back through 1944. In their case report, the patient drank "a single bottle of malt liquor"; unfortunately, the actual quantity and alcohol content of this malt liquor is not delineated. Also, since no urine drug screen was reportedly performed during this patient's evaluation, other drugs of abuse may have been involved and may have precipitated the observed unusual behavior.

The Controversy Over Possible Etiologies of AII

In the last 50 years, a more scientific approach has been applied to understanding AII, and some authors have attempted to delineate specific etiologies of this disorder.

One focus of the more recent investigations has been seizure disorders. Although the relationship between AII and an abnormal EEG need not be relevant or necessary to verify its existence, certain symptoms of AII undoubtedly appear similar to abnormal EEG activity. Primarily, three research studies have addressed this issue (Bach-y-Rita et al. 1970; Greenblatt et al. 1944; Maletzky 1976). All three investigated whether the voluntary ingestion of alcohol under controlled conditions could initiate an AII episode in patients with a supposed history of AII, and whether there are specific EEG changes present during an episode of AII. In these three studies, only a small percentage of patients with reported AII symptoms had temporal spikes on their EEGs, and no specific seizure activity during an AII episode was reported. However, Jacoby and Galanter (1986) made the point that it is quite difficult to attribute the presence of a seizure, even if one is able to be recorded during an AII episode, as a causative factor in the behavioral disturbance.

Greenblatt and colleagues (1944) reported that three of five cases of AII had abnormal EEGs that showed both slow and rapid potentials with no paroxysmal dysrhythmias. Bach-y-Rita and colleagues (1970) reported on 10 patients in whom an intravenous infusion of a 25% solution of alcohol resulted in clinical symptoms of intoxication, yet showed neither seizure activity on the EEG nor symptoms of AII. In Maletzky's (1976) study of EEG recordings during intravenous administration of alcohol, 15 of 22 subjects showed generalized slowing and disorganization with sharp waves in the temporal occipital region. These never organized sufficiently to suggest an epileptic attack, and there were no consistent correlations between AII and EEG activity.

An important feature of these studies was that only high doses of alcohol were successful in eliciting psychotic states similar to AII. The subjects were exposed to the average alcohol content of 8–24 bottles of beer, infused at a rate of 200 cc per hour. (The patients of Bach-y-Rita and colleagues [1970] were infused with an equivalent of 3–6 cans of beer over a 30-minute period and showed no symptoms of AII.) Jacoby and Galanter (1986) concluded after a very thorough review of the literature that the relationship between EEG activity and AII symptoms shows no correlation at the cortical level of activity.

In looking for other etiologies of AII, reports have suggested that it is the concomitant role of head injury or brain damage with alcohol use that predisposes an individual to an outburst similar to AII. Such outbursts may represent a lowered threshold to the stimulating effects of alcohol (Lishman 1978). Fatigue and debilitating illnesses have also been hypothesized to lower tolerance to alcohol in some people and thus predispose them to behavioral outbursts (Perr 1986).

Seelert (in Coid 1979) hypothesized a relationship of PI to hypoglycemia. He noticed the fact that, in healthy nonalcoholic subjects, alcohol can cause increased secretion of insulin. If the increased insulin occurs in the presence of several days of preliminary fasting, hypoglycemia may result. However, Williams (1970) suggested that alcoholic patients and other patients with decreased gluconeogenic reserve may quickly experience symptoms of hypoglycemia after alcohol ingestion, especially in the presence of brain damage or high levels of stress.

The potential role of stress in activating PI episodes has been discussed by some authors. Stress may cause transient excitation of the pituitary-adrenal system, which, when aggravated and potentiated by disinhibiting drugs such as alcohol or barbiturates, might cause certain individuals to experience the PI symptoms. In other words, AII patients may be seen as having a fight or flight reaction as a culmination of a complex interplay of underlying personality structure, predisposing stress, and the trigger of alcohol or barbiturate use (Kosbab and Kuhnley 1978).

Another possible etiology of AII, which is more prominent in the PI literature, is of an underlying psychiatric illness characterized by affective disturbances with hallucinations and illusions of a depressive and persecutory nature, accompanied by significant anxiety (Banay 1944). Bonhoeffer (in Jacoby and Galanter 1986) sometimes described PI as a delirium with faulty perceptions, delusions and anxiety, apprehensive observations, and misinterpretation of reality. These descriptions of AII are consistent with many case reports of PI that have identified underlying psychiatric symptoms (Kosbab and Kuhnley 1978; Skelton 1970).

Factors Complicating the Diagnosis of AII

One of the complicating factors in establishing the specific diagnosis of AII is that self-control is not the hallmark of the intoxicated person. Alcohol intoxication often results in aggressive and antisocial acts in both alcoholic persons and in those who abuse alcohol (Goodwin 1973). Similarly, aggression often occurs in the absence of alcohol ingestion and therefore may not be an important and defining feature of AII. In this vein, the term *episodic dyscontrol syndrome* refers to patients who exhibit aggressive/violent behavior as the only overt symptom of brain injury (Maletzky 1973). Some authors hypothesized that aversive environmental stimuli present during the period of intoxication, including provocative and aggressive behavior within the patient's environment, may also be factors in eliciting the violent and/or psychotic reactions of the patient diagnosed as having AII (Boyatzis 1977). Finally, other environmental stimuli and patterns are also important when evaluating particular AII episodes. These factors can include a family environment with marital discord, alcoholism, and a past history of antisocial behavior.

Another complicating factor, which is rarely mentioned within the AII literature, is the fact that alcohol is usually not the only drug linked to violent behavior, nor is it the only agent for which an idiosyncratic reaction has been reported. For example, another primary drug that has been reported to cause AII-like behavior is secobarbital (Tinklenberg and Woodrow 1974). In addition, amphetamine, psychedelic drugs, and marijuana have likewise been implicated in assaultive behavior (Blum 1969; Goode 1972). These adverse reactions to marijuana and LSD have frequently been called "bad trips." Finally, episodic attacks of violence under the influence of chlordiazepoxide and diazepam have also been reported (Maletzky 1973).

Forensic Implications of AII

The forensic implications of the existence of AII are very complex and highlight the possible etiology of psychopathic traits in some cases of AII. If patients become irrational while under the influence of alcohol, the law requires that they be held responsible for any crime that is committed because they voluntarily placed themselves in a disabling condition (Fingarette and Hasse 1979). On the other hand, if the person suffers from AII, the law appears more lenient (Jacoby and Galanter 1986). As described earlier, however, the literature does not support the fact that a "small amount" of alcohol is sufficient to elicit the symptoms of AII. Furthermore, the best predictor of episodic violent behavior is a history of violent behavior, a behavioral trait that is often associated with antisocial personality disorder and that should be strongly considered in the differential diagnosis of AII.

Edwards (1974) stated that "the type of personality fundamentally lacking in responsiveness to ordinary informal cues or more formal social control (psychopathy, sociopathy, or any of its rephrasings) will probably exhibit the same unresponsiveness in intoxicated and drug-seeking behavior" (p. 181). In fact, earlier authors such as Jellinek (1942) believed that PI occurs predominantly in psychopathic personalities who demonstrate unprovoked fits of rage, even when not drinking. Others hypothesized that suppressed violent, psychotic, and dysphoric symptoms may come to the surface during disinhibiting periods (e.g., when using alcohol or barbiturates). Megargee (1966) suggested that chronically over-controlled persons who rigidly inhibit overt aggressive behavior have such high levels of aggression that a small amount of alcohol will facilitate the expression of these suppressed forces.

Finally, May and Ebaugh (1953) felt that there was an inherent danger in diagnosing PI because a person could, without justification, claim amnesia for crimes committed during the state of intoxication. This concern that sociopathic individuals could undeservedly receive a reduced sentence by claiming the diagnosis of AII is another important reason to consider deleting this diagnosis from DSM-IV, especially considering the lack of evidence for its existence.

Discussion

The literature on AII is entirely anecdotal, filled with inconsistencies, and intertwined with comorbid factors that could account for AII; it contains no clear empirical evidence to support its existence. Numerous scientific studies have failed to reproduce this syndrome in a laboratory setting, and no double-blind, placebo-controlled experiments have been performed that establish the existence of AII.

In determining the validity of AII, the most important issues relate to

1. The concept of a small amount of alcohol.
2. The presence or absence of concomitant mental disorders.

With regard to the first of these points, a thorough review of the literature indicates that only one case report can possibly make the claim that true minimal alcohol intake caused the symptoms of AII, and its validity is questionable (Perr 1986). As for the second point, many authors and case reports suggest the concomitant existence of organic/psychiatric factors with the AII symptoms. Therefore, most, if not all, past cases that are reported as having AII do not meet the criteria for this disorder because they are disqualified from criterion C in the DSM-III-R definition.

Recommendations

It is important to acknowledge the fact that there are some potential reasons for retaining the diagnosis of AII in DSM-IV. First, any decision to delete AII is likely to have an important impact on the legal system because of the long legal history of the diagnosis. It is precisely the longevity of this diagnosis that may make it difficult to persuade the legal community that AII somehow no longer exists. Second, once a diagnosis has been incorporated into the diagnostic manual, any subsequent decision to delete it from the manual should be justified by the same rigorous standards that are being required before any new diagnosis is added to DSM-IV. A third reason to consider maintaining AII is that if the diagnosis is continued into DSM-IV, efforts can be made to collect further data on this matter before the publication of DSM-V. If, as a consequence of this search for further information a decision is made to delete AII from DSM-V, presumably the rigorous standards alluded to above would by then have been fully met.

Although these arguments may have some merit, we recommend that DSM-IV delete the diagnosis of AII for the following reasons:

1. The past literature does not clearly support its existence.
2. There are relatively few case reports published on PI/AII. There have been no new case reports since 1979, and no articles have been published on AII since DSM-III.
3. The symptoms of AII have not been experimentally reproduced. No more than one case report has ever suggested that true minimal alcohol intake has caused the symptoms of AII.

References

American Psychiatric Association: Diagnostic and Statistical Manual: Mental Disorders. Washington, DC, American Psychiatric Association, 1952

American Psychiatric Association: Diagnostic and Statistical Manual of Mental Disorders, 2nd Edition. Washington, DC, American Psychiatric Association, 1968

American Psychiatric Association: Diagnostic and Statistical Manual of Mental Disorders, 3rd Edition. Washington, DC, American Psychiatric Association, 1980

American Psychiatric Association: Diagnostic and Statistical Manual of Mental Disorders, 3rd Edition, Revised. Washington, DC, American Psychiatric Association, 1987

Bach-y-Rita G, Lion JR, Ervin FR: Pathological intoxication: clinical and electroencephalographic studies. Am J Psychiatry 127:698–703, 1970

Banay RS: Pathological reaction to alcohol. Quarterly Journal of Studies on Alcohol 4:580–605, 1944

Blum RH: Crimes of violence, in A Staff Report to the National Commission on the Causes and Prevention of Violence. Edited by Mulvihill R, Tumin MM. Washington, DC, U.S. Government Printing Office, 1969

Boyatzis RE: Alcohol and interpersonal aggression, in Alcohol Intoxication and Withdrawal. Edited by Gross MM. New York, Plenum, 1977

Cohen S: Pathological intoxication. Drug Abuse and Alcoholism Newsletter 10:1–3, 1981

Cohen S: The Substance Abuse Problems, Vol 2: New Issues for the 1980's. New York, Haworth Press, 1985

Coid J: Mania a potu: a critical review of pathological intoxication. Psychol Med 9:709–719, 1979
Edwards G: Drugs, drug dependence and the concept of plasticity. Quarterly Journal of Studies on Alcohol 35:176–195, 1974
Fingarette H, Hasse AF: Mental Disabilities and Criminal Responsibility. Berkeley, CA, University of California Press, 1979
Goode E: Report prepared for marihuana: a signal of misunderstanding. The Technical Papers of the First Report of the National Commission on Marihuana and Drug Abuse. Washington, DC, U.S. Government Printing Office, 1972
Goodwin DW: Alcohol in suicides and homicides. Quarterly Journal of Studies on Alcohol 34:144–156, 1973
Greenblatt M, Levin S, Cori FD: The electroencephalogram associated with chronic alcoholism, alcoholic psychosis and alcoholic convulsions. Archives of Neurology and Psychiatry 52:290–295, 1944
Hollender MH: Pathological intoxication: is there such an entity? J Clin Psychiatry 40:424–426, 1979
Jacoby JH, Galanter M: Alcohol idiosyncratic intoxication and other alcohol-related states of acute behavioral disinhibition, in Psychopathology and Addictive Disorders. Edited by Meyer RE. New York, Guilford, 1986
Jellinek EM: Alcohol Addiction and Chronic Alcoholism. New Haven, CT, Yale University Press, 1942
Kosbab FP, Kuhnley EJ: Pathological intoxication. Psychiatric Opinion 15:35–38, 1978
Langness LL: Hysterical psychosis in the New Guinea highlands: a Bena Bena example. Psychiatry 28:258–277, 1965
Lishman WA: Organic Psychiatry: The Psychological Consequences of Cerebral Disorder. Oxford, Blackwell Scientific Publications, 1978
Maletzky BM: The episodic dyscontrol syndrome. Diseases of the Nervous System 34:178–185, 1973
Maletzky BM: The diagnosis of pathological intoxication. J Stud Alcohol 37:1215–1228, 1976
May PR, Ebaugh FG: Pathological intoxication, alcoholic hallucinosis and other reactions to alcohol. Quarterly Journal of Studies on Alcohol 14:200–227, 1953
Megargee EI: Undercontrolled and overcontrolled personality types in extreme antisocial aggression. Psychological Monographs 80:1–29, 1966
Perr IN: Pathological intoxication and alcohol idiosyncratic intoxication, part I: diagnostic and clinical aspects. J Forensic Sci 31:806–811, 1986
Redlich FC, Freedman DX: The Theory and Practice of Psychiatry. New York, NY, Basic Books, 1966
Skelton WD: Alcohol, violent behavior and the electroencephalogram. South Med J 63:465–466, 1970
Tinklenberg JR, Woodrow KM: Drug use among youthful assaultive and sexual offenders, in Aggression Research Publication (No 52), Association for Research in Nervous and Mental Disease. Edited by Frazier SH. Baltimore, MD, Williams & Wilkins, 1974
Williams RH: Textbook of Endocrinology. Philadelphia, PA, WB Saunders, 1970

Chapter 9

Caffeine Withdrawal, Dependence, and Abuse

John R. Hughes, M.D.

Statement of the Issues

The goal of this review is to determine whether sufficient data exist to warrant inclusion of caffeine withdrawal, dependence, and abuse in DSM-IV. A more detailed review has been published elsewhere (Hughes et al. 1992b).

Significance of the Issues

Caffeine is the most widely used drug in the world. Caffeine can be ingested from brewed coffee (100 mg/6 oz), instant coffee (65 mg/6 oz), tea (40 mg/6 oz), soda (50 mg/12 oz), and over-the-counter analgesics, antihistamines, stimulants, or weight loss aids (50–200 mg/tablet). More than 85% of Americans ingest caffeine daily, and the average caffeine intake is approximately 200 mg/day (Shreiber et al. 1988). Excessive caffeine intake is especially prevalent among psychiatric patients; for example, 22% of psychiatric inpatients use amounts greater than 750 mg/day compared with 9% in the general population (DeFritas and Schwartz 1979).

Methods

The review was based on 1) computerized searches of *Index Medicus* and *Psychological Abstracts* using the term *caffeine* crossed with *drug dependence, drug abuse,* and *withdrawal* (more than 100 articles were generated); 2) references found in the bibliographies of scientific papers (e.g., Griffiths and Woodson 1988a, 1988b); 3) press articles and papers presented at recent conventions; and 4) material supplied by consultants.

Results

Caffeine Withdrawal

In nonhumans, deprivation of caffeine decreases locomotor activity or disrupts operant performance (Griffiths and Woodson 1988a). In humans, cessation of caffeine consistently produced headache, decreased arousal, and fatigue across 14 experimental trials, 5 surveys, and 23 case reports (Griffiths and Woodson 1988a). These symptoms occurred during blind substitution of decaffeinated coffee and were reversed by readministration of caffeine alone. Several other withdrawal symptoms have been reported, including anxiety, nausea, and craving for caffeine, but these have not been as well documented. Whether caffeine deprivation produces psychophysiological changes is debatable. Withdrawal occurred at doses as low as 100 mg/day in one study (Griffiths et al. 1990b). The onset of caffeine withdrawal appears to be 12–24 hours after deprivation, with a peak at 20–48 hours, and a duration of about 1 week (Griffiths and Woodson 1988a).

DSM-III-R (American Psychiatric Association 1987) stated that caffeine withdrawal was not included in prior versions because "although the existence of a caffeine withdrawal headache is well established, the syndrome is usually not severe enough to warrant clinical attention" (p. 138). However, several reports and experimental studies describe individuals in whom the headache, decreased arousal, and fatigue interfered with normal function and at times was incapacitating (Griffiths and Woodson 1988a). Survey studies (Goldstein et al. 1969) suggest that about 10% of coffee drinkers have caffeine withdrawal symptoms of a significant degree. This syndrome is substantial considering the ubiquitous use of caffeine.

Some individuals appear to drink coffee to avoid caffeine withdrawal. For example, experimental studies have found that the onset of withdrawal prospectively predicts the self-administration of caffeinated over decaffeinated coffee (Griffiths et al. 1986b; Hughes et al. 1991a).

Caffeine Dependence and Abuse

At least eight reviews have examined the question of whether caffeine is a drug of abuse or dependence (Bolton and Null 1981; Brecher 1972; Gilbert 1976a; Gilliland and Bullock 1984; Griffiths and Woodson 1988a, 1988b; Holtzman 1990; Hughes et al. 1992a). Two of the principal measures to infer the ability of a drug to produce abuse or dependence are its ability to produce psychoactive effects and to serve as a reinforcer (U.S. Department of Health and Human Services 1988).

The psychoactive effects of caffeine have been tested in nonhumans using the drug discriminative procedure. In this procedure, caffeine partially generalized to the effects of amphetamine (Evans and Johanson 1987; Holloway et al. 1985; Kuhn et al. 1974; Rosen et al. 1986); that is, many, but not all of the animals responded as if caffeine were amphetamine.

In humans, self-reports indicate caffeine can produce slight increases in elation, positive mood, and amphetamine-like reports as well as aversive effects (e.g., increased anxiety and dysphoria). Application of the drug discriminative procedure to humans (Chait et al. 1985; Griffiths et al. 1990a; Stern et al. 1989) produces results concordant with the nonhuman studies; that is, caffeine was labeled similar to amphetamine on a small proportion of tests.

In nonhumans, caffeine is not consistently self-administered at a rate greater than placebo (Griffiths and Woodson 1988b). In humans, two early studies suggested that caffeine in coffee was serving as a reinforcer (Kozlowski 1976; Podboy and Mallory 1977) but lacked adequate controls (e.g., decaffeinated coffee groups). A third study (Stern et al. 1989) found that light caffeine users did not prefer ingesting caffeine capsules (100 mg or 300 mg) over placebo capsules.

Well-controlled studies by Griffiths and colleagues found that a subset of subjects consistently chose to drink caffeinated coffee (100 mg) over decaffeinated coffee (Griffiths et al. 1986a, 1989) or to ingest caffeine capsules (100 mg or 200 mg) over placebo capsules (Griffiths et al. 1986b, 1989) during double-blind tests. Studies by Hughes and colleagues replicated these effects (Hughes et al. 1991a; Oliveto et al. 1992) and extended them to lower doses (25 mg and 50 mg) (Hughes et al. 1992a; Oliveto et al. 1990) and to soda drinkers (Hughes et al. 1991b). In one study, the amount of work to obtain caffeinated coffee, decaffeinated coffee, caffeine capsules, or placebo capsules was increased over time (Griffiths et al. 1989). Self-administration of placebo capsules dropped off quickly, self-administration of caffeinated coffee persisted the longest, and decaffeinated coffee and caffeine capsules were self-administered at an intermediate level. In another study, subjects would make up to 2,500 lever pulls for 2-oz servings of caffeinated coffee (Bickel et al. 1991). In this study, increasing the amount of work to obtain coffee decreased coffee consumption to an extent similar to that when increasing the amount of work to obtain cigarettes.

Discussion

The prior rationale for not including caffeine withdrawal in DSM-III-R (i.e., the symptoms are not severe) may have been premature. Headache, decreased arousal, and fatigue have been shown to be severe withdrawal symptoms in some patients, to be due to the specific deprivation of caffeine, to occur in a substantial proportion of coffee drinkers, to have a characteristic time-limited time course, to occur at moderate caffeine intakes, and to contribute to the self-administration of caffeine.

Furthermore, there could be considerable clinical utility in a specific diagnosis of caffeine withdrawal. For instance, caffeine withdrawal-induced headache, drowsiness, and fatigue could either be mistaken for or aggravate side effects from psychiatric medications or intoxication or withdrawal states from prescribed and nonprescribed psychoactive drugs.

Although I believe the evidence is sufficient for inclusion of caffeine withdrawal, the Substance Use Disorders Work Group had several concerns: 1) only three symptoms of withdrawal have been well validated; 2) two of these (fatigue and drowsiness) are similar; 3) all three symptoms have a high prevalence in the general population; and 4) the symptoms have several noncaffeine withdrawal causes. The Work Group believed these problems would impair the specificity of the diagnosis of caffeine withdrawal such that high false-positive results may be likely.

As for caffeine dependence and abuse, substantial basic research data exist for these disorders; however, a clinical data base is missing. Clinical data that would be necessary for the inclusion of caffeine dependence include empirical evidence that a substantial proportion of coffee drinkers 1) try to stop and cannot, 2) have difficulty switching to decaffeinated coffee, and 3) use caffeine despite knowledge that they have a health problem aggravated by caffeine. Further research into caffeine dependence and abuse is especially important given recent evidence that chronic use of caffeine might potentiate other substance abuse disorders (e.g., alcohol self-administration) (Gilbert 1976b), psychiatric disorders (e.g., panic disorders) (Charney et al. 1985), and anorexia nervosa (Sours 1983).

Recommendations

In summary, although there is substantial basic and clinical evidence to recommend inclusion of caffeine withdrawal into DSM-IV with symptoms of headache, fatigue, and drowsiness, the few number of symptoms and their nonspecificity suggest caffeine withdrawal should not be added to DSM-IV at this point. Similarly, although there are substantial basic research data that suggest that caffeine can serve as a reinforcer in humans, the dearth of evidence on clinical indicators of dependence on caffeine (e.g., inability to stop use, use despite harm) precludes inclusion of the caffeine abuse or dependence categories in DSM-IV.

References

American Psychiatric Association: Diagnostic and Statistical Manual of Mental Disorders, 3rd Edition, Revised. Washington, DC, American Psychiatric Association, 1987

Bickel WK, DeGrandpre RJ, Hughes JR, et al: Behavioral economics of human drug self-administration, II: a unit price analysis of cigarette smoking. J Exp Anal Behav 55: 145–154, 1991

Bolton S, Null G: Caffeine psychological effects, use and abuse. Journal of Orthomolecular Psychiatry 10:202–211, 1981

Brecher EM: Licit and Illicit Drugs. Boston, MA, Little, Brown, 1972

Chait LD, Uhlenhuth EH, Johanson CE: The discriminative stimulus and subjective effects of D-amphetamine in humans. Psychopharmacology (Berlin) 86:307–312, 1985

Charney DS, Heninger GR, Jatlow PI: Increased anxiogenic effects of caffeine in panic disorders. Arch Gen Psychiatry 42:233–243, 1985

DeFritas B, Schwartz G: Effects of caffeine in chronic psychiatric patients. Am J Psychiatry 136:1337–1338, 1979

Evans SM, Johanson CE: Amphetamine-like effects of anorectics and related compounds in pigeons. J Pharmacol Exp Ther 241:817–825, 1987

Gilbert RM: Caffeine as a drug of abuse, in Research Advances in Alcohol and Drug Problems, Vol 3. Edited by Gibbons RJ, Israel Y, Kalant H, et al. New York, Wiley, 1976a

Gilbert RM: Dietary caffeine and alcohol consumption by rats. J Stud Alcohol 37:11–18, 1976b

Gilliland K, Bullock W: Caffeine: a potential drug of abuse, in The Addictive Behaviors. Edited by Shaffer H, Stimmel B. New York, Hawthorne Press, 1984

Goldstein A, Kaizer S, Whitby O: Psychotropic effects of caffeine in man, IV: quantitative and qualitative differences associated with habituation to coffee. Clin Pharmacol Ther 10:489–497, 1969

Griffiths RR, Woodson PP: Caffeine physical dependence: a review of human and laboratory animal studies. Psychopharmacology (Berlin) 94:437–451, 1988a

Griffiths RR, Woodson PP: Reinforcing properties of caffeine: studies in humans and laboratory animals. Pharmacol Biochem Behav 29:419–427, 1988b

Griffiths RR, Bigelow GE, Liebson IA, et al: Human coffee drinking: manipulation of concentration and caffeine dose. J Exp Anal Behav 45:133–148, 1986a

Griffiths RR, Bigelow GE, Liebson IA: Human coffee drinking: reinforcing and physical dependence producing effects of caffeine. J Pharmacol Exp Ther 239:416–425, 1986b

Griffiths RR, Bigelow GE, Liebson IA: Reinforcing effects of caffeine in coffee and capsules. J Exp Anal Behav 52:127–140, 1989

Griffiths RR, Evans SM, Heishman SJ, et al: Low-dose caffeine discrimination in humans. J Pharmacol Exp Ther 252:970–978, 1990a

Griffiths RR, Evans SM, Heishman SJ, et al: Low-dose caffeine physical dependence in humans. J Pharmacol Exp Ther 255:1123–1132, 1990b

Holloway FA, Modrow HE, Michealis RC: Methylxanthine discrimination in the rat: possible benzodiazepine and adenosine mechanisms. Pharmacol Biochem Behav 22:815–824, 1985

Holtzman SG: Caffeine as a model drug of abuse. Trends Pharmacol Sci 11:355–356, 1990

Hughes JR, Higgins ST, Bickel WK, et al: Caffeine self-administration, withdrawal and adverse effects among coffee drinkers. Arch Gen Psychiatry 48:611–617, 1991a

Hughes JR, Oliveto AH, Valliere W, et al: Soda drinkers reliably self-administer caffeine. Paper presented at the Behavioral Pharmacology Society, Chapel Hill, NC, May 1991b

Hughes JR, Hunt WK, Higgins ST, et al: Effect of dose on the ability of caffeine to serve as a reinforcer in humans. Behavioral Pharmacology 3:211–218, 1992a

Hughes JR, Oliveto AH, Helzer JE, et al: Should caffeine abuse, dependence or withdrawal be added to DSM-IV or ICD-10? Am J Psychiatry 149:33–40, 1992b

Kozlowski LT: Effect of caffeine on coffee drinking. Nature 264:354–355, 1976

Kuhn DM, Appel JB, Greenberg I: An analysis of some discriminative properties of D-amphetamine. Psychopharmacologia 39:57–66, 1974

Oliveto AH, Hughes JR, Pepper SL, et al: Low doses of caffeine can serve as reinforcers in humans, in Problems of Drug Dependence, 1990 (NIDA Research Monograph No 105). Edited by Harris LS. Washington, DC, U.S. Government Printing Office, 1990

Oliveto AH, Hughes JR, Higgins ST, et al: Forced-choice vs free-choice procedures: caffeine self-administration in humans. Psychopharmacology 109:85–91, 1992

Podboy JW, Mallory WA: Caffeine reduction and behavior change in the severely retarded. Ment Retard 15:40, 1977

Rosen JB, Young AM, Beuthin FC, et al: Discriminative stimulus properties of amphetamine and other stimulants in lead-exposed and normal rats. Pharmacol Biochem Behav 24:211–215, 1986

Shreiber GB, Maffeo CE, Robins M, et al: Measurement of coffee and caffeine intake: implications for epidemiologic research. Prev Med 17:280–294, 1988

Sours JA: Case reports of anorexia nervosa and caffeinism. Am J Psychiatry 140:235–236, 1983

Stern KN, Chait LD, Johanson CE: Reinforcing and subjective effects of caffeine in normal human volunteers. Psychopharmacology (Berlin) 98:81–88, 1989

U.S. Department of Health and Human Services: The Health Consequences of Smoking: Nicotine Addiction. Washington, DC, U.S. Government Printing Office, 1988

Chapter 10

Anabolic Steroids Withdrawal, Dependence, and Abuse

John W. Tsuang, M.D.

Statement of the Issues

The purpose of this chapter is to review the use and side effects of anabolic steroids and to determine whether sufficient data exist to warrant inclusion of anabolic steroids withdrawal, dependence, and abuse in DSM-IV.

Significance of the Issues

Anabolic steroids have been used by athletes since the 1950s to increase muscle size and strength to improve performance. More recently, not only has anabolic steroids use become more prominent in the athletic world, but use by the lay public has also increased (Bierly 1987; Perry et al. 1990; Schuckit 1988; Windsor and Dumitru 1987; Yesalis et al. 1988). Although data are limited, it has been estimated that the point prevalence of anabolic steroids use in the United States is at approximately one million people (Burkett and Falduto 1984; Taylor 1987). There are reports of increased use of anabolic steroids both in junior high school and at the high school level, and in both male and female athletes and nonathletes. Surveys of adolescents and high school students indicate that the incidence of anabolic steroids use ranges from 3% to 11.1% (Buckley et al. 1988; Johnson et al. 1989; Windsor and Dumitru 1989). More than two-thirds of those who used anabolic steroids began at age 16 or younger, and a significant percentage (10%–42.2%) of use was unrelated to improving athletic performance (Buckley et al. 1988; Johnson et al. 1989; McLain 1989; Pope et al. 1988).

Methods

This review is based on 1) computerized searches of Medline using the term *anabolic steroids* crossed with *dependence, abuse, withdrawal,* and *psychiatric symptoms* (a total of 118 citations was generated); 2) references found in the bibliographies of scientific papers (e.g., Narducci et al. 1990; Pope and Katz 1988); and 3) material supplied by consultants.

Results

Patterns of Use

Anabolic steroids are synthetic derivatives of testosterone that were developed to maximize the anabolic effects of protein synthesis and muscular growth. In general, there are two ways of administering anabolic steroids, with the difference reflecting the type of structural changes to the basic testosterone molecule. One route is the injectable form, which has a delayed absorption made possible by esterification of the 17 beta-hydroxy group. Examples include testosterone cypionate (Andro-Cyp, Andronate) and nandrolone forms (Durabolin and Deca-Durabolin). The other route is the oral form, which has a decreased rate of hepatic breakdown secondary to the alkylation of the 17 alpha position of testosterone. Examples include oxandrolone (Anavar) and methyltestosterone (Android) (Bierly 1987; Schuckit 1988; Windsor and Dumitru 1987). There are various recognized patterns of use, including stacking, pyramiding, cycling, or a combination and variation of these three patterns. Stacking is the simultaneous administration of several different agents, both oral and parental. Pyramiding is the progressive increase in dose of each agent. Cycling involves periods of anabolic steroid consumption ranging from 4 to 18 weeks broken by short periods of abstinence from 4 to 6 weeks (Graham and Kennedy 1990; Haupt and Rovere 1984; Hervey et al. 1976; Lamb 1984; Schuckit 1988; Shepard et al. 1977). The amounts of anabolic steroids ingested each period are usually 10–200 times the approved dosages for legitimate medical indications (Catlin 1987; Graham and Kennedy 1990; Haupt 1989; Haupt and Rovere 1984; Pope and Katz 1988; Yesalis et al. 1988).

Side Effects of Anabolic Steroids

Medical complications. With repeated use of anabolic steroids, there is an increased risk for development of medical problems. Studies have shown that anabolic steroids can elevate levels of low-density lipoprotein and apolipoprotein B, while decreasing levels of high-density lipoprotein and apolipoprotein A1. These lipid profiles have been associated with an increased risk of coronary artery disease (Alen and Rahkila 1984; Alen et al. 1985; Freedman and Srinivasan 1986; Hakkinen and Alen 1986). Indeed, since 1988, five cases of athletes with histories of anabolic steroids use who subsequently developed major vascular events, including two strokes and three myocardial infarctions, have been reported (Bowman et al. 1989; Ferenchick 1990; Frankle et al. 1988; McNutt et al. 1988; Mochizuki and Richter 1988).

Anabolic steroids use has also been linked to a significant rise in systolic and diastolic blood pressures (Freed et al. 1972, 1975; Lenders and Demacker 1988). Despite attempts to reduce its androgenic effects, sexual characteristic changes have been common in those who use anabolic steroids. In males, during anabolic steroids use, the testosterone level is elevated and the follicle-stimulating hormone and the luteinizing hormone are depressed. These hormonal changes can cause testicular atrophy with decreased spermatogenesis, altered sperm morphology and motility, and impotence (Harkness 1975; Schurmeyer et al. 1984). There is an accentuation of male pattern baldness and development of gynecomastia secondary to production of estrogens in the metabolism of anabolic steroids (Aiache 1989; Haupt and Rovere 1984). In females using anabolic steroids, virilization effects have been reported. These include a coarsening and deepening of the voice, reduction in breast size, clitoral hypertrophy, hirsutism, and menstrual irregularity (Hickson et al. 1989; Kibble and Ross 1987; Narducci et al. 1990).

In both sexes, with the enlargement of sebaceous glands and increasing sebum excretion in the skin, acne becomes more problematic (Graham and Kennedy 1990; Kiraly et al. 1987a, 1987b; Narducci et al. 1990). Those who use anabolic steroids may also have abnormal endocrine systems, including low thyroid hormones (Alen et al. 1987) and impaired glucose metabolism due to increased peripheral insulin resistance (Landon and Wynn 1962; Landon et al. 1963; Narducci et al. 1990). Children with anabolic steroids use can have accelerated skeletal growth and early fusion of the epiphyses, which will result in growth retardation (Limbeck et al. 1971).

Finally, those who use anabolic steroids have been reported to have abnormal liver function tests, with increased aspartate aminotransferase, alanine aminotransferase, and lactic acid dehydrogenase as the most commonly reported abnormalities (Graham and Kennedy 1990; Narducci et al. 1990). Three cases of hepatoma have been reported in athletes taking anabolic steroids (Creagh et al. 1988; Goldman 1985; Overly et al. 1984); other malignancies may also be linked to anabolic steroids use (Prat et al. 1965; Roberts and Essenhigh 1986).

Psychiatric complications. The existence of a corticosteroid-induced psychosis has been well documented (The Boston Collaborative Drug Surveillance Program

1972; Clark et al. 1952; Hall et al. 1979; Ling et al. 1981; Ritchie 1956). It is therefore not surprising that people with frequent anabolic steroids use are also at risk for other psychological and psychiatric manifestations. At the initial intake of anabolic steroids, or after a period of abstinence, an enhanced sense of well-being and feelings of euphoria may be reported. However, after a period of anabolic steroids use, feelings of dysphoria, irritability, and lack of energy are common (Schuckit 1988). There have been case reports of weight lifters who developed depressive symptoms with severe dysphoria, insomnia, anorexia, and guilt feelings during or after their anabolic steroids use (Brower et al. 1989a; Pope and Katz 1987, 1988; Schuckit 1988). Meanwhile, manic symptoms with euphoria, labile affect, racing thoughts, hyperactivity, grandiosity, and poor impulse control have also been reported in those who use anabolic steroids (Brower et al. 1989a; Freinhar and Alvarez 1985; Pope and Katz 1988). More impressively, those who use anabolic steroids have developed hallucinations, ideas of reference, paranoid delusions, and bizarre behaviors requiring intense psychiatric treatment (Annitto and Layman 1980; Brower et al. 1989a; Pope and Katz 1987, 1988; Schuckit 1988). Finally, there have been case reports of anabolic steroids use linked to violent crimes, suicide, and even homicide (Brower et al. 1989b; Conacher and Workman 1989; Pope and Katz 1990).

Anabolic Steroids Withdrawal

There are many anecdotal case reports of physical and psychiatric symptoms occurring after withdrawal of medical steroid treatments (The Boston Collaborative Drug Surveillance Program 1972; Clark et al. 1952; Hall et al. 1979; Ling et al. 1981; Ritchie 1956). In a literature review paper on steroid withdrawal psychiatric syndromes, 54.5% of the cases showed evidence of affective symptoms, 27.3% had delirium, and 9.1% demonstrated psychotic and anxiety symptoms (Fricchione et al. 1989). There have been case reports of persons using anabolic steroids who were unable to stop their anabolic steroids use partly because of their withdrawal symptoms. These symptoms included depression, fatigue, decreased sexual drive, insomnia, anorexia, dissatisfaction with body image, and the desire to take more steroids (Brower et al. 1989a; Tennant et al. 1988). In a survey of eight weight lifters, 100% of them had experienced some withdrawal symptoms (Brower et al. 1990). One report postulated that withdrawal from anabolic steroids can be associated with an acute hyperadrenergic syndrome; it pointed out the similarity in symptoms between steroid withdrawal and alcohol or sedative-hypnotic withdrawal (Kashkin and Kleber 1989). Consistent with this postulate are the preclinical findings that suggest a testosterone-benzodiazepine/gamma-aminobutyric acid receptor interaction (Majewsak et al. 1986; Rosse and Deutsch 1990) and the reduction of symptoms in both opioid withdrawal and anabolic steroids withdrawal with the administration of clonidine hydrochloride (an alpha$_2$ agonist) (Gold et al. 1979; Linnoila et al. 1987; Sherwin and Gelfand 1985; Tennant et al. 1988).

Anabolic Steroids Dependence and Abuse

Some researchers have suggested that anabolic steroids may have an addictive potential similar to other drugs of abuse, and others have even postulated an anabolic steroids addiction hypothesis (Cowart 1987; Kashkin and Kleber 1989; Taylor 1987). There are only two detailed case reports and two studies on anabolic steroids dependence. In one case, a noncompetitive weight lifter came for professional help after his own failure to abstain from anabolic steroids use (Brower et al. 1989a). He met the diagnosis for psychoactive substance dependence, having six of nine criteria for a period of greater than 1 month. Specifically, he had an uncontrolled pattern of use, including taking the substance over a longer time period than intended, failing in attempts to cut down, and persisting in use despite adverse consequences. He also suffered from tolerance and withdrawal symptoms, and he continued to take the substance to avoid withdrawal symptoms. In the second case, another weight lifter felt he was addicted to anabolic steroids and could not stop taking them without experiencing withdrawal symptoms, depression, and disabling fatigue (Tennant et al. 1988). Apparently, he also met the criteria for a diagnosis of psychoactive substance dependence.

In one survey study of eight weight lifters, six out of eight subjects seemed to meet the DSM-III-R (American Psychiatric Association 1987) criteria for dependence (Brower et al. 1990). Every subject had two or more symptoms of dependence, including continued use despite adverse consequences and reports of withdrawal effects. In the other study, an epidemiological survey of high school students, a "hard core" group of students was identified (Yesalis et al. 1989). These adolescents initiated anabolic steroids use at a younger age and tended to use more anabolic steroids. They were more likely to report intentions to continue use regardless of long-term health consequences, and they perceived a greater prevalence of anabolic steroids use among their peers than others. The authors of this study argued that by their behaviors, perceptions, and opinions, this group of students met criteria for habituation.

Discussion

There are an increasing number of clinical descriptions of anabolic steroids use causing dependence symptoms such as uncontrolled patterns of use, continued use despite adverse effects, tolerance, and withdrawal. However, no adequate studies have been done to fulfill two of the principal measures used to infer the ability of a drug to produce dependence or abuse. These two measures include the determination of the drug's ability to produce psychoactive effects, as well as the drug's ability to serve as a reinforcer (U.S. Department of Health and Human Services 1988). To test the psychoactive effects of a substance, the drug discriminative procedure is often used. As regards anabolic steroids use, however, the discriminative procedure has not been applied to either animal or human subjects. The reinforcing property of a drug can be tested by using the self-administer procedure. Once again, no such research has been done. Thus, our knowledge regarding anabolic steroids abuse and dependence is based largely on subjective reports, and systematic clinical and animal trials are greatly needed. Similarly, our understanding of anabolic steroids withdrawal syndrome is based on subjective clinical descriptions of symptoms, and no deprivation studies have been undertaken using either animal or human subjects to study anabolic steroids withdrawal. To establish a well-defined anabolic steroids withdrawal syndrome, systematic and preclinical studies are needed to research the effects of anabolic steroids deprivation and the specific characteristics of withdrawal symptoms.

Recommendations

Despite increasing clinical descriptive data on anabolic steroids withdrawal, dependence, and abuse, there are insufficient substantial basic or clinical research data to support the inclusion of these syndromes in DSM-IV at the present time. On the other hand, the data that have accrued are sufficiently important and interesting to warrant mention in the text of DSM-IV. Therefore, it is recommended that anabolic steroids problems should be listed under the category of Other Substance Use Disorders. These issues of anabolic steroids withdrawal, dependence, and abuse should be highlighted as important areas for further research, especially as regards DSM-V.

References

Aiache A: Surgical treatment of gynecomastia in the body-builder. Plast Reconstr Surg 83:61–66, 1989

Alen M, Rahkila P: Reduced high-density lipoprotein-cholesterol in power athletes: use of male sex hormone derivates, an atherogenic factor. Int J Sports Med 5:341–342, 1984

Alen M, Rahkila P, Marniemi J: Serum lipids in power athletes self-administering testosterone and anabolic steroids. Int J Sports Med 6:139–144, 1985

Alen M, Rahkila P, Reinila M, et al: Androgenic-anabolic steroid effects serum thyroid, pituitary and steroid hormones in athletes. Am J Sports Med 15:357–361, 1987

American Psychiatric Association: Diagnostic and Statistical Manual of Mental Disorders, 3rd Edition, Revised. Washington, DC, American Psychiatric Association, 1987

Annitto W, Layman W: Anabolic steroids and acute schizophrenic episode. J Clin Psychiatry 41:143–144, 1980

Bierly J: Use of anabolic steroids by athletes: do the risks outweigh the benefits? Postgrad Med 82:67–74, 1987

The Boston Collaborative Drug Surveillance Program: Acute adverse reactions to prednisone in relation to dosage. Clin Pharmacol Ther 13:694–698, 1972

Bowman S, Tanna S, Fernando S, et al: Anabolic steroids and infarction (letter). BMJ 299:632, 1989

Brower K, Blow F, Beresford T, et al: Anabolic-androgenic steroid dependence. J Clin Psychiatry 50:31–33, 1989a

Brower K, Blow F, Eliopulos G, et al: Anabolic androgenic steroids and suicide (letter). Am J Psychiatry 146:1075, 1989b

Brower K, Eliopulos G, Blow F, et al: Evidence for physical and psychological dependence on anabolic androgenic steroids in eight weight lifters. Am J Psychiatry 147:510–512, 1990

Buckley W, Yesalis C, Friedl K, et al: Estimated prevalence of anabolic steroid use among male high school seniors. JAMA 260:3441–3445, 1988

Burkett LN, Falduto MT: Steroid use by athletes in a metropolitan area. The Physician and Sportsmedicine 12:69–74, 1984

Catlin D: Detection of drug use by athletes, in Drugs and Performance in Sports. Edited by Strauss RH. Philadelphia, PA, WB Saunders, 1987

Clark L, Bauer W, Cobb S: Preliminary observations on mental disturbances occurring in patients under therapy with cortisone and ACTH. N Engl J Med 246:205–216, 1952

Conacher G, Workman D. Violent crime possibly associated with anabolic steroid use (letter). Am J Psychiatry 145:679, 1989

Cowart V: Steroids in sports: after four decades, time to return these genies to bottle? JAMA 257:421–427, 1987

Creagh T, Rubin A, Evans D: Hepatic tumors induced by anabolic steroids in an athlete. J Clin Pathol 41:441–443, 1988

Ferenchick G: Are androgenic steroids thrombogenic? (letter). N Engl J Med 322:476, 1990

Frankle M, Eichberg R, Zachariah S: Anabolic androgenic steroids and a stroke in an athlete: case report. Arch Phys Med Rehabil 69:632–633, 1988

Freed D, Banks A, Longson D: Anabolic steroids in athletics (letter). BMJ 3:761, 1972

Freed D, Banks A, Longson D, et al: Anabolic steroids in athletics: crossover double-blind trial on weightlifters. BMJ 2:471–473, 1975

Freedman D, Srinivasan S: The relation of apolipoproteins A-1 and B in children to parental myocardial infarction. N Engl J Med 315:721–726, 1986

Freinhar J, Alvarez W: Androgen-induced hypomania (letter). J Clin Psychiatry 46:354–355, 1985

Fricchione G, Ayyala M, Holmes F: Steroid withdrawal psychiatric syndromes. Annals of Clinical Psychiatry 1:99–108, 1989

Gold M, Redmond D, Kleber H: Noradrenergic hyperactivity in opiate withdrawal supported by clonidine reversal of opiate withdrawal. Am J Psychiatry 136:100–102, 1979

Goldman B: Liver carcinoma in an athlete taking anabolic steroids (letter). J Am Osteopath Assoc 85:56, 1985

Graham S, Kennedy M: Recent developments in the toxicology of anabolic steroids. Drug Saf 5:458–476, 1990

Hakkinen K, Alen M: Physiological performance, serum hormones, enzymes and lipids of an elite power athlete during training with and without androgens and during prolonged detraining: a case study. J Sports Med Phys Fitness 26:92–100, 1986

Hall R, Popkin M, Stickney S, et al: Presentation of steroid psychoses. J Nerv Ment Dis 167:229–236, 1979

Harkness R: Effects of large doses of anabolic steroids. Br J Sports Med 9:70–73, 1975

Haupt H: Drugs in athletics. Clin Sports Med 8:561–582, 1989

Haupt H, Rovere R: Anabolic steroids: a review of the literature. Am J Sports Med 12:469–484, 1984

Hervey G, Hutchinson I, Knibbs A, et al: "Anabolic" effects of methandienone in men undergoing athletic training. Lancet 2:699–702, 1976

Hickson R, Ball K, Falduto M: Adverse effects of anabolic steroids. Medical Toxicology and Adverse Drug Experience 4:254–271, 1989

Johnson M, Jay M, Shoup B, et al: Anabolic steroid use by male adolescents. Pediatrics 83:921–924, 1989

Kashkin D, Kleber H: Hooked on hormones? an anabolic steroid addiction hypothesis. JAMA 262:3166–3170, 1989

Kibble M, Ross M: Adverse effects of anabolic steroids in athletes. Clin Pharm 6:686–692, 1987

Kiraly C, Alen M, Rahkila P, et al: Effect of androgenic and anabolic steroids on the sebaceous gland in power athletes. Acta Derm Venereol (Stockh) 67:36–40, 1987a

Kiraly C, Collan Y, Alen M: Effect of testosterone and anabolic steroids on the size of sebaceous glands in power athletes. Am J Dermatopathol 9:515–519, 1987b

Lamb D: Anabolic steroids in athletes: how well do they work and how dangerous are they? Am J Sports Med 12:31–38, 1984

Landon J, Wynn V: Effects of anabolic steroid, methandienone on carbohydrate metabolism in man, II: effect of methandienone on response to glucagon, adrenalin, and in insulin in the fasted subject. Metabolism 11:513–523, 1962

Landon J, Wynn V, Samols E: The effects of anabolic steroids on blood sugar and plasma insulin levels in man. Metabolism 12:924–934, 1963

Lenders J, Demacker P: Deleterious effects of anabolic steroids on serum lipoproteins, blood pressure, and liver function in amateur body builders. Int J Sports Med 9:19–23, 1988

Limbeck G, Ruvalcaba R, Mahoney C, et al: Studies on anabolic steroids, IV: the effects of oxandrolone on height and skeletal maturation in uncomplicated growth retardation. Clin Pharmacol Ther 12:793–805, 1971

Ling M, Perry P, Tsuang M: Side effects of corticosteroid therapy: psychiatric aspects. Arch Gen Psychiatry 38:471–477, 1981

Linnoila M, Mefford I, Nutt D, et al: Alcohol withdrawal and noradrenergic function. Ann Intern Med 107:875–889, 1987

Majewsak M, Harrison H, Schwartz R, et al: Steroid hormone metabolites are barbiturate-like modulators of the GABA receptor. Science 232:1004–1007, 1986

McLain L: Anabolic steroids and high school students (abstract). Am J Dis Child 143:412, 1989

McNutt R, Ferenchick G, Kirlin P, et al: Acute myocardial infarction in a 22-year-old world class weight lifter using anabolic steroids (case reports). Am J Cardiol 62:164, 1988

Mochizuki R, Richter K: Cardiomyopathy and cerebrovascular accident associated with anabolic-androgenic steroid use. The Physician and Sportsmedicine 16:108–114, 1988

Narducci W, Wagner J, Hendrickson T, et al: Anabolic steroids: a review of the clinical toxicology and diagnostic screening. Clinical Toxicology 28:287–310, 1990

Overly W, Dankoff J, Wang B, et al: Androgens and hepatocellular carcinoma in an athlete. Ann Intern Med 100:158–159, 1984

Perry P, Yates W, Andersen K: Psychiatric symptoms associated with anabolic steroids: a controlled, retrospective study. Annals of Clinical Psychiatry 2:11–17, 1990

Pope H, Katz D: Bodybuilders' psychosis (letter). Lancet 1:863, 1987

Pope H, Katz D: Affective and psychotic symptoms associated with anabolic steroid use. Am J Psychiatry 145:487–490, 1988

Pope H, Katz D: Homicide and near-homicide by anabolic steroid users. J Clin Psychiatry 51:28–31, 1990

Pope H, Katz D, Champoux R: Anabolic-androgenic steroid use among 1010 college men. The Physician and Sportsmedicine 16:75–82, 1988

Prat J, Gray G, Stolley P, et al: Wilm's tumor in an adult associated with androgen abuse. JAMA 237:464–475, 1965

Ritchie E: Toxic psychosis under cortisone and corticotrophin. The Journal of Mental Science 102:803–837, 1956

Roberts JT, Essenhigh DM: Adenocarcinoma of the prostate in 40-year-old body-builder (letter). Lancet 2:742, 1986

Rosse R, Deutsch S: Hooked on hormones (letter). JAMA 263:2048–2049, 1990

Schuckit M: Weight lifter's folly: The abuse of anabolic steroids. Vista Hill Foundation: Drug Abuse and Alcoholism Newsletter 17, 1988

Schurmeyer T, Belkien L, Knuth U, et al: Reversible azoospermia induced by the anabolic steroid 19-nortestosterone. Lancet 1:417–420, 1984

Shepard R, Killinger D, Fried T: Responses to sustained use of anabolic steroids. Br J Sports Med 11:170–173, 1977

Sherwin B, Gelfand M: Differential symptom response to parenteral estrogen and/or androgen administration in the surgical menopause. Am J Obstet Gynecol 151:153–160, 1985

Taylor W: Synthetic anabolic-androgenic steroids: a plea for controlled substance status. The Physician and Sportsmedicine 15:140–150, 1987

Tennant F, Black D, Voy R: Anabolic steroid dependence with opioid-type features (letter). N Engl J Med 319:578, 1988

U.S. Department of Health and Human Services: The Health Consequences of Smoking: Nicotine Addiction. Washington, DC, U.S. Government Printing Office, 1988

Windsor R, Dumitru D: Anabolic steroid use by athletes: how serious are the health hazards? Postgrad Med 84:37–49, 1987

Windsor R, Dumitru D: Prevalence of anabolic steroid use by male and female adolescents. Med Sci Sports Exerc 21:494–497, 1989

Yesalis C, Herrick R, Buckley W, et al. Self-reported use of anabolic-androgenic steroids by elite power lifters. The Physician and Sportsmedicine 16:91–100, 1988

Yesalis C, Streit A, Vicary J, et al: Anabolic steroid use: indications of habituation among adolescents. J Drug Educ 19:103–116, 1989

Chapter 11

Protracted Abstinence Syndromes in Alcohol, Opioids, and Stimulants

Marc A. Schuckit, M.D.
Thomas Kosten, M.D.
Marian W. Fischman, Ph.D.

Statement of the Issues

This report was commissioned to determine whether an independent diagnosis of protracted withdrawal syndrome should be included in DSM-IV. Alcohol, opioids, and stimulants are reviewed and considered together, because each has a well-described withdrawal syndrome (Kosten et al. 1987; Schuckit 1989).

Significance of the Issues

Before a new diagnosis is incorporated, there should be strong evidence that the syndrome can be defined precisely, has new and important clinical implications, and is clearly distinguished from existing disorders.

For many years, anecdotal reports have documented the persistence of abstinence-type symptoms following acute cessation of alcohol, opioids, and stimulants (e.g., cocaine and the amphetamines). These descriptions of continuing problems are complemented by both animal studies and clinical investigations of emotional and physiological symptoms among recovering alcoholic and drug-addicted persons.

Although the most intense and alarming symptoms associated with withdrawal from stimulants, opiates, and depressants occur in the period immediately following abstinence, both psychological and physiological disturbances are likely to continue for 3–6 or more months following abstinence. These long-term or protracted abstinence syndromes may contribute to general levels of patient discomfort and to craving for the withdrawn substance. The persistence of these syndromes may therefore undermine treatment efforts and increase the likelihood of relapse in detoxified substance-abusing persons. Heightened clinician awareness of persistent abstinence problems may lead to improved patient care and more successful relapse prevention.

Methods

This chapter integrates three separate reports on protracted abstinence in alcohol, opioids, and stimulants. Responsibility for evaluating the data on the three categories of drugs examined is as follows: Marc A. Schuckit (alcohol), Thomas Kosten (opioids), and Marian W. Fischman (stimulants: cocaine and the amphetamines). For the sake of convenience, the evidence from studies of protracted abstinence in cocaine and the amphetamines is treated separately. Although cocaine and the amphetamines differ in both their structure and neurochemical effects, they appear to be quite similar in their behavioral effects. It is likely that any protracted abstinence syndrome existing for one of these drugs will also be found to exist for the other (Gawin and Ellinwood 1988).

The English-language psychiatric and psychological literature was searched for studies containing evidence of a protracted withdrawal syndrome related to the three categories of drugs in humans and animals. The reviews included Medline computer searches using such terms as *alcoholism, opioids, cocaine, amphetamines, abstinence syndromes, withdrawal,* and so on from 1970 to the present.

The automated searches were complemented by a review of articles appearing over the past 5 years in the following journals: *Journal of Studies on Alcohol, British Journal of Addiction, Alcoholism: Clinical and Experimental Research, American Journal of Drug and Alcohol Abuse, Alcoholism, Life Sciences, Archives of General Psychiatry, Journal of Pharmacology and Experimental Therapeutics, Psychopharmacology, Journal of Psychoactive Drugs, Drug and Alcohol Dependence,* and *American Journal of Psychiatry.* Each study was evaluated with respect to the type of subjects, methods of evaluation, number of subjects involved, and the length of follow-up.

Approximately 150 book chapters and journal articles were scanned before focusing on the studies actually referenced in this report.

Results

A Brief Review of the Acute Withdrawal Syndromes

The disturbing psychological and physiological symptoms of acute withdrawal from these three classic substances of abuse make the period immediately following abstinence a crucial time for medical and psychological intervention. Typically, patient discomfort and distress is most intense during the first few days to weeks without the withdrawn substance.

There is ample documentation of the acute withdrawal syndrome regarding alcohol (Schuckit 1989; Sellers 1988). Clinical symptoms are expected to develop within 4–8 hours of a rapid decrease in blood alcohol levels, with symptoms tending to peak in intensity on day 2 or 3 and improving by day 4 or 5. Emotional symptoms of acute withdrawal from alcohol include intense anxiety and deep, sometimes suicidal levels of depression (Brown and Schuckit 1988; Hesselbrock et al. 1985; Schuckit and Monteiro 1988; Schuckit et al. 1990; Smail et al. 1984). These symptoms are likely to be most intense during the first week, with some evidence of continuation of symptoms into weeks 2 and 3 (Brown and Schuckit 1988; Brown et al. 1991). Physiological symptoms include multiple alterations in autonomic nervous system functioning (Drummond and Matthews 1987; Herman et al. 1987; Sellers 1988), electrophysiological abnormalities (Begleiter and Porjesz 1979; Kissin 1979; Porjesz and Begleiter 1983), and sleep disturbances (Gillin et al. 1990).

Similar generalizations can be made regarding the opiates. Although the time course of the acute withdrawal syndrome varies with the half-life of the drug (Schuckit 1989), for most shorter-acting opiates such as heroin the symptoms are likely to be most intense within 8–12 hours of abstention, to peak in intensity on day 2 or 3, and to diminish rapidly by day 4 or 5. Classic psychological symptoms are likely to include a high level of craving for the drug, anxiety, and insomnia. These are complemented by physiological symptoms including sweating, goose bumps on the skin, watering eyes and a runny nose, diarrhea, and intense pain in many body areas including the abdomen, muscles, and bone joints (Gossop et al. 1987; Schuckit 1989).

Abrupt cessation of amphetamines or cocaine is also likely to result in an abstinence syndrome that is, in general, the opposite of the acute effects that the drugs are likely to have on a person first using amphetamines or cocaine (Schuckit 1989). The time course of the acute withdrawal is, once again, likely to include symptoms developing within hours, peaking on day 2 or 3, and diminishing by day 4 or 5. Psychological problems are often described as a "crash" that is characterized by intense craving, depression, feelings of agitation, an increase in appetite, and intense fatigue. Physical pathology is less obvious than for the other two classes of drug, and few diagnostic signs have been described (Gawin and Kleber 1986; Schuckit 1989).

Protracted Abstinence: Evidence From Human Studies

Alcohol. Clinical reports of the maintenance of withdrawal-type symptoms following acute withdrawal from alcohol have appeared in the literature for decades

(Kissin 1979; Segal et al. 1970; Wellman 1954). These accounts consistently support a protracted withdrawal syndrome continuing well beyond the first several weeks of abstinence.

Regarding physiological symptoms, two studies by Roelofs and colleagues used both subjective self-reports and physical measures to gather information about hyperventilation from 37 subjects (Roelofs 1985) and from 15 subjects (Roelofs and Dikkenberg 1987). The first study documented a significant decrease in these symptoms, using both subjective and more objective measures, during the 9 months following abstinence. The second study evaluated the 15 subjects during treatment and again at 17-month follow-up. Of the 9 subjects who maintained either complete or partial abstinence throughout the period, a significant continuing decrease in hyperventilation symptoms was also observed.

Additional direct as well as indirect measures of autonomic nervous system functioning and changes in relevant neurotransmitters have also been documented. In early studies, Kissin and colleagues (1959) related evidence of autonomic dysfunction and possible neuroendocrine abnormalities, together with evidence of increased levels of muscle tension for up to 2 years following the cessation of drinking. These changes tended to revert back to normal with continuing abstinence. Later studies also suggest that autonomic dysfunction continues beyond the acute withdrawal period (Kissin 1979; Segal et al. 1970).

More recent studies have focused on the subjective reports of continuing sleep impairment among alcoholic persons. Several investigators have found that changes in sleep latency as well as altered patterns of changes of sleep stages can often be documented 6 and 12 months following acute withdrawal (Begleiter and Porjesz 1979; Gross and Hastey 1976; Williams and Rundell 1981). Other changes, including the experience of numerous brief arousals during the night, may be observed over longer periods of time, perhaps several years or more (De Soto et al. 1989; Wagman and Allen 1975). Finally, a study of 70 patients abstinent between 2 and 90 days demonstrated that severe sleep impairments were often maintained for at least 5 weeks, with a subsequent likelihood of a decrease in symptomatology over the following 60 days (Alling et al. 1982).

Regarding psychological and emotional symptoms, both clinical lore and formal research demonstrate that the most severe and intense levels of depression and anxiety are likely to disappear within several weeks of abstinence. Evidence suggests, however, that lower levels of symptoms may continue for many months. De Soto and colleagues (1985, 1989) reported both cross-sectional and longitudinal evaluations of as many as 300 alcoholic men and women using the Symptom Checklist—90-R (Derogatis 1983). Both types of studies revealed a continued and persistent slow decrease in anxiety and other symptoms over time, with the most marked changes occurring over the first 12 months, but also continuing beyond that time frame (De Soto et al. 1985, 1989).

These conclusions are consistent with the findings of investigators who have focused on the Minnesota Multiphasic Personality Inventory (Hathaway and McKinley 1943, 1970), showing that over a year there are significant decreases on scores on relevant scales including those relating to hypomania, depression, and psychasthenia (Pettinati et al. 1982; Pokorny et al. 1968; Rohan 1982). Furthermore, the earlier mentioned study by Alling and colleagues (1982) also demonstrated a progressive decrease in fatigability, sadness, and hostility, as well as significant increases in sexual desire. These more formal clinical reports are consistent with an earlier clinical literature dating back to the early 1950s (e.g., Segal et al. 1970; Wellman 1954).

Opioids. The human literature, although somewhat limited, consistently supports a protracted abstinence syndrome lasting for several months after acute withdrawal from opioids. Protracted abstinence was initially described in humans by Himmelsbach (1942). His studies of 21 addicted prisoners led him to believe that 6–9 months of total abstinence was necessary for the complete recovery of "normal" functions. He based this belief on the observation that a wide range of physiological functions—including weight, sleep, basal metabolic rate, temperature, respiration, blood pressure, and blood studies (sedimentation rate, hematocrit)—appeared to be disrupted for several months after acute withdrawal. In a subsequent investigation, Martin and Jasinski (1969) and their colleagues (Eisenman et al. 1969) studied seven morphine-addicted prisoners and also found that a wide range of physiological functions were disrupted for several months after acute withdrawal. They concluded that protracted abstinence persisted for 26–30 weeks, and that 7 weeks represented the transition time between primary withdrawal from morphine and the emergence of secondary or protracted abstinence.

If drug craving is used as an indicator of protracted withdrawal, studies using the opioid antagonist naltrexone should also be considered. In 1976, Meyer and colleagues reported on a study of six heroin-addicted persons with access to heroin in a naltrexone-blocked condition and an unblocked condition. Craving scores were highest during unblocked heroin availability and during acute 7-day methadone detoxification. Naltrexone was then given after a 10-day drug-free interval, and craving scores transiently increased to as high as 50% of maximum craving. However, by day 22 since the last dose of methadone (29 days since last heroin), craving scores were zero. A subsequent outpatient study by Sideroff and colleagues (1978) suggested that protracted withdrawal symptoms, including craving, may last up to 6 weeks. The role of conditioned cues in eliciting drug craving for many months after detoxification has been a clinical observation that deserves further study as a manifestation of protracted abstinence.

The work of Dole (1972) is relevant to these studies of drug craving. Dole is one of the strongest proponents of protracted abstinence and supports methadone maintenance treatment to relieve persistent withdrawal-type symptoms in recovering addicted persons.

Cocaine. Although rather limited, the clinical reports involving cocaine provide further evidence for protracted abstinence. Until quite recently, it was generally believed that repeated use of cocaine did not result in physical dependence (e.g., Jones 1984). In addition, although it has been possible to document the development of acute tolerance to cocaine after repeated dosing, there have not been any demonstrations of protracted abstinence after recurring daily intravenous doses of cocaine 3–4 days per week for 2 weeks (Johanson and Fischman 1989). It is possible, however, that the dosing regimen used was not of sufficient intensity or duration.

Several authors (e.g., Siegel 1982) have observed that depressed mood, fatigue, and prolonged sleep disturbances, lasting for days or weeks, frequently accompany discontinuation of cocaine use. Such observations have generally been unsystematic, based on retrospective reports and clinical judgments. However, through a naturalistic study of 30 long-term cocaine-addicted persons, Gawin and Kleber (1986) developed a three-phase model of abstinence symptomatology. The second phase, withdrawal, can last for up to 10 weeks and is characterized by anhedonia, anergia, anxiety, and high cocaine craving that is exacerbated by conditioned cues. Although there is no general agreement about the separation of a crash and abstinence phase (e.g., Brower and Paredes 1987), most clinical reports of cocaine-addicted persons describe a similar protracted abstinence period.

The amphetamines. The clinical evidence, although limited and mainly observational, appears to support the existence of some protracted abstinence, which can last days or weeks after cessation of amphetamines. Investigators examining physical dependence development to the amphetamines describe a syndrome of "depression, prolonged sleep, and voracious appetite" (LeBlanc et al. 1973, p. 150), which is generally attributed to the substantial fatigue occurring after a period of stimulant use when the person has neither slept nor eaten enough. They consider this pattern of changed behavior as rebound phenomena. Oswald and Thacore (1963) reported changes in rapid-eye-movement (REM) sleep that are compatible with such an explanation. Single-dose amphetamine suppresses REM sleep, but prolonged use diminishes this effect. After cessation of amphetamine use, REM sleep increases substantially for up to a month, but these increases can be eliminated with a dose of amphetamine.

However, Angrist and Sudilovsky (1978) pointed out that this phenomenon also occurs after use of psychotropic substances from a number of different classes and is therefore insufficiently specific to the amphetamines to be used as evidence of an abstinence syndrome. On the other hand, Gossop and colleagues (1982) found that hospitalized amphetamine-dependent patients initially overslept after withdrawal from the drug, but this was followed by a prominent undersleeping phase lasting from days 6 to 20 after cessation of amphetamine.

Smith (1969) reported clinical observations of significant lethargy and sleepiness, as well as severe gastrointestinal cramps, after heavy methamphetamine use. Furthermore, Kramer and colleagues (1967) reported that 12 of the 36 amphetamine-abusing persons they studied had memory and concentration impairments after cessation of use, which lasted for some period of time. This deficit was also reported by Carey and Mandel (1968).

Other evidence for long-term abstinence-related changes is provided by Bell (1973). He described 14 patients in whom psychosis was experimentally induced with only one moderately large dose of amphetamine, and patients in whom a psychosis was reinduced with a single amphetamine dose after they had remained abstinent for some time. Such reinstitution of behavior at doses that were not initially sufficient to elicit the behavior has also been seen in animals (Ellinwood and Kilbey 1977).

Summary: protracted abstinence in human studies. The evidence from human studies and clinical observations, although somewhat limited, is highly suggestive of a clinical phenomenon that might be termed *protracted abstinence from alcohol, opioids, and stimulants* (cocaine and the amphetamines). Uncomfortable and distressing physiological and psychological symptoms may persist for many months after the period immediately following withdrawal.

The symptoms of protracted abstinence from alcohol may include autonomic dysfunction, endocrine abnormalities, sleep impairments, depression, anxiety, and fatigue. The symptoms of protracted abstinence after cessation of opioids may include disturbances in a variety of physiological functions and high craving for the drug. The symptoms of protracted abstinence for cocaine may include sleep disturbances, fatigue, depression, anxiety, and high craving for the drug. Finally, the symptoms of protracted abstinence from amphetamines may include depression, lassitude, general fatigue, prolonged sleep, hyperphagia, and memory and concentration impairments.

Protracted Abstinence: Evidence From Animal Studies

Alcohol. The majority of the data dealing with persisting withdrawal syndromes with alcohol have been generated from clinical samples. This may relate to the emphasis on the more dramatic and more easily measured attributes in humans, including withdrawal seizures (Edmonds et al. 1982). Thus, the major emphasis in this brief report is placed on the human investigations.

Opioids. Several lines of evidence support a protracted abstinence syndrome in animals previously addicted to opioids. For instance, Martin and colleagues (1963) presented data on seven rats abstinent between 4 and 180 days from morphine. The rats exhibited decreased respiration and increases in temperature, weight, metabolism, water intake, and wet dog shakes for up to 4 months after detoxification compared with saline-injected control rats. In addition, Cochin and Kornetsky (1964) observed definite differences in response to morphine between treated rats and control rats up to a year of abstinence.

Other studies have revealed abnormalities in the electroencephalographic and behavioral responses of previously addicted rats to a morphine challenge up to 6 months after opioid detoxification (Khazan and Colasanti 1971; Nash et al. 1973). Related experiments with the opioid antagonist nalorphine in monkeys demonstrated that an increased sensitivity to nalorphine persisted for more than 3 months after detoxification from morphine (Goldberg and Schuster 1969). The monkeys exhibited emesis, excessive salivation, and hyperirritability to doses of nalorphine that produced no effect in control animals not exposed to opioids.

Drug-seeking behavior, which might be considered the animal equivalent of human subjective drug craving, is also sustained for months after detoxification from opioids (Wikler and Pescor 1967; Wikler et al. 1971). This drug-seeking behavior seems to have a limited relationship to conditioning, since drug seeking does not significantly increase in rats with conditioned abstinence compared with control rats. Although the connection between the biological aspects of protracted abstinence and relapse is complicated by the study by Schwartz and Marchok (1976), the consensus appears to be that protracted abstinence is one of several factors making relapse more likely.

Cocaine. Laboratory studies conducted on both rats and rhesus monkeys suggest the possibility of protracted effects after withdrawal from cocaine. For example, Wood and Lal (1987) described rats matching the effects of cocaine withdrawal to the effects of pentylenetetrazole, effects they suggested were anxiety-like. In addition, Woolverton and Kleven (1988) observed that the withdrawal of cocaine produced disrupted responding for food in rhesus monkeys previously maintained on high doses of cocaine. The disrupted pattern of responding lasted for 3–4 days, and the degree of disruption was related to dose and duration of exposure to cocaine. Decreased intake of a sweetened solution after cessation of cocaine maintenance has also been reported in rats (Carroll and Lac 1987). In their 1988 study, Woolverton and Kleven also reported that after initial tolerance development to cocaine in rhesus monkeys, less drug is required for tolerance development during the next maintenance regimen.

The amphetamines. Although the evidence is limited, animal studies do support the existence of some protracted abstinence for amphetamines. For instance, Ellinwood and Kilbey (1977), in a study involving rhesus monkeys and cats, suggested that stimulant-related psychoses may be reinduced after some period of abstinence with doses that were not initially sufficient to elicit the behavior.

In addition, Fischman and Schuster (1977) conducted a study in rhesus monkeys previously maintained on substantial intravenous doses of methamphetamine. After the abrupt substitution of saline for the active drug, no evidence of a withdrawal syndrome was found. However, substantial tolerance developed to the anorectic and performance disrupting effects of the methamphetamine. This tolerance persisted for at least 3 months after cessation of the drug.

Summary: protracted abstinence in animal studies. There are numerous animal studies involving different species that provide further evidence for protracted withdrawal from alcohol, opioids, cocaine, and the amphetamines. The symptoms of protracted abstinence from alcohol in animals include seizures, tremors, temperature changes, and appetite disturbances. Animal studies focusing on opioids document disturbances in an array of physiological functions and prolonged drug-seeking behavior. Studies involving cocaine document anxiety-related responding and disruptions in ongoing food-maintained behavior. Studies focusing on the amphetamines indicate continued tolerance to the anorectic and performance disrupting effects of the drug.

Discussion

This review of the literature demonstrates that there are considerable data supporting the existence of protracted abstinence syndromes for alcohol, opioids, and stimulants. Uncomfortable and distressing physiological and psychological symptoms may clearly persist for many months following the immediate period after withdrawal; furthermore, the prevalence of such symptoms among recovering alcoholic and drug-addicted persons would appear to be relatively high.

Protracted abstinence could be considered for listing as a diagnostic category in DSM-IV. It would be distinguished from remission by the physiological signs and subjective responses that might need specific eliciting stimuli (e.g., conditioned cues such as drug abuse apparatus) to be evident. The time parameters for the syndrome would be about 3 weeks after cessation of the drug up to perhaps

12 months of abstinence. It might justify relapse prevention therapy by providing a more physiological basis for this treatment, although current pharmacological therapies are not easily directed to this specific syndrome.

However, at the present time, there is insufficient documentation of the syndrome to justify its inclusion as a diagnostic subtype in DSM-IV. The clinical significance of the syndrome is more by inference than by direct testing of a causal association between relapse to substance abuse and the range of symptoms labeled protracted abstinence. Because of the current paucity of rigorous, large-scale studies, the parameters of the syndrome are ill-defined, and reliable and valid clinical criteria are lacking. Similarly, there do not appear to be appropriate studies outlining external validators such as demographic characteristics, nor are there appropriate data actually documenting the treatment implications of a label of protracted abstinence. Although we believe that a protracted withdrawal syndrome exists, in our judgment, there are simply not enough data to define the syndrome clearly and to establish its clinical relevance.

Recommendations

On the basis of this review of the literature, the consensus of the Work Group is that there do not appear to be sufficient data to develop specific, reliable criteria appropriate for an independent diagnosis of a protracted withdrawal syndrome at the present time. However, the literature review demonstrates that there are data highly suggestive of a clinical phenomenon that might appropriately be described as protracted withdrawal from alcohol, opioids, and stimulants. Moreover, there appears to be much potential for improvements in the care and treatment of those who are recovering from substance abuse if clinicians gain a heightened understanding of protracted abstinence problems. The potential treatment gains that might accrue from a more complete understanding of this issue certainly warrant further study of protracted abstinence phenomena. Over the next decade, we hope that sufficient data will be generated to allow for the development of reliable diagnostic criteria that justify the inclusion of the syndrome as a diagnostic subtype in DSM-V. In the interim, the phenomenon, although not given a separate number in DSM-IV, should be mentioned in the text.

References

Alling C, Balldin J, Bokstrom K, et al: Studies on duration of a late recovery period after chronic abuse of ethanol. Acta Psychiatr Scand 66:384–397, 1982

Angrist B, Sudilovsky A: Central nervous system stimulants: historical aspects and clinical effects, in Handbook of Psychopharmacology, Vol 11. Edited by Iverson LI, Iverson SD, Snyder SH. New York, Plenum, 1978

Begleiter H, Porjesz B: Persistence of a "subacute withdrawal syndrome" following chronic ethanol intake. Drug Alcohol Depend 4:353–357, 1979

Bell DS: The experimental reproduction of amphetamine psychosis. Arch Gen Psychiatry 29:35–40, 1973

Brower KJ, Paredes A: Cocaine withdrawal (letter). Arch Gen Psychiatry 44:297, 1987

Brown SA, Schuckit MA: Changes in depression among abstinent alcoholics. J Stud Alcohol 49:412–417, 1988

Brown SA, Irwin M, Schuckit MA: Changes in anxiety among abstinent male alcoholics. J Stud Alcohol 52:55–61, 1991

Carey JT, Mandel J: A San Francisco Bay Area "speed" scene. J Health Soc Behav 9:164–174, 1968

Carroll ME, Lac ST: Cocaine withdrawal produces behavioral disruptions in rats. Life Sci 40:2183–2190, 1987

Cochin J, Kornetsky C: Development and loss of tolerance to morphine in the rat after single and multiple injections. J Pharmacol Exp Ther 145:1–10, 1964

Derogatis L: SCL-90-R Manual II. Towson, MD, Clinical Psychometric Research, 1983

De Soto CB, O'Donnell WE, Allred LJ, et al: Symptomatology in alcoholics at various stages of abstinence. Alcoholism: Clinical and Experimental Research 9:505–512, 1985

De Soto CB, O'Donnell WE, De Soto JL: Long-term recovery in alcoholics. Alcoholism: Clinical and Experimental Research 13:693–697, 1989

Dole VP: Narcotic addiction, physical dependence and relapse. N Engl J Med 286:988–992, 1972

Drummond LM, Matthews HP: Single case study: obsessive-compulsive disorder occurring as a complication in benzodiazepine withdrawal. J Nerv Ment Dis 176:688–691, 1987

Edmonds HL, Sytinsky IA, Sylvester DM, et al: Neurochemical, EEG and behavioral correlates of ethanol withdrawal in the rat. Neurobehavioral Toxicology and Teratology 4:33–41, 1982

Eisenman AJ, Sloan JW, Martin WR, et al: Catecholamine and 17-hydroxycorticosteroid excretion during a cycle of morphine dependence in man. J Psychiatr Res 7:19–28, 1969

Ellinwood E, Kilbey MM: Chronic stimulant intoxication models of psychosis, in Animal Models in Psychiatry and Neurology. Edited by Hannan I, Usdin E. Oxford, Pergamon, 1977

Fischman MW, Schuster CR: Long-term behavioral changes in the rhesus monkey after multiple daily injections of D-methylamphetamine. J Pharmacol Exp Ther 201:593–605, 1977

Gawin FH, Ellinwood EH: Cocaine and other stimulants: actions, abuse and treatment. N Engl J Med 318:1173–1182, 1988

Gawin FH, Kleber HD: Abstinence symptomatology and psychiatric diagnosis in cocaine abusers. Arch Gen Psychiatry 43:107–113, 1986

Gillin JC, Smith TL, Irwin M, et al: EEG sleep studies in "pure" primary alcoholism during subacute withdrawal: relationships to normal controls, age, and other clinical variables. Biol Psychiatry 27:477–488, 1990

Goldberg SR, Schuster CR: Nalorphine: increases sensitivity of monkeys formerly dependent on morphine. Science 166:1548–1549, 1969

Gossop MR, Bradley BP, Brewis RK: Amphetamine withdrawal and sleep disturbance. Drug Alcohol Depend 10:177–183, 1982

Gossop M, Green L, Phillips G, et al: What happens to opiate addicts immediately after treatment: a prospective follow-up study. BMJ 294:1377–1380, 1987

Gross MM, Hastey JM: Sleep disturbances in alcoholism, in Alcoholism: Interdisciplinary Approaches to an Enduring Problem. Edited by Tarter RE, Sugerman AA. Reading, MA, Addison-Wesley, 1976

Hathaway SR, McKinley JC: Minnesota Multiphasic Personality Inventory. Minneapolis, MN, University of Minnesota, 1943

Hathaway SR, McKinley JC: Minnesota Multiphasic Personality Inventory, Revised. Minneapolis, MN, University of Minnesota, 1970

Herman JB, Brotman AW, Rosenbaum JF: Rebound anxiety in panic disorder patients treated with shorter-acting benzodiazepines. J Clin Psychiatry 48:22–26, 1987

Hesselbrock MN, Meyer RE, Keener JJ: Psychopathology in hospitalized alcoholics. Arch Gen Psychiatry 42:1050–1055, 1985

Himmelsbach CK: Clinical studies of drug addiction. Arch Intern Med 69:766–772, 1942

Johanson CE, Fischman MW: The pharmacology of cocaine related to its abuse. Pharmacol Rev 41:3–52, 1989

Jones RT: The pharmacology of cocaine, in Cocaine: Pharmacology, Effects and Treatment of Abuse (NIDA Research Monograph No 50). Edited by Grabowski J. Washington DC, U.S. Government Printing Office, 1984

Khazan N, Colasanti B: EEG correlates of morphine challenge in post-addict rats. Psychopharmacologia 22:56–63, 1971

Kissin B: Biological investigations in alcohol research. J Stud Alcohol (Suppl) 8:146–181, 1979

Kissin B, Schenker V, Schenker A: The acute effects of ethyl alcohol and chlorpromazine on certain physiological functions in alcoholics. Quarterly Journal of Studies on Alcohol 20:480–492, 1959

Kosten TR, Rounsaville BJ, Babor T, et al: Substance use disorders in DSM-III-R: evidence for the dependence syndrome across different psychoactive substances. Br J Psychiatry 151:834–843, 1987

Kramer JC, Fischman VS, Littlefield DC: Amphetamine abuse: pattern and effects of high doses taken intravenously. JAMA 201:305–309, 1967

LeBlanc AE, Kalant OJ, Kalant H: The Psychopharmacology of Amphetamine Dependence, in The Amphetamines: Toxicity and Addiction, 2nd Edition. Edited by Kalant OJ. Springfield, IL, Charles C Thomas, 1973

Martin WR, Jasinski DR: Physiological parameters of morphine dependence in man: tolerance, early abstinence, protracted abstinence. J Psychiatr Res 7:9–17, 1969

Martin WR, Wikler A, Eades CG, et al: Tolerance to and physical dependence on morphine in rats. Psychopharmacologia 4:247–260, 1963

Meyer RE, Mirin SM, Altman JL, et al: A behavioral paradigm for the evaluation of narcotic antagonists. Arch Gen Psychiatry 33:371–377, 1976

Nash P, Colasanti B, Khazan N: Long-term effects of morphine on the electroencephalogram and behavior of the rat. Psychopharmacologia 29:271–276, 1973

Oswald I, Thacore VR: Amphetamine and phenmetrazine addiction: physiological abnormalities in the abstinence syndrome. BMJ 2:427–431, 1963

Pettinati HM, Sugerman AA, Maurer HS: Four year MMPI changes in abstinent and drinking alcoholics. Alcoholism: Clinical and Experimental Research 6:487–494, 1982

Pokorny AD, Miller BA, Cleveland SE: Response to treatment of alcoholism: a follow-up study. Quarterly Journal of Studies on Alcohol 29:364–381, 1968
Porjesz B, Begleiter H: Brain dysfunction and alcohol, in The Biology of Alcoholism, Vol 7: The Pathogenesis of Alcoholism: Biological Factors. Edited by Kissin B, Begleiter H. New York, Plenum, 1983
Roelofs SM: Hyperventilation, anxiety, craving for alcohol: a subacute alcohol withdrawal syndrome. Alcohol 2:501–505, 1985
Roelofs SM, Dikkenberg GM: Hyperventilation and anxiety: alcohol withdrawal symptoms decreasing with prolonged abstinence. Alcohol 4:215–220, 1987
Rohan WP: MMPI changes in hospitalized alcoholics: a second study. J Stud Alcohol 33:65–76, 1982
Schuckit MA: Drug and Alcohol Abuse: A Clinical Guide to Diagnosis and Treatment, 3rd Edition. New York, Plenum, 1989
Schuckit MA, Monteiro MG: Alcoholism, anxiety and depression. Br J Addict 83:1373–1380, 1988
Schuckit MA, Irwin M, Brown S: The history of anxiety symptoms among 171 primary alcoholics. J Stud Alcohol 51:34–41, 1990
Schwartz AS, Marchok PL: Persistence of relapse of morphine-seeking behavior in rats: the relative role of certain biological variables. Psychopharmacologia 47:149–152, 1976
Segal BM, Kushnarev VM, Urakov IG, et al: Alcoholism and disruption of the activity of deep cerebral structures: clinical-laboratory research. Quarterly Journal of Studies on Alcohol 31:587–601, 1970
Sellers EM: Alcohol, barbiturate and benzodiazepine withdrawal syndromes: clinical management. Can Med Assoc J 139:113–123, 1988
Sideroff SI, Charuvastra VC, Jarvik ME, et al: Craving in heroin addicts maintained on the opiate antagonist naltrexone. Am J Drug Alcohol Abuse 5:415–423, 1978
Siegel RK: Cocaine smoking. J Psychoactive Drugs 14:271–359, 1982
Smail P, Stockwell T, Canter S, et al: Alcohol dependence and phobic anxiety states, II: a retrospective study. Br J Psychiatry 144:53–57, 1984
Smith DE: Physical vs psychological dependence and tolerance in high-dose methamphetamine abuse. Clinical Toxicology 2:99–103, 1969
Wagman AM, Allen RP: Effects of alcohol ingestion and abstinence on slow wave sleep of alcoholics. Adv Exp Med Biol 59:453–466, 1975
Wellman M: The late withdrawal symptoms of alcohol addiction. Can Med Assoc J 70:526–529, 1954
Wikler A, Pescor FT: Classical conditioning of a morphine abstinence phenomenon, reinforcement of opioid-drinking behavior and "relapse" in morphine-addicted rats. Psychopharmacologia 10:255–284, 1967
Wikler A, Pescor FT, Miller D, et al: Persistent potency of a secondary (conditioned) reinforcer following withdrawal of morphine from physically dependent rats. Psychopharmacologia 20:103–117, 1971
Williams HL, Rundell OH: Altered sleep physiology in chronic alcoholics: reversal with abstinence. Alcoholism: Clinical and Experimental Research 5:318–325, 1981
Wood DM, Lal H: Anxiogenic properties of cocaine withdrawal. Life Sci 41:1431–1436, 1987
Woolverton WL, Kleven MS: Evidence for cocaine dependence in monkeys following a prolonged period of exposure. Psychopharmacology (Berlin) 94:288–291, 1988

Chapter 12

Familial Alcoholism

Marc A. Schuckit, M.D.

Statement and Significance of the Issues

The process of revising DSM-III-R (American Psychiatric Association 1987) highlights the need to use the best available data to develop carefully structured criteria for major psychiatric disorders. In this context, changes in the diagnostic scheme should be considered when information can be marshaled to show that they enhance communication, the clinical utility, or the predictive validity of the diagnostic process.

Among the changes that can be made for DSM-IV is the identification of clinically relevant subgroups of established categories. These might highlight patients with unique clinical conditions that were developed in response to specific etiologic factors. I outline the results of a literature review concerning the potential clinical relevance of diagnoses of *familial alcoholism,* a term that indicates an individual with alcohol abuse or dependence who has at least one similarly diagnosed close relative.

The potential clinical importance of identifying alcoholic persons with alcoholic close family members was first discussed almost 50 years ago (Penick et al. 1987). Subsequently, Goodwin and colleagues (1971) presented the possibility that such individuals might be relatively distinct from other alcoholic persons, suggesting that the family history of alcohol-related life problems might indicate a relevant subdiagnosis. These alcoholic persons with a family history of alcoholism were felt to have an earlier onset of problems and a more severe clinical course (Goodwin 1983; Hesselbrock et al. 1985). The purpose of this review is to ascertain the support existing within the research literature for a familial subtype of alcoholism.

Methods

A search was conducted of the psychiatric and psychological literature for empirical studies concerned with a familial history of alcoholism. The review included a

Medline computer search using such terms as *alcoholism, family,* and *genetic,* covering 1970 to the present. The computer search was confined to journal articles published in the English language and to research concerned with human subjects. The reference lists of seven journals—*Journal of Studies on Alcohol, British Journal of Addiction, Alcoholism: Clinical and Experimental Research, American Journal of Drug and Alcohol Abuse, Alcoholism, Archives of General Psychiatry,* and *American Journal of Psychiatry*—over the past 5 years were reviewed for more recent papers. The reference lists of recent review articles (e.g., Rounsaville 1987) and studies (e.g., Buydens-Branchey et al. 1989) were also reviewed, and researchers were solicited for papers in press or under editorial review.

Studies that did not compare "alcoholics" with a familial history of alcohol abuse and/or dependence with "alcoholics" with no familial history were excluded. In addition, the review was confined to those studies that provided data on clinical course, treatment, and external validators that were associated with a family history of alcohol abuse and/or dependence. No studies were excluded on the basis of their definition of alcoholism, alcohol abuse, or alcohol dependence, but the criteria provided in each study were recorded. Studies that provided identical or overlapping data sets were excluded.

Each study was cataloged with respect to the number of alcoholic subjects included in the analysis, the criteria for alcoholism, the setting in which the data were collected (e.g., inpatient Veterans Administration hospital), the percentage of male subjects, the criteria for family history (e.g., first-degree relatives), and the percentage of the sample that was considered to have a family history of alcohol abuse/dependence. Each of these is presented in Table 12–1.

In addition, each study was coded with respect to whether the findings suggested that the alcoholic subjects with a family history, in comparison with those without, had 1) an earlier age at onset of alcoholism, 2) a greater severity of alcohol abuse/dependence symptomatology, 3) increased social-occupational consequences of the alcohol use, 4) a family history for another major mental disorder (e.g., depression), 5) an increased history of childhood conduct disorder symptomatology, 6) more current antisocial personality disorder symptomatology, 7) an association with a biological correlate of alcohol abuse/dependence, and 8) a distinct responsivity to treatment. The results are presented in Table 12–2.

Results

The Prevalence of Familial Alcoholism

The exact prevalence of alcoholic persons with a family history of alcoholism differs depending on the research methods used. Some studies insist that careful diagnostic

Table 12–1. Familial alcoholism studies: design features

Study	N[a]	Diagnostic criteria	Setting (inpatient)	Men (%)	Familial criteria[b]	Familial alcoholism (%)[c]
Hasin et al. 1988	111	RDC	Medical center	73	First degree	61
Schuckit 1984	453	DSM-III	VA	100	Parents	44
Penick et al. 1978	155	None	VA	100	Parents/grandparents	39
Hesselbrock et al. 1985	169	DSM-III	Mixed	100	First degree	62
McKenna and Pickens 1981	1,930	"Chronic"	Public hospital	79	Parents	22
Frances et al. 1980	7,064	None	Navy	100	First degree	49
Penick et al. 1990	212	DSM-III	VA	100	First degree	55
Stabenau 1984	210	DSM-III	Mixed	74	Parents/sibling of parents	85

Note. RDC = Research Diagnostic Criteria (Spitzer et al. 1978). VA = Veterans Administration.
[a]Number of alcoholic patients.
[b]Criteria for family history.
[c]Percentage of sample considered to have a family history of alcohol abuse/dependence.

Table 12–2. Familial alcoholism studies: findings

Study	Alcohol symptomatology			Comorbid			External	
	Age at onset	Severity[a]	Consequences[b]	Family other[c]	History CD[d]	ASP[e]	Biological correlates	Treatment reponsivity
Hasin et al. 1988	NE	–	–	NE	–/+	–	NE	NE
Schuckit 1984	+	+	+/–	–	+	+	NE	NE
Penick et al. 1978	+	+	+	NE	NE	NE	NE	NE
Hesselbrock et al. 1985	+	+	+	NE	+	+	NE	NE
McKenna and Pickens 1981	+	–	+	NE	+	NE	NE	NE
Frances et al. 1980	NE	+/-	+/-	+	+	+	NE	NE
Penick et al. 1990	+	+	–/+	NE	NE	–	NE	NE
Stabenau 1984	+	+	+	NE	NE	+	NE	NE

Note. NE = not examined.
[a]Of alcohol symptomatology.
[b]Social-occupational consequences of alcohol.
[c]Family history of other major mental disorder.
[d]History of childhood conduct disorder symptoms
[e]Comorbid antisocial personality disorder symptomatology.

criteria for alcoholism be applied to personal interviews with multiple family members; others allow for less restrictive criteria as reported by one informant only. In some investigations only alcoholism in biological parents is considered relevant; other studies describe individuals as having familial alcoholism when any first-degree relative demonstrates this disorder (i.e., usually parents, siblings, or children). Yet other investigations accept the criterion of alcoholism in grandparents or blood-related aunts and uncles (i.e., second-degree relatives) as well.

Using the most restrictive criteria, between 20% and 35% of alcoholic persons who enter treatment have an alcoholic father and/or mother (McKenna and Pickens 1981). Estimates of the prevalence of alcoholic first-degree relatives (including full siblings) have varied from approximately 45%, using DSM-III (American Psychiatric Association 1980) criteria, to 55% of alcoholic men and women who are considered family history positive with less restrictive criteria (Hasin et al. 1988; Jones-Saumity et al. 1980; Penick et al. 1990; Vrasti and Olteanu 1988). When familial alcoholism is defined based on alcohol-related major life problems in either first-degree or second-degree relatives, almost two-thirds of alcoholic persons entering treatment would be considered to have a familial form of the disorder (Frances 1984; Penick et al. 1987, 1990; Stabenau 1984), with some studies reporting rates as high as 80%.

The potential clinical importance of familial versus nonfamilial alcoholism has been discussed for many years. Although the prevalence of this potential subtype varies with definitions and methodological approaches, it is likely that approximately one half of alcoholic men and women appearing for treatment have at least one alcoholic close relative (Frances et al. 1980; Goodwin 1983).

Clinical Characteristics Associated With Familial Alcoholism

In general, alcoholic persons with a family history of alcoholism and those with no family history of alcoholism tend to be similar in occupation, education, and income (Penick et al. 1978). However, most studies indicate that those with alcoholic close relatives have an earlier onset of drinking, more alcohol-related life problems, and a younger age at admission for inpatient treatment (Schuckit 1984; Vrasti and Olteanu 1988). Furthermore, prior to the onset of major life problems related to alcohol use, those men and women with family histories of alcoholism are more likely to experience difficulties with truancy and incorrigibility (Frances et al. 1980; Hasin et al. 1988). Although the two groups based on family history generally report similar frequencies of drinking, and some studies show no differences on the days per month on which intoxication occurs (Jones-Saumity et al. 1980; Vrasti and Olteanu 1988), there is a possibility of a greater number of drinks per drinking day for those with alcoholic family histories (Vrasti and Olteanu 1988).

Most studies agree that alcoholic persons with a family history of alcoholism are likely to have an increased rate of alcohol-related life problems (Frances 1984; Frances et al. 1980; Hasin et al. 1988; Jones-Saumity et al. 1980; Stabenau 1984). These include a possible greater likelihood of blackouts and more reports of an inability to stop drinking once intake has begun (Penick et al. 1987). Associated with this pattern is likely to be an enhanced past history of alcohol-related job losses and arrests, as well as evidence of more intense withdrawal symptoms (Frances et al. 1980; Latchman 1985; Penick et al. 1987; Schuckit 1984). Although there is disagreement, other studies indicate that alcoholic persons with and without familial alcoholism are relatively similar on levels of cognitive functioning, driving arrests or accidents, health problems, and drug use patterns (Jones-Saumity et al. 1980; Penick et al. 1987; Schuckit 1984). It is possible that those individuals with alcoholism on both the maternal and paternal sides of the family might demonstrate a more severe clinical course than those whose alcoholism is unilineal (McKenna and Pickens 1981; Stabenau 1984).

In summary, alcoholic persons with a family history of alcoholism are reported to develop their alcohol-related problems earlier and to demonstrate more intense symptoms of physical dependence on alcohol and are likely to show more severe social consequences of their drinking in some (but not all) areas than those without a family history of alcoholism.

Possible Mechanisms Contributing to the Clinical Course of Familial Alcoholism

Despite the above findings, however, it appears as if the intensity of the clinical differences between alcoholic persons with and without familial alcoholism is considerably diminished when additional factors are considered. Two such factors include the impact of any psychiatric disorder in the family (not just alcoholism) and a notation of an established diagnostic entity, namely the antisocial personality disorder.

Research shows that alcoholic persons with a family history of alcoholism are likely to demonstrate increased rates of other psychiatric diagnoses among their family members (Penick et al. 1987). For example, in one study the evaluation of 377 carefully defined alcoholic men demonstrated that those with close family members with depressive disorders were also likely to demonstrate more severe alcohol-related clinical syndromes (Zisook and Schuckit 1987). This raises the possibility that a family history of any major psychiatric disorder, not just alcoholism, might increase the likelihood of an earlier onset and more severe course of alcohol-related problems. This could occur through the effects of stresses encountered during childhood that are associated with an ill family member or via an enhanced genetic loading toward psychopathology in general. In either event, it is not clear that a family history of alcoholism uniquely contributes to the clinical picture that has been described.

Another specific psychiatric syndrome may explain much of the difference between familial and nonfamilial alcoholism. One characteristic of the typical alcoholic person with a family history of alcoholism is relatively severe antisocial life problems in childhood, difficulties that often predate alcohol-related life problems (Frances et al. 1980; McKenna and Pickens 1981; Schuckit 1984; Stabenau 1984). When evaluated closely, significantly more of those with a family history of alcoholism than those lacking family histories of this disorder fulfill criteria for a clearly preexisting antisocial personality disorder. For example, in one careful study, 34% of those alcoholic subjects with but only 5% of those without familial alcoholism were classified as having antisocial personality disorder by research criteria (Penick et al. 1987, 1990). Once the possible importance of antisocial personality disorder is controlled, the remaining familial and nonfamilial alcoholic subjects appear to be much more similar than dissimilar on age at onset and clinical course (McKenna and Pickens 1981; Penick et al. 1987; Stabenau 1984). Consistent with this conclusion is a report indicating that evaluation of more middle-class and higher-functioning alcoholic persons, a group for whom prior antisocial personality disorder would be expected to be less prevalent, reported few impressive differences between familial and nonfamilial alcoholic subjects (Hasin et al. 1988).

Discussion

Alcoholic persons come in all shapes and sizes and demonstrate diverse backgrounds. It makes clinical sense that in treating any individual with any disorder, their prior life experiences, level of education, intelligence, and medical condition could have an impact on both clinical course and treatment needs.

The data described earlier document the potential clinical importance of also determining the family history of major psychiatric disorders. This information may help the clinician identify alcoholic patients more likely to have had chaotic childhood experiences and those for whom alcohol-related life problems might be more severe.

At first glance, the notation of familial alcoholism might appear to meet some of the criteria for change for DSM-IV. For example, regarding potential *clinical utility,* the notation of a familial subtype would encompass one-half or more of inpatients. A number of clinicians in their writings have not only called for identification of alcoholic subgroups, but have specifically cited the familial rubric as having possible importance. In addition, the rate of a family history of alcoholism also appears to be relatively *consistent.* Although the level of agreement probably differs with the definitions and methods used, similar results have been cited across different studies for the prevalence of this characteristic.

However, it is the criterion of *validity* where major difficulties become apparent. As described above, the apparent ability of this diagnostic scheme to predict the clinical course is considerably weakened when other important variables are considered. These include the impact of any psychiatric disorder in the family (not just alcoholism) and the importance of the notation of an established diagnostic entity, the antisocial personality disorder. Once the potential importance of these issues is considered, the notation of familial alcoholism might add little specific information relevant to a diagnosis that might be highlighted in DSM-IV.

As a result of these considerations, it is not likely that *external validators* such as demographic characteristics and treatment implications would support the general usefulness of this proposed diagnostic subtype.

Recommendations

The process of determining the potential relevance of diagnoses and diagnostic subtypes for DSM-IV has set forth specific criteria that must be met in order for changes in the diagnostic scheme to be seriously considered. In light of these guidelines, although familial alcoholism does indicate some useful information about the future clinical course, once additional factors are controlled, it does not appear as if there is sufficient reason to incorporate a diagnosis of familial alcoholism within the new diagnostic manual. On the other hand, the potential relevance of a family history of alcoholism in attempting to understand the probable clinical course of a specific alcoholic individual might be worthy of several sentences or a paragraph in the accompanying text. Perhaps more appropriately controlled studies in the future might justify reconsidering this issue for DSM-V.

References

American Psychiatric Association: Diagnostic and Statistical Manual of Mental Disorders, 3rd Edition. Washington, DC, American Psychiatric Association, 1980

American Psychiatric Association: Diagnostic and Statistical Manual of Mental Disorders, 3rd Edition, Revised. Washington, DC, American Psychiatric Association, 1987

Buydens-Branchey L, Branchey MH, Noumair D: Age of alcoholism onset, I: relationship to psychopathology. Arch Gen Psychiatry 46:225–230, 1989

Frances RJ: Outcome study of familial and nonfamilial alcoholism. Am J Psychiatry 141:1469–1471, 1984

Frances RJ, Stephen T, Steven B: Studies of familial and nonfamilial alcoholism. Arch Gen Psychiatry 37:564–566, 1980

Goodwin DW: Familial alcoholism: a separate entity? Substance and Alcohol Actions/Misuse 4:129–136, 1983

Goodwin DW, Crane JB, Guze SB: Felons who drink: an 8-year follow-up. Quarterly Journal of Studies on Alcohol 32:136–147, 1971

Hasin DS, Bridget GF, Endicott J: Severity of alcohol dependence and social occupational problems: relationship to clinical and familial history. Alcoholism: Clinical and Experimental Research 12:660–664, 1988

Hesselbrock VM, Hesselbrock MN, Stabenau JR: Alcoholism in men patients subtyped by family history and antisocial personality. J Stud Alcohol 46:59–64, 1985

Jones-Saumity DJ, Oscar AP, Marjorie SF: Familial alcoholism, drinking behavior, and neuropsychological performance in alcoholic women. Alcohol Technical Reports 9:29–34, 1980

Latchman RW: Familial alcoholism: evidence from 237 alcoholics. Br J Psychiatry 147:54–57, 1985

McKenna T, Pickens R: Alcoholic children of alcoholics. J Stud Alcohol 42:1021–1029, 1981

Penick EC, Read MR, Crowley PA, et al: Differentiation of alcoholics by family history. J Stud Alcohol 39:1944–1948, 1978

Penick EC, Powell BJ, Bingham SF, et al: A comparative study of familial alcoholism. J Stud Alcohol 48:136–146, 1987

Penick EC, Nickel EJ, Powell BJ, et al: A comparison of familial and nonfamilial male alcoholic patients without a co-existing psychiatric disorder. J Stud Alcohol 51:443–447, 1990

Rounsaville BJ: Substance use disorders, in An Annotated Bibliography of DSM-III. Edited by Skodol AE, Spitzer RL. Washington, DC, American Psychiatric Press, 1987

Schuckit MA: Relationship between the course of primary alcoholism in men and family history. J Stud Alcohol 45:334–338, 1984

Spitzer RL, Endicott J, Robins E: Research Diagnostic Criteria: rationale and reliability. Arch Gen Psychiatry 35:773–782, 1978

Stabenau JR: Implications of family history of alcoholism, antisocial personality, and sex differences in alcohol dependence. Am J Psychiatry 141:1178–1182, 1984

Vrasti R, Olteanu I: The difference between biological heredity and cultural heredity: preliminary findings in assessment of parental rearing practice in primary alcoholism. Neurol Psychiatr (Bucur) 26:171–178, 1988

Zisook S, Schuckit MA: Male primary alcoholics with and without family histories of affective disorder. J Stud Alcohol 48:337–344, 1987

Chapter 13

Cocaine and Amphetamine

Psychostimulant Abuse

Michael R. Irwin, M.D.

Statement of the Issues

Abuse of amphetamine and of cocaine are separated into two categories in DSM-III-R (American Psychiatric Association 1987). In this review I appraise the utility of combining abuse of amphetamine and cocaine into the same category in DSM-IV. The similarities and differences of the two drugs are addressed through an examination of their biochemical actions, pharmacologic properties (both behavioral and physiologic), and associated psychiatric complications.

Significance of the Issues

A review of the history and epidemiology of use of amphetamine and cocaine is necessary to understand why separate diagnostic categories were created for drugs that act pharmacologically in a similar manner and produce an identical spectrum of acute intoxicating effects and psychiatric complications following chronic use.

Prior to the mid-1980s, cocaine was claimed to be a relatively safe, nonaddicting euphoriant agent (Grinspoon and Bakalar 1980). Cocaine dependence was dismissed as a moralistic exaggeration (Lewin 1924; Maier 1926), and the absence of research on cocaine addiction was misinterpreted to mean that cocaine, as compared with amphetamine, was not addictive. In fact, national commissions on drug abuse reported that amphetamine, but not cocaine, caused substantial morbidity (National Commission on Marihuana and Drug Abuse 1973; Strategy Council on Drug Abuse 1973), even though studies in animals showed a close similarity between cocaine and amphetamine.

Amphetamine and cocaine do not usually have concurrent abuse histories, and it appears that over the last 40–50 years they have alternated in popularity (Fischman 1987). Amphetamine abuse began to appear in the early 1940s (Brill and Hirose 1969), peaked in the mid-1960s (Angrist and Sudilovsky 1978), and reached a general decline by the late 1970s (Newmeyer 1979). In contrast, cocaine use showed a relatively low prevalence and comparable stability until 1976 (Abelson and Miller 1985), at which time a dramatic increase occurred, progressing to the highest rate ever of cocaine use (17%) for a population of high-school seniors during 1985 (Fischman 1987). It is now well recognized that cocaine abuse produces severe medical and social problems identical to those reported to be caused by amphetamine and methamphetamine in the early 1950s and late 1960s. Combining amphetamine and cocaine abuse into one diagnostic category may help remind clinicians that even though these two drugs alternate in popularity, they produce very similar and severe medical and psychiatric complications.

Methods

The English-language psychiatric and psychological literature was searched for studies containing evidence of classification of stimulant drugs based on data from humans and animals. The reviews included Medline computer searches using such terms as *cocaine, amphetamines, abstinence syndromes,* and *withdrawal* from the period of 1970 to the present.

The automated searches were complemented by a review of articles appearing over the past 5 years in the following journals: *Journal of Studies on Alcohol, British Journal of Addiction, Alcoholism: Clinical and Experimental Research, American Journal of Drug and Alcohol Abuse, Alcoholism, Archives of General Psychiatry, Journal of Psychoactive Drugs, Drug and Alcohol Dependence,* and *American Journal of Psychiatry.* Approximately 100 book chapters and journal articles were scanned before focusing on the studies actually referenced in this report.

Results

Biochemical Actions

Similarities. Cocaine and amphetamine are neuropharmacologically similar (Fischman 1987; Gawin and Ellinwood 1988). They cannot be distinguished as different by long-term cocaine-addicted persons during blinded laboratory administration (Fischman et al. 1976). Both amphetamine and cocaine increase concentrations of dopaminergic and noradrenergic transmitters at the neuron synapse—cocaine mainly by blocking reuptake and amphetamine by both augmenting release and blocking reuptake (Woolverton 1984).

Differences. Cocaine and amphetamine are structurally dissimilar. Cocaine is an ester of benzoic acid, whereas amphetamine is a phenylpropyl amine (Gawin and Ellinwood 1988). Cocaine is isolated from the plant *Erythroxylon coca* (Grabowski 1984) and is a naturally occurring anesthetic. Amphetamine, on the other hand, was first synthesized as part of a program for the manufacture of aliphatic amines and was used as a bronchial dilator (Caldwell 1980).

Furthermore, cocaine is a less potent inhibitor of the uptake of norepinephrine and dopamine than amphetamine (Glowinski and Axelrod 1965; Heikkila et al. 1975; Langer and Enero 1974; Ross and Renyi 1967). Cocaine neither affects the accumulation of intraventricularly administered tritiated norepinephrine (Carr and Moore 1970), nor does it enhance the efflux of this amine into cerebral perfusates as compared with amphetamine (Heikkila et al. 1979). Cocaine appears to be 10- to 20-fold less potent than amphetamine in facilitating dopaminergic transmission (Fung and Uretsky 1980). Cocaine injected intrastriatally in animals with unilateral nigrostriatal 6-hydroxy-dopamine lesions does not induce circling in mice but does prevent circling induced by systemically administered amphetamine (Fung and Uretsky 1980). Finally, cocaine appears to affect vesicular pools of dopamine, whereas amphetamine appears to interact mainly with extravesicular or newly synthesized pools of the neurotransmitter (Gawin and Ellinwood 1988).

Pharmacologic Properties: Behavioral Effects

Similarities. In animals, cocaine resembles amphetamine in inducing enhanced locomotor activity at lower doses and focused stereotypies at higher doses (Langer and Enero 1974). In humans, a single moderate dose of either cocaine or amphetamine produces a decrease in food intake and fatigue and an increase in activity, talkativeness, and reports of euphoria and general well-being (Fischman 1987; Gawin and Ellinwood 1988). Both amphetamine and cocaine are capable of reversing, at least partially, fatigue-induced decrements in performance. When subjects are deprived of sleep for either 24 or 48 hours and then inhale 96 mg of cocaine, a reversal of the 24-hour–induced decrement is found (Johanson et al. 1976). Likewise, amphetamine has also been shown to have mental effects on performance in sleep-deprived subjects. Thus, moderate doses of either stimulant are generally successful in reversing decrements in performance that are a result of fatigue and sleep deprivation. At higher doses, both stimulants acutely produce repetitive motor activity and, with further increases, convulsions, hyperthermia, coma, and death (Kilbey and Sannerud 1985).

Repeated administration or use of these drugs is the usual manner in which they are taken (Fischman 1987). Thus, studies in behavioral pharmacology have been extended from acute- to repeated-dose paradigms.

Studies in animals have demonstrated that repeated administration of psychomotor stimulants induces sensitization for a number of dependent variables including activity, stereotypy, startle response, seizures, and brain stimulation (Post and Contel 1983). Increased sensitivity to the effects of psychomotor stimulant drugs occurs after intermittent repetitive administration (Gunne 1977). Regardless of the regimen of administration, studies have demonstrated that repeated doses of both amphetamine and cocaine result in enhancement of stereotyped behaviors and locomotor stimulant effects. Patterns of characteristic stereotyped behavior have been reported for both humans and animals (Post 1981). Such behaviors generally occur during the first 8 hours after injection.

Sensitization elicited by one psychomotor stimulant drug such as amphetamine generalizes to others such as cocaine (Leith and Kuczenski 1981) and persists for long periods of time after administration is terminated (Demellweek and Goudie 1983; Ellinwood and Kilbey 1977). Thus, it has been suggested that amphetamine and cocaine are interchangeable in their ability to sensitize and induce increases in locomotor activity as well as other behavioral manifestations. However, it is not currently clear whether sensitization, produced by repeated doses of amphetamine or cocaine, occurs by similar mechanisms (Schuster et al. 1966).

Cross-tolerance between cocaine and amphetamine is also seen. In animal studies, tolerance to drug administration results in a decrease in reinforcement density (Schuster and Johanson 1981). In addition, both cocaine and amphetamine produce similar tolerance effects on anorexia (Fischman et al. 1985; Woolverton et al. 1978).

In humans, there is also acute tolerance development to the subjective effects of both cocaine and amphetamine (Sherer et al. 1985). For example, when constant cocaine blood levels were maintained in human volunteers for a period of 4.5 hours, tolerance to the subjective effects of the drug rapidly appeared (Leith and Kuczenski 1981). Tolerance development is also seen in volunteer research subjects who are allowed to self-administer the drug repeatedly within a 1-hour session (Gawin and Kleber 1986). Thus, there is clear evidence that the positive mood-enhancing properties of cocaine appear to decrease with repeated dosing. A similar finding has also been demonstrated for the action of amphetamine (Post 1981). The pattern of steadily increasing doses of amphetamine during a binge produces an inability to obtain a level of positive subjective effects achieved earlier in that drug-taking occasion (Martin et al. 1971).

In summary, the subjective effects of cocaine and amphetamine are identical; experienced drug-using persons given a variety of stimulant drugs cannot differentiate between cocaine and amphetamine, both of which appear to have similar profiles of action (Fischman et al. 1976; Jones 1985). Both cocaine and amphetamine produce changes in a number of scales including fatigue, elation, friendliness, arousal, and positive mood. Similarities between the two drugs are impressive given the fact that many studies have controlled for neither administration nor dose.

Differences. The main difference in behavioral action between cocaine and amphetamine concerns the duration of action of the two drugs (Gawin and Ellinwood 1988). Amphetamine's plasma half-life is 4–8 times longer than that of cocaine's (only 90 minutes) (Gunne and Anggard 1973). Thus, although both cocaine and amphetamine produce a dynamic tachyphylaxis, resulting in a rapidly declining effect despite the continued presence of the stimulant in plasma, cocaine's elicited euphoria is often less than 45 minutes (Gawin and Kleber 1985), whereas the duration of euphoria following amphetamine can last for up to 2 hours or longer (Kramer et al. 1967). This difference in duration of action produces differences in the typical schedule of administration used by persons abusing the two drugs. For example, cocaine binges are characterized by readministration of the drug up to every 10 minutes, causing rapid and frequent mood changes. Such binges can last as long as 7 consecutive days, although the average length is often only 12 hours (Fischman 1984). Amphetamine binges can often last more than 24 hours, with 1 to several hours between readministration of the drug (Tewes and Fischman 1982). Despite these differences in the amount and duration of use of cocaine versus amphetamine, it is again important to emphasize that the psychiatric sequelae resulting from use of these two drugs are indistinguishable.

Usual routes of administration of cocaine differ from those of amphetamine. Cocaine can be smoked when it is chemically altered to form a cocaine base. Such a base makes it readily available for diffusion across the pulmonary area and absorption for delivery to the brain. Comparable smoking of amphetamine has not been reported.

Despite the striking similarity in the behavioral effects of amphetamine and cocaine, the two drugs do differ in their ability to interfere with the acquisition of new behavior patterns. In individual research subjects, it has been found that doses (32 mg) of intravenous cocaine, but not amphetamine, interfered with the acquisition of new behavior patterns, increasing the error rate without affecting response rate (Resnick et al. 1977). However, this differential effect between the two drugs may be due to the fact that only one amphetamine dose was tested.

Pharmacologic Properties: Physiologic Effects

Similarities. Cardiovascular changes are seen following the administration of either cocaine or amphetamine. Although both drugs cause dose-related increases in heart rate and blood pressure (Fischman et al. 1976; Rechtschaffen and Maron 1964), intravenous cocaine has not been shown to have any effect on the electrocardiogram (Fischman et al. 1976) or on the respiratory rate as compared with changes induced by amphetamine (Connell 1969).

Both amphetamine and cocaine have a suppressive effect on rapid eye movement sleep and total sleep (Smith 1969).

Differences. Cocaine, as stated earlier, is a local anesthetic and has been used in surgery of the upper respiratory tract because of its unique blood vessel constriction properties. Amphetamine shows neither anesthesia nor significant local blood vessel constriction following administration.

Psychiatric Complications: Acute Intoxication

Similarities. High-dose binge use of either cocaine or amphetamine can produce inhibition, impaired judgment, grandiosity, impulsiveness, hypersexuality, hypervigilance, compulsively repeated actions, and extreme psychomotor activation (Gawin and Kleber 1986; Gold et al. 1985; Smith 1984; Tewes and Fischman 1982). Such marked behavioral changes may lead to accidents, illegal acts, or atypical sexual behavior. These social complications of psychostimulant abuse occur in up to 80% of those who regularly use cocaine and 75%–80% of those who abuse amphetamines. Furthermore, as the binge lengthens, anxiety, hyperactivity, and irritability become mixed with euphoria and a stimulant-associated paranoia (Gawin and Ellinwood 1988). Again, both drugs can induce a paranoia that is so severe that reality testing becomes markedly impaired, and, in extreme cases, homicide results.

Differences. Substantial differences in the acute intoxication complications of amphetamine and cocaine are not well recognized.

Psychiatric Complications: Abstinence Syndromes

Similarities. Both amphetamine and cocaine can produce the typical stimulant abstinence syndrome characterized by a three-phase pattern of crash, withdrawal, and extinction (Citron et al. 1970; Kleber and Gawin 1987; Kloss et al. 1984). Following the discontinuation of either stimulant, there is an intense depression, agitation, anxiety, and then craving for sleep. The severe neurovegetative symptoms, consistent with the clinical depression-withdrawal symptoms, are the inverse of the acute effects of stimulants. Although these symptoms are often mildest immediately after the crash, decreased energy, limited interest in the environment, and anhedonia increase in intensity during the next 12–96 hours following drug withdrawal (Kleber and Gawin 1987). Symptoms often fluctuate and are often neither constant nor severe enough to meet psychiatric diagnostic criteria for a major mood disorder. Sustained abstinence for 6–18 weeks produces an amelioration of the anhedonia, fatigue, and dysphoria (Gold et al. 1985; Kleber and Gawin 1987; Smith 1984).

Differences. The acute abstinence symptoms are not substantially different between amphetamine and cocaine.

Psychiatric Complications: Toxicity

Similarities. Clinical and experimental evidence suggests that irreversible morphological and behavioral toxicity result from repeated high doses of either cocaine or amphetamine (Rumbaugh et al. 1971; Seiden et al. 1975; Weiss et al. 1981). For example, necrotizing angiitis is found frequently in those who abuse methamphetamines (Rumbaugh et al. 1971). In a laboratory study involving rhesus monkeys, 1.5 mg/kg of amphetamine was given intravenously every other day for 2 weeks (Weiss et al. 1981). Extensive neurologic effects were identified, including petechial hemorrhages and cerebral edema. Furthermore, it has been found that amphetamine produces an irreversible reduction of up to 70% in caudate dopamine levels (Vilensky 1982). Similar studies have not been carried out using cocaine.

Differences. Toxic effects due to differences in the route of administration are found in those who abuse cocaine versus those who abuse amphetamines. Cocaine freebase smoking produces an impaired pulmonary gas exchange (Weiss et al. 1981). Inhalation of cocaine leads to chronic rhinitis or sinusitis and necrosis and perforation of the nasal septum (Vilensky 1982). Those who use amphetamines primarily use the drug intravenously and suffer complications of those who use other intravenous drugs such as hepatitis, septicemia, endocarditis, and acquired immunodeficiency syndrome.

Discussion

Amphetamine and cocaine are strikingly similar in terms of their biochemical effects, pharmacologic profile of action on behavioral and physiologic measures, and induction of psychiatric complications. However, differences in the time course of action and typical route of administration do exist between the two drugs.

Separation of cocaine abuse and amphetamine abuse highlights the fact that the two drugs differ in their typical schedule of administration. However, other classes of drugs such as sedatives, hypnotics, and anxiolytics or hallucinogens also differ in the time course of action and patterns of administration, yet DSM-III-R has grouped these classes of drugs together on the basis of profile of action rather than administration and dosage schedules. Thus, the single diagnostic label of Psychostimulant Abuse would be consistent with the classification of other drugs of abuse and would emphasize that both amphetamine and cocaine can produce similar severe medical and psychiatric morbidity.

Recommendation

On the basis of an extensive review of the literature, it is recommended that amphetamine abuse and cocaine abuse be combined into a single diagnostic category in DSM-IV.

References

Abelson HI, Miller JD: A decade of trends in cocaine use in the household population, in Cocaine Use in America: Epidemiologic and Clinical Perspectives (NIDA Research Monograph No 61). Edited by Kozel NJ, Adams EH. Washington, DC, U.S. Government Printing Office, 1985

American Psychiatric Association: Diagnostic and Statistical Manual of Mental Disorders, 3rd Edition, Revised. Washington, DC, American Psychiatric Association, 1987

Angrist B, Sudilovsky A: Central nervous system stimulants: historical aspects and clinical effects, in Handbook of Psychopharmacology, Vol 11. Edited by Iversen LL, Iversen SD, Snyder SH. New York, Plenum, 1978

Brill H, Hirose T: Rise and fall of a methamphetamine epidemic: Japan 1945–55. Seminars in Psychiatry 1:179–194, 1969

Caldwell J: Amphetamines and related stimulants: some introductory remarks, in Amphetamines and Related Stimulants: Chemical, Biological, Clinical, and Sociological Aspects. Edited by Caldwell J. Boca Raton, FL, CRC Press, 1980

Carr L, Moore K: Release of norepinephrine and normetanephrine from rat brain by central nervous system stimulants. Biochem Pharmacol 19:2671–2675, 1970

Citron BP, Halpern M, McCarron M, et al: Necrotizing angiitis associated with drug abuse. N Engl J Med 283:1003–1011, 1970

Connell PH: Some observations concerning amphetamine misuse: its diagnosis, management, and treatment with special reference to research needs, in Drugs and Youth. Edited by Wittenborn JR, Brill H, Smith JP, et al. Springfield, IL, Charles C Thomas, 1969

Demellweek C, Goudie AJ: Behavioral tolerance to amphetamine and other psychostimulants: the case for considering behavioral mechanisms. Psychopharmacology (Berlin) 80:287–307, 1983

Ellinwood E, Kilbey MM: Stimulant abuse in man: the use of animal models to assess and predict behavioral toxicity, in Predicting Dependence Liability of Stimulant and Depressant Drugs. Edited by Thompson T, Unna KR. Baltimore, MD, University Park Press, 1977

Fischman MW: The behavioral pharmacology of cocaine in humans, in Cocaine: Pharmacology, Effects, and Treatment of Abuse (NIDA Research Monograph No 50). Edited by Grabowski J. Washington, DC, U.S. Government Printing Office, 1984

Fischman MW: Cocaine and the amphetamines, in Psychopharmacology: The Third Generation of Progress. Edited by Meltzer HY. New York, Raven, 1987

Fischman MW, Schuster CR, Resnekov L, et al: Cardiovascular and subjective effects of intravenous cocaine administration in humans. Arch Gen Psychiatry 33:983–989, 1976

Fischman MW, Schuster CR, Javaid J, et al: Acute tolerance development to the cardiovascular and subjective effects of cocaine. J Pharmacol Exp Ther 235:677–682, 1985

Fung YK, Uretsky NJ: The effect of dopamine uptake blocking agents on the amphetamine-induced circling behavior in mice with unilateral nigro-striatal lesions. J Pharmacol Exp Ther 214:651–656, 1980

Gawin FH, Ellinwood EH Jr: Cocaine and other stimulants: actions, abuse, and treatment. N Engl J Med 318:1173–1182, 1988

Gawin FH, Kleber HD: Cocaine use in a treatment population: patterns and diagnostic distinctions, in Cocaine Use in America: Epidemiologic and Clinical Perspectives (NIDA Research Monograph No 61). Edited by Kozel NJ, Adams EH. Washington, DC, U.S. Government Printing Office, 1985, pp 182–192

Gawin FH, Kleber HD: Abstinence symptomatology and psychiatric diagnosis in cocaine abusers: clinical observations. Arch Gen Psychiatry 43:107–113, 1986

Glowinski J, Axelrod J: Effects of drugs on the uptake release and metabolism of ^{3}H-norepinephrine in the rat brain. J Pharmacol Exp Ther 149:43–49, 1965

Gold MS, Washton AM, Dackis CA: Cocaine abuse: neurochemistry, phenomenology, and treatment, in Cocaine Use in America: Epidemiologic and Clinical Perspectives (NIDA Research Monograph No 61). Edited by Kozel NJ, Adams EH. Washington, DC, U.S. Government Printing Office, 1985, pp 130–150

Grabowski J (ed): Cocaine: Pharmacology, Effects, and Treatment of Abuse (NIDA Research Monograph No 50). Washington, DC, U.S. Government Printing Office, 1984

Grinspoon L, Bakalar JB: Drug dependence: non-narcotic agents, in Comprehensive Textbook of Psychiatry, 3rd Edition. Edited by Kaplan HI, Freedman AM, Sadock BJ. Baltimore, MD, Williams & Wilkins, 1980

Gunne LM: Effects of amphetamines in humans, in Drug Addiction II: Amphetamine, Psychotogen, and Marihuana Dependence. Edited by Martin WR. Berlin, Springer-Verlag, 1977

Gunne LM, Anggard E: Pharmacokinetic studies with amphetamines: relationship to neuropsychiatric disorders. J Pharmacokinet Biopharm 1:481–495, 1973

Heikkila RE, Orlansky H, Cohen G: Studies on the distinction between uptake inhibition and release of ^{3}H-dopamine in rat brain tissue slices. Biochem Pharmacol 24:847–852, 1975

Heikkila RE, Felicitas S, Manzino L, et al: Rotational behavior induced by cocaine analogs in rats with unilateral 6-hydroxydopamine lesions of the substantia nigra: dependence upon dopamine uptake inhibition. J Pharmacol Exp Ther 211:189–194, 1979

Johanson CE, Balster RL, Bonese K: Self-administration of psychomotor stimulant drugs: the effects of unlimited access. Pharmacol Biochem Behav 4:45–51, 1976

Jones RT: The pharmacology of cocaine, in Cocaine: Pharmacology, Effects, and Treatment of Abuse (NIDA Research Monograph No 50). Edited by Grabowski J. Washington, DC, U.S. Government Printing Office, 1985, pp 34–53

Kilbey MM, Sannerud CA: Models of tolerance: do they predict sensitization to the effects of psychomotor stimulants, in Behavioral Pharmacology: The Current Status. Edited by Seiden LS, Balster RL. New York, Alan R Liss, 1985

Kleber HD, Gawin FH: Cocaine withdrawal (letter). Arch Gen Psychiatry 44:298, 1987

Kloss MW, Rosen GM, Rauckman EJ: Cocaine-mediated hepatotoxicity: a critical review. Biochem Pharmacol 33:169–173, 1984

Kramer JC, Fischman VS, Littlefield DC: Amphetamine abuse: pattern and effects of high doses taken intravenously. JAMA 201:305–309, 1967

Langer SZ, Enero M: The potentiation of responses to adrenergic nerve stimulation in the presence of cocaine: its relationship to the metabolic fate of released norepinephrine. J Pharmacol Exp Ther 191:431–443, 1974

Leith NJ, Kuczenski R: Chronic amphetamine: tolerance and reverse tolerance reflect different behavioral actions of the drug. Pharmacol Biochem Behav 15:399–404, 1981

Lewin L: Phantastica. Berlin, Verlag von Georg Stilke, 1924

Maier HW: Der Kokainismus. Leipzig, Georg Thieme Verlag, 1926

Martin WR, Sloan JW, Sapira JD, et al: Physiologic, subjective, and behavioral effects of amphetamine, methamphetamine, ephedrine, phenmetrazine, and methylphenidate in man. Clin Pharmacol Ther 12:245–258, 1971

National Commission on Marihuana and Drug Abuse: Drug Use in America: Problem in Perspective. Second Report of the National Commission on Marihuana and Drug Abuse. Washington, DC, National Institute on Drug Abuse, 1973

Newmeyer JA: The epidemiology of amphetamine use, in Amphetamine Use, Misuse and Abuse: Proceedings of the National Amphetamine Conference, 1978. Edited by Smith DE, Wesson DR, Buxton ME, et al. Boston, MA, G.K. Hall, 1979

Post RM: Central stimulants: clinical and experimental evidence on tolerance and sensitization, in Research Advances in Alcohol and Drug Problems, Vol 6. Edited by Israel Y, Glaser FB, Kalant H, et al. New York, Plenum, 1981

Post RM, Contel NR: Human and animal studies of cocaine: implications for development of behavioral pathology, in Stimulants: Neurochemical, Behavioral, and Clinical Perspectives. Edited by Creese I. New York, Raven, 1983

Rechtschaffen A, Maron L: The effect of amphetamine on the sleep cycle. Electroencephalogr Clin Neurophysiol 16:438–445, 1964

Resnick RB, Kestenbaum RS, Schwartz LK: Acute systemic effects of cocaine in man: a controlled study by intranasal and intravenous routes. Science 195:696–698, 1977

Ross SB, Renyi A: Inhibition of the uptake of tritiated catecholamines by antidepressant and related agents. Eur J Pharmacol 2:181–186, 1967

Rumbaugh CL, Bergeron RT, Scanlan RL, et al: Cerebral vascular changes secondary to amphetamine abuse in the experimental animal. Radiology 101:345–351, 1971

Schuster CR, Johanson CE: Environmental variables affecting tolerance development to anorectic drugs, in Anorectic Agents: Mechanisms of Action and Tolerance. Edited by Garratini S, Samanin R. New York, Raven, 1981

Schuster CR, Dockens WS, Woods JH: Behavioral variables affecting the development of amphetamine tolerance. Psychopharmacologia 9:170–182, 1966

Seiden LS, Fischman MW, Schuster CR: Long-term methamphetamine induced changes in brain catecholamines in tolerant rhesus monkeys. Drug Alcohol Depend 1:215–219, 1975

Sherer M, Kumor K, Thompson L, et al: Psychopharmacologic and cardiovascular responses after two methods of cocaine administration: cocaine bolus versus cocaine bolus with continuous infusion. Paper presented at the Annual Meeting of the American College of Neuropsychopharmacology, 1985

Smith DE: The characteristics of dependence in high-dose methamphetamine abuse. Int J Addict 4:453–459, 1969

Smith DE: The spectrum of cocaine abuse and its treatment. J Clin Psychiatry 45:18–23, 1984

Strategy Council on Drug Abuse: Federal Strategy for Drug Abuse and Drug Traffic Prevention 1973. Washington, DC, U.S. Government Printing Office, 1973

Tewes PA, Fischman MW: Effects of D-amphetamine and diazepam on fixed-interval, fixed-ratio responding in humans. J Pharmacol Exp Ther 221:373–383, 1982

Vilensky W: Illicit and licit drugs causing perforation of the nasal septum. J Forensic Sci 27:958–962, 1982

Weiss RD, Goldenheim PD, Mirin SM, et al: Pulmonary dysfunction in cocaine smokers. Am J Psychiatry 138:1110–1112, 1981

Woolverton WL: Pharmacological analysis of the discriminative stimulus properties of D-amphetamine in rhesus monkeys (abstract). Pharmacologist 26:161, 1984

Woolverton WL, Kandel D, Schuster CR: Tolerance and cross-tolerance to cocaine and D-amphetamine. J Pharmacol Exp Ther 205:525–535, 1978

Section II

Delirium, Dementia, and Amnestic and Other Cognitive Disorders

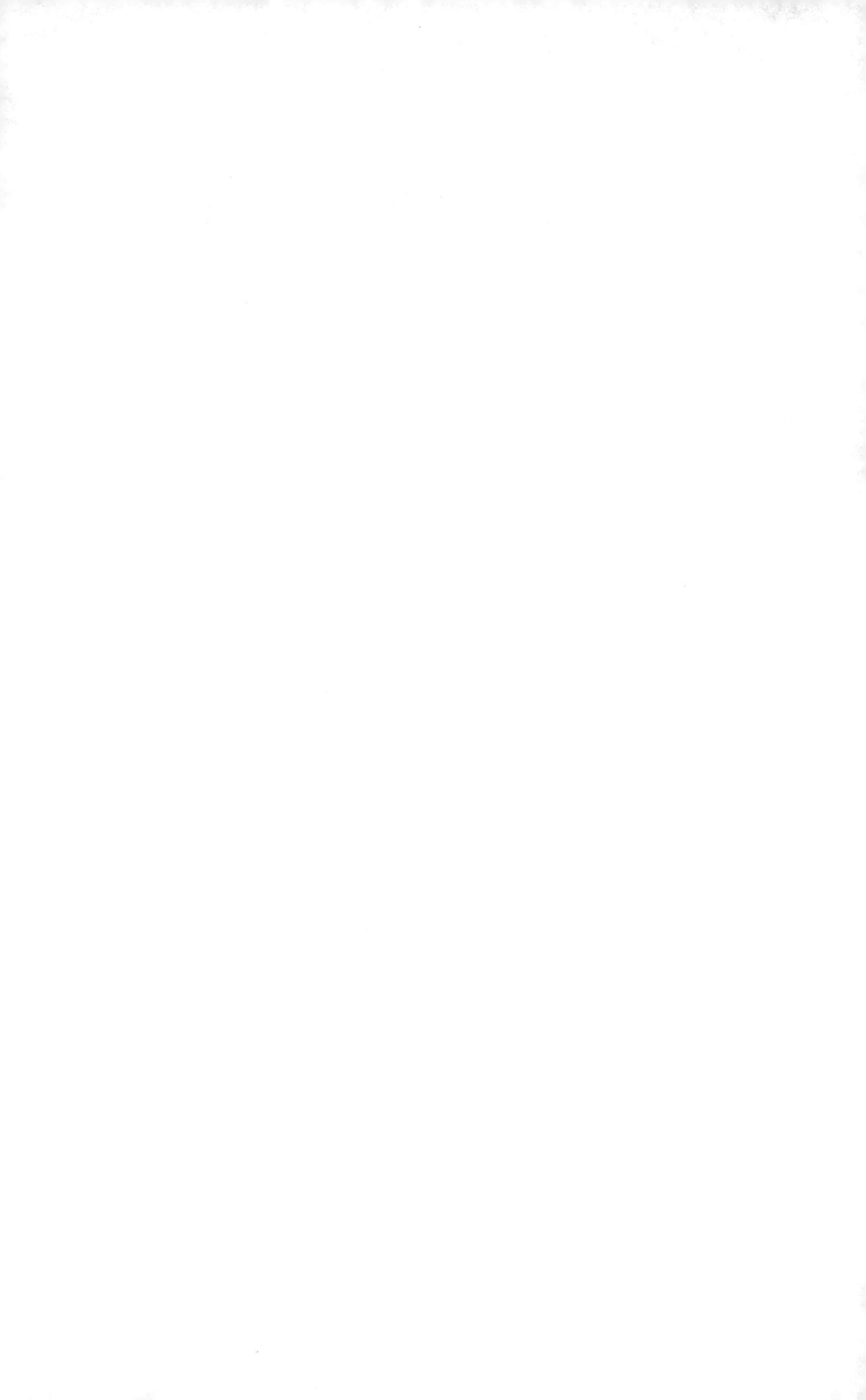

Contents

Introduction to Section II

Delirium, Dementia, and Amnestic and Other Cognitive Disorders

Gary J. Tucker, M.D., Eric D. Caine, M.D.
Michael K. Popkin, M.D.

The suggested changes for the Organic Mental Disorders section of DSM-III-R (American Psychiatric Association 1987) represent, perhaps, the most sweeping theoretical and practical changes made for any options in DSM-IV. Briefly, the main suggested changes—as discussed in detail in the *DSM-IV Options Book* (American Psychiatric Association 1991)—are as follows:

1. Eliminate the distinction between "Organic" and "Non-organic" (or functional) by relabeling this category "Cognitive Impairment Disorders," thereby eliminating the implication that the non-organic label applies to the remaining diagnostic categories in DSM-IV. "Amnestic Disorders," "Delirium," and "Dementia" would be grouped under the new category of "Cognitive Impairment Disorders."
2. All other syndromes currently within the Organic Mental Disorders section of DSM-III-R would be placed within the major diagnostic category with which they share phenomenology. For example, Organic Mood Disorder would move to the Mood Disorders section and be renamed "Secondary Mood Disorder Due to a General Medical Condition," and so on. (Note: In the *Options Book, Secondary Disorder Due to a General Medical Condition* is used. However, after the publication of the *Options Book,* it was subsequently decided to refer to such disorders in DSM-IV simply as "Disorders Due to General Medical Conditions.")
3. New categories of "Postconcussional Disorder," "Secondary Catatonic Disorder," "Secondary Dissociative Disorder," "Secondary Sexual Dysfunction," "Secondary Sleep Disorder," "Aging-Associated Cognitive Decline," and

"Mild Cognitive Disorder" were recommended for inclusion in DSM-IV. The category of secondary disorders emphasizes the need for differential diagnosis as well as etiological identification. As mild cognitive disorders are included in ICD-10 (World Health Organization 1992), we may include it in the Appendix of DSM-IV.

4. All suggested changes have been based as much as possible on data rather than expert opinion alone, particularly changes recommended for specific diagnostic criteria.

Background

The widespread nature of the changes recommended in DSM-IV must be considered as a reflection of the state of psychiatry at the current time. Their sweeping nature can be understood only in reference to the previous diagnostic and statistical nomenclatures (see Table 1). The first DSM (American Psychiatric Association

Table 1. Diagnostic and statistical nomenclature

DSM-I (1952)	*DSM-III-R (1987)*
Acute Brain Disorder	Added:
(e.g., infection, trauma, drugs, tumor)	Multi-infarct
Chronic Brain Disorder	Dementia
(e.g., infection, trauma, drugs, tumor)	Dementia Alzheimer Type
DSM-II (1968)	Changed some diagnostic criteria
Psychotic Organic Brain Syndromes	*DSM-IV*
Senile	Cognitive Disorders
Alcoholic	Delirium
Infection	Dementia
Other	Amnestic
Non-Psychotic Organic Brain Syndromes	Postconcussional
(e.g., infection, trauma, drugs, tumor)	Mild Cognitive Disorder
DSM-III (1980)	Cognitive Disorders Not Otherwise Specified
Organic Brain Syndromes	Secondary Disorders
Delirium	Psychotic
Dementia	Catatonic
Senile	Mood
Presenile	Anxiety
Amnestic	Personality
Delusional	Dissociative
Hallucinosis	Sleep
Affective	Sexual
Personality	Condition (R Code)
Intoxication/Withdrawal	Aging-Associated Memory Decline

1952) reflected many early attempts at nomenclature and the experience of World War II. The major criteria for the symptoms of an organic mental disorder were rooted clearly in Bleuler's (1924) concept of an organic "psychosyndrome." The symptoms that he cited as characteristic of this syndrome were included in DSM-I and DSM-II (American Psychiatric Association 1968) as the major criteria for the diagnosis of an organic mental disorder. They include defects in orientation, memory, intellectual functions, judgment, and labile or shallow affect, and have become the deficits most often associated with central nervous system dysfunctions. It is interesting that Bleuler probably developed these specific criteria to contrast and highlight the distinctions he made with schizophrenia and other diagnostic categories. DSM-I divided the Organic Disorders into "Acute Brain Disorders" and "Chronic Brain Disorders." DSM-II in 1968 changed "Disorder" to "Syndrome" and made the major categorical distinctions "Psychotic" and "Non-Psychotic Conditions." Reversibility of those disorders was regarded as a specific criteria to be noted.

Interestingly, none of these classifications included the specific categories of Dementia, Amnestic Disorder, or Delirium. One can only speculate that the above criteria were so meager because the practice of psychiatry was based in outpatient settings and had little exposure to those who were cognitively impaired. Perhaps most of the psychiatrists involved in the creation of these manuals were not involved in hospital care and, certainly, not general hospital psychiatric care. How the distinctions in DSM-I and DSM-II were determined remains an interesting historical question.

The changes of DSM-III (American Psychiatric Association 1980) were a radical shift. One can wonder, as well, if these changes did not reflect the movement of psychiatry into general hospital settings and an awareness of the types of psychiatric and behavioral conditions confronting psychiatrists who now worked in general hospitals. Consequently, we see the recognition of Delirium, Dementia, and Amnestic Syndromes as well as the addition of four syndromes that do not primarily have the traditional symptoms outlined by Bleuler (1924), but rather have mainly behavioral symptoms with little or no associated cognitive dysfunction. Therefore, we see the addition of "Organic Delusional Syndrome," "Organic Hallucinosis," "Organic Affective Syndrome," and "Organic Personality Syndrome." The distinctions between "Acute" and "Chronic," and "Psychotic" and "Non-Psychotic" were completely dropped.

In a similar way, the changes proposed for DSM-IV probably also relate to the current practice of psychiatry. A particular impetus for these changes has been the development of specially funded centers for the study of specific conditions such as Alzheimer's disease and increased studies of dementia. Secondly, the role of the central nervous system in all types of behavior has become more delineated. We have found evidence of central nervous system dysfunction in affective disorders, schizophrenia, obsessive-compulsive disorder, and so on. Many of these investigations have been made possible by the availability of techniques for investigating the in vivo functioning of the central nervous system such as neuropsychological testing, cerebral blood flow measures, new imaging techniques, and new and more sophisticated electroencephalography. Lastly, as medicine in general becomes more technological, we have become more aware of behavioral disturbances created by various procedures (e.g., transplants). There has also been increased survival in people with central nervous system disorders. With these developments came a tremendous interest in doing away with the distinction between "Organic" and "Non-organic." In the evaluation of DSM-III and DSM-III-R, Taylor (1987) noted the potential importance of doing away with this distinction. In early discussions of the Task Force, all cited concern about this. These concerns were crystallized in the proposal by Spitzer et al. (1989).

"Organic Mental Disorders" to "Cognitive Impairment Disorders"

Although changing "Organic Mental Disorders" to "Cognitive Impairment Disorders" and "Secondary Disorders Due to . . . " seems like a semantic shift, it is really a conceptual shift. These changes imply that there are no clear a priori etiological implications for any diagnostic category in the nomenclature, thus allowing the full brunt of scientific and clinical data to clarify specific etiology. Through much searching for other names, it was determined that disruptions of cognition represent the predominant feature of the conditions Delirium, Dementia, and Amnestic Disorders. "Secondary" was identified as most explicitly stating the symptomatic relationship between primary etiological disorders and their behavioral manifestations. It contrasted most clearly with the designation of primary (idiopathic) psychiatric disorders. Although many other terms were sought, none seemed to characterize these conditions as well. No other suggestion for DSM-IV has created more controversy than this suggestion. There have been at least seven articles (Lipowski 1990a; Popkin et al. 1989; Spitzer et al. 1989, 1992; Tucker 1991, 1993; Tucker et al. 1990) published about this recommended change and other aspects of the suggestions, as well as at least seven letters to the editor (Golden 1991; Lipowski 1990b, 1991; Liptzin 1991; Pies 1991; Spitzer 1991; Spitzer et al. 1991).

Consultation-liaison psychiatrists particularly felt that "Cognitive Impairment Disorders" would not convey the appropriate information to our medical colleagues and that, although all could understand that this is an organic condition, nonpsychiatrists would become confused about the meaning of "Cognitive Impairment Disorders." Psychiatrists who were particularly interested in psychopathology noted that cognitive changes took place in affective disorders and schizophrenia also. However, these are educational problems. Also, the cognitive changes in most psychopathological syndromes are not the predominant and defining symptoms that they are in the disorders in these categories.

Alternative names for this section were also considered, such as simply using the triple heading of "Delirium, Dementia, and Amnestic Disorder." An alternative to this suggestion was to let each of these categories stand on its own. In other words, there would be a category for "Delirium" (Liptzin and colleagues, Chapter 14), a category for "Dementia" (Rebok and Folstein, Chapter 15), and a category for "Amnestic Disorders" (Caine, Chapter 16) much as there is a category for "Mood Disorders," "Anxiety Disorders," and so on. However, if each of these entities is not to stand alone, then some overarching title for these categories will be necessary. Exactly what this section will be called is still an open question to be decided by the entire Task Force.

Secondary Disorders

Initially, "Symptomatic" was recommended for these entities, but because of concerns about the degree of certainty of any relationship and the specificity this term implied, it was changed to a "Secondary Disorder Due to . . . . " The suggestion to place these conditions within the diagnostic categories with which they share phenomenology was based on the premise that clinicians tend to think in terms of diagnostic categories. When they see a patient with a mood disorder, they tend to think of the differential diagnosis of the mood disorder. Consequently, moving these conditions to the major psychopathological category they most resemble and calling them "Secondary Conditions" would be more consistent with clinical thinking. However, this simple change raised two major questions.

1. The first major question concerns how closely does the condition have to match the diagnostic criteria for the parent category. For example, if one talks about a Secondary Mood Disorder, does it have to meet all the criteria for Major Depressive Disorder? Or does it have merely to meet the "sounds like" or "similarity" criteria. We settled on the latter as most do not meet full DSM-IV diagnostic criteria. Often, the symptom can be part of the medical symptoms or illness, or the symptoms are too few to meet full diagnostic criteria, but a predominant symptom such as depressive affect is present and correlates with the physical condition.
2. The second major question concerns the relationship and strength of the relationship in implicating the medical condition as the cause of the Secondary

Disorder. One will see from the review of the literature by Popkin and Tucker (Chapter 17) that these associations have varying degrees of certainty, and few of them are very strong. Many of our consultants were also concerned about this problem, which typifies the entire question of the relationship of Axis I disorders to Axis III disorders. We are in the process of developing some specific recommendations for determining this association. (Note: In the *Options Book, Secondary Disorder Due to a General Medical Condition* is used. However, after the publication of the *Options Book,* it was subsequently decided to refer to such disorders in DSM-IV simply as "Disorders Due to General Medical Conditions.")

Other Deliberations of the Work Group

Since psychiatrists seem to be dealing more with disturbances of the central nervous system, the question arose of how we should deal with neurological conditions. Some suggested that we include various neurological categories such as aphasia and apraxia. Based on our literature reviews, we decided that this would be premature. However, we could no longer overlook movement disorders, particularly those related to neuroleptic medication. A group of consultants was selected to review these issues and make recommendations.

Another area of concern was how much laboratory data would be required for the diagnosis of these conditions. For example, how much neuropsychological test data is required for the diagnosis of Dementia? Would electroencephalogram data be necessary for the diagnosis of Delirium? The issue of including laboratory data in diagnostic classification rules was a general problem for all work groups, but most apparent for this one, as more etiologically related data are potentially available. We recommend putting the pertinent laboratory tests into the text of DSM-IV rather than in the criteria themselves. However, the one possible exception is Mild Cognitive Impairment, which would call for neuropsychological or clinical cognitive testing as part of the criteria set, although the latter can be performed by the psychiatric clinician.

The correlation between the changes recommended for DSM-IV and ICD-10 is good. ICD-10 is often more specific, whereas DSM-IV uses more broad, over-arching categories. However, in general, most categories are covered in both nomenclatures.

Consultants who have been very involved in responding to the work of this group are F. Benson, J. Cummings, B. Fogel, R. Heaton, Z. Lipowski, A. Lishman, R. Mayeux, M. Mesulam, V. Neppe, M. Raskind, B. Reisberg, M. Roth, R. Schiffer, M. Taylor, L. Teri, and R. Veith.

Specific Disorders

Amnestic Disorders

The Amnestic Disorder category as proposed includes

1. Amnestic Disorder Due to a General Medical Condition
2. Substance-Induced Amnestic Disorder
3. Amnestic Disorder Due to Unknown Etiology
4. Amnestic Disorder Not Otherwise Specified

Previously in DSM-III-R, Amnestic Disorder was listed in two different sections of the classification: "Psychoactive Substance-Induced Organic Mental Disorders" and "Organic Mental Disorders Associated With Axis III Physical Disorders or Conditions." We felt it would be easier to group these entities together and remove the distinction between "Amnestic Syndrome" and "Amnestic Disorder." We attempted to clarify the major diagnostic criteria for Amnestic Disorders by proposing to state the major criteria as "development of memory impairment as manifested by the inability to learn new information and the inability to recall previously learned knowledge or past events." We feel this is a clearer and more operational definition. An impairment criterion would also be added. We feel that the Amnestic Disorders do deserve to be placed in a distinct category since they can be differentiated from the other syndromes of Dementia and, certainly, Delirium. From the literature review, it was noted that memory impairment is the most prominent feature of Amnestic Disorders; although other associated cognitive deficits may be present, they are not the prominent features.

Two clarifying terms related to the course of the Amnestic Disorder were also proposed: "Transient" and "Persistent." This would cover transient global amnesia. In light of the literature review, it is clear that transient global amnesia does exist, most often associated with transient cerebral ischemia.

Delirium

The Delirium category as proposed includes

1. Delirium Due to a General Medical Condition
2. Substance-Induced Delirium
3. Delirium Due to Multiple Etiologies
4. Delirium Due to Unknown Etiology
5. Delirium Not Otherwise Specified

Again, in DSM-III-R, Delirium was listed in two different sections of the classification: "Psychoactive Substance-Induced Organic Mental Disorders" and "Organic Mental Disorders Associated With Axis III Physical Disorders or Conditions." It is proposed that these be grouped together in one category.

A number of changes are recommended for the specific diagnostic criteria in order to return to DSM-III criteria (which many preferred) and to make them more compatible with ICD-10. The core concept of impairment of consciousness as the key diagnostic criterion for Delirium would be restored as it was in DSM-III. In DSM-III-R, the major criteria are related to attention rather than to consciousness.

Another recommendation was to subsume the specific symptoms (e.g., disorganized thinking, perceptual disturbances) under the more general and global "changes in cognition," adding a comment that these are "not better accounted for by a preexisting, established, or evolving dementia," thus allowing a patient with a preexisting Dementia to be diagnosed as also having Delirium. It was noted that certain specific symptoms listed in DSM-III-R were sometimes hard to assess, such as language difficulty in a mute patient or sleep disturbance and psychomotor retardation in a medically ill patient. We also felt it would be important to have the criteria reflect a change from a previous condition and not just rely on the cross-sectional symptom stipulation.

The proposed options for Delirium were based on several data reanalyses that are reviewed in Volume 4 of the Sourcebook. Using the results of these data-based studies, the Work Group has recommended that the criteria for Delirium be based on core symptoms that can be operationalized. The emphasis on core symptoms would allow the clinician to define the disorder in a clearer fashion that might allow physicians to diagnose these patients more consistently. Associated symptoms such as conceptual disorganization, perceptual disturbances, sleep disturbance, and psychomotor retardation or agitation would be described in the text of DSM-IV but would not be required for making the diagnosis. The "change" criterion for cognitive function should be useful for diagnosing Delirium in the presence of Dementia and allow for the recognition of concurrent diagnoses as well. With these criteria, Delirium could now be diagnosed independently of Dementia. Although it is recognized that some education will be necessary to familiarize clinicians with these new criteria, operationalizing them will allow for greater precision in research and eventually improved communication.

Another proposed new category is "Delirium Due to Multiple Etiologies." It was noted that it is quite common to encounter Delirium associated with more than one etiological factor—for example, medication side effects (as an example of a Substance-Induced Delirium) and renal failure. In the conditions due to multiple etiology and in Substance-Induced Delirium, it would be important to specify the agent responsible for the Delirium.

Dementia

The Dementia category as proposed includes

1. Dementia of the Alzheimer's Type
2. Vascular Dementia
3. Dementia Due to Other General Medical Conditions (e.g., Pick's disease, Creutzfeldt-Jakob disease, Huntington's disease, Parkinson's disease, human immunodeficiency virus disease, and other)
4. Substance-Induced Persisting Dementia
5. Dementia Due to Multiple Etiologies
6. Dementia Due to Unknown Etiology
7. Dementia Not Otherwise Specified

In DSM-III-R, Dementia was cited in three different areas: "Dementias Arising in the Senium and Presenium," "Psychoactive Substance-Induced Organic Mental Disorders," and "Organic Mental Disorders Associated With Axis III Physical Disorders or Conditions." It was proposed that the criteria for "Dementia of the Alzheimer's Type" be revised in DSM-IV to accomplish several things: 1) to clarify the central construct of Dementia (i.e., the development of multiple cognitive deficits) and to ensure that individuals with memory loss and some mild personality change would be diagnosed as having the more appropriate Amnestic Disorder rather than Dementia and 2) most importantly, to reconcile DSM-IV diagnostic criteria with the criteria established by the National Institute of Neurological and Communicative Disorders and Stroke and by the Alzheimer's Disease and Related Disorders Association. We also thought we should remove "Primary Degenerative Dementia" from the name and simply label it "Dementia of the Alzheimer's Type."

Recommended diagnostic criterion A delineates the associated multiple cognitive and memory impairments needed for the diagnosis of Dementia. From the data analysis, it was noted that there are two types of onset of Alzheimer's Dementia: one early and one later. It would now be possible to specify these. What was most lacking in the nomenclature, however, were the reasons that psychiatrists frequently saw these patients: that is, the behavioral conditions associated with Dementia. New specifications were therefore proposed that would allow the clinician to stipulate or specify behavioral features of Dementia, such as "depressed mood," "delusions," "hallucinations," "perceptual disturbance," "behavioral disturbance" (violence), "communication disturbance," "motor skill disturbance," "mixed" (where one can specify several of the above), and "not otherwise specified." It was clear from both the literature review and the data reanalysis that these behavioral criteria were the ones most needed by psychiatrists as descriptors of patients with Dementia. In the past, we were not able to specify these behavioral and psychiatric symptoms. This change would greatly increase our understanding of the reasons for treating these patients as well as the difficulties involved.

We also attempted to clarify the difference between "impairment" and "disability." Consequently, "impairment" would be included as part of the diagnostic criteria but could probably be further operationalized, whereas "disability" would be determined as part of the multiaxial approach. It was noted that distinctions are made in the literature between the cortical and subcortical Dementias; however, it was felt that at our current state of knowledge, there were not enough data to warrant inclusion of these terms. There also did not seem to be any compelling reason as yet, from the literature review, to include any kind of data about the stages of Alzheimer's.

The concept of Vascular Dementia, called "Multi-Infarct Dementia" in DSM-III-R, presented two problems that were not really clarified by the literature. The first was related to the course of Vascular Dementia. The following three options have been proposed: Option 1 would be to omit any mention of "Course"; Option 2 would be to describe the course as being "characterized by sustained periods of clinical stability punctuated by sudden significant cognitive and functional losses"; and Option 3 would be to retain the DSM-III-R characterization, or a "Stepwise deteriorating course with 'patchy' distribution of deficits." The second major problem concerned the addition of laboratory evidence as a way of documenting focal neurological damage, thus broadening the way the neurological deficit could be diagnosed.

Secondary Disorders

The proposal for Secondary Disorders includes

1. Secondary Psychotic Disorder
2. Secondary Catatonic Disorder
3. Secondary Mood Disorder
4. Secondary Anxiety Disorder
5. Secondary Dissociative Disorder
6. Secondary Personality Change
7. Secondary Sleep Disorder
8. Secondary Sexual Dysfunction

As described previously, one of the major additions to DSM-III was the addition of conditions that did not have the primary cognitive changes associated with known or presumed damage to the central nervous system, but did have a clear association with such conditions. We propose expanding the DSM-III categories by the addition of four more conditions and by collapsing Organic Hallucinosis and Organic Delusional Disorder into one category of "Secondary Psychotic Disorder."

As one can see from the review of the literature of these syndromes, the data supporting the relationship between behavioral syndromes and medical and neurological disorders are variable and mostly weak. The stipulation of "due to" or "secondary to" in terms of specifying an etiological relationship is often a difficult one. Most of the proposed associations rest on case reports, but these anecdotes occur often enough to include them in the nomenclature both for clinical utility and for future study. However, it is important to note that in those conditions where there is overt evidence of central nervous system disturbance, a stronger and consistent relationship between the behavioral syndrome and the lesion is evident.

It is also clear that all of the secondary disorders may not present the exact diagnostic symptoms for the disorders with which they are phenomenologically grouped. However, when the diagnostic symptoms do coincide with specific criterion symptoms, the more defined classification should be used. It is particularly important to recognize that the symptoms of the physical illness will frequently confound the ability to use the strict criteria. For example, in the diagnosis of Secondary Mood Disorder, differentiating vegetative signs of a depressive process from symptoms of a patient's medical illness may be almost impossible at times.

In general, the proposed format would require "evidence from history, physical examination, or laboratory findings of a general medical condition judged to be etiologically related to the disturbance." This is merely a means of citing an association, and at this point it is extremely difficult to impute etiology or the strength of the etiological relationship. However, including these categories may allow these data to be more firmly related etiologically in the future.

Attempts have been made to allow a greater specification of these conditions; for example, it is proposed that for Secondary Psychotic Disorders, one could specify with "delusions," with "hallucinations," or with "mixed features." In a similar way for the Secondary Mood Disorders, there would be specifications of types with a "Manic Episode," with a "Major Depressive Episode," with "manic features," with "depressive features," and with "mixed features," which would allow the clinician to use the major criteria if they are present, but if they are not, to have more flexible criteria for a mood disturbance secondary to some medical condition.

This same approach would be used for Anxiety Disorders, where the clinician could specify types "with generalized anxiety," "with panic attacks," "with obsessive-compulsive symptoms," "with social phobic symptoms," or "with agoraphobic symptoms."

Because of the results of the literature reviews and also to parallel ICD-10, it was proposed to include "Secondary Catatonic Disorder," "Secondary Sexual

Dysfunction," "Secondary Sleep Disorder," and "Secondary Dissociative Disorder." Interestingly, the "Secondary Sexual Dysfunctions" are stipulated with a different code because they are encompassed in the Genital-Urinary section of ICD-10.

The discussion of Organic Personality Syndromes in DSM-III-R clearly delineated the fact that there was little question that structural central nervous system injury as well as other neurological disorders such as epilepsy can and will give rise to alterations and disturbances of personality. This led to the proposal for a new category in DSM-IV entitled "Personality Change Disorders." The personality dysfunctions are covered in Popkin and Tucker's review of secondary disorders (Chapter 17) and in Tucker's review of regional syndromes (Chapter 18). Although the literature is frequently full of anatomical descriptions of personality syndromes—such as the "Temporal Lobe Personality," the "Frontal Lobe Personality," and "Parietal Lobe Personality"—when one reviews the literature, the data supporting the distinctness of these regional syndromes are rather weak. The causal correlation of a specific behavior with injury to a specific brain region is not high, and other locations are often as likely to cause the same behavior. However, it was apparent that there are clusters of behavioral symptoms that predominate from many anatomical sites; these symptom clusters would therefore be better stipulated without reference to anatomical site (e.g., as "apathetic" or "labile").

This would allow broader criteria to be used for the diagnosis of personality change since the major criterion would now become "a persistent personality disturbance that represents a change from the individual's previous personality characteristics." The types suggested for specification include "labile," "disinhibited," "aggressive," "apathetic," "paranoid," "other," "combined" (more than one feature predominates in the clinical picture), and "unspecified."

There was a recommendation that a longitudinal dimension be added for paroxysmal or episodic conditions, but this was not included because there were little data in the literature on the longitudinal course of these conditions. Another difficulty related to the age of the patient, since it was not clear how these personality changes would be related to children in terms of the variable effect of cerebral insults on different age groups.

Proposed New Categories

Clinicians are dealing more and more with patients with head injuries. The overwhelming data from reviewing the literature show that there is a Postconcussional Disorder (Brown and Grant, Chapter 20). The criteria suggested in the Sourcebook literature review are at some variance with the proposal described in the *Options*

Book. The *Options Book* criteria are closely aligned to ICD-10 and are less specific than the criteria recommended in Chapter 20. The inclusion of Postconcussional Disorder in ICD-10 was also an important motivation to include it in the *Options Book*; however, the data alone would seem to warrant inclusion.

Recommendations were made that two proposed categories, "Mild Neurocognitive Disorders" (Gutierrez et al., Chapter 19) and "Aging-Associated Memory Decline" (Caine, Chapter 21), should be recognized. With regard to mild cognitive conditions, we recognize the problem of determining when symptoms become an illness or a disorder. What is the threshold for diagnosis? Certainly, many medical conditions such as pulmonary disease, various metabolic abnormalities, and various infectious disorders are associated with mild cognitive impairment. These conditions do not often reach the status of either a Dementia or a Delirium, and in fact most of the evidence for them is based on subtle deviations in neuropsychological test data. Mild cognitive changes can even be noted with various medication use. Consequently, it is clear that this is an area that needs future consideration and one that rests less on clinical evaluation than on laboratory substantiation. As a result, how laboratory data will be treated in future nomenclature is very important to the fate of this category.

The category "Aging-Associated Memory Decline" would attempt to capture the cognitive alterations experienced by many as they grow older. If there are normatively defined intellectual changes associated with aging, is it appropriate to label these using a clinical diagnosis as a description usually reserved for medically defined disease processes? The question of labeling becomes very important if it is predictive of future negative outcome or future significant functional interference. As yet, there are no data suggesting that these mild changes are forbearers of more serious illness. Moreover, there has been insufficient research to establish the degree of normative changes that are associated with aging, precluding the present possibility of establishing valid diagnostic standards.

Summary and Conclusions

The changes proposed for DSM-IV with regard to dysfunctions of the central nervous system are major recommendations for change in theory and practice. Conceptually, they reflect the evolution of knowledge about how the central nervous system affects behavior. Practically, we have attempted to base them as much as possible on data and literature reviews. When there were no data, we used our experience as clinicians and researchers to support our recommendations. We hope that after reading the Sourcebook, one will be able to discern when recommendations were based on data and when they were based on clinical judgment.

References

American Psychiatric Association: Diagnostic and Statistical Manual: Mental Disorders. Washington, DC, American Psychiatric Association, 1952

American Psychiatric Association: Diagnostic and Statistical Manual of Mental Disorders, 2nd Edition. Washington, DC, American Psychiatric Association, 1968

American Psychiatric Association: Diagnostic and Statistical Manual of Mental Disorders, 3rd Edition. Washington, DC, American Psychiatric Association, 1980

American Psychiatric Association: Diagnostic and Statistical Manual of Mental Disorders, 3rd Edition, Revised. Washington, DC, American Psychiatric Association, 1987

American Psychiatric Association: DSM-IV Options Book: Work in Progress 9/9/91. Washington, DC, American Psychiatric Association, 1991

Bleuler E: Textbook of Psychiatry. New York, MacMillan, 1924

Golden SZ: Concerns and issues of the diagnostic category of organic mental disorders in the DSM-IV. Psychosomatics 32:112, 1991

Lipowski ZJ: Is "organic" obsolete? Psychosomatics 31:342–344, 1990a

Lipowski ZJ: Task Force on DSM-IV: organic disorders. Am J Psychiatry 147:947, 1990b

Lipowski ZJ: Dr. Lipowski replies. Am J Psychiatry 148:396, 1991

Liptzin B: Dr. Liptzin replies. Am J Psychiatry 148:1612, 1991

Pies R: The organic disorders. Hosp Community Psychiatry 42:199, 1991

Popkin MK, Tucker GJ, Caine E, et al: The fate of organic mental disorders in DSM-IV: a progress report. Psychosomatics 30:438–441, 1989

Spitzer RL: Revising diagnostic criteria for delirium. Am J Psychiatry 148:1611–1612, 1991

Spitzer RL, Williams JBW, First M, et al: A proposal for DSM-IV: solving the "organic/nonorganic" problem. Journal of Neuropsychiatry and Clinical Neurosciences 2:126–127, 1989

Spitzer RL, First M, Tucker GJ: Organic mental disorders and DSM-IV. Am J Psychiatry 148:396, 1991

Spitzer RL, First MB, Williams JBW, et al: Now is the time to retire the term "Organic Mental Disorders." Am J Psychiatry 149:240–244, 1992

Taylor MA: DSM-III organic mental disorders, in Diagnosis and Classification in Psychiatry. Edited by Tischler G. Cambridge, MA, Cambridge University Press, 1987, pp 147–174

Tucker GJ: DSM-IV: proposals for revision of diagnostic criteria for delirium. International Psychogeriatrics 3:197–208, 1991

Tucker GJ: The DSM-IV criteria for organic disorders, in Current Psychiatric Therapy. Edited by Dunner DL. Philadelphia, PA, WB Saunders, 1993, pp 57–59

Tucker GJ, Popkin MK, Caine ED, et al: Reorganizing the "organic" disorders. Hosp Community Psychiatry 41:722–724, 1990

World Health Organization: The ICD-10 Classification of Mental and Behavioural Disorders: Clinical Descriptions and Diagnostic Guidelines. Geneva, World Health Organization, 1992

Chapter 14

Delirium

Benjamin Liptzin, M.D.
Sue E. Levkoff, Sc.D.
Gary L. Gottlieb, M.D., M.B.A.
Jerry C. Johnson, M.D.

Statement of the Issues

The diagnostic category of "Delirium" presents some special problems in current classification schemes. Although there are no specific criteria for Delirium in ICD-9 (World Health Organization 1977) or ICD-10 (World Health Organization 1992), DSM-III (American Psychiatric Association 1980) did recognize this disorder and provided specific criteria. These criteria were based on extensive clinical experience, particularly the experience of general hospital psychiatrists. Although no phenomenologic studies were published between the time of introduction of DSM-III and its revision DSM-III-R (American Psychiatric Association 1987), the diagnostic criteria for Delirium were altered substantially. Changes were made after extensive discussion and the development of consensus among recognized experts but without data from field testing or clinical research. Key changes included 1) the addition of "disorganized thinking, as indicated by rambling, irrelevant, or incoherent speech" as a required criterion; 2) the separation of the attentional deficit from reduced level of consciousness, with the former becoming a required criterion and the latter in the group of six symptoms of which two are required; and 3) the shifting of disorientation and memory impairment from required to the group of six symptoms. The requirement of a short time course and fluctuation during the day was maintained from DSM-III but no specific directions are given on how to interpret some symptoms (e.g., memory impairment) that may have been present for a long time. The requirement in DSM-III for a specific etiologic factor was broadened to include the presumption of an etiologic organic factor if nonorganic mental disorders could be excluded.

In this review, we summarize the studies done since the introduction of explicit criteria in DSM-III and identify limitations that are inherent in the application of the DSM-III and DSM-III-R criteria. Additionally, we present data from two large studies of Delirium that operationalized diagnostic criteria for Delirium and examined the utility of current classification systems. Finally, options for DSM-IV are presented.

Significance of the Issues

The absence of agreed on diagnostic criteria has led to widely varying estimates of the prevalence of Delirium (Levkoff et al. 1991b). Furthermore, the presence of Delirium in demented patients may be underrecognized because of the overlap between the syndromes. The requirement for a known or presumed specific etiologic factor has emphasized unitary rather than multiple etiologies for Delirium. Frequent changes in criteria have made it difficult to compare studies.

Methods

A search was conducted of the medical, psychiatric, and psychological literature looking for empirical studies of Delirium. A computer search was done in 1989 with Medline using terms such as *delirium, confusion,* and *acute confusional state.* The search was confined to journal articles published in English. The reference lists of recent review articles or chapters (e.g., Beresin 1988; Liston 1989) were also reviewed. Researchers who participated in a conference on Delirium sponsored by the National Institute of Mental Health in June 1989 were also asked for most recent references.

Following the conference, a review paper on the epidemiology of delirium was prepared summarizing studies published through 1990 (Levkoff et al. 1991a).

In addition to the literature review, data collected from two prospective studies of delirium in medically hospitalized older adults were analyzed. The first study (Johnson et al. 1990) was a prospective study of delirium at the Hospital of the University of Pennsylvania (HUP) that explicitly operationalized DSM-III criteria as a component of evaluation by a single psychiatrist as the "gold standard" for diagnosis. The frequency and severity of DSM-III symptoms were collected for all patients evaluated, and patients with delirium were compared to nondelirious control subjects. The second study (Levkoff et al. 1991a) was the Harvard Study of Acute Confusion in which data on specific symptoms were collected by research assistants without requiring that patients meet DSM-III or DSM-III-R criteria. Neither of these studies excluded patients with dementia. The options for DSM-IV presented in this chapter draw heavily on these data sets since no other published studies have operationalized the diagnostic criteria as explicitly nor tested them in large populations.

Results

The literature of the past decade regarding delirium and its diagnosis is dominated by reviews synthesizing the state of the art in diagnosis, evaluation of associated medical disorders, and clinical management (Beresin 1986, 1988; Levkoff et al. 1986; Lipowski 1983, 1984, 1987, 1989; Liston 1982, 1989). Although these reviews address many of the limitations in the knowledge base regarding this disorder and are helpful clinical teaching tools, they do not provide any empirical data for better defining the syndrome. Additionally, despite associated morbidity and mortality rates and potential reversibility, physician recognition of this disorder is notoriously poor (McCartney and Palmateer 1985; Trzepacz et al. 1985). Lipowski (1983) blamed a lack of progress in recognition, management, and clinical research in delirium on inconsistency and lack of clarity in terminology and on the absence of stable diagnostic criteria. This lack of consistent and specific terminology has contributed to underrecognition of the disorder and to substantial clinical uncertainty. Consistent nomenclature and reliably applicable diagnostic criteria are necessary to identify homogeneous patient populations and for more effective research, teaching, and clinical efforts.

Several investigators have examined risk factors and morbidity associated with delirium in populations selected because of presumed vulnerability to development of this syndrome (Gustafson et al. 1988; Levkoff et al. 1988; Rogers et al. 1989; Trzepacz et al. 1985). Unfortunately, none of these studies described how diagnostic criteria were employed or the ease or difficulty of using the diagnostic classification system selected.

Rabins and Folstein (1982) compared morbidity and mortality in hospitalized patients with delirium and dementia referred for psychiatric consultation. Determination of clouding of consciousness was based on a psychiatrist's interpretation of the patient's "mental state along a continuum from inaccessible to accessible" (p. 149). A vague definition of accessibility was used and "any impairment of consciousness" (p. 149) was considered to be abnormal. The authors recognized the limitations in this diagnostic assessment. They suggested evaluation of the importance of the other DSM-III criteria in making the diagnosis of delirium.

The ability of the Mini-Mental State Exam (Folstein et al. 1975) to identify cases of dementia and delirium among hospitalized patients was confirmed by an analysis of these data (Anthony et al. 1982). However, the authors concluded that the Mini-Mental State Exam could not reliably distinguish patients with delirium from those with dementia. Using a psychiatrist's clinical evaluation as a gold standard, Anthony and colleagues (1985) found that a standardized rating of global accessibility was 90% sensitive and 95% specific in screening for delirium. The importance of the other diagnostic criteria described in DSM-III and DSM-III-R was not described.

Growing recognition of the importance of delirium has generated several epidemiologic studies that have employed standard diagnostic criteria. However, most of these studies do not describe how or by whom diagnostic criteria were applied. Erkinjuntti and colleagues (1986), Cameron and colleagues (1987), and Rockwood (1989) all used DSM-III criteria to screen for delirium in hospitalized patients. None of these investigators described how criteria were applied. Additionally, psychiatrists' evaluations using these criteria were not used as diagnostic gold standards or correlated with screening instruments as has been suggested by other investigators (Anthony et al. 1985; Rabins and Folstein 1982). Cameron and colleagues attempted to "test the Diagnostic and Statistical Manual III Criteria on Medical Inpatients." They reported that "delirium could be readily and reliably detected using the DSM-III criteria" (p. 1009). However, the authors did not describe how they trained their observers to rate each symptom or whether the diagnosis was made on a more global impression. Furthermore, although they reported a kappa statistic for interrater reliability of 0.62, this was based on only 56 of the 133 patients in the cohort. They did not describe whether those 56 patients were selected based on likelihood of having delirium. Furthermore, they did not describe the interrater reliability of individual symptoms or symptom domains (e.g., clouding of consciousness) or the relationship of individual domains to the overall judgment of whether delirium was present or not. The study makes clear that the DSM-III criteria do not include operational definitions of symptoms such as clouding of consciousness.

Trzepacz and colleagues (1988) recognized the multifaceted nature of delirium and the importance of distinguishing delirium from other psychiatric and neurological disorders. They developed the Delirium Rating Scale (DRS). The DRS defines 10 areas that are associated with delirium in DSM-III and throughout the literature. Each of the DRS items is measured for presence and severity, with an explicit description of presentation required for scoring. Each symptom (e.g., temporal onset of symptoms or perceptual disturbance) is given a severity rating, and item ratings are summed to provide a total score. Interestingly, disorientation and attentional disturbances are lumped in one item on "cognitive status" with a possible maximum of 4, whereas perceptual disturbances and hallucination type are separate items with a maximum score of 3 each. The authors evaluated the DRS in a small field trial of medically hospitalized patients referred for psychiatric evaluation and in small control groups who were diagnosed with dementia, schizophrenia, or with no psychiatric disorder. The DRS distinguished delirious patients from individuals with other psychiatric disorders and from nonpsychiatric control subjects. Interrater reliability between two independent raters yielded an intraclass correlation coefficient of .97. Although the authors noted that their rating scale could be valuable in research regarding the phenomenology of delirium, the frequency and severity of each of the symptoms in delirious and nondelirious patients were not reported. Additionally, some of the DSM-III criteria are not included in the DRS. However, this study represented an important advance in the measurement of symptoms and in characterization of delirium on the basis of numerous aspects of clinical presentation but has not been used in subsequent published studies.

Francis and colleagues (1990) reported a prospective study of delirium in hospitalized elderly but did not use explicit operationalized criteria. They also excluded patients with severe dementia and patients from nursing homes. A minority of patients with delirium in this study had a single identifiable etiologic factor.

The prospective study of delirium in medically hospitalized older adults at HUP (Johnson et al. 1990) and the Harvard Study of Acute Confusion (Levkoff et al. 1991a) used different methods to operationalize DSM-III criteria for delirium. Both studies evaluated their methods prospectively in large populations of acutely ill patients. The HUP study used a single psychiatrist to apply operationalized criteria as a gold standard for diagnosis. The Harvard study developed an effective screening instrument administered by research assistants after a field trial validating assessments with those performed by a psychiatrist or a neurologist (Albert et al. 1992). These studies are unique in their examination of the application of DSM-III criteria in delirious and nondelirious populations of older adults and in analyses of the frequency and severity of observed symptoms in both populations. A review of findings from these studies is useful in synthesizing recommendations for evolution of the diagnostic approach to this disorder. The HUP study examined only the application of the DSM-III criteria and focused deliberately on a detailed operationalization of symptoms as they could be elicited by a psychiatrist. The more flexible approach of the Harvard study allowed an evaluation of the DSM-III, the DSM-III-R, and the ICD-10 research criteria (Liptzin et al. 1991).

The HUP delirium study attempted to apply widely accepted and well-standardized clinical behavioral measures, used commonly in psychiatric and cognitively impaired populations, to define and rate specifically each of the DSM-III criteria. In areas like clouding of consciousness, where standard instruments are not used widely, measures were used that had been evaluated previously in delirious populations (e.g., the accessibility scale [Anthony et al. 1985]). This approach allowed for reproducibility of methods and ensured reliability. The approach to defining DSM-III criteria was somewhat arbitrary. However, it was based on limited examples of operational criteria for delirium in the literature (Trzepacz et al. 1988; Williams et al. 1985). Historical evidence for dementia prior to admission was sought in all patients. The characteristics of the patients, the prevalence of delirium, and associated medical disorders are described in detail elsewhere (Johnson et al. 1990).

Using the methods described, of 235 patients screened, 48 subjects (20%) were delirious at some point during the hospital stay; 38 subjects (16%) were delirious on admission; and 10 other patients (4%) developed delirium after the first hospital day. Using a case-control model, the frequency of DSM-III symptoms was compared in the delirious and nondelirious groups. By definition, all of the required DSM-III symptoms were present in 100% of the delirious subjects. However, because of the age of the population, a substantial number of individuals had a history of impairment in cognition or a previous diagnosis of dementia prior to the study period: 13.8% of the patients without delirium had a history of memory impairment for greater than 6 months, and 7.3% of the nondelirious group had a previous diagnosis of dementia. In contrast, 65.9% and 41.9% of the patients with delirium had histories of these conditions, respectively. Of the patients without delirium, 34% had some impairment in orientation, and 64% of this group had difficulty with memory.

All of the nonrequired DSM-III symptoms had a significant association with delirium ($P < .0001$). Perceptual disturbances were found in 75% of the delirious patients and 3% of the nondelirious patients. Incoherence was exhibited by 76% of the delirious patients and 6% of the nondelirious patients. A disorder in the sleep-wake cycle was demonstrated in 96% of the delirious patients and 65% of the nondelirious patients. Measurable changes in psychomotor function were exhibited by 93% of the delirious patients and 40% of the nondelirious patients.

The major methodological departure of this study was a careful description of the observations that were used to establish each of the DSM-III criteria, which should improve diagnostic reliability. Assurance of validity is hindered by the lack of gold standards for criterion validity. The content validity of this approach is based solely on the judgment of the clinical experts who established the DSM-III criteria.

Impairment in cognition is ubiquitous among older adults, even in the community (Evans et al. 1989). When hospitalized, older adults may appear to be more impaired cognitively than they are at baseline. Memory impairment and disorientation are significantly associated with delirium, but are not specific markers for the disorder. Close to two-thirds of the control patients in this population exhibited impairment in memory, and more than a third of the nondelirious patients also showed impairment in orientation. Clearly, when examining hospitalized older adults, clinicians should not rely on impairment in cognition alone when distinguishing delirium from dementia or from normal aging. As mentioned, DSM-III-R "reduced" disorientation and memory impairment to nonexplicit criteria status. Therefore, it is now possible for individuals to have no impairment in cognition and meet criteria for delirium. Previous studies in this area contradict this notion. Because the HUP investigators used impairment of cognition as evidenced by an Mini-Mental State Exam score of less than 24 as a screening criterion, they could not effectively evaluate the effect of this change in the criterion.

Among the nonrequired criteria, perceptual disturbance and incoherence appeared to have the highest specificity in diagnosing delirium among non-psychiatric medically infirm older adults. Further understanding of the phenomenology of delirium should allow for better recognition of the specific types of thought process and content disorders associated with this disorder. This should facilitate the design of measurement tools that more specifically measure frequency and severity of the symptoms most likely to be associated with this disorder. For example, tangentiality and circumstantiality may be associated frequently with dementia as well as delirium. It is conceivable that other forms of derailment may be more specifically associated with delirium.

Disturbances of the sleep-wake cycle, although associated more frequently with delirium, were also seen in about two-thirds of the patients who were not delirious. In a hospital setting, where patients are confined to bed, medicated with central nervous system toxic drugs and frequently awakened during the night for procedures, disturbances of the sleep-wake cycle are ubiquitous. Additionally, older adults are likely to be less comfortable in a strange environment, and the medical disorders associated with hospitalization may be important risk factors for sleep disorder. A gross measure of sleep-wake disturbance was not useful in distinguishing patients with delirium from other medically hospitalized older adults. Finer measures that describe activity level during the daytime, functional ability, and the ability to initiate and terminate sleep would be more useful. DSM-III-R accepts reduced level of consciousness (e.g., difficulty keeping awake during examination) as a nonexplicit criterion for delirium. This provision may increase specificity regarding changes in sleep-wake function.

Overall, the HUP study found that the required and nonrequired symptoms for the diagnosis of DSM-III delirium constitute an identifiable syndrome clinically and statistically. They describe a group of patients with clear deficits in attention, cognition, function, and behavior.

The Harvard Study of Acute Confusion operationalized the criteria for delirium and field tested the Delirium Symptom Interview (Albert et al. 1992) in 50 elderly hospitalized patients. In the development of the Delirium Symptom Interview, several issues emerged. Some of the criteria in DSM-III or DSM-III-R were inherently problematic to rate. For example, as discussed earlier, "insomnia" is very difficult to judge in a general hospital population. Any of the factors associated with sleep disorder and its treatment may cause delirium but do not necessarily indicate the presence of delirium. Similarly, decreased psychomotor activity may be present because the patient is physically ill and confined to bed rather than because the patient is delirious. Rating speech as rambling, irrelevant, or incoherent may be impossible in an ill or hard-of-hearing patient who does not produce much speech. In rating disorientation or memory impairment, there are no specific directions in DSM-III or DSM-III-R whether to count as positive these symptoms if due to an underlying dementia. If they are counted as positive, the rate of delirium would clearly be higher in demented patients because they already met some of the criteria. This raises the whole issue of the overlap of symptoms of dementia with those of delirium, which makes it difficult to know how to use or rate the requirement for acuteness and fluctuation. What if some features fluctuate but others are more consistently present even over long periods? Moreover, the DSM-III and DSM-III-R criteria require a specific etiologic factor. Similar to Francis and colleagues (1990), in many or most cases, it was impossible to implicate any individual factor when a patient had multiple physical impairments and was receiving multiple medications.

In a prospective study of delirium in hospitalized elderly, the Delirium Symptom Interview was used to rate symptoms of delirium so that diagnoses could be derived retrospectively using any combination of symptoms rated. The number of patients diagnosed as delirious using DSM-III or DSM-III-R or ICD-10 criteria were compared (Liptzin et al. 1991). Of the 125 cases that met DSM-III criteria, 26 did not meet DSM-III-R criteria. Of the 104 patients who met DSM-III-R criteria, 8 did not meet DSM-III criteria. The mean age for both the DSM-III and the DSM-III-R delirious groups was 86 years and the mean length of stay was 20 and 19 days, respectively, not a significant difference. Similarly, the mortality rates at 6 months in the two groups were not significantly different (23% versus 26%, respectively). This suggests that both criteria sets identified overlapping groups of patients who were clearly delirious but that DSM-III criteria were more inclusive and therefore preferable because they missed fewer clearly delirious patients than DSM-III-R criteria.

Data were also analyzed to address the relationship of preexisting diagnosis of dementia to the development of delirium and to see whether it is preferable to have a diagnosis of "dementia with delirium" as opposed to diagnosing both conditions independently. Table 14–1 presents the data comparing delirious patients with and without preexisting dementia and shows that the two groups are not significantly different in age, sex, residence, length of stay, or mortality. Other analyses confirmed the widely held view that dementia or preexisting cognitive impairment is a major risk factor for the development of delirium (Schor et al. 1992). Any study that ignores or excludes this group of patients is missing the majority of patients with delirium in a hospital setting. Furthermore, the criterion in DSM-III or DSM-III-R that symptoms develop over a short period of time is problematic since

Table 14–1. Characteristics of patients with Delirium who also had or did not have Dementia

Characteristics	Dementia ($n = 58$)	No Dementia ($n = 67$)	Total ($N = 125$)
Age (years)	87.5	84.8	86.1
Men (%)	36.2	38.8	37.6
HRCA (%)	63.8	55.2	59.2
Length of stay (days)	19.5	18.1	18.8
Mortality in hospital (%)	6.9	4.5	5.6
Mortality within 6 months (%)	27.6	19.4	23.2

Note. HRCA = Hebrew Rehabilitation Center for the Aged.

some cognitive symptoms may be preexisting.

Table 14–2 demonstrates that the symptom patterns are virtually identical for the patients who met DSM-III criteria for delirium who had a diagnosis of dementia and those who did not. These findings suggest that delirium may not be phenomenologically different in these two groups and therefore the two diagnoses should be made independently.

Discussion

Several options are available for DSM-IV.

Option 1: Keep the DSM-III-R Criteria

Advantages. This option represents the least change for clinicians and investigators who are just becoming familiar with DSM-III-R criteria. It also preserves the specific examples that begin to operationalize the criteria.

Disadvantages. The DSM-III-R criteria may miss a substantial number of patients who most clinicians would agree have delirium. In the Harvard study, of 26 patients who met DSM-III but not DSM-III-R criteria, 7 had sparse speech, and this made it impossible to judge whether their thinking was disorganized. This problem could be corrected by adding the phrase "if testable" after disorganized thinking. Another 7 cases had all of the symptoms of DSM-III-R delirium at some point in their hospital stay but not all within the same 24-hour period. This problem could be addressed by expanding the window for having all the symptoms from 24

Table 14–2. Pattern of symptoms of patients with DSM-III Delirium and with or without Dementia: number and percentage with new symptoms in each DSM-III domain

	Dementia ($n = 58$)		No Dementia ($n = 67$)		Total ($N = 125$)	
Symptoms	*n*	%	*n*	%	*n*	%
Disorientation[a]	43	74	55	82	98	78
Disturbance of consciousness[b]	58	100	67	100	125	100
Sleep disturbance	41	71	55	82	96	77
Perceptual disturbance	29	50	19	28	48	38
Speech disturbance	54	93	62	93	116	93
Psychomotor disturbance	54	93	62	93	116	93
Fluctuating behavior	20	34	27	40	47	38

[a]If a patient was disoriented when first seen, a new symptom of disorientation was not required for making the diagnosis of delirium.
[b]All patients were required to have a new disturbance of consciousness for the DSM-III diagnosis of delirium.

to 72 hours. The Harvard study required that the symptoms occur within the same 24-hour period but DSM-III and DSM-III-R have no such requirement. However, even with both of these changes, a large number of patients with symptoms of delirium who do not meet these criteria but would be diagnosed with delirium using ICD-10 (which does not have explicit criteria) would be excluded. Both the Harvard and the HUP studies suggest that sleep disturbance and psychomotor retardation are heavily confounded in a hospital setting and do not add to the specificity of the diagnosis.

Option 2: Eliminate Any Explicit Criteria

Advantages. This is the approach taken in ICD-10. It recognizes the paucity of available data and would provide the most opportunity for ongoing phenomenologic research into the syndrome of delirium.

Disadvantages. This approach provides no guidance to clinicians or investigators in defining the syndrome of delirium. It represents a step backward from the overall DSM thrust toward use of explicit diagnostic criteria. Lack of a clear description of the syndrome could perpetuate the underdiagnosis by physicians and nurses who might have too restrictive a definition or one that focuses on a particular subtype, namely the hyperactive, agitated, or hallucinating delirious patient.

Option 3: Revert to the DSM-III Criteria

Advantages. Since most clinicians have some familiarity with the criteria used in DSM-III, this change would not be too disruptive. These criteria clearly define a group of delirious patients and a syndrome comprised of well-correlated symptoms that most clinicians would agree are reasonable.

Disadvantages. This change would raise many questions about how or why the DSM-III-R changes were made. It also drops the useful attempt in DSM-III-R to provide some examples that help operationalize the criteria (although these could be added). This change would not be consistent with ICD-10. The requirement for cognitive impairment rather than a change in cognitive function is a sensitive but not a specific marker for this disorder, particularly in the elderly. As noted under the disadvantages of Option 1, sleep disturbance and psychomotor retardation are difficult to rate because they are heavily confounded in a hospitalized population.

Option 4: Use New Criteria

Advantages. Table 14–3 provides proposed criteria. This approach would focus on the core symptoms that define the syndrome rather than the associated symptoms that could be included in the text. It would encourage clinicians to recognize patients with these disturbances. The core symptoms can be operationally defined and reliably rated, as shown in two large-scale studies. The etiology would be defined in the title.

Table 14–3. Proposed DSM-IV diagnostic criteria for Delirium due to a nonpsychiatric medical condition

A. Impairment of consciousness (i.e., reduced clarity of awareness of the environment) with reduced ability to focus, sustain, or shift attention.

B. Change in cognition (such as memory deficit, disorientation, language disturbance, perceptual disturbance) that is not better accounted for by a preexisting, established, or evolving dementia.

C. The disturbance develops over a short period of time (usually hours to days) and tends to fluctuate over the course of the day.

D. There is evidence from the history, physical examination, or laboratory findings of a general medical condition judged to be etiologically related to the disturbance. (In the absence of evidence that either a specific general medical condition or a specific substance is etiologically related to the delirium, the condition should be coded as "Delirium due to unknown etiology" if it cannot be better accounted for by another Axis I disorder, e.g., Manic episode.)

Disadvantages. Clinicians and investigators would have to become familiar with new criteria. This change would be based on a limited data base. Additionally, the need to query for misperceptions and thought process disorder, found to be relatively specific markers for delirium in the HUP study, might be lost, particularly by nonpsychiatric clinicians.

Recommendations

Based on the synthesis of the data and experience of the HUP study of delirium in hospitalized elderly and the Harvard study, the recommended option is number 4. It provides explicit criteria that can be operationalized and rated reliably and that define the essence of what clinicians and investigators mean by delirium. Key associated symptoms (i.e., conceptual disorganization, perceptual disturbances, sleep disturbance, and psychomotor retardation or agitation) would be described in the text but not required for making the diagnosis. Change in cognitive function, not merely its presence, will be useful in distinguishing delirium from dementia and allow recognition of concurrent diagnoses. Delirium will be diagnosed independently of dementia. Etiology will be defined in the title. Maintaining the use of explicit criteria will help educate clinicians and encourage them to make the diagnosis more frequently. Finally, this approach allows for the broadest possible ongoing phenomenologic research.

References

Albert MS, Levkoff SE, Reilly C, et al: The delirium symptom interview: an interview for the detection of delirium in hospitalized patients. J Geriatr Psychiatry Neurol 5:14–21, 1992

American Psychiatric Association: Diagnostic and Statistical Manual of Mental Disorders, 3rd Edition. Washington, DC, American Psychiatric Association, 1980

American Psychiatric Association: Diagnostic and Statistical Manual of Mental Disorders, 3rd Edition, Revised. Washington, DC, American Psychiatric Association, 1987

Anthony JC, LeResche L, Niaz U, et al: Limits of the Mini-Mental State as a screening test for dementia and delirium among hospital patients. Psychol Med 12:397–408, 1982

Anthony JC, LeResche LA, Vonkorff MR, et al: Screening for delirium on a general medical ward: the tachistoscope and a global accessibility rating. Gen Hosp Psychiatry 7:36–42, 1985

Beresin E: Delirium, in Inpatient Psychiatry: Diagnosis and Treatment, 2nd Edition. Edited by Sederer LI. Baltimore, MD, Williams & Wilkins, 1986

Beresin EV: Delirium in the elderly. J Geriatr Psychiatry Neurol 1:127–143, 1988

Cameron DJ, Thomas RI, Mulvihill M, et al: Delirium: a test of the Diagnostic and Statistical Manual III criteria on medical inpatients. J Am Geriatr Soc 35:1007–1010, 1987

Erkinjuntti T, Wikstrom J, Palo JU, et al: Dementia among medical inpatients: evaluation of 2000 consecutive admissions. Arch Intern Med 146:1923–1926, 1986

Evans DA, Funkenstein HH, Albert MS, et al: Prevalence of Alzheimer's disease in a community population of older persons: higher than previously reported. JAMA 262:2551–2556, 1989

Folstein MF, Folstein SE, McHugh PR: "Mini-Mental State": a practical method for grading the cognitive state of patients for clinicians. J Psychiatr Res 12:189–198, 1975

Francis J, Martin D, Kapoor WN: A prospective study of delirium in hospitalized elderly. JAMA 263:1097–1101, 1990

Gustafson Y, Berggren D, Brannstrom B, et al: Acute confusional states in elderly patients treated for femoral neck fracture. J Am Geriatr Soc 36:525–530, 1988

Johnson JC, Gottlieb GL, Sullivan E, et al: Using DSM-III criteria to diagnose delirium in elderly general medical patients. The Journals of Gerontology: Medical Sciences 45:113–119, 1990

Levkoff SE, Besdine R, Wetle T: Acute confusional states (delirium) in the hospitalized elderly, in Annual Review of Gerontology and Geriatrics, Vol 6. Edited by Eisdorfer C. New York, Springer, 1986, pp 1–25

Levkoff SE, Safran C, Cleary PD, et al: Identification of factors associated with the diagnosis of delirium in elderly hospitalized patients. J Am Geriatr Soc 36:1099–1104, 1988

Levkoff SE, Cleary P, Liptzin B, et al: Epidemiology of delirium: an overview of research issues and findings. International Psychogeriatrics 3:149–167, 1991a

Levkoff SE, Liptzin B, Cleary PD, et al: Review of research instruments and techniques used to detect delirium. International Psychogeriatrics 3:253–271, 1991b

Lipowski ZJ: Transient cognitive disorders (delirium, acute confusional states) in the elderly. Am J Psychiatry 140:1426–1436, 1983

Lipowski ZJ: Acute confusional states (delirium) in the elderly, in Clinical Neurology of Aging. Edited by Albert ML. Boston, MA, Oxford University Press, 1984

Lipowski ZJ: Delirium (acute confusional states). JAMA 258:1789–1792, 1987

Lipowski ZJ: Delirium in the elderly patient. N Engl J Med 320:578–582, 1989

Liptzin B, Levkoff SE, Cleary PD, et al: An empirical study of diagnostic criteria for delirium. Am J Psychiatry 148:454–457, 1991

Liston EH: Delirium in the aged. Psychiatr Clin North Am 5:49–66, 1982

Liston EH: Delirium, in Treatments of Psychiatric Disorders. Edited by Karasu TB. Washington, DC, American Psychiatric Association, 1989, pp 804–815

McCartney JR, Palmateer LM: Assessment of cognitive deficit in geriatric patients. J Am Geriatr Soc 33:467–471, 1985

Rabins PV, Folstein MF: Delirium and dementia: diagnostic criteria and fatality rates. Br J Psychiatry 140:149–153, 1982

Rockwood K: Acute confusion in elderly medical patients. J Am Geriatr Soc 37:150–154, 1989

Rogers MP, Liang MH, Daltroy LH, et al: Delirium after elective orthopedic surgery: risk factors and natural history. Int J Psychiatry Med 19:109–121, 1989

Schor JD, Levkoff SE, Lipsitz LA, et al: Risk factors for delirium in hospitalized elderly. JAMA 267:827–831, 1992

Trzepacz PT, Teague GB, Lipowski ZJ: Delirium and other organic mental disorders in a general hospital. Gen Hosp Psychiatry 7:101–106, 1985

Trzepacz PT, Baker RW, Greenhouse J: A symptom rating scale for delirium. Psychiatr Res 23:89–97, 1988

Williams MA, Campbell EB, Raynor WJ, et al: Predictors of acute confusional states in hospitalized elderly patients. Res Nurs Health 8:31–40, 1985

World Health Organization: International Classification of Diseases, 9th Revision. Geneva, World Health Organization, 1977

World Health Organization: The ICD-10 Classification of Mental and Behavioural Disorders: Clinical Descriptions and Diagnostic Guidelines. Geneva, World Health Organization, 1992

Chapter 15

Dementia

George W. Rebok, Ph.D.
Marshal F. Folstein, M.D.

Statement of the Issues

The importance of accurately diagnosing dementia, estimating its severity, and monitoring its course has led to the development of a number of assessment methods including neuropsychological test batteries and new imaging procedures. One major purpose of the present review is to evaluate the reliability (reproducibility) and validity of the DSM-III-R (American Psychiatric Association 1987) criteria and other standard antemortem clinical diagnostic criteria for dementia in light of the methods used to operationalize these criteria. These methods must be sufficiently reliable and valid to ensure accuracy of diagnosis and staging.

Since dementia can be caused by several different diseases, it also is important to determine if the pattern of dysfunction observed is characteristic of Alzheimer's disease, multi-infarct dementia, Huntington's disease, or another pathology. One distinction that has proven useful clinically for making these discriminations is the distinction between cortical and subcortical dementia (Albert et al. 1974; Cummings 1986; S. E. Folstein et al. 1990; McHugh and Folstein 1973). Although the clinical validity of the cortical-subcortical distinction has yet to be established, it is increasingly clear that cortical dementias present with a distinctly different cluster of symptoms than do subcortical dementias. The second purpose of the present review is to examine the usefulness of the cortical-subcortical distinction as a valid discriminator of subtypes of dementia and the adequacy of DSM-III-R criteria for making these discriminations. Currently, the criteria are more appropriate for diagnosing cortical dementia syndromes than subcortical syndromes. For example, the clinical evidence for memory impairment relies on recall (retrieval) deficits rather than recognition memory deficits, which show different patterns in cortical dementia (both recall and recognition impaired) and subcortical dementia (recall impaired, recognition spared) (Brandt 1991). In addition, current criteria do not adequately reflect the mental slowing and absence of frank aphasia, apraxia, and agnosia that characterize subcortical dementia.

Significance of the Issues

The term *dementia* replaces older terms such as *chronic brain syndrome, senility,* or *hardening of the arteries.* Dementia is a psychological syndrome of a deterioration of multiple cognitive functions in clear consciousness. It also is classified according to pathology such as dementia of the Alzheimer's type or dementia due to Huntington's disease. Each pathological type is classified according to etiology such as genetic and sporadic forms.

A major advance occurred in 1980 with the publication of DSM-III (American Psychiatric Association 1980), which defined dementia in terms of observable clinical criteria and incorporated clinical features not present in other diagnostic schemes (e.g., ICD-9 [World Health Organization 1978]). The DSM-III-R further specified the diagnostic criteria and differentiated among some of the best known types of dementia. In 1984, a special work group established by the National Institute of Neurological and Communicative Disorders and Stroke (NINCDS) and the Alzheimer's Disease and Related Disorders Association (ADRDA) defined a set of clinical criteria for the diagnosis of possible, probable, and definite Alzheimer's disease (McKhann et al. 1984). Currently, the ICD-10 (World Health Organization 1989) system is being developed with the aim of providing a more complete description of the main clinical features of dementia and other disorders and a set of diagnostic guidelines indicating the number and balance of symptoms required for a confident diagnosis.

Although clinical diagnostic criteria for dementia have improved markedly over the past decade, further refinements and improvements should be considered for several reasons. First, more accurate diagnostic schemes would be helpful to clinicians in their day-to-day practice since the human cost of misdiagnosing dementia and of missing any conditions that might be arrested or reversed is quite high (Forette et al. 1989). Second, increased specification of diagnostic criteria would provide a more accurate means of comparing the results of research involving different patient populations, types of dementia, and methodologies. Third, the evaluation of the current therapeutic trials and the epidemiological studies of prevalence and incidence of dementia could be improved by improving the criteria and accuracy of diagnosis (National Institutes of Health 1988). Finally, more accurate diagnostic criteria are important for genetic considerations and family counseling, even though the exact inheritance patterns of many dementing illnesses are under active investigation.

At the present time, diagnosis of many of the most important dementing illnesses can be confirmed or denied with certainty only at autopsy, the current "gold standard" of accuracy of the clinical diagnosis (Berg et al. 1984; Khachaturian 1985; Marks et al. 1988; McKhann et al. 1984; Tierney et al. 1988). While awaiting the identification of pathognomonic proteins that lead to accurate antemortem diagnosis, further refinements in the clinical criteria might be warranted (National Institutes of Health 1988). Even in cases such as Huntington's disease, where the identification of an abnormal gene is expected, patients and social agencies such as employers and insurance companies will still need a classification that indicates that the abnormal chemistry manifests itself in disabling symptoms. More precise identification of the full range of cognitive and noncognitive symptoms (including depression, delusions, hallucinations, and behavior disorders) will lead to more comprehensive assessments of the severity of the dementia for disability assessment and possibly will indicate subtypes of different prognosis (Stern et al. 1990). Reliable means of documenting mild, moderate, and severe forms of dementia will assist in planning and reimbursing care (Erkinjuntti et al. 1986, 1988; Jorm and Henderson 1985).

One of the major goals of the DSM-IV revision is to achieve greater compatibility between the diagnostic criteria in DSM-IV and ICD-10 (Frances et al. 1989). Table 15–1 provides a direct comparison of criteria for dementia that appear in DSM-III-R and in the most recent draft of ICD-10. Criteria in both systems include impairments of memory and in abstract thinking ability that are sufficient to interfere with daily activities and that occur in clear consciousness. DSM-III-R further specifies criteria for severity of dementia, whereas ICD-10 proposes that the symptoms should have at least 6 months' duration. In addition, the DSM-III-R system describes criteria for dementias arising in the senium and presenium (primary degenerative dementia of the Alzheimer type and multi-infarct dementia) and various psychoactive substance-induced organic mental disorders. The ICD-10 system provides specific diagnostic guidelines for Alzheimer's disease (including early and late onset Alzheimer's disease), vascular dementia (including vascular dementia of acute onset, multi-infarct vascular dementia, and mixed cortical and subcortical vascular dementia), Creutzfeldt-Jakob disease, Huntington's disease, Parkinson's disease, human immunodeficiency virus infection, and dementia in other diseases (World Health Organization 1989). Comparisons of the DSM-III-R and ICD-10 diagnostic criteria to NINCDS/ADRDA criteria for probable Alzheimer's disease also are presented in Table 15–1.

Methods

A search was conducted of the psychiatric, psychological, geriatric, gerontological, and epidemiological literature for research studies dealing with the diagnosis of dementia. The review included a computer search with Medline of the English-language literature covering the period 1980 to 1990. Index terms such as *dementia, diagnostic criteria, Alzheimer's disease,* and *imaging techniques* were used to conduct the search, and a total of 141 citations were generated. The reference lists of relevant articles from the following journals for the period 1985 to 1990 also were reviewed: *Annals of Neurology, Archives of Neurology, Alzheimer's Disease and Associated Disorders—An International Journal, Psychological Medicine, Journal of the American Geriatrics Society, International Journal of Geriatric Psychiatry, Journal of Gerontology, Neurology, American Journal of Psychiatry, British Journal of Psychiatry,* and *Journal of Clinical and Experimental Neuropsychology.* Abstracts of original articles as they appear in *Alzheimer's Disease and Associated Disorders* also were reviewed. The identified publications were reviewed, and references to other articles on dementia were obtained. The reference lists of comprehensive reviews (e.g., Wragg and Jeste 1989) and chapters (e.g., Katzman et al. 1988) were reviewed, and researchers were solicited for papers in press and/or under editorial review. Pre-1980 publications were included where appropriate.

The review focused on studies that provided data on the prevalence, symptoms, diagnosis, and clinical course of dementia and that employed DSM-III-R, ICD-9, NINCDS/ADRDA, or other standard diagnostic criteria. The review particularly focused on studies that distinguished among various types of dementia (e.g., Alzheimer's disease, multi-infarct dementia, Huntington's disease) rather than studies that failed to subdivide the dementia syndrome. A partial list of studies

Table 15–1. Comparison of diagnostic criteria for Dementia

Criteria	DSM-III-R	ICD-10	NINCDS/ADRDA
Memory impairment	R	R	R
Impairment of additional area of cognition (e.g., language, construction, praxis, or personality change)	R	R	D
Confirmed on mental status tests			R
Impaired social or occupational function	R	R	
State of consciousness unclouded	R	R	R
Evidence of specific organic factor etiologically related to the disorder or absence of conditions other than organic mental syndrome	R	R	
Duration of symptoms specified		R	

Note. NINCDS = National Institute of Neurological and Communicative Disorders and Stroke. ADRDA= Alzheimer's Disease and Related Disorders Association. R = required. D = desirable/not required.
Source. Adapted from Katzman et al. (1988).

reviewed, point prevalence rates, diagnostic criteria employed, and types of dementia is shown in Table 15–2 and Table 15–3. Each study was categorized according to the number of demented subjects in the study sample, their average ages, the criteria for dementia, average duration of illness, severity of the dementia, and the reliability and validity of the diagnosis. To explore the diagnostic utility of the cortical-subcortical distinction, we surveyed review articles (e.g., Cummings 1986)

Table 15–2. Prevalence of dementia and severe cognitive impairment

Study	Population	Ages	Diagnoses	Point prevalence
Molsa et al. 1982	Finland	45–54	Degenerative dementia, by exclusion	0.02
		55–64		0.07
		65–74		0.4
		75–84		1.9
		≥ 85		6.3
M. Kramer et al. 1985	U.S. urban	65–74	Severe cognitive impairment, DIS/DSM-III	3.0
		> 75		9.3
Kay et al. 1985	Australia	≥ 70	Mild dementia, moderate dementia, severe dementia, DSM-III	17.5
				5.5
				0.4
Sulkava et al. 1985	Finland	30–64	Multi-infarct dementia	0.08
		65–74		1.4
		75–84		4.3
		> 85		2.5
Schoenberg et al. 1985	U.S. rural	≥ 40	Primary chronic progressive dementia, interview by neurologist	0.5
Larson et al. 1985	U.S. outpatients with suspected dementia	> 60	Alzheimer's disease, drug-induced, alcohol-related, multi-infarct dementia	64.5
				5.0
				4.0
				1.0
Kokmen et al. 1989	U.S. urban	0–54	Alzheimer's disease	0.0
		55–59		0.09
		60–64		0.05
		65–69		0.43
		70–74		1.1
		75–79		3.4
		80–84		7.0
		> 85		12.7
Evans et al. 1989	U.S. urban	65–74	Alzheimer's disease	3.0
		75–84		10.3
		≥ 85		47.2

(continued)

Table 15–2. Prevalence of dementia and severe cognitive impairment *(continued)*

Study	Population	Ages	Diagnoses	Point prevalence
Rocca et al. 1990	Italy urban and rural	60–69	Dementia of all types, DSM-III	0.6
		70–74		3.6
		75–79		8.1
		80–84		17.6
		85–89		40.0
		90–94+		
Heyman et al. 1991	U.S. rural	≥ 65	Dementia of all types, DSM-III, NINCDS/ADRDA	16.0
M. F. Folstein et al. 1991	U.S. urban	65–74	Alzheimer's disease	0.3
		75–84		3.7
		85+		8.2
		65–74	Multi-infarct dementia	0.7
		75–84		1.0
		85+		15.5
		65–74	Mixed	0.2
		75–84		0.6
		85+		1.9
		65–74	Dementia of all types, DSM-III	0.2
		75–84		5.3
		85+		25.6

Note. DIS = Diagnostic Interview Schedule (Robins et al. 1981). NINCDS = National Institute of Neurological and Communicative Disorders and Stroke. ADRDA = Alzheimer's Disease and Related Disorders Association.

and empirical articles (e.g., Heindel et al. 1989) reporting differential patterns of neuropsychological performance between various cortical and subcortical dementias. Data from the Alzheimer's Disease Research Center and the Baltimore Huntington's Disease Project at The Johns Hopkins Hospital also were analyzed for information on the clinical course of dementia and for evidence of cortical and subcortical patterns.

Results

Prevalence and Incidence of Dementia

The results of epidemiological surveys of the prevalence of dementia show a remarkably consistent rate of about 5% for the prevalence of moderate and more

Table 15–3. Reliability and validity of diagnostic criteria in Dementia studies

Study	Population	Ages	Duration	Criteria	Reliability/ validity
Molsa et al. 1982	28 AD	NE	NE	Clinical exam	.69 SN .72 SP
	19 MID				.70 SN .75 SP
	5 CD				.17 SN .91 SP
	Other				.46 SN 1.00 SP
Klein et al. 1985	72 demented 144 nondemented	72 66	NE	DSM-III, MMSE, family report	.88 SN .88 SP (with 5-item decision rule)
Huff et al. 1987b	79 AD 86 controls	67.4 62.6	NE	NINCDS/ADRDA, MMSE, HIS, clinical exam, CT, EEG	.96 SN .86 SP 1.00 SN .89 SP
Martin et al. 1987	11 AD	64.9	3.9	NINCDS/ADRDA, MMSE, CT, EEG	1.00 SN 1.00 SP
Wade et al. 1987	38 AD 10 mixed AD 6 MID 11 other (PSP, Pick's, Creutzfeldt-Jakob, PD)	69.6 74.8 62.5 63.1	8.9 6.6 9.5 5.6	CT, clinical exam, HIS	.87 SN .78 SP
Morris et al. 1988	26 AD 2 controls	72.0 75.8 75.8 77.5	4.3 5.6 8.8	NINCDS/ADRDA, CDR	1.00 SN .65 SP
Kukull and Larson 1989	20 AD 9 mixed AD	71.9	NE	DSM-III, HIS, relative report	.93 SN .43 SP
Forette et al. 1989	55 patients with suspected cognitive impairment	74.4	NE	DSM-III, HIS, CT, clinical exam, MMSE, SCAG, family report	.95 1-year follow-up reliability
Kukull et al. 1990	27 AD 12 mixed AD 4 other	76.0	NE	DSM-III, NINCDS/ ADRDA, ECRDC	.55 reliability .64 (kappa) .37

Note. AD = Alzheimer's disease. NE = not examined. SN = sensitivity. SP = specificity. MID = multi-infarct dementia. CD = combined dementia. MMSE = Mini-Mental State Exam. NINCDS = National Institute of Neurological and Communicative Disorders and Stroke. ADRDA = Alzheimer's Disease and Related Disorders Association. HIS = Hachinski Ischemic Scale. CT = computed tomography. EEG = electroencephalogram. PSP = progressive supranuclear palsy. PD = Parkinson's disease. CDR = Clinical Dementia Rating. SCAG = Sandoz Clinical Assessment Geriatric. ECRDC = Eisdorfer and Cohen Research Diagnostic Criteria.

severe dementia in the age 65 years and over population (Henderson 1983; Kokmen et al. 1989; Rocca et al. 1986) (see Table 15–2). In contrast, the rate of mild dementia has varied from roughly 2% to more than 50% (Henderson and Huppert 1984; Kay et al. 1985). However, these studies have relied on different diagnostic criteria and nonstandardized methods, which contribute to marked variation in prevalence rates.

Several groups of investigators have identified Alzheimer's disease to be the most common of the dementias, accounting for 50%–75% of older patients with dementia seen in psychiatric practice (Kaszniak 1986; Larson et al. 1986; Loeb and Gandolfo 1983). An additional 10%–25% are reported to have multi-infarct dementia, either alone or in combination with Alzheimer's disease (Barclay et al. 1985; Cummings 1987; Kase 1991). Under age 75, the prevalence of Alzheimer's disease and multi-infarct dementia is approximately equal; by age 85 and over Alzheimer's disease is six times more common than multi-infarct dementia (Sulkava et al. 1985). A survey of probable Alzheimer's disease in a community population in East Boston, Massachusetts, reported a prevalence rate of over 47% among those age 85 years and older (Evans et al. 1989). This prevalence rate is much higher than that found in previous studies of severe dementia but similar to those reporting mild impairment (Pfeffer et al. 1987).

There have been very few incidence studies of dementia. In an analysis of available studies, Mortimer (1983) reported that investigators generally report an incidence of approximately 1% per year for the elderly population. Incidence rates for dementia in general, and Alzheimer's disease in particular, have been found to rise dramatically with age (Schoenberg et al. 1987).

Accuracy of Diagnosis Using Current Clinical Criteria

Much current research into the presentation and progression of the dementias in general, and Alzheimer's disease in particular, depends on the accuracy of clinical diagnosis. It is difficult to offer a precise diagnosis early in the course of dementing illness because many are of insidious onset and gradual progression so that the patient and family are unaware of onset, and the full pattern of symptoms develops only over a period of years. The onset of many types of dementia is characterized by memory impairment, but later, as the pathology spreads in the brain, a more distinctive pattern emerges. The diagnosis becomes more certain as the disease progresses and as impairments become more severe. Two small series have reported 100% accuracy of diagnosing Alzheimer's disease following NINCDS/ADRDA criteria (Martin et al. 1987; Morris et al. 1988). A larger series has shown an 80% accuracy rate (Boller et al. 1989), a figure consistent with most published reports that indicate 50%–80% agreement between clinical diagnosis and neuropathological findings (Forette et al. 1989; Sulkava et al. 1983; Wade et al. 1987). Neuropathological confirmation rates of Alzheimer's disease may be lower in cases of presenile onset dementia. In one study (Risse et al. 1990), an 86% accuracy rate was reported in diagnosing patients with senile (i.e., over age 65 years) onset, but only a 61% accuracy rate was obtained in diagnosing presenile onset dementia. Other studies have used longitudinal follow-up as a way of evaluating the accuracy of the diagnosis of dementia (Berg et al. 1988; Forette et al. 1989; Huff et al. 1987a, 1987b; Kaszniak et al. 1986; Rubin et al. 1989). Using cognitive deficits found on neuropsychological tests to evaluate the clinical diagnosis of Alzheimer's disease, Huff and colleagues (1987b) concluded that at 1-year follow-up, NINCDS/ADRDA criteria have a sensitivity of 100% and a specificity of 89%. Forette and colleagues (1989) found an interrater reliability of 95% for clinical diagnosis of dementia a year after initial evaluation using diagnostic criteria comparable to the NINCDS/ADRDA criteria for Alzheimer's disease.

Because no diagnostic test to identify dementia noninvasively has been found, much effort has gone into neuroradiological data—computed tomography (CT), magnetic resonance imaging (MRI), positron-emission tomography (PET), and single photon emission computed tomography (SPECT)—that might assist in the evaluation of dementia. It is thought that atrophy is more evident in dementing illness, and it seems likely that premortem assessment of atrophy can assist in diagnosing Alzheimer's disease, multi-infarct dementia, and other dementias more confidently. Efforts to identify mild Alzheimer's disease using CT, however, have been disappointing; demented patients can have a normal CT scan, and nondemented elderly persons can have significant atrophy (Freedman et al. 1984). Measures of ventricular size most consistently separate groups of Alzheimer's disease from elderly controls without dementia and from patients with other dementing conditions on CT scan (Luxenberg et al. 1987; Mendez et al. 1992), and the rate of ventricular enlargement is correlated with rate of cognitive deterioration. CT studies can reliably validate the Hachinski Ischemic Scale score and are appropriate for identifying focal neurologic signs in multi-infarct dementia (Loeb and Gandolfo 1983; Luxenberg et al. 1987). The use of MRI holds promise because its improved neuroimaging ability has been shown to enhance diagnostic accuracy and to assist in differentiating normal aging from dementia (Bondareff et al. 1988; Filley et al. 1989). Several studies also have demonstrated the utility of PET scans for differentiating Alzheimer's disease from other forms of dementia and from normal aging (Jorm 1985; Small et al. 1989). The SPECT scanning technique may provide a more economical and widely available technique than PET since it does not require a local cyclotron as a positron source. Preliminary work with this technique suggests that it may have an adjunctive role in the diagnosis of dementia in the presence of moderate or severe dementia, but may be less useful for mild cases (DeKosky et al. 1990). SPECT does not seem to be ready for routine use in distinguishing between Alzheimer's disease and multi-infarct dementia (Weinstein et al. 1991).

Olfactory testing may be useful in the diagnostic evaluation of early dementia (Corwin et al. 1986; Serby et al. 1991). Significant deficits in olfactory identification have been reported in the earliest stages of Alzheimer's disease.

Clinical Characteristics Associated With Dementia

Cognitive. The earliest cognitive symptoms of dementia usually appear in the form of subjective complaints of memory deficit, such as forgetting where one has placed familiar objects or forgetting names of familiar people (Reisberg et al. 1982). Difficulties in recent memory, word finding and confrontation naming, and orientation and concentration are manifest during the early stages of the illness. Later stages are characterized by severe disorientation; abnormalities of language, perception, and praxis; disorganization of executive functions such as planning; and slowed rate of information processing (Kaszniak 1986). The relative sparing of language functions in Huntington's disease and Parkinson's disease is in marked contrast to abnormalities of memory, executive abilities, and visuospatial performance.

Behavioral. Evidence suggests that dementing disorders frequently are accompanied by multiple disruptive behaviors, including aggression, angry outbursts, assaultiveness, wandering, repetitive manipulation of objects, and vegetative disorders such as disturbed sleep and incontinence (Rabins et al. 1982; Teri et al. 1989). These behaviors often overshadow cognitive decline as the most critical management problem, but have, until recently, attracted little investigative attention (Cohen-Mansfield et al. 1989; Reisberg et al. 1987; Swearer et al. 1988). It has been reported that about 60% of patients with progressive dementia develop agitated and self-centered behaviors (Reisberg et al. 1987; Rubin et al. 1987), and almost 90% exhibit passive behavior (Rubin et al. 1987). The occurrence and severity of behavioral problems are associated with the severity of dementia and the rapidity of its course (Swearer et al. 1988; Teri et al. 1990). Teri and colleagues (1990) reported that Alzheimer's disease patients with various behavioral problems, in particular agitation, declined at a rate between 1.4 and 5 times faster than patients without such problems.

Affective changes and psychotic symptoms. Accompanying cognitive and behavioral changes in dementia are psychiatric abnormalities, including affective changes, particularly depression, and psychotic symptoms such as delusions and hallucinations (Rubin and Kinscherf 1989). No consensus yet exists about the prevalence, phenomenology, and implications of these symptoms in Alzheimer's disease and other dementing illnesses (Berrios 1985).

The frequency of depressed mood in patients with Alzheimer's disease ranged from 0% to 87% in 30 studies reviewed by Wragg and Jeste (1989). Higher frequencies (42%–55%) tended to occur in samples drawn from acute care facilities, whereas lower frequencies (0%–17%) were noted among dementia patients from research clinics. Depressive symptoms were more common than depressive disorders. In two additional studies reviewed here, estimates of the prevalence of clinical depression in dementia were 17% (Rovner et al. 1989) and 40% (Lazarus et al. 1987). Variation between studies may be attributable to differences in sampling procedures, assessment methods, diagnostic criteria, and length of follow-up as well as lifetime prevalence estimates (Wragg and Jeste 1989). The rate of depression appears to increase dramatically—fourfold in one report (Mackenzie et al. 1989)—if diagnosis based on data from the patient interview is replaced with diagnosis based on information supplied by the family.

Depression also is a common complication of multi-infarct dementia. In two studies prevalence rates of 25% (Reding et al. 1985) and 30% (Bucht et al. 1984) were reported. Depression is commonly found in Huntington's disease and Parkinson's disease as well (S. E. Folstein et al. 1990; Kaszniak 1986).

Among outpatients with dementia, estimated incidence of delusions or paranoias has ranged from 21% to 57%, and from 12% to 30% for hallucinations (Patterson et al. 1990). Persecutory delusions are the most commonly observed psychotic symptom in dementia (Wragg and Jeste 1989). Although reported frequencies for Alzheimer's disease patients who had experienced delusions at some time in the course of their illness ranged from 10% to 73%, the greatest number of studies reviewed by Wragg and Jeste had clusters between 30% and 38% (median – 33.5%). Delusions were found in 40% of patients with multi-infarct dementia at the time of examination compared with 30% of patients with Alzheimer's disease (Cummings et al. 1987). The reports reviewed by Wragg and Jeste suggested that hallucinations of any type occurred only slightly less frequently than other psychotic symptoms in Alzheimer's disease (median = 28%, range 21%–49%). Higher frequencies were observed in patients in acute care settings, whereas lower frequencies were seen in patients referred for outpatient care. Visual hallucinations occurred more often (median = 22%) than did auditory hallucinations (median = 13%) in patients with Alzheimer's disease. One study that directly compared the frequency of hallucinations in Alzheimer's disease with that of other dementias found the frequencies to be essentially the same (Cummings et al. 1987), but both auditory and visual hallucinations were more common in multi-infarct dementia than in Alzheimer's disease.

Systems for Staging Dementia

In addition to an accurate description of diagnostic criteria, it is useful for clinical and research purposes to develop systems for staging patients with dementing disorders. Three methods have been proposed for patients with Alzheimer's disease. In the earliest attempt, Sjögren and colleagues (1952) used particular symptoms to describe three stages—the first showing amnestic disturbances, lack of spontaneity and initiative, and a rapidly progressive disorientation; the second showing progressive dementia and increasingly apparent focal symptoms in the form of aphasia, apraxia, and agnosia; and the third, or terminal stage, showing profound dementia, progressive deterioration of speech, and rapid physical decline. The focal symptoms in the second stage are thought to begin after an interval of 1–3 years following onset, with a clear language disorder marking the beginning of the second stage. Clinical analysis of a group of probands followed for several years provided strong support for the three stages of Sjögren and colleagues.

More recently, means for staging the severity of Alzheimer's disease have been proposed by Reisberg and colleagues (1986, 1989) and by Berg (1984; Botwinick et al. 1986). On the basis of clinical observations, Reisberg and colleagues (1982) described the Global Deterioration Scale (GDS), with seven major, clinically distinguishable stages ranging from normality to severe degenerative dementia: GDS 1, "normal," neither subjective nor objective evidence of cognitive deficit in a clinical interview; GDS 2, "forgetfulness," subjective evidence of cognitive deficit only; GDS 3, "early confusional," deficit manifest but subtle in a clinical interview; GDS 4, "late confusional," deficit readily manifest in a clinical interview; GDS 5, "early dementia," deficit sufficient to interfere with independent survival and functioning; GDS 6, "mid-dementia," deficit sufficient to interfere with activities of daily living; and GDS 7, "late dementia," deficit sufficient to interfere with all activities of daily living. Current data on the reliability of this staging procedure show high correlations between the GDS and mental status questionnaires (.89 with the Mini-Mental State Exam [M. F. Folstein et al. 1975] and .83 with the Mental Status Questionnaire). Similarly high relationships are observed between global GDS assessments and a psychometric deterioration score. Weaker relationships are reported between structural measures of brain change and global deterioration (*r* s = .33 and .31, respectively, for CT assessments and progressive ventricular dilatation). A similar method for staging the severity of Alzheimer's disease is the clinical dementia rating (Berg 1984). The clinical dementia rating is based on clinician evaluations of cognitive abilities in the areas of memory, orientation, judgment and problem solving, community affairs, home and hobbies, and personal care. Both the reliability of the clinical dementia rating (Burke et al. 1988) and validity of the diagnosis by this procedure (Morris et al. 1988) have been demonstrated by neuropathological confirmation in a consecutive series of 31 autopsies.

To examine the staging issue further, G. W. Rebok and M. F. Folstein (unpublished study, 1990) analyzed the data from 181 outpatients participating in a longitudinal study of Alzheimer's disease at the Johns Hopkins Alzheimer's Disease Research Center. Mini-Mental State Exam (M. F. Folstein et al. 1975) scores and psychiatrist ratings of behavioral symptoms, depression, delusions, and hallucinations for each patient were obtained at the time of the initial visit to the research center. Among the Alzheimer's disease patients, the most pronounced deficits in the first 3 years of the disease were seen on the recall and calculation items; deteriorative changes also occur on time and place orientation items, a result supporting earlier observations of Sjögren and colleagues (1952) and those of Reisberg and colleagues (1986, 1989). The results also lend support to the findings of an item analysis of the Mini-Mental State Exam, which showed a differential pattern of loss in 86 possible and probable Alzheimer's disease patients, with memory and calculation items showing the earliest loss, followed by time and place orientation items (Ashford et al. 1989). Increasingly progressive declines in more focal abilities such as registration, naming, repetition, following a command, reading, writing, and copying begin to occur around years 3 and 4, a result also supporting Sjögren, Reisberg, and the item analysis results (Ashford et al. 1989).

At the time of their initial evaluation, 40.9% of the Alzheimer's disease patients displayed wandering behavior, 56.4% apathy, 64.6% irritability, 50.3% social withdrawal, 16.0% physical violence, 30.4% crying spells, 14.9% incontinence, and 39.2% insomnia. About 7.6% of the Alzheimer's disease patients had major depression, 24.7% delusions, and 12.0% hallucinations. Thus, behavioral and psychiatric problems appear to be quite common in Alzheimer's disease. There appears to be considerable variability in the pattern of symptoms by duration of illness, although the behavioral symptoms of wandering, apathy, irritability, and insomnia and the psychiatric symptoms of depression and delusions tend to be found in higher percentages of patients as duration increases. Reisberg and colleagues (1986) also have shown that most behavioral measures demonstrate significant deterioration in performance between stages of the GDS from levels 2 to 6. The relationship of psychiatric symptoms to the clinical stage of Alzheimer's disease is equivocal, with some studies reporting symptoms occurring early in the course of the disease, and other studies reporting symptoms as more common in the advanced stages (Wragg and Jeste 1989).

The GDS and the clinical dementia ratings discussed earlier include progressive functional changes (Berg 1984; Reisberg et al. 1986). By definition, dementia implies cognitive impairment that is severe enough to interfere with social and occupational role functioning. G. W. Rebok and M. F. Folstein (unpublished study,

1990) examined functional changes by examining the percentage of perfect activities of daily living scores for Alzheimer's disease patients by duration of illness and found that functional abilities decreased with duration of dementia. However, cognitive losses and functional impairments seem to be two distinct aspects of dementia severity that must be assessed separately (Reed et al. 1989).

Validity of the Cortical/Subcortical Distinction

The term *subcortical dementia* was used by McHugh and Folstein (1973) to describe cognitive impairments in patients with Huntington's disease. Later the term was extended to other disorders as well, including progressive supranuclear palsy, Wilson's disease, Parkinson's disease, spinocerebellar degeneration, lacunar state, traumatic injuries, and multiple sclerosis (Cummings 1986). Dementia also has been observed in patients with acquired immunodeficiency syndrome (AIDS) (Goethe et al. 1989; Navia et al. 1986b; Van Gorp et al. 1989), and neuropathological studies indicate that the subcortical regions of the brain are most affected, with the cortical regions being relatively spared. The exact sites of neuropathological involvement in AIDS-related dementia, however, remain controversial (Navia et al. 1986a).

The features distinguishing subcortical dementia from cortical dementia have been elaborated by several investigators (Albert et al. 1974; Cummings 1986; S. E. Folstein et al. 1990; McHugh and Folstein 1973). Subcortical dementia has been characterized by marked slowness of mental processing, forgetfulness (failure of retrieval), apathy and depressed mood, and relative lack of disorders of acquired knowledge (e.g., aphasia, apraxia, and agnosia). These patients often have disorders of gait and movement early in the disease course. Cortical dementia, on the other hand, is characterized by amnesia (storage deficit), aphasia, constructional apraxia, agnosia, and emotional alteration in the form of emotional indifference, emotional lability, and paranoia. Fine motor movements and gait are preserved until late in the disease.

The validity of the two dementia categories has been challenged on neuroanatomical grounds (Whitehouse 1986). Most dementing diseases are neither *purely* cortical nor subcortical. Analysis of neuropathological changes has not supported a broad cortical-subcortical distinction. For example, subcortical changes in the nucleus basalis of Meynert are seen in both Alzheimer's disease (a cortical dementia) and Parkinson's disease (a subcortical dementia).

In contrast, when specific neuropsychological measures have been used, the two dementia subtypes can be differentiated, and such a distinction may be clinically meaningful (Cummings 1986). For example, semantic memory disruptions differ in Alzheimer's disease and Huntington's disease patients (Butters et al. 1988; Troster et al. 1989). Huntington's disease patients have selective deficits in the perception of personal, or egocentric, space, whereas Alzheimer's disease patients have difficulties with the perception of extrapersonal spatial relations (Brouwers et al. 1984). However, Huntington's disease patients are as distinguishable from subcortically demented Parkinson's disease patients as they are from cortically demented Alzheimer's disease patients in their verbal learning performance (J. H. Kramer et al. 1990). These latter results indicate the difficulty of using Parkinson's disease as an exemplar of the subcortical condition.

To explore further the utility of the cortical dementia and subcortical dementia distinction, G. W. Rebok and M. F. Folstein (unpublished study, 1990) compared the Mini-Mental State Exam scores of the previously discussed sample of 181 Alzheimer's disease patients with those of 55 Huntington's disease patients. The Huntington's disease patients were enrolled in the Baltimore Huntington's Disease Project at The Johns Hopkins Hospital. Rebok and Folstein also collapsed the data across years of illness and compared the Mini-Mental State Exam scores of the Alzheimer's disease and Huntington's disease patients with those of nondemented older adult control subjects. Because duration is not necessarily the most sensitive index of disease severity, Brandt and colleagues (1988) grouped their data according to overall Mini-Mental State Exam score using a different sample of Alzheimer's disease and Huntington's disease patients. Three major findings emerged from these two separate analyses. First, Alzheimer's disease results in a more severe global dementia than Huntington's disease, as shown by scores on the Mini-Mental State Exam. Second, impairment of recall memory is particularly severe in Alzheimer's disease patients compared to Huntington's disease patients in all but the most severe cases of dementia. Third, Huntington's disease patients show relatively more difficulty with tests of attention.

The literature reviewed above and the G. W. Rebok and M. F. Folstein (unpublished study, 1990) analyses support the utility of the cortical-subcortical division for characterizing various dementia subtypes. Subcortical dementia also is seen in cases of severe depression but is not necessarily associated with depression.

Discussion

Although the differential diagnosis of dementing illness has improved considerably, inaccuracy in antemortem diagnosis of Alzheimer's disease and related disorders is common, ranging as high as 45% (Morris et al. 1988; Rocca et al. 1986). There appears to be a need to develop more sensitive and specific clinical criteria for the diagnosis of dementia during life. Improvements in accuracy of the diagnostic process are essential for educating families and caregivers about the nature of dementia and the manner in which disabilities are manifested as well as for evaluating the efficacy of various treatments. Certain treatments or management approaches may lead to global improvements; others may improve cognition but not psychiatric or behavioral symptoms; and others may improve certain symptoms at the expense of other symptoms.

We also need to identify dementia subgroups and subtypes, beginning with the broad distinction between cortical and subcortical dementia (Brandt et al. 1988; Brouwers et al. 1984; Cummings 1986; J. H. Kramer et al. 1990). Individual variation is evident in the presentation of dementia and in the rate and intensity of its progression (Folstein 1989; Jorm 1985; Kaszniak et al. 1986), which has led to greatly increased interest in longitudinal follow-up assessment (Boller et al. 1991; Burns et al. 1991; Grady et al. 1988; Knesevich et al. 1985; Rebok et al. 1990).

Recommendations

The diagnostic criteria in DSM-IV could be expanded beyond the cognitive symptoms of DSM-III-R to include psychiatric symptoms such as depression, delusions, and hallucinations found in early and late-stage dementia. Symptoms of behavioral disturbance, including violence, insomnia, wandering, dependency, and incontinence, also should be included as part of the diagnostic criteria. In DSM-III-R, dementia is diagnosed only when loss of cognitive function is sufficient to interfere with social or occupational functioning. It is suggested that these criteria be modified to state that "The disturbance in A and B has produced a significant deterioration in work or usual social activities or relationships with others." For the criterion involving delirium, we suggest including "alertness," "responsiveness," and "problems in attention" in addition to consciousness. Problems in attention refer to "the inability to focus, maintain, and direct attention." The cognitive criteria for mild dementia should include documented memory loss greater than the normative values for age, some difficulties with time and space orientation, difficulties in reasoning and planning, and maintenance of social judgment. For moderate dementia, the criteria should include severe memory loss with memory for overlearned material intact, full disorientation to time and partial disorientation to space, severe difficulties solving complex problems, and impairments in social judgment. The criteria for severe dementia should include severe memory loss for new and familiar material, orientation to person only, and inability to make judgments or solve problems. Because the pattern of symptoms of different pathologies such as Alzheimer's disease and Huntington's disease differ, staging of dementia should be disease-specific.

The severity of dementia should include the multiaxial approach. Thus dementia could be one of mild impairment but of severe disability for some patients who depend on intellect in their occupations.

DSM-III-R includes criteria for the diagnosis of multi-infarct dementia, which can be distinguished from Alzheimer's disease by its history of onset, clinical features, and subsequent course. These criteria include "stepwise deteriorating course with 'patchy' distribution of deficits. . . . focal neurologic signs and symptoms. . . . evidence from history, physical examination, or laboratory tests of significant cerebrovascular disease" (p. 123). Few patients have been found to meet these criteria exactly (Katzman et al. 1988). The scoring system introduced by Hachinski and colleagues (1975) and modified by Rosen and colleagues (1980) has been more useful in differential diagnoses, but the sensitivity and specificity of these criteria are under study. MRI techniques also aid in distinguishing multi-infarct dementia from other dementing illnesses but the specificity of these findings are not yet established. Criteria for multi-infarct dementia should be established by a clinical examination, documented by the modified Hachinski scale, and confirmed by CT or MRI, and ultimately by neuropathological examination.

Criteria for AIDS-related dementia are under development and are not yet ready for publication.

Behavioral and psychiatric symptoms have not received adequate attention in the diagnostic assessment of dementia and should be included as part of the diagnostic criteria. However, the behavioral measures currently used are largely new and of unknown reliability. There also is a heavy reliance on caregivers for measures of psychiatric and behavioral symptoms. More refined guidelines are still needed for the use of data from multiple sources in the diagnosis of dementia.

It is necessary to distinguish between impairment of functioning and disability, since impairment need not imply disability. However, there is no consensus about the degree of functional disability needed to qualify for a diagnosis of dementia or the scales to be used for determining deterioration (Katzman et al. 1988; Stern et al. 1990). Finally, the cortical-subcortical dichotomy, although clinically useful, may be overly simplistic. Its utility may be limited to certain dementia subtypes that exhibit the expected patterns of deficits such as AIDS, hydrocephalus, and Huntington's disease.

References

Albert ML, Feldman RG, Willis AL: The "subcortical dementia" of progressive supranuclear palsy. J Neurol Neurosurg Psychiatry 37:121–130, 1974

American Psychiatric Association: Diagnostic and Statistical Manual of Mental Disorders, 3rd Edition. Washington, DC, American Psychiatric Association, 1980

American Psychiatric Association: Diagnostic and Statistical Manual of Mental Disorders, 3rd Edition, Revised. Washington, DC, American Psychiatric Association, 1987

Ashford JW, Kolin P, Colliver JA, et al: Alzheimer patient evaluation and the mini-mental state: item characteristic curve analysis. J Gerontol 44:P139–P146, 1989

Barclay LL, Zemcov A, Blass JP, et al: Survival in Alzheimer's disease and vascular dementias. Neurology 35:834–840, 1985
Berg L: Clinical dementia rating. Br J Psychiatry 145:339, 1984
Berg L, Danziger WL, Storandt M, et al: Predictive features in mild senile dementia of the Alzheimer type. Neurology 34:563–569, 1984
Berg L, Miller JP, Storandt M, et al: Mild senile dementia of the Alzheimer type, 2: longitudinal assessment. Ann Neurol 23:477–484, 1988
Berrios GE: Presbyophrenia: clinical aspects. Br J Psychiatry 147:76–79, 1985
Boller F, Lopez OL, Moosy J: Diagnosis of dementia: clinicopathological correlations. Neurology 29:76–79, 1989
Boller F, Becker JT, Holland AL, et al: Predictors of decline in Alzheimer's disease. Cortex 27:9–17, 1991
Bondareff RC, Raval J, Colletti PM, et al: Quantitative magnetic resonance imaging and the severity of dementia in Alzheimer's disease. Am J Psychiatry 145:853–856, 1988
Botwinick J, Storandt M, Berg L: A longitudinal behavioral study of senile dementia of the Alzheimer type. Arch Neurol 43:1124–1127, 1986
Brandt J: Cognitive impairments in Huntington's disease: insights into the neuropsychology of the striatum, in Handbook of Neuropsychology, Vol 5. Edited by Boller F, Grafman J. Amsterdam, Elsevier Science, 1991, pp 241–266
Brandt J, Folstein SE, Folstein MF: Differential cognitive impairment in Alzheimer's disease and Huntington's disease. Ann Neurol 23:555–561, 1988
Brouwers P, Cox C, Martin A, et al: Differential perceptual-spatial impairment in Huntington's and Alzheimer's dementias. Arch Neurol 41:1073–1076, 1984
Bucht G, Adolfson R, Winblad B: Dementia of the Alzheimer type and multi-infarct dementia: a clinical description and diagnostic problems. J Am Geriatr Soc 32:491–497, 1984
Burke WJ, Miller J, Rubin E, et al: The reliability of the Washington University Clinical Dementia Rating. Arch Neurol 45:31–32, 1988
Burns A, Jacoby R, Levy R: Progression of cognitive impairment in Alzheimer's disease. J Am Geriatr Soc 39:39–45, 1991
Butters N, Salmon DP, Heindel W, et al: Episodic, semantic, and procedural memory: some comparisons of Alzheimer and Huntington disease patients, in Aging and the Brain, Vol 32. Edited by Terry RD. New York, Raven, 1988, pp 63–87
Cohen-Mansfield J, Marx MS, Rosenthal AS: A description of agitation in a nursing home. J Gerontol 44:M77–M84, 1989
Corwin J, Serby M, Rostrosen J: Olfactory deficits in AD: what we know about the nose. Neurobiol Aging 7:580–581, 1986
Cummings JL: Subcortical dementia: neuropsychology, neuropsychiatry, and pathophysiology. Br J Psychiatry 149:682–697, 1986
Cummings JL: Multi-infarct dementia: diagnosis and management. Psychosomatics 28:117–126, 1987
Cummings JL, Miller B, Hill MA, et al: Neuropsychiatric aspects of multi-infarct dementia and dementia of the Alzheimer type. Arch Neurol 44:389–393, 1987
DeKosky ST, Shih W-J, Schmitt FA, et al: Assessing utility of single photon emission computed tomography (SPECT) scan in Alzheimer's disease: correlation with cognitive severity. Alzheimer Dis Assoc Disord 4:14–23, 1990
Erkinjuntti T, Laaksonen R, Sulkava R, et al: Neuropsychological differentiation between normal aging, Alzheimer's disease, and vascular dementia. Acta Neurol Scand 74:393–403, 1986

Erkinjuntti T, Haltia M, Palo J, et al: Accuracy of the clinical diagnosis of vascular dementia: a prospective clinical and post-mortem neuropathological study. J Neurol Neurosurg Psychiatry 51:1037–1044, 1988

Evans DA, Funkenstein H, Albert MS, et al: Prevalence of Alzheimer's disease in a community population of older persons: higher than previously reported. JAMA 262:2551–2556, 1989

Filley CM, Davis KA, Schmitz SP, et al: Neuropsychological performance and magnetic resonance imaging in Alzheimer's disease and normal aging. Neuropsychiatry, Neuropsychology, and Behavioral Neurology 2:81–91, 1989

Folstein MF: Heterogeneity in Alzheimer's disease. Neurobiol Aging 10:434–435, 1989

Folstein MF, Folstein SE, McHugh PR: Mini-Mental State: a practical method for grading the cognitive status of patients for the clinician. J Psychiatr Res 12:189–198, 1975

Folstein MF, Bassett SS, Anthony JC, et al: Dementia: case ascertainment in a community survey. J Gerontol 46:M132–M138, 1991

Folstein SE, Brandt J, Folstein MF: Huntington's disease, in Subcortical Dementia. Edited by Cummings JL. New York, Oxford University Press, 1990, pp 87–107

Forette F, Henry JF, Orgogozo JM, et al: Reliability of clinical criteria for the diagnosis of dementia: a longitudinal multicenter study. Arch Neurol 46:646–648, 1989

Frances AJ, Widiger TA, Pincus HA: The development of DSM-IV. Arch Gen Psychiatry 46:373–375, 1989

Freedman M, Knoefel J, Naeser M, et al: Computerized axial tomography in aging, in Clinical Neurology of Aging. Edited by Albert ML. New York, Oxford University Press, 1984, pp 139–148

Goethe KE, Mitchell JE, Marshall DW, et al: Neuropsychological and neurological function of human immunodeficiency virus seropositive asymptomatic individuals. Arch Neurol 46:129–133, 1989

Grady CL, Haxby JV, Horwitz B, et al: Longitudinal study of the early neuropsychological and cerebral metabolic changes in dementia of the Alzheimer type. J Clin Exp Neuropsychol 10:576–596, 1988

Hachinski VC, Iliff LD, Zilhka E, et al: Cerebral blood flow in dementia. Arch Neurol 32:632–637, 1975

Heindel WC, Salmon DP, Shults CW, et al: Neuropsychological evidence for multiple implicit memory systems: a comparison of Alzheimer's, Huntington's, and Parkinson's disease patients. J Neurosci 9:582–587, 1989

Henderson AS: The coming epidemic of dementia. Aust N Z J Psychiatry 17:117–127, 1983

Henderson AS, Huppert FA: The problem of mild dementia. Psychol Med 14:5–11, 1984

Heyman A, Fillenbaum G, Prosnitz B, et al: Estimated prevalence of dementia among elderly black and white community residents. Arch Neurol 48:594–598, 1991

Huff FJ, Growdon JH, Corkin S, et al: Age at onset and rate of progression of Alzheimer's disease. J Am Geriatr Soc 35:27–30, 1987a

Huff FJ, Becker JT, Belle SH, et al: Cognitive deficits and clinical diagnosis of Alzheimer's disease. Neurology 37:1119–1124, 1987b

Jorm AF: Subtypes of Alzheimer's dementia: a conceptual analysis and critical review. Psychol Med 15:543–553, 1985

Jorm AF, Henderson AS: Possible improvements to the diagnostic criteria for dementia in DSM-III. Br J Psychiatry 147:394–399, 1985

Kase CS: Epidemiology of multi-infarct dementia. Alzheimer Dis Assoc Disord 5:71–76, 1991

Kaszniak AW: The neuropsychology of dementia, in Neuropsychological Assessment of Neuropsychiatric Disorders. Edited by Grant I, Adams KM. New York, Oxford University Press, 1986, pp 172–220

Kaszniak AW, Wilson RS, Fox JH, et al: Cognitive assessment in Alzheimer's disease: cross-sectional and longitudinal perspectives. Can J Neurol Sci 13:420–423, 1986

Katzman R, Lasker B, Berstein N: Advances in the diagnosis of dementia: accuracy of diagnosis and consequences of misdiagnosis of disorders causing dementia, in Aging and the Brain, Vol 32. Edited by Terry RD. New York, Raven, 1988, pp 17–61

Kay DWK, Henderson AS, Scott R, et al: Dementia and depression among the elderly living in the Hobart community: the effect of the diagnostic criteria and the prevalence rates. Psychol Med 15:771–788, 1985

Khachaturian ZS: Diagnosis of Alzheimer's disease. Arch Neurol 42:1097–1105, 1985

Klein LE, Roca RP, McArthur J, et al: Diagnosing dementia: univariate and multivariate analyses of the Mental Status Examination. J Am Geriatr Soc 33:483–488, 1985

Knesevich JW, Toro F, Morris JC, et al: Aphasia, family history, and the longitudinal course of senile dementia of the Alzheimer type. Psychiatry Res 14:255–263, 1985

Kokmen E, Beard CM, Offord KP, et al: Prevalence of medically diagnosed dementia in a defined United States population: Rochester, Minnesota, January 1, 1975. Neurology 39:773–776, 1989

Kramer JH, Levin BE, Brandt J, et al: Differentiation of Alzheimer's, Huntington's, and Parkinson's disease patients on the basis of verbal learning characteristics. Neuropsychology 3:111–120, 1990

Kramer M, German PS, Anthony JC, et al: Patterns of mental disorder among the elderly residents of eastern Baltimore. J Am Geriatr Soc 33:236–245, 1985

Kukull WA, Larson EB: Distinguishing Alzheimer's disease from other dementias: questionnaire responses of close relatives and autopsy results. J Am Geriatr Soc 37:521–527, 1989

Kukull WA, Larson EB, Reifler BV, et al: Interrater reliability of Alzheimer's disease diagnosis. Neurology 40:257–260, 1990

Larson EB, Reifler BV, Sumi SM, et al: Diagnostic evaluation of 200 elderly outpatients with suspected dementia. J Gerontol 40:536–543, 1985

Larson E, Reifler BV, Sumi SM, et al: Diagnostic tests in the evaluation of dementia: a prospective study of 200 elderly outpatients. Arch Intern Med 146:1917–1921, 1986

Lazarus LW, Newton N, Cohler B, et al: Frequency and presentation of depressive symptoms in patients with primary degenerative dementia. Am J Psychiatry 144:41–45, 1987

Loeb C, Gandolfo C: Diagnostic evaluation of degenerative and vascular dementia. Stroke 14:399–401, 1983

Luxenberg JS, Haxby JV, Creasey H, et al: Rate of ventricular enlargement in dementia of the Alzheimer type correlates with rate of neuropsychological deterioration. Neurology 37:1135–1140, 1987

Mackenzie TB, Robiner WN, Knopman DS: Differences between patient and family assessments of depression in Alzheimer's disease. Am J Psychiatry 146:1174–1178, 1989

Marks WA, Shuman RM, Leech RW, et al: Cerebral degenerations producing dementia: importance of neuropathologic confirmation of clinical diagnoses. J Geriatr Psychiatry Neurol 1:187–198, 1988

Martin EM, Wilson RS, Penn RD, et al: Cortical biopsy results in Alzheimer's disease: correlation with cognitive deficits. Neurology 37:1201–1204, 1987

McHugh PR, Folstein MF: Subcortical dementia. Address to the American Academy of Neurology, Boston, MA, April 1973

McKhann G, Drachman D, Folstein M, et al: Clinical diagnosis of Alzheimer's disease: report of the NINCDS-ADRDA Work Group under the auspices of Department of Health and Human Services Task Force on Alzheimer's disease. Neurology 34:939–944, 1984

Mendez MF, Mastri AR, Zander BA, et al: A clinicopathological study of CT scans in Alzheimer's disease. J Am Geriatr Soc 40:476–478, 1992

Molsa PK, Marttila RJ, Rinne UK: Epidemiology of dementia in a Finnish population. Acta Neurol Scand 65:541–552, 1982

Morris JC, McKeel DW, Fulling K, et al: Validation of clinical diagnostic criteria for Alzheimer's disease. Ann Neurol 24:17–22, 1988

Mortimer JC: Alzheimer's disease and senile dementia: prevalence and incidence, in Alzheimer's Disease. Edited by Reisberg B. New York, Free Press, 1983, pp 141–148

National Institutes of Health: Differential diagnosis of dementing diseases. Alzheimer Dis Assoc Disord 2:4–15, 1988

Navia BA, Jordan BA, Price RW: The AIDS dementia complex, I: clinical features. Ann Neurol 19:517–524, 1986a

Navia BA, Cho ES, Petito CK: The AIDS dementia complex, II: neuropathology. Ann Neurol 19:525–535, 1986b

Patterson MB, Schnell AH, Martin RJ, et al: Assessment of behavioral and affective symptoms in Alzheimer's disease. J Geriatr Psychiatry Neurol 3:21–30, 1990

Pfeffer RI, Afifi AA, Chance JM: Prevalence of Alzheimer's disease in a retirement community. Am J Epidemiol 125:420–436, 1987

Rabins PV, Mace NL, Lucas MJ: The impact of dementia on the family. JAMA 248:333–335, 1982

Rebok GW, Brandt J, Folstein M: Longitudinal cognitive decline in patients with Alzheimer's disease. J Geriatr Psychiatry Neurol 3:91–97, 1990

Reding M, Haycox J, Blass J: Depression in patients referred to a dementia clinic. Arch Neurol 42:894–896, 1985

Reed BR, Jagust WJ, Seab JP: Mental status as a predictor of daily function in progressive dementia. Gerontologist 29:804–807, 1989

Reisberg B, Ferris SH, de Leon MJ, et al: The Global Deterioration Scale for assessment of primary degenerative dementia. Am J Psychiatry 139:1136–1139, 1982

Reisberg B, Ferris SH, Shulman E, et al: Longitudinal course of normal aging and progressive dementia of the Alzheimer's type: a prospective study of 106 subjects over a 3.6 year mean interval. Prog Neuropsychopharmacol Biol Psychiatry 10:571–578, 1986

Reisberg B, Borenstein J, Salob SP, et al: Behavioral symptoms in Alzheimer's disease: phenomenology and treatment. J Clin Psychiatry 48 (suppl):9–15, 1987

Reisberg B, Ferris SH, Kluger A, et al: Symptomatic changes in CNS aging and dementia of the Alzheimer type: cross-sectional, temporal, and remediable concomitants, in Diagnosis and Treatment of Senile Dementia. Edited by Bergener M, Reisberg B. Berlin, Springer-Verlag, 1989

Risse SC, Raskind MA, Nochlin D, et al: Neuropathological findings in patients with clinical diagnoses of probable Alzheimer's disease. Am J Psychiatry 147:168–172, 1990

Robins LN, Helzer JE, Croughan J, et al: National Institute of Mental Health Diagnostic Interview Schedule: its history, characteristics, and validity. Arch Gen Psychiatry 38:381–389, 1981

Rocca WA, Amaducci LA, Schoenberg BS: Epidemiology of clinically diagnosed Alzheimer's disease. Ann Neurol 19:415–424, 1986

Rocca WA, Bonaiuto S, Lippi A, et al: Prevalence of clinically diagnosed Alzheimer's disease and other dementing disorders: a door-to-door survey in Appignano, Macerata Province, Italy. Neurology 40:626–631, 1990

Rosen WG, Terry RD, Fuld PA, et al: Pathological verification of Ischemic Score in differentiation of dementia. Ann Neurol 7:486–488, 1980

Rovner BW, Broadhead J, Spencer M, et al: Depression and Alzheimer's disease. Am J Psychiatry 146:350–353, 1989

Rubin EG, Kinscherf DA: Psychopathology of very mild dementia of the Alzheimer type. Am J Psychiatry 146:1017–1021, 1989

Rubin EH, Morris JC, Berg L: The progression of personality changes in senile dementia of the Alzheimer's type. J Am Geriatr Soc 35:721–725, 1987

Rubin EH, Morris JC, Grant EA, et al: Very mild senile dementia of the Alzheimer type, I: clinical assessment. Arch Neurol 46:379–382, 1989

Schoenberg BS, Anderson DW, Haerer AF: Severe dementia: prevalence and clinical features in a biracial US population. Arch Neurol 42:740–743, 1985

Schoenberg BS, Kokmen E, Okazaki H: Alzheimer's disease and other dementing illnesses in a defined United States population: incidence rates and clinical features. Ann Neurol 22:724–729, 1987

Serby M, Larson P, Kalkstein D: The nature and course of olfactory deficits in Alzheimer's disease. Am J Psychiatry 148:357–360, 1991

Sjögren T, Sjögren H, Lindgren AGH: Morbus Alzheimer and morbus Pick. Acta Psychiatrica et Neurologica Scandinavica 82 (suppl):1–152, 1952

Small GW, Kuhl DE, Riege WH, et al: Cerebral glucose metabolic patterns in Alzheimer's disease: effect of gender and age at dementia onset. Arch Gen Psychiatry 46:527–532, 1989

Stern Y, Hesdorffer D, Sano M, et al: Measurement and prediction of functional capacity in Alzheimer's disease. Neurology 40:8–14, 1990

Sulkava R, Haltia M, Paetau A, et al: Accuracy of clinical diagnosis in primary degenerative dementia: correlation with neuropathological findings. J Neurol Neurosurg Psychiatry 46:9–13, 1983

Sulkava R, Wikstrom J, Aromaa A, et al: Prevalence of severe dementia in Finland. Neurology 35:1025–1029, 1985

Swearer JM, Drachman DA, O'Donnell BF, et al: Troublesome and disruptive behaviors in dementia: relationships to diagnosis and disease severity. J Am Geriatr Soc 36:784–790, 1988

Teri L, Borson S, Kiyak A, et al: Behavioral disturbance, cognitive dysfunction, and functional skill: prevalence and relationship in Alzheimer's disease. J Am Geriatr Soc 37:109–116, 1989

Teri L, Hughes JP, Larson EB: Cognitive deterioration in Alzheimer's disease: behavioral and health factors. J Gerontol 45:P58–P63, 1990

Tierney MC, Fisher RH, Lewis AJ, et al: The NINCDS-ADRDA work group criteria for the clinical diagnosis of probable Alzheimer's disease: a clinicopathologic study of 57 cases. Neurology 38:359–364, 1988

Troster AI, Salmon DP, McCullough D, et al: A comparison of category fluency deficits associated with Alzheimer's disease and Huntington's disease. Brain Lang 37:500–513, 1989

Van Gorp WG, Mitrushina M, Cummings JL, et al: Normal aging and the subcortical encephalopathy of AIDS: a neuropsychological comparison. Neuropsychiatry, Neuropsychology, and Behavioral Neurology 2:5–20, 1989

Wade JPH, Mirsen TR, Hachinski VC, et al: The clinical diagnosis of Alzheimer's disease. Arch Neurol 44:24–29, 1987

Weinstein HC, Haan J, van Royen EO, et al: SPECT in the diagnosis of Alzheimer's disease and multi-infarct dementia. Clin Neurol Neurosurg 93:39–43, 1991

Whitehouse PJ: The concept of subcortical and cortical dementia: another look. Ann Neurol 19:1–6, 1986

World Health Organization: Mental disorders and guide to their classification in accordance with the ninth revision of the International Classification of Diseases. Geneva, World Health Organization, 1978

World Health Organization: Mental and behavioral disorders of psychological development: 1989 draft of chapter 5. Geneva, World Health Organization, 1989

Wragg RE, Jeste DV: Overview of depression and psychosis in Alzheimer's disease. Am J Psychiatry 146:577–587, 1989

Chapter 16

Amnestic Disorders

Eric D. Caine, M.D.

Statement and Significance of the Issues

The diagnostic criteria for amnestic disorder in DSM-III-R (American Psychiatric Association 1987) are generally satisfactory, although they require simplification to highlight the central feature of the condition—that is, the inability to learn and subsequently to recall new information. DSM-III-R also fails to provide any criterion for defining the degree of impairment necessary for diagnosing a disorder. Defining such a criterion is necessary in light of the known changes in cognitive functioning associated with normal aging processes, where memory efficiency (one among several alterations) may decline, although not to an extent that is impairing socially or vocationally (see Caine, Chapter 21, this volume).

Within the context of the amnestic disorder literature review, two additional issues emerge as relevant for consideration in the revision of DSM-III-R. First, it is uncertain whether objective criteria exist to differentiate amnestic disorders from dementing disorders. At the extremes, clinicians can effectively distinguish individuals with isolated, severe memory problems (in the absence of other cognitive abnormalities) from patients suffering multiple intellectual deficits, including not only memory, but language, visuospatial processing, "executive" functions, and so on. It is the intermediate forms that present difficulties. Second, should transient global amnesia be included in DSM-IV? It is essential to establish whether sufficient diagnostic clarity exists, as well as understanding whether this is, indeed, a truly distinct phenomena. Additionally, it is important to consider whether this disorder is so infrequently seen by psychiatrists to preclude useful inclusion in psychiatric nosology.

Methods

A Medline search covering the years from 1984 to 1989 identified more than 300 papers dealing with memory disorders. Only 3 were directly or indirectly pertinent to the question of separating amnestic disorder from dementia; 18 concerned transient global amnesia.

Results

Amnesia Versus Dementia

Corkin and colleagues (1985) and Squire and Shimamura (1986) accepted the notion that "amnestic disorders" are focal rather than globally affecting multiple cognitive functions. However, neither group grappled specifically with the question of how much nonmemory cognitive impairment is allowable before the concept of an isolated memory disorder is no longer tenable. Indeed, one gains the impression that these authors would broadly define amnestic disorders, as long as memory impairment is, by far, *predominant* relative to other possible impairments. This was particularly true for Corkin and colleagues, where they included disorders that can cause a variety of nonmemory impairments (e.g., closed head injury, anoxia, herpes simplex encephalitis).

Jacobson and Lishman (1987) attempted to examine the issue specifically in 38 patients with alcoholic Korsakoff's syndrome (amnestic disorder). They utilized the National Adult Reading Test to provide an estimate of premorbid verbal intelligence and compared these estimated premorbid IQ scores with results obtained using the Wechsler Adult Intelligence Scale. Memory impairment was assessed using the Wechsler Memory Scale, and the degree of memory decline versus overall cognitive decline was based on a comparison of current full scale IQ minus memory quotient versus premorbid estimated IQ minus current IQ. Using this methodology, Jacobson and Lishman suggested that the population of Korsakoff patients was characterized by considerable variation, with a transition from pure memory loss to global intellectual deficits indicative of dementia. They suggested an arbitrary standard for separating the groups and confirmed that Korsakoff's syndrome with isolated memory disorder does exist, as does alcoholic dementia, but patients often fall into a heterogeneous middle ground. This study had several methodological limitations, including the tests that were used to characterize the patients' current cognitive state, the exclusive use of the National Adult Reading Test to estimate premorbid intelligence, and the use of a one standard deviation (15 point) discrepancy level for the standard of impairment (i.e., when comparing premorbid versus current IQ, current IQ versus current memory quotient).

Transient Amnesia

The phenomena of transient amnesia was presented in greatest detail by Fisher and Adams in 1964, when they described a disorder they termed *transient global amnesia.* At the outset of their monograph they wrote:

> Not infrequently the neurologist or psychiatrist is confronted with the problem of determining the cause of episodes of temporary amnesia. The best known of these occur in relation to cerebral trauma, epilepsy (especially from foci in the temporal lobe) or an unbearable maladjustment in social relations—hysteria, neurosis, psychosis or malingering. (p. 7)

They described patients who had a

> history of having experienced a sudden episode of temporary amnesia, usually of a few hours' duration, after which there was complete restoration to the previous state of health. . . . the clinical manifestations of the attack consisted for the most part of a disorder of mentation in which a defect of memory, involving the events of the recent past and the present but leaving personal identification intact, was the most definite feature. (p. 7)

Although Fisher and Adams did not determine the pathogenesis of these disorders, they indicated that they might "represent a special type of focal cerebral seizure" (p. 7).

This work stimulated an interest in transient amnesias; publications have been produced at a slow but steady pace, almost exclusively in the neurological literature. Heathfield and colleagues (1973) supported the conclusions of Fisher and Adams (1964) regarding the characteristic nature of transient global amnesia and noted that hysterical fugue ends abruptly with the patient's

> sudden awareness of a long period for which he has no memory. In transient global amnesia, however, the retrograde amnesia characteristically shortens as the patient recovers so that when recovery is complete amnesia persists only for the period of the attack itself, during which registration of ongoing events has not occurred. (pp. 733–734)

Heathfield and colleagues pointed to clear evidence of temporal lobe disease in their patients; in many cases, damage appeared to be bilateral. In addition to the classic form of transient global amnesia, they described other patients with transient amnesia suffering from temporal lobe epilepsy, migraine, or encephalitis, as well as hysterical fugues. Although Fisher and Adams had noted that most of their patients suffered only a single episode, 8 of the 19 patients with transient global amnesia described by Heathfield and colleagues had recurrent events, and 9 had evidence of a vascular cause.

Interest in electroencephalographic abnormalities related to transient global amnesia arose originally from the work of Fisher and Adams (1964) and was pursued further in subsequent years (Rowan and Protass 1979; Steinmetz and Vroom 1972). However, more recent data with electroencephalographic records at the time of onset have indicated that an epileptic discharge is not necessary for the development of transient global amnesia (Cole et al. 1987). A variety of causes have been noted, including arterial embolism (Shuttleworth and Wise 1973), limbic and pituitary tumors (Boudin et al. 1975; Hartley et al. 1974), and mild head trauma (Haas and Ross 1986). However, the majority of findings support a cerebrovascular etiology (Cattaino et al. 1984; Hinge et al. 1986; Kushner and Hauser 1985; Matias-Guiu et al. 1986; Miller et al. 1987). Careful large-scale studies (Hinge et al. 1986; Miller et al. 1987) have revealed that the syndrome typically occurs after age 50 years, and approximately one-third of the patients had antecedent events or were physically active at the time of onset. The incidence in Rochester, Minnesota, was found to be 5.2 cases per 100,000 per year (Miller et al. 1987), and although approximately one-quarter of the patients in that study of 277 individuals followed for an average of 80 months had recurrent episodes, there was no increased risk for subsequent stroke. In a Danish multicenter investigation (Hinge et al. 1986), the observed rates of death and cerebrovascular morbidity were similar to those in the Danish population as a whole; 22% of the 74 patients had recurrent episodes. These investigators stated that transient global amnesia was a relatively benign disorder, one most probably caused by a "functional cerebral disturbance unrelated to cerebrovascular disease in general" (p. 673).

Neuropsychological studies have been conducted during and following episodes (Donaldson 1985; Hodges and Ward 1989; Kritchevsky et al. 1988; Regard and Landis 1984). During the episode, patients experienced a partial retrograde amnesia and complete anterograde amnesia. Objective recovery tended to be slower than what was experienced subjectively. Typically there was preservation of other neuropsychological functions such as language, motor praxis, right-left orientation, and constructional or visual praxis. One article (Kritchevsky et al. 1988) noted some cognitive impairment in addition to amnesia, but this was relatively minor. Additionally, these authors found that one patient had patchy recall from the first 2 hours of the episode. Most authors noted no change in personality during the episodes, although in one article the patient was described as "perplexed" (Donaldson 1985), whereas in another, three of five were said to have "exhibited passive, quiet personalities during TGA [transient global amnesia]" (Kritchevsky et al. 188, p. 216), a feature that had also been noted by Fisher and

Adams (1964). In any case, there were no instances of bizarre or grossly disturbed behavior.

Discussion and Recommendations

The results of Jacobson and Lishman (1987) indicated a useful direction for suggesting changes in DSM-IV. Insufficient data are available for making any recommendations regarding diagnostic criteria; however, textual changes may prove beneficial for refining the diagnosis of amnestic disorder. Beyond recommending corollary neuropsychological testing, we should indicate in DSM-IV that other cognitive deficits (when present) are not sufficiently severe to contribute to substantial functional impairment. Where a patient's functional impairment is the reflection of more than a memory disorder (i.e., manifesting two or more clinically significant domains of deficit), a diagnosis of dementia should be considered. However, continuing uncertainty will involve cognitive functions such as those typically subsumed under the designations of "executive" or "frontal lobe" function, as these are difficult to demonstrate objectively on relatively short cognitive assessments. Moreover, the lack of initiative, planning, organizing, and sustained motivation that is common in many amnestic patients may contribute to their apparent apathy or unconcern regarding their memory deficiencies.

With respect to transient global amnesia, it seems appropriate to consider including in DSM-IV the category of transient amnesia, which may be due to a variety of etiologies, but is most typically related to transient cerebral ischemia. Where appropriate, the terminology *transient global amnesia* should be employed for those episodes that are characterized by a dense, transitory inability to learn new information (i.e., to form longer-term memories), with a variable (ultimately shrinking on recovery) retrograde amnesia; the episode is followed by restoration to a completely intact cognitive state. There are no data to suggest that this is associated in any way with disturbed or abnormal behavior, beyond mild confusion or perplexity, which may be manifest during the episode.

References

American Psychiatric Association: Diagnostic and Statistical Manual of Mental Disorders, 3rd Edition, Revised. Washington, DC, American Psychiatric Association, 1987

Boudin G, Pepin B, Mikol J, et al: Gliome du systeme limbique posterieur, revele par une amnesie globale transitoire. Rev Neurol (Paris) 131:157–163, 1975

Cattaino G, Querin F, Pomes A, et al: Transient global amnesia. Acta Neurol Scand 70:385–390, 1984

Cole AJ, Gloor P, Kaplan R: Transient global amnesia: the electroencephalogram at onset. Ann Neurol 22:771–772, 1987
Corkin S, Cohen NJ, Sullivan EV, et al: Analyses of global memory impairments of different etiologies. Ann N Y Acad Sci 444:10–40, 1985
Donaldson IM: "Psychometric" assessment during transient global amnesia. Cortex 21:149–152, 1985
Fisher CM, Adams RD: Transient global amnesia. Acta Neurol Scand (suppl 9) 40:1–82, 1964
Haas DC, Ross GS: Transient global amnesia triggered by mild head trauma. Brain 109:251–257, 1986
Hartley TC, Heilman KM, Garcia-Bengochea F: A case of a transient global amnesia due to a pituitary tumor. Neurology 24:998–1000, October 1974
Heathfield KWG, Croft PB, Swash M: The syndrome of transient global amnesia. Brain 96:729–736, 1973
Hinge HH, Jensen TS, Kjaer M, et al: The prognosis of transient global amnesia: results of a multicenter study. Arch Neurol 43:673–676, 1986
Hodges JR, Ward CD: Observations during transient global amnesia: a behavioural and neuropsychological study of five cases. Brain 112:595–620, 1989
Jacobson RR, Lishman WA: Selective memory loss and global intellectual deficits in alcoholic Korsakoff's syndrome. Psychol Med 17:649–655, 1987
Kritchevsky M, Squire LR, Zouzounis JA: Transient global amnesia: characterization of anterograde and retrograde amnesia. Neurology 38:213–219, 1988
Kushner MJ, Hauser WA: Transient global amnesia: a case-control study. Ann Neurol 18:684–691, 1985
Matias-Guiu J, Colomer R, Segura A, et al: Cranial CT scan in transient global amnesia. Acta Neurol Scand 73:298–301, 1986
Miller JW, Petersen RC, Metter EJ, et al: Transient global amnesia: clinical characteristics and prognosis. Neurology 37:733–737, 1987
Regard M, Landis T: Transient global amnesia: neuropsychological dysfunction during attack and recovery in two "pure" cases. J Neurol Neurosurg Psychiatry 47:668–672, 1984
Rowan AJ, Protass LM: Transient global amnesia: clinical and electroencephalographic findings in 10 cases. Neurology 29:869–872, 1979
Shuttleworth EC, Wise GR: Transient global amnesia due to arterial embolism. Arch Neurol 29:340–342, 1973
Squire LR, Shimamura AP: Characterizing amnesic patients for neurobehavioral study. Behav Neurosci 100:866–877, 1986
Steinmetz EF, Vroom FQ: Transient global amnesia. Neurology 22:1193–1200, 1972

Chapter 17

Mental Disorders Due to a General Medical Condition and Substance-Induced Disorders

Mood, Anxiety, Psychotic, Catatonic, and Personality Disorders

Michael K. Popkin, M.D.
Gary J. Tucker, M.D.

Statement of the Issues

Although the term *organic* has enjoyed a firm place in psychiatric classification for decades, its connotations and boundaries have increasingly become points of concern. For many, the presence of a separate section of the diagnostic manual identified as "organic mental disorders" carries the implication that the remainder of the manual consists of nonorganic or "functional" mental disorders. In years past, this functional-organic dichotomy was often invoked by clinicians, and particularly by nonpsychiatric physicians arriving at a psychiatric diagnosis by the exclusion of physical or organic factors. Advances in neuroscience and brain imaging have steadily made apparent that a range of psychiatric disorders have structural or pathophysiologic underpinnings (e.g., a significant biological component in their etiology) and that "organic" contributions to psychiatric conditions are in the future likely to be shown to be the rule rather than the exception. Accordingly, a major question confronting those charged with the development of

The authors wish to express their appreciation for the thoughtful review and commentary of Drs. Thomas Wise, Robert Robinson, Richard Hall, and Roger Kathol. Special thanks to Janet Polich and Sandra Rizzo for all of their assistance in the preparation of this manuscript.

DSM-IV has been whether the term *organic* has outlived its usefulness and should be deleted. Companion issues are the renaming of these conditions and their disposition or placement in a revised diagnostic framework.

The DSM-IV Organic Mental Disorders Work Group (renamed the Cognitive Impairment Disorders Work Group) has proposed 1) that the term *organic* be discarded; 2) that the general organic category (including delirium, dementia, and amnestic disorders) be retitled Cognitive Impairment Disorders; 3) that the term *secondary disorders*[1] due to an Axis III condition be used to designate the remaining conditions of the current organic mental disorders section (organic mood, organic anxiety, organic delusional, and organic personality); 4) that the group of secondary conditions expand to include secondary catatonic disorder, secondary dissociative disorder (both of which are listed in ICD-10 [World Health Organization 1992]), secondary sleep disorder, and secondary sexual dysfunction; and 5) that these "secondary conditions" be placed in their respective phenomenological home groups (e.g., mood, psychotic, or anxiety disorders).

In the effort to gauge the merits of the last three proposals, a careful review of literature was instituted. The objective of the review was to document and specify the strength of the relationship between the major proposed secondary conditions (e.g., secondary mood, psychotic, anxiety, catatonic, and personality disorders) and the purported etiological factor(s) (e.g., medical-neurological illnesses, drugs). What evidence substantiates, especially statistically, that these secondary disorders exist as discrete entities? What characteristics of each entity have been delineated and what of drug-induced syndromes?

Significance of the Issues

DSM-III (American Psychiatric Association 1980) introduced what Lipowski (1984) characterized as a "radically novel approach to the organic mental disorders" (p. 542). This included a liberalization of the concept of organicity; cognitive or intellectual impairment was no longer a sine qua non for the diagnosis. With this particular shift, three new categories were added in DSM-III to the roster of organic mental disorders. These were organic affective syndrome, organic delusional syndrome, and organic personality syndrome. Lipowski (1978) proposed

[1]The term *Secondary Disorder* was used in the *DSM-IV Options Book* (American Psychiatric Association 1991). However, it was decided after publication of the *Options Book* to refer to these disorders simply as "Disorders Due to a General Medical Condition." This chapter was written to review the proposals given in the *Options Book* and uses the term *Secondary.*

that these three be called "symptomatic functional syndromes" (p. 320). After DSM-III was published, the categories were frequently referred to as "functional equivalents." Labeling aside, they drew sharp criticism from Roth (1981). He objected that the relationship between the organic lesion and the psychiatric features was "obscure and uncertain" (p. 56) for these three entities. He argued that the revisionist DSM-III format blurred the usual boundaries between organic and functional psychopathology.

Despite these objections, DSM-III-R (American Psychiatric Association 1987) added a fourth category, organic anxiety syndrome, to the "liberalized" construct of organic mental disorder. In addition, organic affective syndrome was retitled organic mood syndrome, and the diagnostic criteria were modified and simplified for each of the original three categories. However, DSM-III-R did not address the challenging question of explicit criteria or guidelines to satisfy the etiological requirement unique to organic mental disorders.

In early dialogue regarding DSM-IV, many observers expressed concern regarding the diagnostic imprecision and vagueness associated with the four "functional equivalents" (or the "organic syndromes with little or no cognitive impairment"). It was noted that few studies had examined these categories since their DSM-III inception; little data regarding reliability or validity had emerged. Publications addressing the organic mental disorders (as set forth in DSM-III) had focused largely on dementia; very few had taken the liberalized organic mental disorder construct as a point of systematic study. Confronted with this situation, numerous advisers urged that these four entities be returned to their phenomenological home bases in DSM-IV. Spitzer and colleagues (1989) proposed that the term *secondary* be used as a generic marker for these conditions, signaling the organic etiology. They contend that this will facilitate differential diagnosis by grouping phenomenologically similar disorders in the same diagnostic class. Lipowski (1990) argued for maintaining the term *organic* and the constructs associated with it.

Methods

In an attempt to address the questions enumerated, a literature review was conducted. Three sources were utilized: 1) a Medline search for *Organic Mental Disorder* citations from 1980 to 1989; 2) an organic mental disorder bibliography compiled by the DSM-III-R Task Force; and 3) the author's consultation-liaison service files, which are maintained and updated via weekly review of *Current Contents* for clinical medicine. Studies using structured interviews for psychiatric diagnoses of medically or neurologically ill patients were particularly sought and emphasized. The resultant review is selective rather than comprehensive.

Results

Secondary and Drug-Induced Mood Disorders

Mood disturbances emerging in patients with medical or neurological illness have received increasing attention in the past few years. Yet few studies have been couched in DSM-III or DSM-III-R terms of *organic affective* or *organic mood syndrome.* Investigators have avoided these labels and questions of causality; they focused on depression or depressive constellations in patients with specific medical or neurological illnesses. Most often such studies have sidestepped the diagnostic dilemmas posed by "medical depression," relying on symptom rating scales. Several investigators have offered lists of medical illnesses that induce or cause depressive states (Hall 1980; Jefferson and Marshall 1981). Fava and colleagues (1988) identified 17 conditions "clearly associated with organic affective syndromes" (p. 92). Robinson (1989) emphasized that four types of mood disorders *may be found* in patients with chronic medical illness: major depression, dysthymic depression, adjustment disorder with depression, and organic mood syndrome. Although the final group (those *due* to the physical illness) is the stated principal object of this review, it is important to recognize the other diagnostic options that are at hand in dealing with medically ill patients. Few investigators have made serious effort to separate medically ill patients by the four categories reviewed by Robinson.

Clayton and Lewis (1981) reviewed the features of secondary depressions—following Research Diagnostic Criteria (RDC) (Spitzer et al. 1978) and including those depressions emerging in the setting of severe or life-threatening medical illness. They noted that secondary depressions 1) were phenomenologically similar to primary conditions, 2) had a male predominance, 3) had earlier onset, 4) had an increased familial history of alcoholism, and 5) had normal rapid-eye-movement latency. In studies to date concerning depression in medically ill patients, the absence of a gender predominance (or the slight male predominance noted by Clayton and Lewis) is among the strongest points for the prospect of secondary mood disorder as a discrete entity.

Kathol and Petty (1981) and Klerman (1981) noted the difficulties inherent in diagnosing affective disorder in the face of major medical-surgical illness. The clinician must decide whether depressive syndromes in medically ill patients are reactions to the experience and impact of physical illness or whether they are manifestations of the intrinsic pathologic process (Popkin et al. 1987). Another problem is that an association of depression and medical illness need not imply an etiological relationship. These fundamental dilemmas have seriously impeded past efforts to investigate depression due to medical illness (or what will be identified as "secondary mood syndromes"). This has been the case though mood disturbances have been long identified as features or facets of medical illnesses ranging from endocrinopathies to malignancies to cardiovascular disease.

Early studies (Moffic and Paykel 1975; Schwab et al. 1967; Stewart et al. 1965) estimated the prevalence of depression in medically ill patients to range between 20% and 30%. Using varied methodologies, these studies examined heterogeneous groups of medically ill patients. Current work has increasingly addressed the prevalence of depression in specific medical or neurological disorders; the focus has therefore been on homogeneous samples (which eventually may be compared with one another). Using a different tact, Wells and colleagues (1988) studied the Epidemiologic Catchment Area (Regier et al. 1984) data regarding psychiatric disorders and eight chronic medical conditions. They found significantly increased 6-month and lifetime rates of psychiatric disorders in medically ill patients (25% over 6 months and 42% lifetime in persons with psychiatric disorders versus 17% and 33%, respectively, in persons with no medical condition). Nearly 13% of those with a chronic medical condition had a lifetime diagnosis of affective disorder versus 8% of those without a chronic medical condition.

Neurological Diseases

Of available studies focusing on a single disease, perhaps the most systematic and formidable investigations have involved patients with neurological disorders. The prevalence and features of depression have been vigorously examined/described in neurological patients with Parkinson's disease, Huntington's disease, multiple sclerosis, and cerebrovascular accidents. Attention to mood disturbances in patients with human immunodeficiency virus (HIV) and with Alzheimer's is likewise growing.

Of prospective, nonbiased studies in Parkinson's disease, frequency of depression has "consistently found to be around 40%" (Starkstein and Robinson 1989b, p. 214). The latter investigators concluded that more than 50% of Parkinson's disease patients will show symptoms of affective disorder (major or minor) during the evolution of the disease. This depression appears independent of gender, is not related to the motor impairment, and is independent of familial affective disorder. It appears linked to low levels of 5-hydroxyindoleacetic acid (5-HIAA) in cerebrospinal fluid (Mayeaux et al. 1984) and has cognitive impairment associated with it, particularly in the late stages of the disease (Starkstein et al. 1988). Other investigators have suggested that subgroupings of Parkinson's disease patients, categorized by the pattern of clinical symptoms, may differ with respect to severity of depression. Huber and colleagues (1988) reported that patients without depression had significantly more extensive tremor compared with those who were depressed.

In Huntington's disease, Folstein and colleagues (1983a) found 41% of patients in a consecutive case series with the Diagnostic Interview Schedule (Robins et al. 1981) to have a lifetime history of major affective disorder (9% bipolar, 32%

major depressive disorder). Numerous authors have noted that episodes of depression may appear years before the onset of chorea and dementia (and before people recognize their risk). Folstein and colleagues (1983a) noted that mania also occurs in Huntington's disease and "is not an understandable reaction to the prospect of Huntington's disease" (p. 541). The association of affective disorder and Huntington's disease may be confined to certain families (Folstein et al. 1983b). Caine and Shoulson (1983) reported dysthymia or major depression in 11 of 30 patients (37%) using the Schedule of Affective Disorders and Schizophrenia (Endicott and Spitzer 1978). They observed that antidepressants improved sleep, energy, and humor in five or six with major depressive disorder but did not alleviate hopelessness, helplessness, and dysphoria. The possible link between location of lesions and affective disorder is an open question.

In some of the most formidable studies to date regarding mood and neurological disease, Robinson, Starkstein, and colleagues (Robinson and Starkstein 1990; Robinson et al. 1984; Starkstein and Robinson 1989a) at Johns Hopkins published extensively on depression emerging after stroke. In a review (Starkstein and Robinson 1989a), they observed that empirical studies have demonstrated major and minor depressive disorders occur in 30%–50% of stroke patients and last more than a year without treatment. "These disorders are not strongly associated with severity of impairment, demographic characteristics, social supports or prior personal history" (p. 170). However, lesion location may account for more than 50% of the variance as regards the association of stroke and depression (Robinson et al. 1984). Starkstein and Robinson (1989a) suggested that major depression is often associated with left frontal or left basal ganglia lesions and that left posterior lesions often evoke a minor but persistent depressive constellation. Whereas the major depressive episodes resolve within months, the minor constellations are more intractable, often lasting longer than 1 year. Mania is an infrequent sequela of stroke, which is apparently linked to right hemisphere lesions "in a limbic connected area" (p. 170) and "a second predisposing factor such as genetic loading for affective disorder, pre-existing subcortical atrophy or seizure disorder" (p. 170). Mechanisms are unknown, but may involve changes in biogenic amines and limbic system input.

Eastwood and colleagues (1989) found 10% with major depression and 40% with minor depression in a series of stroke patients studied with rating scales and a diagnostic instrument. "Depression scores were negatively correlated with the distance from the frontal pole and the amount of brain tissue infarcted. These findings support the specificity of lesion hypothesis" (p. 199).

The nature of mood disorder in patients with multiple sclerosis has long been a point of controversy. Is the mood disturbance, previously estimated at a prevalence of from 11% to 50% (Schiffer and Babigian 1984; Surridge 1969), an intrinsic part of the pathophysiologic process of demyelination (Whitlock and Siskind 1980) or is it largely a reactive response to the progression of the disease (Wells and Duncan 1980)? Unlike the other neurological disorders already discussed, in multiple sclerosis euphoria is found in nearly equal degree as depression. Schiffer and colleagues (1988) suggested three clusters of patients with multiple sclerosis: 1) those with a family history of affective disorder—these patients are usually female and with bipolar disorder; 2) those patients with affective disorder but no family history—these are usually females with unipolar disorder; and 3) those without affective disorder—equally likely to be male or female and without family history of affective disorder. Schiffer and colleagues (1983) found depression in multiple sclerosis to be more common than in "neurological controls." Rabins and colleagues (1986) confirmed observations of Schiffer and colleagues (1983), finding higher rates of depressive episodes in multiple sclerosis patients with brain involvement versus those with spinal cord only involvement. A family history of depression and a history of depression prior to the onset of multiple sclerosis are risk factors for developing depression in multiple sclerosis (Rabins 1989); Rabins concluded that the available "data suggest that depression in multiple sclerosis patients can be both 'reactive' and 'endogenous' in nature" (p. 231).

Depression in Alzheimer's disease has been reported to range between 15% and 55% (Kral 1983; Liston 1979), but most studies have had sharp methodological limitations (Rovner and Morriss 1989). Although often thought to be a "psychological reaction," depression in Alzheimer's disease may be the product of neuroanatomic and neurochemical interrelationships (e.g., loss of ascending noradrenergic and cholinergic cortical projects) (Liston et al. 1987). Rovner and Morriss (1989) suggested unpublished data indicated that approximately 20% of demented outpatients met DSM-III criteria for major depressive disorder. The clinical features that best distinguished Alzheimer's disease cases with depression, from those without depression, were psychomotor retardation, ideas of worthlessness, recurrent thoughts of death, and early morning awakening. The depressed Alzheimer's disease patients had greater cognitive dysfunction, were more disabled, and were more likely to have had a prior psychiatric history than Alzheimer's disease patients without depression. It has been suggested that some Alzheimer's disease patients may have a genetic vulnerability to mood disorder, inherited separately from Alzheimer's disease, which is expressed or precipitated (Rovner and Morriss 1989) by the Alzheimer's disease brain changes.

Depressive symptoms and constellations occur frequently in patients with HIV infection. Early studies have found rates of major depression between 7% and 15% in HIV seropositive patients (Becker et al. 1988) and hospitalized patients with acquired immunodeficiency syndrome (Dilley et al. 1985). However, Marotta and Perry (1989) called attention to methodological limitations of existing studies (e.g., especially regarding staging of the disease). Schaerf and Miller (1989) reviewed the various depressive syndromes emerging in conjunction with HIV-1 infection. More systematic studies are in progress including "organic mood disorder" linked to medications.

Although the various neurological studies do not form a totally consistent picture of mood disorder due to a general medical condition, a number of common features are suggested for these conditions with direct involvement of the central nervous system (CNS) or structural lesions of the CNS. The prevalence of affective disorder seems to range from 30% to 50+% in these conditions (except for multiple sclerosis, possibly due to noncerebral disease), is largely independent of the severity of the neurological disease, and may (except for multiple sclerosis and Alzheimer's disease) be independent of demographics. However, subgroups of "younger" or early-onset patients with a family history of depression and depressive episode prior to the onset of neurological disease may be at greater risk. Lesion location in the CNS may play a critical role in the association with mood disorder and the neurological disease. Temporal relationships vary widely; in some instances affective disorder may antedate the appearance of the neurological process—in others it follows (in prompt or slow fashion) the disease's onset.

Krauthammer and Klerman (1978) described secondary mania and reviewed known etiologies for this condition. Cassem (1987) and Cummings (1986) presented in tabular form reported causes of secondary mania. With the possible exception of a few metabolic conditions and drug-induced manias, almost all known etiologies entail processes that directly compromise the structural integrity or normal physiology of the brain.

Medical Illness

Looking to secondary mood disorders in medical or systemic illness, the literature is less instructive than with the neurological conditions. A brief review of observations regarding selected endocrine disorders, end-stage renal disease, coronary artery disease, and cancer is in order, since a small number of formal studies apply in these areas. As Rodin and Voshart (1986) noted, many studies of depression in medically ill patients are difficult to gauge due to problems, including 1) poor case definition, 2) absence of assessment measures standardized in medically ill patients, 3) selection bias, 4) heterogeneity of subject populations, and 5) absence of control groups. They also noted the limitations of self-reporting measures. Although Hall (1980) identified 61 medical conditions commonly presenting with depression, "the evidence for a specific link with depression is lacking for most of these disorders" (Rodin and Voshart 1986, p. 698).

Although the association of psychiatric disorders and primary disorders of the neuroendocrine system is well recognized clinically, Haskett and Rose (1981) stated that "there is a dearth of systematic research. There has been little use of criterion-based diagnostic systems or quantitative measures of psychiatric symptomatology to clearly define the psychopathology which occurs in patients with endocrine dysfunction. Much of the relevant literature is anecdotal" (p. 245). They also noted that "the etiological relationship between endocrinopathies and psychiatric complications is no better understood" (p. 245). Reviews of the psychopathology associated with neuroendocrine dysfunction have highlighted these points (Brown 1975; Ettigi and Brown 1978; Popkin and Mackenzie 1980; Sachar and Rose 1981; Smith et al. 1972). Gottlieb and Greenspan (1989) updated prior reviews; they focused on the role of the hypothalamic-pituitary-thyroid axis.

Of the few studies that have taken a systematic approach, Haskett and colleagues (1979) used the Research Diagnostic Criteria and identified 67% of a series of patients with Cushing's syndrome as depressed. Lability, loss of energy, anhedonia, and impaired concentration were common features of these depressions. Earlier studies suggested depression to occur in one-third of cases of hypercortisolism (Popkin and Mackenzie 1980). In patients with diabetes mellitus, Lustman and colleagues (1986) used the Diagnostic Interview Schedule and reported lifetime prevalence rates of 33% for affective disorder in Type I and Type II diabetic patients. Popkin and colleagues (1988) studied the lifetime prevalence of psychiatric disorder in 75 consecutive Type I candidates for pancreas transplantation; 24% met Diagnostic Interview Schedule criteria for major depression. In neither the data of Lustman and colleagues (1986) nor the data of Popkin and colleagues (1988) were the diagnostic frequencies of mood changes correlated with duration of illness or severity of complications. Lustman and colleagues (1988) subsequently report a 5-year follow-up and found that the depressed cohort experienced multiple recurrences independent of complications. "These data suggest the natural course of depression in diabetes is malevolent, possibly more so than depression in the medically well" (p. 605). As a counterpoint, Breslau's (1990) review of chronic physical illness in children noted "recent studies are unanimous in finding little evidence for psychiatric sequelae in children with diabetes" (p. 377).

As regards depressive syndromes in patients with end-stage renal disease, Smith and colleagues (1985) administered the Schedule for Affective Disorders and Schizophrenia to 60 randomly selected patients; 5% met criteria for major depression. However, 47% were classified as depressed by the Beck Depression Inventory (Beck et al. 1961). Using the Diagnostic Interview Schedule, Craven and colleagues (1987) found 8% of 99 dialysis patients to meet criteria for major depression. Somatic symptoms of weight loss and anorexia were more common in the dialysis patients with depression versus the rest of the sample. Henrickson and colleagues (1989) found a 6.5% prevalence of major depression and 17.7% minor depression in 124 patients with end-stage renal disease on hemodialysis.

Carney and colleagues (1988) studied 75 patients undergoing diagnostic coronary angiography: 26% met criteria for lifetime prevalence of major depression (using DSM-III-R criteria with a modified Diagnostic Interview Schedule). Patients were reevaluated 1 year later, and Diagnostic Interview Schedule depression proved a better predictor of the occurrence of major cardiac events than traditional cardiovascular risk factors. The effect was independent of severity of coronary artery disease and impairment of functional capacity of the heart.

The prevalence of depression among patients with cancer has been an area of controversy. The association has been carefully reviewed by Petty and Noyes (1981) and Noyes and Katho (1986). In a review, Greenberg (1989) stated that "recent studies have suggested that major affective disorder is only a little more common among cancer patients than among other medical patients or even among the normal population" (pp. 105–106). A collaborative study of new admissions to oncology treatment programs found 6% with major affective disorder and 25% with adjustment disorder with depressed mood (Derogatis et al. 1983). However, Bukberg and colleagues (1984) found 42% of a series of oncology patients (with various malignancies) to be currently depressed using a "modified DSM-III depression criteria scale." None were psychotic, nor did any meet criteria for melancholia. "Suicidal ideation in the group as a whole was uncommon" (p. 209). The factor most clearly associated with depression was physical performance status as measured by the Karnofsky (1968) scale. Poor social support was also associated with depression. Pancreatic carcinoma has long been recognized to evoke depression, almost invariably heralding other symptoms. This is assumed to be a paraneoplastic phenomenon involving neuropeptides. It merits attention because it mitigates arguments of depression as a "reactive response" in physical illness.

In sum, there appears far more variability in the reported prevalence rates of depression in patients with medical illness versus those with neurological disease. Although hypercortisolism may be the exception, overall rates of depression apparently are lower than those in neurological illness. Perhaps this reflects the impact of direct structural change of the CNS in the former illnesses. Cognitive impairment is seldom mentioned (although decreased concentration is commonly reported). Finally, drug treatments (e.g., steroids, chemotherapy agents) and irradiation constitute risk factors for depression in at least subgroups of patients with malignancy, end-stage renal disease, and coronary artery disease.

Are mood disorders due to general medical condition discrete entities? Undoubtedly, affective disorders emerge in neurologically and medically ill patients at rates that are significantly greater than in the general population. However, prevalence rates and "comorbidity" (Schulberg et al. 1987) do not clarify the etiology of these mood changes. It may, at present, be necessary to view the neurological and medical illnesses somewhat differently. In the former, a more consistent picture emerges (Table 17–1), possibly reflecting the common feature of structural change of the brain and CNS. Not only have these conditions been more vigorously studied, but the brain involvement offers a ready basis for judging the mood disturbance as "due to" the physical illness.

In contrast, mood disturbances arising in the setting of medical illness have received less extensive investigation in terms of structured interviews, causality, and so on. Although the medical illnesses listed in Table 17–2 can compromise brain function and integrity, they will not invariably do so. In the absence of such change, the diagnosis of a secondary mood disorder is often a point of discussion (or more difficult to establish). The picture emerging from Table 17–2 is more varied, less consistent than in the neurological illnesses. What suffices to establish that a mood disorder is due to a medical illness remains unresolved. This could entail factors such as the temporal relationship of the physical illness and the psychiatric features, the resolution of psychiatric symptoms with correction or treatment of the physical illness, and other demonstrations of the interrelationship of the two processes (versus their independence from one another). Available studies of depression in medically ill patients have not addressed such issues systematically.

Old literature often characterized depressions in medically ill patients as largely "reactive" in nature. Many are still inclined to view mood disorders in the medically and neurologically ill as "reactive responses" to the physical illness as stressor. However, data are increasingly accumulating to suggest that this explanation is limited in its usefulness or at least unsatisfactory on several counts; for example, the findings regarding cerebrospinal fluid 5-HIAA levels in Parkinson's disease; the link to lesion location in cerebrovascular accidents; depression's independence of disease severity in numerous disorders; and depressive constellations (like that in pancreatic carcinoma) that antedate the emergence of the physical illnesses' central features, and the emergence of mania in several physical illnesses (which is harder to explain as a psychologically mediated response). Even the previously enumerated differences in medical versus neurological diseases suggest that physical factors are crucial in the genesis of these mood disorders and that they are distinct from primary major depressive disorder. Attention to risk factors is likewise instructive: there is no evidence of the usual female preponderance in affective illness; rather the incidence of depression in medically ill patients appears independent of gender. Although not within the scope of this review, treatment outcome suggests secondary disorders may be discrete (Fava et al. 1988; Popkin et al. 1987). Likewise, the course of some secondary disorders may be more "malevolent" (Lustman et al. 1986). Suicide rates, which vary according to different medical illnesses, also imply secondary disorders are "different."

Associations between mood disorder and physical illness have long been recognized, but few studies have distinguished those psychiatric syndromes that

Table 17–1. Secondary depressive disorders in selected neurological disease

Neurological disease	Lifetime prevalence of depression	Risk factors for depression	Key clinical features of depression
Parkinson's disease	40%–50%	Low 5-HIAA in CSF. Subgroup with younger age at onset of motor symptoms, family history of affective disorder, and depression episode prior to Parkinson's disease	Independent of motor impairment; cognitive impairment frequent in late stages
Huntington's disease	40% (approximately)	Confined to "certain" families with Huntington's disease (subgroup)	Depression may antedate chorea by years; mania also occurs
Cerebrovascular accidents	30%–50% (includes major and minor depressions)	Lesion location (left frontal, left basal ganglia); independent of demographics	Not associated with severity of impairment; major and minor constellations; mania also occurs
Multiple sclerosis	10%–50%	Cerebral involvement (versus spinal); ? temporal lobe involvement; family history of depression; depressive episode prior to onset of multiple sclerosis	Euphoria in approximately 25%; often associated with cognitive impairment
Alzheimer's disease	15%–55%	Prior psychiatric history; younger onset of Alzheimer's; subgroup with "genetic" risk?	Psychomotor retardation, early morning awakening; ideas of worthlessness; increased cognitive dysfunction; decreased ADL; greater neuronal loss in locus coeruleus

Note. 5-HIAA = 5-hydroxyindoleacetic acid. CSF = cerebrospinal fluid. ADL = activities of daily living.

Table 17–2. Secondary (comorbid?) depressive disorders in selected medical illnesses

Illness	Lifetime prevalence of depression	Risk factors for depression	Key clinical features of depression
Cushing's syndrome	33%–67%	??	Often preceding hirsutism, striae; anergia, anhedonia, decreased concentration
Type I/Type II diabetes mellitus	19%–33%	Independent of gender, severity of complications	Refractory to traditional treatment (?)
End-stage renal disease	5%–8% (18% minor depression)	Drugs (steroids)	Presence of a death wish, suicidal intent; decreased concentration
Coronary artery disease	26%	Drugs (?)	Predictive of increased combined mortality and morbidity in 1-year follow-up; effect independent of severity of coronary artery disease
Cancer (heterogeneous and single disease type)	6%–42% (current prevalence only)	Decreased physical performance status; poor social support; drugs (chemotherapy); radiation	Seldom psychotic or melancholic; suicide risk varies by malignancy; "reactive in nature"

are caused by the physical illness from those arising in response to the illness or merely coincident with it. At present, the case for secondary mood disorder seems more clear-cut in the neurological diseases. The data at hand hint that secondary mood constellations may differ in various ways, dependent on the presence of demonstrable lesions or change in the CNS and possibly dependent on the nature and status of the physical illness.

Drug-Induced Mood Disorders

More than 100 medications have been reported to give rise to depression as an adverse drug reaction (Zelnick 1978). Major medications that have been reported to evoke depressive constellations include alpha-methyldopa, reserpine, propanolol, guanethidine, clonidine, thiazide diuretics, digitalis, oral contraceptives, L-dopa, adrenocorticotropic hormone (ACTH) and glucocorticoids, anabolic steroids, benzodiazepines, cimetidine, ranitidine, cyclosporin, neuroleptics, nonsteroidal anti-inflammatory agents, ethambutol, cycloserine, disulfiram, sulfonamides, baclofen, metoclopramide, cocaine, and amphetamines (compiled from Cassem 1987; Fava et al. 1988; Hall 1980; Pascually and Veith 1989). Pascually and Veith (1989) detailed the numerous methodological limitations of existing literature on depression as adverse drug reaction. Consisting of largely anecdotal reports, the literature seldom uses explicit criteria for depression and fails to distinguish drug response from possible underlying primary mood disorder. In addition, it does not address psychosocial stressors, baseline prevalence of major depression in the study population, the complexities of multiple drug protocols, or preceding personal or familial history of depression.

Pascually and Veith (1989) concluded that available data suggest "that a high index of suspicion should be maintained that such agents as reserpine, alpha methyldopa, and propanolol induce depression in a moderate number of patients or those predisposed to depression by a family or personal history of depression" (p. 147). They viewed data regarding other agents as "too limited or conflicting" (p. 147) to allow firm conclusions.

Secondary and Drug-Induced Anxiety Disorders

Although mood disorders in medically ill patients have drawn considerable attention in the past few years, anxiety disorders due to medical or neurological disease have all but been ignored. The ubiquity of anxiety or anxious symptomatology in medically ill patients may explain a good part of this seeming disinterest. Although DSM-III-R introduced the category of organic anxiety syndrome (Mackenzie and Popkin 1983), studies utilizing the category have been almost exclusively confined to case reports. A few studies have explored relationships between anxiety and specific medical conditions such as mitral valve prolapse; these have not been designed in terms of organic anxiety syndrome. All the criticisms and methodological limitations cited previously regarding studies of mood disorder due to a general medical condition are applicable to the available literature regarding anxiety disorders due to medical illness. With these concerns in mind, and recognizing the paucity of systematic studies, the available literature is briefly reviewed.

Hall (1980) reported in a comprehensive review of earlier work that neurological and endocrine disorders accounted for approximately half of the medical causes of anxiety. He identified chronic infections (12%), rheumatic-collagen vascular disorders (12%), circulatory disorders (12%), and an array of assorted other illnesses (14%) as etiologically responsible for "medically induced" anxiety constellations. Hall suggested that organic anxiety could be differentiated from psychogenic anxiety by 1) its characteristic fluctuations in severity and duration, and 2) its onset before age 18 or after age 35 in patients with negative personal and familial psychiatric histories. Hall also suggested that psychogenic anxiety patients often had other psychiatric symptoms (e.g., phobias, conversion symptoms) and a recent major psychosocial stressor. Finally he suggested that a duration of 2 or more years of symptoms implied a psychological origin rather than an organic one.

Numerous investigators have estimated or reported the prevalence of anxiety or symptoms of anxiety among medical outpatients and inpatients. These estimates have usually ranged from 10% to approximately 30% (Lader and Marks 1971; Sheehan 1978). Wells and colleagues (1988) studied Epidemiologic Catchment Area data on psychiatric disorders and eight chronic medical conditions. In a sample of 2,554, they found persons with a chronic medical condition had a significantly higher adjusted lifetime prevalence of anxiety disorders ($F = 3.00$, 2,550 df, $P < .01$). The results were statistically significant for recent anxiety disorder after adjustment for multiple comparisons ($F = 3.64$, 2,550 df, $P < .005$). "More than 11% of the persons with chronic medical conditions had a recent anxiety disorder" (p. 979).

The prevalence rates of anxiety or symptoms of anxiety per se do not clarify those instances in which the medical illness *caused* (in a physiological fashion) the psychiatric symptomatology versus those in which the anxiety represents reactive response to the "stress" of illness or those in which an anxiety disorder antedated the physical illness. Rosenbaum and Pollack (1987) presented a three-page table titled, "Medical Causes of Anxiety"; they commented that "the number of medical illness . . . that may generate or exacerbate anxiety symptoms obviously renders an exhaustive evaluation for each of them impractical" (p. 163). Schuckit (1983) reported that between 10% and 40% of medical patients with anxiety had organic etiologies for their psychiatric symptoms. Starkman and colleagues (1990) found that 17 patients with pheochromocytoma displayed anxiety that differed *qualitatively* from primary anxiety disorders; few of their subjects met criteria for panic disorder or generalized anxiety disorder. In the 17 patients with pheochromocytoma, there were no significant correlations of anxiety symptoms with peripheral norepinephrine or epinephrine levels. In comparison groups, consisting of hypertensive patients and panic disorder patients, anxiety correlated significantly with plasma norepinephrine but not with plasma epinephrine. Starkman and colleagues suggested that "the effects of catecholamines in the periphery derived from a source independent of nervous system control are not sufficient to elicit an anxiety disorder meeting DSM-III criteria" (p. 129).

Jefferson and Marshall (1981) identified a small number of medical disorders in which anxiety is an integral part of the illness. After first acknowledging substance-induced anxiety and anxiety attendant to withdrawal, they listed medical disorders often mistaken for a primary anxiety disorder: hyperthyroidism, hypoglycemia, pheochromocytoma, and hyperadrenalism. Hall (1980) observed that thyroid disorders are the most common endocrine cause of episodic anxiety. Anxiety can be caused by a full gamut of endocrine problems (Popkin and Mackenzie 1980): hypothyroidism and hyperthyroidism, hypocortisolism and hypercortisolism, hypoparathyroidism and hyperparathyroidism, virilization syndromes, hypopituitarism and hyperpituitarism, and diabetes mellitus. Of these conditions, only hypercortisolism and diabetes have been recently systematically studied with structured psychiatric interviews. In a sample with type I and II diabetic patients, Lustman and colleagues (1986) used the Diagnostic Interview Schedule and reported lifetime prevalence rates of 26.5% for phobic disorders and 41% for generalized anxiety disorders. Data regarding other anxiety disorders in medical illnesses are needed. Hall (1980) contended that neurological diseases are major contributors to secondary anxiety syndromes. In his review, he observed that cerebral vascular insufficiency is the most common neurological cause of anxiety. He further listed encephalitis, multiple sclerosis, Wilson's disease, Huntington's disease, closed head injury, polyneuritis, myasthenia gravis, cerebral syphilis, combined systems disease, and tumors of the CNS as neurological conditions with associated or induced anxiety. Sato and Takeichi (1987) described a case of organic anxiety secondary to a chronic subdural hematoma extending from the right frontal lobe to the temporal lobe.

The relationship of mitral valve prolapse and anxiety disorder, specifically panic disorder, has been investigated; however, the nature of the association remains an open question (Venkatesh et al. 1981; Wooley 1983, 1987). This points to the possibility of an underlying autonomic dysregulation or impairment in patients with anxiety, independent of medical illness. This construct recalls early work (Frohlich et al. 1966) exploring the links between hyperdynamic beta-adrenergic state and anxiety-panic syndromes. In turn, this led to studies with lactate infusion, and so on (Pitts and McClure 1967).

Drug-induced anxiety disorders or anxious symptoms include aspirin intolerance, drug intoxications (drugs of abuse), caffeinism, withdrawal from CNS depressant drugs, steroids, behavioral toxicity from drugs, procarbazine, hydralazine, nicotinic acid, ethosuximide, sympathomimetics, bronchodilators (theophylline, Alupent), cholinergic blocking agents, insulin, thyroid preparations, estrogens, antihistamines, L-dopa, and digitalis (based on Hall 1980).

DSM-III-R does not offer explicit criteria or guidelines by which to establish an organic etiology for an anxiety syndrome. (This is left to the clinician's personal judgment.) If correction or effective treatment of the medical condition or problem resolves the psychiatric disturbance, it seems reasonable to conclude retrospectively that the medical illness was the causal factor. If, for example, a patient with Graves' disease is restored to a euthyroid state by ^{131}I treatment and her anxiety disturbance resolves in short order, an organic etiology seems a fair judgment (although some might argue that she was "psychologically" relieved). In some instances, medical intervention may be unable or too late to achieve full restitution—such situations make it more difficult to confirm the organic etiology.

In sum, secondary anxiety disorders have been overlooked. Although numerous investigators have addressed the issues of treating anxiety in specific medical illnesses (e.g., chronic obstructive pulmonary disease, irritable bowel, cardiac disease, asthma), the approach has really not centered on anxiety *induced* in a physiological fashion by the medical disease. This oversight needs correction, and there is indication that this will occur in the early years of the coming decade.

Secondary and Drug-Induced Psychotic Disorders

A wide range of neurological and medical disorders, including toxic-metabolic disturbances, have been reported to cause psychotic states (Cummings 1985; Davison 1983; Davison and Bagley 1969). In earlier literature, these presentations were often called "schizophrenia-like psychoses"; DSM-III and DSM-III-R categorized them as organic delusional syndromes, focusing on delusions as their prominent clinical features. For this category, DSM-III listed exclusion criteria of delirium, dementia, hallucinosis, and organic affective disorder; DSM-III-R eliminated this hierarchical approach and required only that the delusional disorder not occur exclusively during delirium. Noting these conditions to be common, Cummings (1986) said that "there has been relatively *little systematic evaluation* of the frequency, clinical characteristics, or treatment responsiveness of these disorders" (p. 293, italics added). Only the psychoses emerging in association with epilepsy have been the subject of much study (and controversy). Despite the limitations noted above, there are some instructive points from available work.

Both Davison and Bagley (1969) and Cummings (1985) reviewed numerous physical disorders that have been reported to give rise to psychosis. Lipowski (1984) observed that "intoxication with drugs, such as amphetamine or cocaine, appears to be the commonest cause of this syndrome" (p. 545) (e.g., organic delusional syndrome). Cummings (1985) offered a list of specific delusions and their reported "organic causes"; he included delusions of thought control, Capgras syndrome, Fregoli syndrome, intermetamorphosis syndrome, Othello syndrome, delusions of infestation, lycanthropy, heutoscopy, and de Clerambault syndrome. Cummings also identified delusions "uniquely associated with specific neurological defects" (p. 188); for example, Anton's syndrome (denial of blindness), which is encountered with bilateral posterior cerebral artery occlusion. Davison (1983) noted that "the association of many organic cerebral disorders with schizophrenia exceeds chance expectations" (p. 1). These reviews, despite the acknowledged limitations of the studies in question, demonstrate the variety of physical conditions thought capable of evoking psychoses and call attention to the importance of the location or site of the CNS lesion and the nature of the pathologic process in the resultant psychiatric configurations.

With regard to site of lesion, Cummings (1986) observed that "diseases affecting *subcortical* (basal ganglia, thalamus and midbrain) and *limbic* structures produce the highest frequency of delusions" (p. 294, italics added). Prevalence rates for delusions and psychosis have been previously reported at >50% in Huntington's disease (Dewhurst et al. 1969); less than 25% in postencephalitic Parkinson's disease (Bromberg 1930; Fairweather 1947); and >50% in idiopathic basal ganglia calcification (Cummings 1985). In Alzheimer's disease, Larsson and colleagues (1963) found 18% of the patients to be delusional. In a study on psychopathology in multi-infarct dementia, Tomonasa and colleagues (1982) reported nearly 60% were psychotic.

"Limbic system lesions also produce a high frequency of psychosis" (Cummings 1986). Although the question of psychosis associated with epilepsy will be detailed later, it should be noted that considerable controversy has surrounded the issues of 1) temporal lobe epilepsy and the frequency of attendant psychosis, and 2) right-sided versus left-sided temporal lobe lesions in regard to psychosis. Regarding location of CNS lesions, Cummings (1986) concluded that "in disorders involving only one hemisphere, psychosis appears to be more common with left sided lesions." As for toxic-metabolic conditions, prevalence of organic psychoses are not to my knowledge available; however, Lipowski (1980) noted that between 40% and 100% of delirious patients will display delusional thinking.

In perhaps the one available prospective study, Cummings (1985) examined 20 consecutive patients referred for neurobehavioral evaluation with organic delusions. He observed four general types of delusions in the study population: 1) simple persecutory delusions, 2) complex persecutory delusions, 3) grandiose delusions, and 4) delusions related to specific neurological deficits. Cummings observed that cognitive integrity was necessary for complex delusional thinking; those with dementia manifested simple, loosely held persecutory beliefs that were often transient. Older age at onset appeared to distinguish the organic delusional patients from those with idiopathic delusions. Simple delusions responded more favorably to neuroleptics; the complex delusions, occurring in patients with subcortical or limbic lesions, were more resistant to treatment. Cummings found laterality effects among the limbic lesions—with left-sided lesions more likely to yield schizophrenic-like presentations. In a study titled, "Late life paraphrenia: an organic delusional syndrome," Miller and colleagues (1986) reported five patients with late-life onset of delusional thought in whom occult illnesses were subsequently identified as probable "organic" etiologies.

Levine and Grek (1984) studied patients manifesting delusions after right cerebral infarction. No particular site or size of lesion was associated with particular delusions; however, there was a relationship between delusions and all measures of brain atrophy. Levine and Grek concluded that the emergence of delusions depended on brain atrophy; they argued that the state of the left hemisphere determined the response to right cerebral infarction.

In the absence of much formal epidemiologic inquiry regarding "secondary psychotic disorders," the work of Hall and colleagues (1980) offers an interesting perspective regarding the frequency and nature of psychotic presentations of medical illness. Using exhaustive medical evaluation of 1,000 psychiatrically disturbed subjects of lower socioeconomic strata admitted to a research ward, Hall and colleagues found that 46% of these psychotic patients had a physical illness accounting for or contributing significantly to their psychiatric disturbance. Of this group, one-third had a schizophreniform presentation, and another third presented with affective features. The study by Hall and colleagues underscores that secondary disorders are often unrecognized as such and that clinicians need to direct more vigor to possible medical explanations for psychiatric constellations.

Psychotic Disorders in Epilepsy

It is interesting to recall that Kraepelin (1922) divided major psychiatric illness into three groups: manic-depressive insanity, dementia-praecox, and epileptic insanity.

The psychoses of epilepsy have been recognized for centuries (Trimble 1985) but they remain a point of controversy and heated exchanges in the literature (Parnas et al. 1982; Stevens 1975; Trimble 1981). Despite large numbers of publications concerning the relationship between epilepsy and psychosis, the area remains poorly explored and ill defined (Neppe and Tucker 1988a, 1988b). The current classification of epilepsy by the International League Against Epilepsy has been reviewed by Neppe and Tucker (1988a, 1988b). This classification uses partial (focal, local) seizures versus generalized seizures. Partial includes *simple* with motor, somatosensory, autonomic, or psychic symptoms, and *complex* with impairment of consciousness. (Note that temporal lobe epilepsy is not included as such.) The psychoses of epilepsy may be grouped as peri-ictal versus interictal (Trimble 1985) or brief versus persistent (McKenna et al. 1985).

Two hypothetical constructs have been raised regarding psychosis and epilepsy. One proposes that psychosis and epilepsy are antagonistic to each other. A second notion is the *affinity* hypothesis: the belief that epilepsy predisposes to the development of a schizophrenia-like psychosis (Hermann and Whitman 1984). In their review of psychotic syndromes in epilepsy, McKenna and colleagues (1985) divided the relevant clinical pictures into 1) brief psychotic episodes—short-lived confusional and nonconfusional states; and 2) persistent psychotic states in epilepsy. Many of the former are "ictal or postictal confusional states" with generalized changes on the electroencephalogram. Dongier (1959/1960), Ervin and colleagues (1955), and Tucker and colleagues (1986) reported on patients with these transient psychotic episodes. Landolt (1958) argued that forced normalization constituted brief, self-limited nonconfusional psychoses that were not ictal or postictal events.

However, most attention in the literature has been directed to the chronic psychotic states or the interictal psychoses.

A critical question in examining the association of epilepsy and chronic psychosis concerns what the reported prevalence of psychosis is in epileptic populations. Studies to date have reported rates varying from 0% in a general practice survey (Taylor 1972) to 27% (Jensen and Larsen 1979) of patients proceeding to temporal lobectomy. Of available work, Gudmundsson's (1966) data are the most satisfactory. He surveyed the entire epileptic population of Iceland and found that 7.1% were currently psychotic or had been at some time. The prevalence of epilepsy among patients in psychiatric hospitals has been reported at 2%–3% (Pincus and Tucker 1985) versus 0.5% in the general population. Together, "these figures would place the risk of psychosis for persons with epilepsy at about 10% over a thirty year period, whereas the lifetime risk for schizophrenia is about 0.8%" (Neppe and Tucker 1988b, p. 267).

Slater and colleagues (1963) reactivated interest in the relationship between psychosis and epilepsy. They described in clinical detail 69 cases of psychosis in epilepsy. Slater and colleagues observed the following features: these psychoses emerged a mean of 14 years after the epilepsy had begun; most of the patients had temporal lobe epilepsy; and the psychosis resembled schizophrenia but differed in *subtle* but important ways. These differences included the maintenance of a warm affect, the absence of any clearly defined premorbid personality style (schizoid), a presentation with intense affective symptoms, and the lack of a family history of schizophrenia. Perez and Trimble (1981) found that 12 of 23 patients with epilepsy and chronic psychosis had a Present State Examination (Wing et al. 1974) yielding a diagnosis of schizophrenia; this was significantly associated with temporal lobe epilepsy. (Psychoses other than schizophrenia were found in 5 of 16 patients with temporal lobe epilepsy.) "The idea that schizophrenia in epilepsy shows a *lack of negative features* and runs a benign course" (McKenna et al. 1985, p. 899, italics added) is also common in the literature.

In his review, Trimble (1985) observed that

> the schizophreniform psychoses . . . have many of the presenting features of process schizophrenia, with some notable exceptions. The majority of patients develop an illness with so-called positive symptoms, mainly delusions and hallucinations; and Schneiderian first rank symptoms are common. Delusions of persecution and religious delusions are often reported, although hebephrenic deterioration and catatonic phenomena are rare. (p. 215)

Temporal lobe epilepsy. Is psychosis occurring in epilepsy selectively associated with temporal lobe epilepsy? Neppe and Tucker (1988b) reviewed the issues confounding the question of whether behavioral disturbances are more common in patients with temporal lobe epilepsy versus those with seizure disorders in general. They noted that these issues "argue against our current ability to stipulate that the behavioral changes associated with seizure disorders are specific to localization in the temporal lobes" (p. 266). Hermann and Whitman (1984) reviewed 64 studies published since 1962 dealing with temporal lobe epilepsy and psychosis, general psychopathology, and so on. They also identified multiple methodological problems hindering a clear understanding of the relationship between epilepsy and psychopathology. For example, they called attention to the almost totally ignored issue of the base rate of temporal lobe epilepsy in the patient population from which the psychotic individuals were drawn. They cited Stevens (1975) in this regard. Hermann and Whitman concluded "that a multitude of variables other than seizure type are associated with increased psychological risk" (p. 451), and they offered a list of 19 such risk factors for psychosis (p. 478). Neppe (1985) specified eight elements that may be responsible for aberrant behavior in a patient with epilepsy: ictal firing, subictal firing, medication effects, focus of firing, incidental predisposition, kindling-like phenomena, other cerebral abnormalities, and epilepsy as a complication.

How might a temporal lobe focus predispose to psychosis? Flor-Henry (1979) suggested that the *laterality* of the focus might be crucial to the nature of an epileptic psychosis. Several studies have found that left-sided or dominant lesions are more frequently associated with schizophreniform presentations and right-sided lesions evoke affective changes. Trimble (1985) reviewed nine such studies; however, Neppe and Tucker (1988a) disagreed, specifically stating, "such conclusions are rather premature and possibly flawed" (p. 395). "A possibly less controversial finding has been that, in patients with TLE [temporal lobe epilepsy], presence of bilateral or multiple foci seems especially to increase the likelihood of psychosis" (McKenna et al. 1985, p. 900). In an editorial, Reynolds (1983) concluded that "much psychopathology in TLE may be due to the interaction of multiple factors. Patients with partial seizures . . . tend to have more frequent attacks, take more drugs and suffer more adverse psychosocial stresses than patients with generalized seizure" (pp. 3–4).

Undoubtedly patients with seizure disorders have a greater incidence of psychopathology than the general population, with "psychosis" as a major subgroup of presentation. However, questions regarding the relationship of temporal lobe epilepsy and psychosis and laterality remain to be resolved by further study.

Drug-Induced Psychotic Disorders

Cummings (1986) detailed in tabular form drugs, metals, and withdrawal states associated with delusional disorders. Table 17–3 lists the categories he identified. (There were two to eight agents specified per category.)

Curiously, steroids (including anabolic steroids) were not included—but certainly can evoke psychosis. Likewise, Hall (1980) presented in tabular form psychiatric side effects of medical drugs.

Secondary Catatonic Disorder

First described by Karl Kahlbaum in 1874, catatonia was identified as "a symptom complex," characterized by psychotic negativism, catalepsy, mutism, stereotypy,

Table 17–3. Categories of drugs, metals, and withdrawal states associated with delusional disorders

Dopaminergic agents	Minor tranquilizers and hypnotics
Anticholinergic agents	Endocrine agents
Antituberculous agents	Psychostimulants
Antimalarial drugs	Nonsteroidal anti-inflammatory agents
Anticonvulsants	Appetite suppressants
Antidepressants	Cardioactive drugs
Antihypertensive agents	Pulmonary drugs
Metal intoxication	Drug withdrawal
Antibiotics	Miscellaneous drugs/toxins
Hallucinogens/euphoriants	

Source. Categories from Cummings 1986.

posturing, muscular rigidity, and verbigeration. Noting parallels between catatonia and general paresis, Kahlbaum (1874/1972) anticipated that the etiology of the condition would eventually be shown to lie in pathologic changes of brain structure. Kraepelin (1919/1971) included catatonia together with paranoia and hebephrenia as subtypes of the deteriorating mental illness he named "dementia praecox." Kraepelin (1919/1971) and Bleuler (1911/1950) both recognized that isolated catatonic signs existed in other illnesses, including manic-depressive disease, the postictal state of epilepsy, and focal brain disease (Gelenberg 1976). However, as Gelenberg noted, "most teaching and clinical practice since Kraepelin has tended to overlook the pleomorphic causes of this syndrome" (p. 1339). A curious footnote to this history is Marsden's observation (Mahendra 1981) that looking back on Kahlbaum's cases, "it is evident that a number are of neurological, possibly post-encephalitic, origin" (p. 669).

"That catatonic phenomena occasionally have an organic basis has never been in dispute" (Mahendra 1981, p. 669). In 1976, Gelenberg proposed that catatonia be treated as a syndrome resulting from a diverse number of possible causes. He reviewed an extensive roster of physical causes for the syndrome reported in earlier literature; he emphasized the need for medical investigation to uncover the probable cause. Stoudemire (1982) and Weddington and colleagues (1980) also reviewed organic etiologies for catatonia. Carroll (1992) reviewed catatonic presentations in the medical-surgical setting.

Gelenberg's (1976) review (to which the interested reader is directed) detailed catatonia as a manifestation of various neurological disorders involving the basal ganglia, the limbic system and temporal lobes, the diencephalon, and a range of other lesions of the brain (vascular, infectious, traumatic, and malignant). Gelenberg further identified citations describing catatonia as a concomitant of several metabolic derangements (e.g., diabetes, hypercalcemia, hepatic, encephalopathy, homocystinuria). Likewise numerous drugs noted to induce catatonic reactions include aspirin, ACTH, neuroleptics, disulfiram, mescaline, amphetamines, ethyl alcohol, and phencyclidine. Catatonia has also resulted from toxic agents including illuminating gas and organic fluorides.

Little in the literature to date suggests that the phenomenology of the catatonic constellation varies substantially whether the etiology be a physical-structural cause or one presumed to be psychogenic. Particularly puzzling is the problem of "lethal catatonic" in which patients may die from cardiovascular collapse (Lechtenberg 1982). Autopsy rarely shows abnormalities sufficient to explain death. "Symptoms indistinguishable from those in lethal catatonia occur with general paresis, viral encephalitis, and brainstem strokes" (Lechtenberg 1982, p. 65). Following work by Morrison (1973), it is now thought that catatonic states of excitement and stupor are quite distinct in their course and prognosis. Some investigators group catatonic presentations as phasic and nonphasic. Included in the former (alternating hyperkinetic and akinetic phases) are "cycloid" affective disorders, those linked to limbic kindling, the on-off of treated Parkinsonism, and acute drug- and toxin-related conditions. The nonphasic catatonias (akinetic-hypertonic only) include Parkinson syndrome, lesions of the globus pallidus, and other lesions productive of catalepsy (drug, neurological, and metabolic).

In a 1981 editorial titled, "Where have all the catatonics gone?" Mahendra suggested that the decline in catatonic symptomatology may be explained by a decline of some infective disorder—perhaps viral. Mahendra closed by warning not to reify disease concepts and symptomatology prematurely. With this in mind, it should be noted that DSM-III-R has no condition corresponding to secondary catatonic disorder. However, such a disorder is listed in ICD-10. The proposed inclusion of secondary catatonic disorder (like dissociative disorder due to a general medical condition, which is not discussed here) corrects the prior omissions of the manual.

At present, the clinician encountering a catatonic syndrome with negativism, mutism, rigidity, and catalepsy is obligated to explore carefully both medical and neurological as well as nonmedical psychiatric etiologies for the presentation. Prospective studies could clarify incidence, course, treatment, and so on.

Secondary Personality Disorders

The DSM-III and DSM-III-R category of organic personality syndrome traced its origins to the 19th century recognition of behavioral change in end-stage neurosyphilis (Popkin 1986). The encephalitis epidemic of 1918 and the large number of brain injuries in World War I subsequently led to study of the changes in personality and behavior following CNS insult. Like the other "secondary syndromes," the category of organic personality syndrome has since 1980 received a minimum of formal investigation. The clinical use of the category (organic personality syndrome) has largely been restricted to patients with epilepsy, closed head injury and other structural insults to the CNS, or the early stages of dementing illnesses. Some have noted that the DSM-III-R category (organic personality syndrome) shared surprisingly little with any of the 12 personality disorders coded on Axis II.

The construct of a global or general "epileptic personality" has not been substantiated (Hermann and Whitman 1984). However, interest has remained in the notion that certain personality characteristics bear a relationship to temporal lobe epilepsy (e.g., sudden religious conversion, increased philosophical interest, humorlessness [Hermann and Whitman 1984]). In his review, Taylor (1987) identified the most common personality syndrome associated with epilepsy as "adhesive"; "a second interictal personality is characterized by a profound deepening of the patient's emotional responses" (p. 151). Following work by Waxman and Geschwind (1975), Bear and Fedio (1977) proposed 18 personality traits associated with temporal lobe epilepsy. The Bear-Fedio Personality Inventory and its findings have been substantially criticized on methodological grounds (Hermann and Whitman 1984). Among others, Mungas (1982) argued that the inventory was a nonspecific measure of overall psychopathology and not specific for temporal lobe epilepsy. However, others (Mendez 1988) look to the possibility "that a *subgroup* develop traits such as circumstantiality and viscosity in their interactions and excessive seriousness in their affect, preoccupations, and interests" (p. 200, italics added). This theme of an affected subgroup has been echoed by Garyfallos and colleagues (1988). Using clinical interviews, they found 13 of 101 epileptic patients met DSM-III criteria for Organic Personality Syndrome. All 13 came from the temporal lobe epilepsy cohort in the study (as did the 8 receiving the diagnosis of Organic Delusional Syndrome). The authors contended that the subgroup "seem to be differentiated from the rest of the epileptics, temporal lobe epilepsy and non-temporal lobe epilepsy, who had quite 'benign' psychological problems if at all" (p. 87).

At present, a consistent picture has yet to emerge regarding epilepsy and purported personality change. Extensive, if anecdotal, clinical observations have not been systematically objectified in formal investigations.

Although epilepsy may constitute an open question, the literature leaves no doubt that lesions or damage to the brain will evoke striking alterations in personality. Insult to the frontal lobe is well known to yield such changes (Benson 1984). Lishman (1966) described 1) lack of judgment, foresight; 2) facetiousness; 3) disinhibition; and 4) euphoria in patients sustaining frontal injury. Lishman (1987b) noted that the clinical features emerging after damage to the frontal lobes "are not unique to frontal lobe pathology but are seen more regularly and perhaps more strikingly than after damage to other cerebral regions" (p. 68). Blumer and Benson (1975) proposed two discrete frontal lobe personality syndromes—a "pseudoretarded state" following medial, frontal polar, or convexity damage; and a "pseudopsychopathic state" with orbital frontal injury. Blumer and Benson noted that in addition to localization, the nature of the lesion is important, suggesting that frontal personality disorders result from destructive lesions, whereas temporal personality changes are the product of irritative disorders. Although the temporal lobe changes are moot (see earlier), Blumer and Benson also cautioned that "in most cases of frontal lobe disorder, pathology fails to respect anatomical boundaries" (p. 169). Benson (1984) concluded that frontal personality changes are characterized by "abnormalities of both drive and cognitive control affecting emotional responses" (p. 34).

Further testimony to the link between structural CNS insult and personality change is seen in the work of Motomura and colleagues (1988), who studied patients with right hemisphere strokes. These investigators found organic personality syndromes (per DSM-III-R) in 33% of a series of consecutive patients with right hemisphere injury. Personality change was strongly associated with unilateral spatial neglect, anosognosia, hemiasomatagnosia, extinction, constructional disturbance, and motor impersistence.

Disinhibition or reduced impulse control is well recognized as a concomitant of brain insult and head injury and indeed is a central characteristic of what have been previously termed *organic mental disorders* in DSM-III-R. The symptom of reduced control over aggression following brain insult or injury may deserve special consideration (Lishman 1987a, 1987b). Yudofsky and Silver (1985) argued for a discrete category "organic aggressive syndrome" (p. 147) to describe patients with neurological problems etiologically associated with "organic dyscontrol of aggressive behaviors" (p. 147).

Finally, it should be noted that personality alterations are often part of the clinical picture of evolving dementing illnesses. For example, in dementia of the Alzheimer's type, subtle changes in personality may be among the earliest presenting signs (Heston and White 1983). DSM-III-R notes that these changes "may involve either an alteration or an accentuation of premorbid traits" (p. 104). These concerns likewise apply to HIV. Marotta and Perry (1989) reviewed the challenging problems associated with neuropsychological dysfunction in patients with HIV infection. Changes in personality may emerge before the full impact of a dementia is appreciated.

Change in personality can undoubtedly be evoked by a wide range of medical drugs. Most systematic investigation, however, has focused on disturbances of mood, thought, or arousal rather than personality per se. Personality change secondary to use of substances such as marijuana is an open question.

In sum, there can be little question that structural CNS injury (epilepsy aside) can and will give rise to alterations and disturbances of personality.

Discussion and Recommendations

The available literature addressing psychiatric disturbances of mood, anxiety, thought, catatonia, and personality "due to" medical-neurological illnesses or drug effects is highly variable in nature. Systematic studies with diagnostic rigor and careful attention to demonstrating the etiological relationship are few (at best). A wealth of older literature, often consisting of case reports and small series, has examined the associations of physical and psychiatric illnesses; but few studies have distinguished psychiatric disorders that are *caused* by the physical illness from those arising in response to the illness or merely coincident with it. Previously "secondary" psychotic disorders and personality alterations have drawn the majority of attention in this area; recent focus has somewhat shifted to the "secondary" mood disorders. Here prevalence rates of depression in medically and neurologically ill patients have increasingly been studied, but establishing the etiological link has been bypassed—left an open question.

In an overview of all of the proposed secondary categories, it appears that the most straightforward and strongest cases for these disorders as discrete clinical entities are those involving structural injury or insult to the CNS. In these instances, the location of the lesion and its nature appear crucial to the resultant psychiatric configuration. Without such overt CNS involvement, determining that a psychiatric presentation is due to a physical illness is more difficult, more challenging, and open to interpretation. In these instances, the nature and status of the physical illness appear instrumental.

On balance the literature appears to justify the construct of secondary disorders as discrete entities whose etiological relationships are to date variably demonstrated. Within the literature are numerous indications that these secondary conditions may not be precisely the same as disturbances with which they are phenomenologically consistent or similar. The literature suggests that some of these disturbances may differ in terms of factors, including gender distribution, genetic risk, treatment responsivity, and even course. Clearly further study of these conditions is needed to resolve the open questions. Changes in the nosology should facilitate such study.

Unquestionably DSM-IV must address the criteria that govern or define the etiological relationships of the mental disorders due to a general medical condition. Unlike DSM-III and DSM-III-R, DSM-IV cannot remain silent on what suffices to link Axis I and Axis III, and proposed changes in the pertinent criterion speak to this point. The proposed general format for the criterion requires "evidence from history, physical examination or laboratory findings" of an Axis III condition that is thought to cause the disturbance. Whether the term *secondary* proves helpful to clinicians, the proposal to incorporate the Axis III condition directly within the Axis I diagnosis using the phase "due to" seems an important step forward—one that makes the presumed connection unmistakable.

To what extent the proposed categories will resolve the problem of the confounding of psychiatric signs by medical-neurological illnesses remains at issue. This is most apparent in the case of secondary mood disorders and the difficulty in gauging vegetative signs of a depressive process in the face of physical illness. It may be that the inclusion of subtypes to increase specificity of phenomenological description will surmount this long-standing dilemma. In practice, the severity of the change in mood is the critical determinant; if marked, clinical intervention is usually judged to be indicated (even recognizing that symptoms are possibly confounded).

Finally the proposed addition of categories such as secondary catatonic disorder and secondary dissociative disorder is consistent with the structure of ICD-10, although no corresponding disorders are operative in DSM-III-R. It should also be noted that the construct of disorders "secondary to an Axis III condition" is proposed to encompass both secondary sleep disorders and secondary sexual dysfunctions.

The proposed changes are substantial, but hopefully will help investigators and clinicians alike in the effort to understand this group of conditions that bridge mental and physical illness.

References

American Psychiatric Association: Diagnostic and Statistical Manual of Mental Disorders, 3rd Edition. Washington, DC, American Psychiatric Association Press, 1980

American Psychiatric Association: Diagnostic and Statistical Manual of Mental Disorders, 3rd Edition, Revised. Washington, DC, American Psychiatric Association, 1987

American Psychiatric Association: DSM-IV Options Book: Work in Progress 9/9/91. Washington, DC, American Psychiatric Association, 1991

Bear DM, Fedio P: Quantitative analysis of interictal behavior in TLE. Arch Neurol 34:454–467, 1977

Beck A, Ward CH, Mendelson M, et al: An inventory for measuring depression. Arch Gen Psychiatry 4:561–571, 1961

Becker JT, Schaerf FW, Dew MA, et al: No relationship between affective disorders, neuropsychological function and HIV-1 seropositive status in healthy homosexual men: MACS. Abstract presented at IV International Conference on AIDS, Stockholm, Sweden, June 1988

Benson DF: The neurology of human emotion. Bull Clin Neurosci 49:23–42, 1984

Bleuler E: Dementia Praecox or the Group of Schizophrenias (1911). Translated by Zinkin J. New York, International Universities Press, 1950

Blumer D, Benson DF: Personality changes with frontal and temporal lobe lesions, in Psychiatric Aspects of Neurologic Disease. Edited by Benson DF, Blumer D. New York, Grune & Stratton, 1975, pp 151–170

Breslau N: Chronic physical illness, in Handbook of Studies in Child Psychiatry. Edited by Burrows GS. New York, Elsevier Science Publishing, 1990, pp 371–384

Bromberg W: Mental states in chronic encephalitis. Psychiatr Q 4:537, 1930

Brown GM: Psychiatric and neurological aspects of endocrine disease. Hosp Pract [Off] 10:71–79, 1975

Bukberg J, Penman D, Holland JC: Depression in hospitalized cancer patients. Psychosom Med 46:199–212, 1984

Caine ED, Shoulson I: Psychiatric syndromes in Huntington's disease. Am J Psychiatry 140:728–733, 1983

Carney RM, Rich M, teVelde A, et al: Major depressive disorder predicts cardiac events. Psychosom Med 50:627–633, 1988

Carroll BT: Catatonia on the consult service. Psychosomatics 33:310–315, 1992
Cassem NH: Depression, in the MGH Handbook of General Hospital Psychiatry, 2nd Edition. Edited by Hackett TP, Cassem NH. Littleton, MA, PSG Publishing, 1987
Clayton PJ, Lewis CE: The significance of secondary depression. J Affective Disord 3:25–35, 1981
Craven JL, Rodin GM, Johnson L, et al: The diagnosis of depression in renal dialysis patients. Psychosom Med 49:482–492, 1987
Cummings JL: Organic delusions: phenomenology, anatomical correlations and review. Br J Psychiatry 146:184–197, 1985
Cummings JL: Organic psychoses: delusional disorders and secondary mania. Psychiatr Clin North Am 9:293–312, 1986
Davison K: Schizophrenia-like psychoses associated with organic cerebral disorders: a review. Psychiatr Dev 1:1–34, 1983
Davison K, Bagley CR: Schizophrenia-like psychoses associated with organic disorders of the CNS: a review of the literature. Br J Psychiatry 4:113, 1969
Derogatis LR, Morrow GR, Fetting J, et al: The prevalence of psychiatric disorders among cancer patients. JAMA 249:751–757, 1983
Dewhurst K, Oliver J, Trick KLK, et al: Neuropsychiatric aspects of Huntington's disease. Confinia Neurologica 31:258, 1969
Dilley JW, Ochitill HN, Perl M, et al: Findings in psychiatric consultations with patients with AIDS. Am J Psychiatry 142:82–86, 1985
Dongier S: Statistical study of clinical and electroencephalographic manifestations of 536 psychotic episodes occurring in 516 epileptics between clinical seizures. Epilepsia 1:117–142, 1959/1960
Eastwood MR, Rifat SL, Nobbs H, et al: Mood disorder following CVA. Br J Psychiatry 154:195–200, 1989
Endicott J, Spitzer RL: A diagnostic interview: the Schedule for Affective Disorders and Schizophrenia. Arch Gen Psychiatry 35:837–844, 1978
Ervin F, Epstein FW, King HE: Behavior of epileptic and nonepileptic patients with "temporal spikes." Archives of Neurology and Psychiatry 74:488–497, 1955
Ettigi PG, Brown GM: Brain disorders associated with endocrine dysfunction. Psychiatr Clin North Am 1:117–136, 1978
Fairweather DS: Psychiatric aspects of the postencephalitic syndrome. Journal of Mental Sciences 93:201, 1947
Fava GA, Sonino N, Wise TN: Management of depression in medical patients. Psychother Psychosom 49:81–102, 1988
Flor-Henry P: On certain aspects of the localization of the cerebral systems regulating and determining emotion. Biol Psychiatry 14:677–698, 1979
Folstein SE, Abbott MH, Chase GA, et al: The association of affective disorder with Huntington's disease in a case series and in families. Psychol Med 13:537–542, 1983a
Folstein SE, Franz ML, Jensen BA: Conduct disorder and affective disorder among the offspring of patients with Huntington's disease. Psychol Med 13:45–52, 1983b
Frohlich ED, Tasazi RC, Dustan HP: Hyperdynamic beta-adrenergic circulatory state. Arch Intern Med 117:614–619, 1966
Garyfallos G, Manos N, Adamopoulou A: Psychopathology and personality characteristics of epileptic patients: epilepsy, psychopathology and personality. Acta Psychiatr Scand 78:87–95, 1988
Gelenberg AJ: The catatonic syndrome. Lancet 1:1339–1341, 1976

Gottlieb G, Greenspan D: Depression and endocrine disorders, in Aging and Clinical Practice: Depression and Co-Existing Disease. Edited by Robinson RG, Rabins PV. New York, Igaku-Shoin, 1989, pp 83–102

Greenberg DB: Depression and cancer, in Aging and Clinical Practice: Depression and Co-Existing Disease. Edited by Robinson RG, Rabins PV. New York, Igaku-Shoin, 1989, pp 103–115

Gudmundsson G: Epilepsy in Iceland—a clinical and epidemiological investigation. Acta Neurol Scand Suppl 25:1–124, 1966

Hall RCW (ed): Psychiatric Presentations of Medical Illness. New York, Spectrum, 1980

Hall RCW, Gardner ER, Stickney SK, et al: Physical illness manifesting as psychiatric disease, II: analysis of a state hospital inpatient population. Arch Gen Psychiatry 37:989–995, 1980

Haskett RF, Rose RM: Neuroendocrine disorders and psychopathology. Psychiatr Clin North Am 4:239–252, 1981

Haskett RF, Schteingart DE, Starkman MN, et al: Use of RDC criteria in Cushing's syndrome (Program Abstracts). Park City, UT, 10th Congress of International Society of Psychoneuroendocrinology, August 1979, p 12

Henrickson GA, Lieberman JA, Pollack S, et al: Depression in hemodialysis patients. Psychosomatics 30:284–285, 1989

Hermann BP, Whitman S: Behavioral and personality correlates of epilepsy: a review, methodologic critique and conceptual model. Psychol Bull 95:451–497, 1984

Heston LL, White JA: Dementia: A Practical Guide to Alzheimer's Disease and Related Illness. New York, WH Freeman, 1983

Huber SJ, Paulson GW, Shuttleworth EC, et al: Depression in Parkinson's disease, in Neuropsychiatry, Neuropsychology and Behavioral Neurology 1:47–51, 1988

Jefferson JW, Marshall JR (eds): Neuropsychiatric Features of Medical Disorders. New York, Plenum Medical, 1981

Jensen I, Larsen JK: Mental aspects of temporal lobe epilepsy: follow up of 74 patients after resection of a temporal lobe. J Neurol Neurosurg Psychiatry 42:256–265, 1979

Kahlbaum K: Catatonia (1874). Translated by Levis Y, Pridan T. Baltimore, MD, Johns Hopkins University Press, 1972

Karnofsky PA: Clinical evaluation of anticancer drugs, in Cancer Chemotherapy. Edited by Goklin A. Tokyo, Japan, Japanese Cancer Association, 1968

Kathol RG, Petty F: Relationship of depression to medical illness. J Affective Disord 3:111–121, 1981

Klerman GL: Depression in the medically ill. Psychiatr Clin North Am 4:301–317, 1981

Kraepelin E: Dementia Praecox and Paraphrenia (1919). Translated by Barclay RM. Edited by Robertson GM. New York, RE Krieger, 1971

Kraepelin E: Psychiatre, Vol 3, 8th Edition. Leipzig, Johan Abrosius Barth, 1922

Kral VA: The relationship between senile dementia (Alzheimer type) and depression. Can J Psychiatry 28:304–306, 1983

Krauthammer C, Klerman GL: Secondary mania. Arch Gen Psychiatry 35:1333–1339, 1978

Lader M, Marks I: Clinical Anxiety. London, Heinemann Medical, 1971

Landolt H: Serial electroencephalographic investigations during psychotic episodes in epileptic patients and during schizophrenic attacks, in Lectures on Epilepsy. Edited by de Haas L. London, Elsevier, 1958

Larsson T, Sjögren T, Jacobson G: Senile dementia. Acta Psychiatr Scand Supp 167:1–259, 1963

Lechtenberg R: Catatonia: psychiatric and neurologic, in The Psychiatrist's Guide to Diseases of the Nervous System. New York, Wiley, 1982, pp 62–66

Levine DN, Grek A: The anatomic basis of delusions after right cerebral infarction. Neurology 34:577–582, 1984

Lipowski ZJ: Organic brain syndromes: a reformulation. Compr Psychiatry 19:309–322, 1978

Lipowski ZJ: Delirium. Springfield, IL, Charles C Thomas, 1980

Lipowski ZJ: Organic mental disorders: an American perspective. Br J Psychiatry 144:542–546, 1984

Lipowski ZJ: Organic mental disorders and DSM-IV (letter). Am J Psychiatry 147:947, 1990

Lishman WA: Psychiatric disability after head injury: the significance of brain damage. Proclamation of the Royal Society of Medicine 59:261–266, 1966

Lishman WA: Head injury, in Organic Psychiatry: The Psychological Consequences of Cerebral Disorder. Edited by Lishman WA. Oxford, Blackwell Scientific Publications, 1987a, pp 137–186

Lishman WA: Symptoms and syndromes with regional afflictions: head injury, in Organic Psychiatry: The Psychological Consequences of Cerebral Disorder. Edited by Lishman WA. Oxford, Blackwell Scientific Publications, 1987b, pp 21–77

Liston EH: Clinical findings in presenile dementia: a report of 50 cases. J Nerv Ment Dis 167:337–342, 1979

Liston EH, Jarvik LF, Gerson S: Depression in Alzheimer's disease: an overview of adrenergic and cholinergic mechanisms. Compr Psychiatry 28:444–457, 1987

Lustman PJ, Griffith LS, Clouse ER, et al: Psychiatric illness in diabetes mellitus: relationship to symptoms and glucose control. J Nerv Ment Dis 174:736–742, 1986

Lustman PJ, Griffith LS, Clouse RE: Depression in adults with diabetes: results of a 5 year follow-up study. Diabetes Care 11:605–612, 1988

MacKenzie TB, Popkin MK: Organic anxiety syndrome. Am J Psychiatry 140:342–344, 1983

Mahendra E: Where have all the catatonics gone? Psychol Med 11:669–671, 1981

Marotta R, Perry S: Early neuropsychological dysfunction caused by HIV. Journal of Neuropsychiatry 1:225–234, 1989

Mayeaux R, Stein Y, Cote L, et al: Altered serotonin metabolism in depressed patients with Parkinson's disease. Neurology 34:642–646, 1984

McKenna PJ, Kane JM, Parrish K: Psychotic syndromes in epilepsy. Am J Psychiatry 142:895–904, 1985

Mendez MF: Psychopathology in epilepsy: prevalence, phenomenology and management. Int J Psychiatry Med 18:193–210, 1988

Miller BL, Benson F, Cummings JL, et al: Late life paraphrenia: an organic delusional syndrome. J Clin Psychiatry 47:204–207, 1986

Moffic HS, Paykel ES: Depression in medical inpatients. Br J Psychiatry 126:346–353, 1975

Morrison JR: Catatonia, retarded and excited types. Arch Gen Psychiatry 28:39–41, 1973

Motomura N, Sawada T, Inoue N: Neuropsychological and neuropsychiatric findings in right hemisphere damaged patients. Jpn J Psychiatry Neurol 42:747–752, 1988

Mungas D: Interictal behavior abnormality in TLE: a specific syndrome or non-specific psychopathology. Arch Gen Psychiatry 39:108–111, 1982

Neppe VM: Epilepsy and psychiatry: essential links. Psychiatric Insights 2:28–40, 1985

Neppe VM, Tucker GJ: Modern perspectives on epilepsy in relation to psychiatry: behavioral disturbances of epilepsy. Hosp Community Psychiatry 39:389–396, 1988a

Neppe VM, Tucker GJ: Modern perspectives on epilepsy in relation to psychiatry: classification and evaluation. Hosp Community Psychiatry 39:263–271, 1988b

Noyes R, Kathol RG: Depression and cancer. Psychiatr Dev 2:77–100, 1986

Parnas J, Korsgaard S, Krautwald O, et al: Chronic psychosis in epilepsy: a clinical investigation of 29 patients. Acta Psychiatr Scand 66:282–293, 1982

Pascually M, Veith RC: Depression as an adverse drug reaction, in Aging and Clinical Practice: Depression and Co-Existing Disease. Edited by Robinson RG, Rabins PV. New York, Igaku-Shoin, 1989, pp 132–151

Perez MM, Trimble MR: Epileptic psychosis: diagnostic comparison with process schizophrenia. Br J Psychiatry 137:245–249, 1981

Petty F, Noyes R: Depression secondary to cancer. Biol Psychiatry 16:1203–1220, 1981

Pincus JH, Tucker GJ: Behavioral Neurology, 3rd Edition. London, Oxford University Press, 1985

Pitts FN Jr, McClure JN: Lactate metabolism in anxiety neuroses. N Engl J Med 277:1328–1336, 1967

Popkin MK: Organic brain syndromes with little or no cognitive impairment, in Medical Psychiatry. Edited by Winokur G, Clayton P. Philadelphia, PA, WB Saunders, 1986, pp 29–38

Popkin MK, Mackenzie TB: Psychiatric presentations of endocrine dysfunction, in Psychiatric Presentations of Medical Illness. Edited by Hall RCW. New York, Spectrum, 1980, pp 139–156

Popkin MK, Callies AL, Colón EA: A framework for the study of medical depression. Psychosomatics 28:27–33, 1987

Popkin MK, Callies AL, Lentz RD, et al: Prevalence of major depression, simple phobia, and other psychiatric disorders in patients with longstanding Type I diabetes mellitus. Arch Gen Psychiatry 45:64–68, 1988

Rabins PV: Depression and multiple sclerosis, in Aging and Clinical Practice: Depression and Co-Existing Disease. Edited by Robinson RG, Rabins PV. New York, Igaku-Shoin, 1989, pp 226–233

Rabins PV, Brooks BR, O'Donnell P, et al: Structural brain correlates of emotional disorder in multiple sclerosis. Brain 109:585–597, 1986

Regier DA, Myers JK, Kramer M, et al: The NIMH Epidemiologic Catchment Area program: historical context, major objectives, and study populations characteristics. Arch Gen Psychiatry 41:934–941, 1984

Reynolds EH: Interictal behavior in TLE. BMJ 286:918–919, 1983

Robins LN, Helzer JE, Croughan J, et al: National Institute of Mental Health Diagnostic Interview Schedule: its history, characteristics, and validity. Arch Gen Psychiatry 38:381–389, 1981

Robinson RG: Introduction to depression and chronic medical illness, in Aging and Clinical Practice: Depression and Co-Existing Disease. Edited by Robinson RG, Rabins PV. New York, Igaku-Shoin, 1989

Robinson RG, Starkstein SE: Current research in affective disorders following stroke. Journal of Neuropsychiatry 2:1–14, 1990

Robinson RG, Kubos KL, Starr LB, et al: Mood disorders in stroke patients: importance of location of lesion. Brain 107:81–93, 1984

Rodin G, Voshart K: Depression in the medically ill: an overview. Am J Psychiatry 143:696–705, 1986

Rosenbaum JF, Pollack MH: Anxiety, in the MGH Handbook of General Hospital Psychiatry, 2nd Edition. Edited by Hackett TP, Cassem NH. Littleton, MA, PSG Publishing, 1987, pp 154–183

Roth M: Discussion of "Classification of late life organic states and the DSM-III" by Clayton PJ, Martin R, in Clinical Aspects of Alzheimer's Disease and Senile Dementia (Aging, Vol 15). Edited by Miller NE, Cohen GD. New York, Raven, 1981, pp 55–59

Rovner BW, Morriss RK: Depression and Alzheimer's disease, in Aging and Clinical Practice: Depression and Co-Existing Disease. Edited by Robinson RG, Rabins PV. New York, Igaku-Shoin, 1989, pp 202–212

Sachar EJ, Rose RM: Psychoendocrinology, in the Textbook of Endocrinology. Edited by Williams RH. Philadelphia, PA, WB Saunders, 1981

Sato T, Takeichi M: A case of chronic subdural hematoma with anxiety states and concomitant regression-like symptoms. Jpn J Psychiatry Neurol 41:663–667, 1987

Schaerf FW, Miller RR: Depression and HIV-1 infection, in Aging and Clinical Practice: Depression and Co-Existing Disease. Edited by Robinson RG, Rabins PV. New York, Igaku-Shoin, 1989, pp 169–185

Schiffer RB, Babigian HM: Behavioral disorders in multiple sclerosis, TLE and ALS: an epidemiologic study. Arch Neurol 41:1067–1068, 1984

Schiffer RB, Caine ED, Bamford KA, et al: Depressive episodes in patients with multiple sclerosis. Am J Psychiatry 140:1498–1500, 1983

Schiffer RB, Weitkamp LR, Wineman M, et al: Multiple sclerosis and affective disorders. Arch Neurol 45:1345–1346, 1988

Schuckit MA: Anxiety related to medical disease. J Clin Psychiatry 44:31–37, 1983

Schulberg HC, McClelland M, Burns BJ: Depression and physical illness: prevalence, causation and diagnosis of co-morbidity. Clinical Psychology Review 7:145–167, 1987

Schwab JJ, Bialow M, Brown JM, et al: Diagnosing depression in medical inpatients. Ann Intern Med 67:695–707, 1967

Sheehan DV: Extreme manifestations of anxiety in the general hospital, in the MGH Handbook of General Hospital Psychiatry. Edited by Hackett TP, Cassem WH. St. Louis, CV Mosby, 1978

Slater E, Beard AW, Glithero E: The schizophrenia-like psychoses of epilepsy. Br J Psychiatry 109:95–150, 1963

Smith CK, Barish J, Correa J, et al: Psychiatric disturbance in endocrinologic disease. Psychosom Med 34:69–86, 1972

Smith MD, Hong BA, Robson AM: Diagnosis of depression in patients with endstage renal disease. Am J Med 79:160–166, 1985

Spitzer RL, Endicott J, Robins E: Research Diagnostic Criteria: rational and reliability. Arch Gen Psychiatry 35:773–782, 1978

Spitzer RL, Williams JBW, First M, et al: A proposal for DSM-IV: solving the organic-nonorganic problem. Journal of Neuropsychiatry 1:126–127, 1989

Starkman MN, Cameron OG, Nesse RM, et al: Peripheral catecholamine levels and the symptoms of anxiety: studies in patients with and without pheochromocytoma. Psychosom Med 52:129–142, 1990

Starkstein SE, Robinson RG: Affective disorders and cerebral vascular disease. Br J Psychiatry 154:170–182, 1989a

Starkstein SE, Robinson RG: Depression and Parkinson's disease, in Aging and Clinical Practice: Depression and Co-Existing Disease. Edited by Robinson RG, Rabins PV. New York, Igaku-Shoin, 1989b, pp 213–225

Starkstein SE, Bolduc PL, Prezioski TJ, et al: Cognitive impairment in different stages of Parkinson's disease. Journal of Neuropsychiatry 1:243–248, 1988

Stevens JR: Interictal clinical manifestations of complex partial seizures, in Advances in Neurology, II. Edited by Penry JK, Daly DD. New York, Raven, 1975, pp 85–112

Stewart JA, Drake F, Winokur G: Depression among medically ill patients. Diseases of the Nervous System 26:479–485, 1965

Stoudemire A: The differential diagnosis of catatonic states. Psychosomatics 23:245–252, 1982

Surridge D: An investigation into some psychiatric aspects of multiple sclerosis. Am J Psychiatry 115:749–764, 1969

Taylor DC: Mental state and temporal lobe epilepsy: a correlative account of 100 patients treated surgically. Epilepsia 13:727–765, 1972

Taylor MA: DSM-III organic mental disorders, in Diagnosis and Classification in Psychiatry. Edited by Tischler G. Cambridge, MA, Cambridge University Press, 1987, pp 147–174

Tomonasa M, Yamanouchi H, Tokyi H, et al: Clinicopathologic study of progressive subcortical vascular encephalopathy (Binswanser type) in the elderly. J Am Geriatr Soc 30:524–529, 1982

Trimble MR: The Psychopathology of Epilepsy. Horsham, West Sussex, Geigy, 1981

Trimble MR: The psychoses of epilepsy and their treatment. Clin Neuropharmacol 8:211–220, 1985

Tucker GJ, Price TRP, Johnson VB, et al: Phenomenology of temporal lobe dysfunction: a link to atypical psychoses: a series of cases. J Nerv Ment Dis 174:348–356, 1986

Venkatesh A, Pauls DL, Crowe R, et al: MVP in anxiety neurosis (panic disorder). Am Heart J 37:1361–1365, 1981

Waxman SG, Geschwind N: The interictal behavior syndrome of TLE. Arch Gen Psychiatry 32:1580–1588, 1975

Weddington WW, Marks RC, Verghese P: Disulfiram encephalopathy as a cause of the catatonia syndrome. Am J Psychiatry 137:1217–1219, 1980

Wells CE, Duncan GS: Other neurologic disorders important for the psychiatrist, in Neurology for Psychiatrists. Edited by Wells CE, Duncan GS. Philadelphia, PA, FA Davis, 1980, pp 203–222

Wells KB, Golding JM, Burnham MA: Psychiatric disorder in a sample of the general population with and without chronic medical conditions. Am J Psychiatry 145:976–981, 1988

Whitlock FA, Siskind MM: Depression as a major symptom of multiple sclerosis. J Neurol Neurosurg Psychiatry 43:861–865, 1980

Wing JK, Cooper JE, Sartorius N: The Measurement and Classification of Psychiatric Symptoms. New York, Cambridge University Press, 1974

Wooley CF: The mitral valve prolapse syndrome. Hosp Pract [Off] 18:163–174, 1983

Wooley CF: From irritable heart to mitral valve prolapse: World War I—the US experience and the origin of neurocirculatory asthenia. Am J Cardiol 59:1183–1186, 1987

World Health Organization: The ICD-10 Classification of Mental and Behavioural Disorders: Clinical Descriptions and Diagnostic Guidelines. Geneva, World Health Organization, 1992

Yudofsky SC, Silver JM: Psychiatric aspects of brain injury: trauma, stroke and tumor, in Psychiatry Update: American Psychiatric Association Annual Review, Vol 4. Edited by Hales RE, Frances AJ. Washington DC, American Psychiatric Press, 1985, pp 142–158

Zelnick T: Depressive effects of drugs, in the Presentations of Depressions and Depressive Symptoms in Medical and Other Psychiatric Disease. Edited by Cameron O. New York, Wiley Interscience, 1978, pp 382–3830

Chapter 18

Regional Syndromes

Gary J. Tucker, M.D.

Statement of the Issues

In DSM-III-R (American Psychiatric Association 1987) the primary conditions related to dysfunction of the central nervous system are delirium and dementia. However, for many years clinicians have identified syndromes in which behavior disturbance secondary to central nervous system damage was the paramount clinical feature rather than either delirium or prominent dementia. Often these behaviors have been named for the supposed anatomical region that has been damaged (e.g., frontal lobe, temporal lobe) or more globally organic personality syndromes. The purpose of this review is to see whether there is a data base to support the specific designation of such behavioral syndromes in DSM-IV.

At present, there are five major behavioral syndrome areas that seem clinically relevant but are not currently covered in DSM-III-R: 1) disinhibited syndrome, 2) apathetic syndrome, 3) paroxysmal syndromes, 4) various akinetic states, and 5) movement disorder secondary to neuroleptics. (Disinhibited syndrome and apathetic syndrome are often grouped together as frontal lobe syndrome.)

The major question remains, does the state of our knowledge warrant stipulation of such categories or are they best subsumed under the existing categories as is currently done. If these syndromes are clear and not covered by existing categories, then there would be great clinical utility in including them as well as providing more precision to the diagnostic process for clinical diagnosis, treatment, and research.

Significance of the Issues

It would be extremely important to include more diagnostic categories if there are data to warrant them in order to make treatment, particularly, more precise. For

I thank Drs. F. Benson, J. Cummings, and M. Mesulum for their review of this chapter.

example, in using the concept of "frontal lobe syndrome," one is often confronted with two distinct syndromes (e.g., a disinhibited state and an apathetic state). The treatment for both of these conditions is probably quite different, and the attendant management and care issues are also quite different. Consequently, for concerns about reimbursement and difficulty in the care of patients, it might be extremely important to distinguish between these conditions. Also, each of these states may very well represent a continuum of behavior as an illness progresses. Without the possibility of stipulating this, it might be missed. Lastly, the research implications are extremely important. It is important to note that ICD-10 (World Health Organization 1992) is much more generous in the use of categories for various behavioral conditions related to damage of central nervous system dysfunction (e.g., various types of dementia, human immunodeficiency virus, Parkinson's disease, postencephalitic syndromes).

Methods

Frequently, these syndromes have been labeled by the anatomical region of the brain that seems to have been injured (e.g., frontal, parietal, temporal). Perhaps most important to this discussion, however, is to recall that most of the anatomical regions of the brain have been delineated on the basis of their gross anatomy and not necessarily on their function, although to some extent the gross anatomical descriptions and function have some rough correlation.

The concept of specific regional syndromes has existed in the literature for a long time; however, it is based mostly on case reports. We have limited this review to studies that employed control subjects and used standardized test batteries. Another potential source of data is the large number of studies done on psychiatric patients who had frontal lobotomies; these are cited but not used as part of the data base because it is confusing to compare brain-damaged patients without psychopathology to brain-damaged patients with existing serious psychopathology.

Results

Syndromes such as we are considering are characterized by the classic case of Phineas Gage (Harlow 1868). Similar classic case examples have been described by Brickner (1936), Hebb and Penfield (1940), Ackerly and Benton (1947), and Stuss and Benson (1986). Damasio (1979) reviewed these case reports and concluded that the patients share the following similar features:

> lack of originality and creativity; inability to organize future activity, hold gainful employment, and be fully independent; inability to focus attention (distractibil-

> ity); recent memory vulnerable to interference; tendency to present a favorable view of themselves often to the point of boastfulness; stereotyped but pleasant manners in nonthreatening situations; tendency to display inappropriate emotional reaction; diminished ability to experience pleasure and probably also to react to pain; diminished sexual and exploratory drives; lack of motor, sensory, or communication deficits; overall intelligence scale within average for age and education. (p. 377)

However, Damasio (1979) and others cited the difficulty with attempts to localize functions to specific anatomical areas in light of the following specific factors: 1) the types of lesions vary; 2) the age of the individual when injured is critical to the development of compensatory functions; and 3) the nature of the lesion in terms of extent of cerebral involvement and complications vary (e.g., intercranial hypertension). These factors are particularly evident when one moves from case reports to the few large-scale studies that have been done on patients with frontal lobe injuries. Hecaen (1964) reported on 131 patients with frontal lobe tumors. He compared these to 359 patients with tumors not in the frontal lobes. He described two states in the frontal lobe tumors. In one, there was a confused state with dementia; this was present in 67% of the cases. These patients showed slowing, both of psyche and movement, apathy, mutism and inertia, decreased attention and decreased memory, as well as indifference, somnolence, and childlike behavior. Of these patients with dementia, 37%–41% showed mood and character changes manifested by irritability, euphoria, depression, emotional instability, increases in "instinctive" behavior (e.g., bulimia and changes in sexual activity), and hallucinations. Hecaen stated that similar symptoms have been found in other studies and cited 300–400 cases of frontal lobe damage where the patients show symptomatology similar to the two syndromes that he described. However, Hecaen noted that although these syndromes occur more frequently with frontal lobe damage, they can also occur with damage to other brain regions, and often the symptoms lack specificity with regard to anatomical location.

Reitan (1964) reported on a series of 112 patients equally divided between those who had anterior (frontal) and posterior brain damage as well as those who had diffuse as opposed to focal damage. Although many of the patients behaviorally fell into the two syndromes delineated by Hecaen (1964), he noted that an experienced neuropsychologist could make inferences about localization but no statistical difference could be made on a basis of the test results using the Halstead-Reitan Neuropsychological Test Battery (Reitan 1979). He stated in summary:

> Although we have carefully studied several thousand patients during the past 11 years, each having taken the same battery of psychological tests, we had barely

> enough material to fill out the cells. . . . We do not yet have nearly enough patients to set up adequate samples of differently localized lesions within the lesion categories in order to study the problem properly. We may be able to accumulate large enough groups within the next 20 years but we would hope by that time the tests might have lost their significance. (p. 305)

However, it is clear that 25 years later the tests are still used, and the data are not yet available.

Milner (1963, 1964) studied patients with seizure disorders using the Wisconsin Card Sorting Test (Heaton 1985) and showed that patients with frontal lobe damage had difficulty in shifting tasks or set. However, Teuber (1964) also used the Wisconsin Card Sorting Test but studied patients with gunshot wounds to the frontal region, and he could not confirm Milner's findings. Also Rosvold (1972) showed that in lobotomized patients similar deficits as Milner found on the card sort test were present postoperatively but seemed to disappear over time. Classic studies by Luria (1965, 1966, 1969) of patients with frontal lobe damage also demonstrated poor ability to change set and problems with word fluency. Similar behavioral deficits in maintaining sets and attending to tasks have been cited in animal models (Fulton and Jacobson 1935) as well.

A large literature on lobotomy patients that confirms the above behavioral findings also exists (Lewis et al. 1956; Mettler 1949, 1952; Tow 1955). Again, these studies lend some credence to specific dysfunctions in frontal lobe injury but often these are not specific to frontal lobe injury. However, the same dysfunctions have been reported in patients with lesions in other brain regions as well.

Discussion

From this review it is apparent that there are clinical syndromes that exist both in large series of well-studied patients and in individual detailed clinical reports that manifest noticeable and consistent behavior change as the major features and where deficits in intelligence (cognitive functioning) or memory are much less prominent. Although the evidence does not support a regional specificity for these syndromes, there does seem to be clinical evidence that these syndromes exist. Consequently, the current DSM nomenclature is without characterization for these syndromes, which are common to everyday clinical practice. We propose that the following neurobehavioral conditions be considered for inclusion in the psychiatric nomenclature as they are partially included in ICD-9 (World Health Organization 1977) and proposed, in part, for ICD-10.

- *Apathetic syndrome.* This syndrome usually includes an apathetic condition, indifference, and some diminished activity, often with motor perseveration and cognitive perseveration. The patients often fail to initiate, persevere in activity, and lose interest easily.
- *Disinhibited syndrome.* These patients are impulsive, inappropriate, often with a euphoric and jocular affect (Witzelsucht). They have emotional lability, very poor judgment and insight, and are easily distractible. They frequently show a loss of previous social behaviors and an inability to modulate their affect.

It is important to note that these conditions can exist, usually without prominent memory and cognitive deficits. Although memory and cognitive deficits certainly can be detected, the major facet of the syndrome is the change in behavior. Also it is quite clear that these symptoms can and often do overlap; however, there seems to be a predominance of symptoms that group together into clear-cut syndromes. Although inferences can be made that certain behaviors are due to specific frontal lobe, temporal lobe, or parietal lobe dysfunctions, it is quite clear that these anatomical designations are inferential. These symptoms are common in many nonlocalized as well as localized neurologic disorders and probably represent general responses (that may be either genetically determined or related to stages of disease) to central nervous system damage. There are many functional neurophysiologic loops connecting the cortex with most other brain regions that highlight the difficulty in correlating a precise anatomical lesion with a behavior, as the newer theories of neurofunction cite dual simultaneous processing as important mediators of most responses or behaviors (Goldman-Rakic et al. 1984; Stuss and Benson 1986). Consequently, to specify anatomical locations for the behavioral syndromes is probably not warranted by our current state of knowledge.

Distinct Disorder Versus Personality Disorder

Although there seem to be good data to show that there are two syndromes that we could label *disinhibited* and *apathetic*, the question immediately arises as to why these should not be labeled as a personality disorder. The fact is that they could be labeled as a personality disorder or a specific syndrome. In fact, ICD-10 does just this, citing under organic personality disorder (F07.0) "frontal lobe syndrome" and also citing organic and emotionally labile or asthenic disorder (F06.5) as a specific syndrome.

Apathetic or disinhibited changes can certainly occur as a prolonged habitual way of relating to the world. They certainly would meet the criteria that a personality disorder is an "enduring pattern of perceiving, relating to, and thinking about the environment and oneself" (American Psychiatric Association 1987, p. 335).

However, this does not answer the question of whether lability and apathy are personality traits or symptoms. It would be more appropriate if we could use the personality diagnosis for changes in personality traits of a persistent nature, such as a mild-mannered person who becomes aggressive, or someone who is used to being rather passive becoming aggressive in dealing with problems, or someone who is hyposexual becoming hypersexual over a prolonged period of time. ICD-10 stipulates symptoms must be present for 6 months. One could look at the symptoms attendant with organic damage like lability and apathy as moderating influences on an already existing personality. In fact, they are major symptoms associated with all types of brain damage. In this sense, we would then have to classify the apathy and energy in a depressed patient as "affective personality disorder." In part, these symptoms are the symptoms that make the diagnosis, and by putting them as a personality disorder, they become more than symptoms. In this respect, a patient with senile dementia Alzheimer's type could then have several diagnoses: "organic affective disorder," "organic personality disorder," and "organic anxiety disorder." A factor in favor of retaining a diagnostic entity for these conditions unrelated to personality disorder would also relate to the fact that many of these changes are transient, and in 6 months to a year, many are reversible by treating the organic condition. Often, many of these traits respond to medication better than what we consider most personality traits; therefore, one would have to consider the personality and the phenomena itself. The personality traits induced by organicity are often the epiphenomena that moderate existing personality traits.

We could also consider apathetic or disinhibited as stipulations to the diagnosis of dementia or delirium, but if the symptoms of dementia or delirium are not prominent, then it would be difficult to fit them in, using the current nomenclature.

Paroxysmal or Episodic Conditions

An increasing number of patients who have recurrent paroxysmal behavioral disturbances related most often to seizure disorders and other cerebral pathology have been described (Blumer et al. 1988; Himmelhoch 1984; McKenna et al. 1985; Monroe 1982; Neppe and Tucker 1988; Tucker et al. 1985; Wells 1975). These paroxysmal attacks can take the form of amnesia, lapses, automatisms, hallucinations, delusional thoughts, affective disturbance, and suicidal ideation. These symptoms are often so ego-alien that the patient experiences them for brief periods of time (hours to weeks) and then returns to normal with no behavioral residual. The electroencephalogram is often abnormal and of a paroxysmal nature; however, it can also be normal as well. The chief characteristics of this condition are the paroxysmal nature of the symptoms and the return to normalcy.

There is excellent evidence in the literature that supports the occurrence of brief psychotic episodes, which are indistinguishable from schizophrenia, in patients with seizure disorders. These psychotic states are not related to delirious or confusional episodes but occur in clear consciousness. Perez and Trimble (1980, 1985) have shown with standardized rating scales that these psychotic states are indistinguishable in large part from schizophrenia. Landholt (1953, 1958) described 51 patients with similar conditions. Dongier (1959) described 516 patients with such conditions; of course, there are also the classic cases described by Slater and colleagues (1963). Whether these psychotic states are peri-ictal, ictal, or postictal is as yet unclear, but it is clear that psychotic states can mimic schizophrenic episodes. These patients, in most part, do not have a family history of schizophrenia.

However, these conditions can be stipulated in current use by citing the primary medical condition that causes them. They do not form a distinct category associated with nonspecific central nervous system damage but are more specific to the underlying condition.

Movement Disorders

There are a small number of patients who, after various insults to the central nervous system, develop an akinetic state. These patients manifest a paucity of spontaneous movement, sparse verbal output, and motor weakness (specifically of the lower extremity). These patients must be differentiated from patients with catatonia, seizure disorders, and drug-induced conditions. ICD-10 has a category for these patients called organic catatonic disorder (F06.1). Perhaps we should consider using this as well or at least referring to it.

We also considered the possibility of including categories for the various movement disorders that are secondary to psychotropic substances (e.g., dystonias, pseudo-parkinsonian, akathisia, and tardive dyskinesia).

Recommendations

1. Include three syndrome types—Personality Change Disorders under Secondary Personality Change due to a nonpsychiatric medical condition:
   A. *Apathetic Type.* This syndrome usually includes an apathetic condition, indifference, some diminished activity often with motor perseveration and cognitive perseveration. The patients often fail to initiate and persevere in activity and frequently lose interest easily.
   B. *Disinhibited Type.* These patients are impulsive, inappropriate, often with a euphoric and jocular affect (Witzelsucht). They have emotional lability, very poor judgment and insight, and are easily distractible. They

frequently show a loss of previous social behavior and an inability to modulate their affect.

C. *Labile Type.* This is manifested by an episodic course of any of the above symptoms.

If this is not deemed possible, then consider these categories as stipulations for the dementias.

2. Cite in text various categories for movement disorders cited in neurology portion of ICD-10, such as:

   Neuroleptic Malignant Syndrome (G21.0)
   Medication-Induced Parkinsonianism (G21.1)
   Medication-Induced Akathisia (G21.8)
   Medication-Induced Dyskinesia (G24.01)
   Medication-Induced Dystonia (G24.02)
   Medication-Induced Tremor (G25.1)
   Medication-Induced Movement Disorder Not Otherwise Specified (G25.9)

References

Ackerly S, Benton A: Report of a case of bilateral frontal lobe defect. Association for Research in Nervous Mental Diseases 27:479–504, 1947

American Psychiatric Association: Diagnostic and Statistical Manual of Mental Disorders, 3rd Edition, Revised. Washington, DC, American Psychiatric Association, 1987

Blumer D, Heilbronn M, Himmelhoch J: Indications for carbamazepine in mental illness: atypical psychiatric disorder or temporal lobe syndrome? Compr Psychiatry 29:108–122, 1988

Brickner RM: The Intellectual Function of the Frontal Lobes. New York, MacMillan, 1936

Damasio A: The frontal lobes, in Clinical Neuropsychology. Edited by Heilman K, Valenstein E. New York, Oxford University Press, 1979, pp 360–412

Dongier S: Statistical study of clinical and EEG manifestations of 536 psychotic episodes occurring in 516 epileptics between clinical seizures. Epilepsia 1:117–142, 1959

Fulton J, Jacobson C: The functions of the frontal lobe. Advanced Medical Biology 4:113–123, 1935

Goldman-Rakic P, Seleman L, Schwartz M: Dual pathways connecting the dorsilateral prefrontal cortex with the hippocampal formation and parahippocampal cortex in the rhesus monkey. Neuroscience 12:719–743, 1984

Harlow J: Recovery after severe injury to the head. Massachusetts Medical Society 2:327–346, 1868

Heaton R: Wisconsin Card Sorting Test. Odessa, TX, Psychological Assessment Resources, 1985

Hebb D, Penfield W: Human behavior after extensive bilateral removal from frontal lobes. Archives of Neurology and Psychiatry 44:421–438, 1940
Hecaen H: Mental symptoms associated with tumors of the frontal lobe, in Frontal Granular Cortex and Behavior. Edited by Warren J, Akert K. New York, McGraw-Hill, 1964, pp 335–352
Himmelhoch JM: Major mood disorders related to epileptic changes, in Psychiatric Aspects of Epilepsy. Edited by Blumer D. Washington, DC, American Psychiatric Press, 1984, pp 271–294
Landholt H: Some clinical EEG correlations in epileptic psychosis. Electroencephalogr Clin Neurophysiol 5:121, 1953
Landholt H: Serial electroencephalographic investigations during psychotic episodes in epileptic patients and during schizophrenic attacks, in Lectures on Epilepsy. Edited by Lorentz de Haas AM. Amsterdam, Elsevier, 1958, pp 91–133
Lewis N, Landis C, Kuig H: Studies in Topectomy. New York, Grune & Stratton, 1956
Luria A: Two kinds of motor perseveration in massive injury of the frontal lobes. Brain 88:1–10, 1965
Luria A: Higher Cortical Functions in Man. New York, Basic Books, 1966
Luria A: Frontal lobe syndromes, in Handbook of Clinical Neurology. Edited by Vinker P, Bruzer G. Amsterdam, North Holland, 1969, pp 725–757
McKenna P, Kane JM, Parrish K: Psychiatric syndromes in epilepsy. Am J Psychiatry 142:895–904, 1985
Mettler FA (ed): Selective Partial Ablation of the Frontal Cortex. New York, Columbia Greystroke Associates, 1949
Mettler FA: Psychological Problems. Philadelphia, PA, Blakiston, 1952
Milner B: Effects of different brain lesions on card sorting: the role of the frontal lobes. Arch Neurol 9:90–100, 1963
Milner B: Some effects of frontal lobectomy in man, in Frontal Granular Cortex and Behavior. Edited by Warren J, Akert K. New York, McGraw-Hill, 1964, pp 313–334
Monroe R: Limbic ictus and atypical psychosis. J Nerv Ment Dis 170:711–716, 1982
Neppe VM, Tucker GJ: Modern perspectives on epilepsy in relation to psychiatry: behavioral disturbances of epilepsy. Hosp Community Psychiatry 39:389–396, 1988
Perez M, Trimble MR: Epileptic psychosis diagnostic comparison with process schizophrenia. Br J Psychiatry 137:245–249, 1980
Perez M, Trimble MR: An evaluation of PSE profiles. Br J Psychiatry 146:155–164, 1985
Reitan R: Psychological deficits resulting from cerebral lesions in man, in Frontal Granular Cortex and Behavior. Edited by Warren J, Akert K. New York, McGraw-Hill, 1964, pp 295–312
Reitan RM: Halstead-Reitan Neuropsychological Test Battery. Tucson, AZ, Neuropsychology Laboratory, University of Arizona, 1979
Rosvold H: The frontal lobe system. Acta Neurobiol Exp (Warsz) 32:439–460, 1972
Slater E, Beard AW, Glithro E: The schizophrenia-like psychoses of epilepsy. Br J Psychiatry 109:95–150, 1963
Stuss D, Benson F: The Frontal Lobes. New York, Raven, 1986
Teuber H: The riddle of frontal lobe function in man, in The Frontal Granular Cortex and Behavior. Edited by Warren J, Akert K. New York, McGraw-Hill, 1964, pp 410–444
Tow P: Personality Changes Following Frontal Leukotomy. London, Oxford Press, 1955
Tucker G, Price T, Johnson V: Phenomenology of temporal lobe dysfunction. J Nerv Ment Dis 174:348–356, 1985

Wells C: Transient ictal psychosis. Arch Gen Psychiatry 32:1201–1203, 1975

World Health Organization: International Classification of Diseases, 9th Revision. Geneva, World Health Organization, 1977

World Health Organization: The ICD-10 Classification of Mental and Behavioural Disorders: Clinical Descriptions and Diagnostic Guidelines. Geneva, World Health Organization, 1992

Chapter 19

Mild Neurocognitive Disorder

A Needed Addition to the Nosology of Cognitive Impairment (Organic Mental) Disorders?

Rosben Gutierrez, M.D.
J. Hampton Atkinson, M.D.
Igor Grant, M.D.

Statement of the Issues

In this review, we address the question of whether DSM-IV should include a new organic mental disorder diagnosis.[1] This diagnosis would consider disturbances in cognition related to an Axis III disorder, but the severity or qualitative features of which fail to meet DSM criteria for delirium, dementia, or other specific organic mental disorder. What exists in the current DSM (and proposed DSM-IV) nomenclature for organic mental syndromes and disorders (cognitive impairment disorders) is essentially a dichotomy of "normal," that is, a condition failing to meet diagnostic criteria, versus a demented or delirious state. Interestingly, ICD-10 (World Health Organization 1992) has recognized the importance of the omission of such disorders from its earlier versions and now proposes a category of mild cognitive disorder.

Information presented here also appears in the *Journal of Neuropsychiatry and Clinical Neurosciences* 5:161–177, 1993.

[1] DSM-IV proposes to use the term *Cognitive Impairment Disorders* as a replacement for *Organic Mental Disorders.* These terms are used interchangeably in this chapter.

Significance of the Issues

Organic mental syndromes and disorders, primarily dementia and delirium, are widely recognized in medically ill patients (Golinger and Fedoroff 1989; Wise and Taylor 1990; Wragg and Jeste 1989). Although dementia and delirium are two conditions that are clinically and diagnostically well characterized, they represent only one extreme end of the cognitive spectrum. Many individuals may present with substantial cognitive dysfunction, but the degree of this impairment is not severe enough to warrant a diagnosis of dementia or delirium. Clinicians, particularly those working in consultation-liaison settings, often observe patients who exhibit neurocognitive symptoms thought to be related to disturbances in central nervous system structure or function, but for which there is no readily applicable DSM diagnosis. Nonetheless, this "milder" cognitive impairment may have significant implications for everyday functioning (Heaton and Pendleton 1981). As evidence accumulates that milder organic mental syndromes or disorders are common in an even larger proportion of medically ill patients, more descriptive nosology is needed to enhance specificity in diagnosis and eventual treatment (Dickson and Ranseen 1990; Kendler 1990; Silver et al. 1990). Up to this time, however, reports of these milder findings have not been systematically reviewed in the context of neuropsychological assessment and level of cognitive impairment.

Features distinguishing this proposal from other specific organic mental syndromes or disorders will include a reliably documented neurocognitive impairment that fails to reach criteria for delirium or dementia coupled with a known or strongly suspected Axis III etiology. This proposal defines diagnostic criteria that should be usable in clinical practice.

Methods

We utilized the MELVYL system's search of the medical catalog at the University of California, San Diego. A comprehensive search sought recent citations that described standardized neuropsychological assessment in medical, neurological, and substance use disorders. Additionally, major recent review articles in areas such as alcohol use disorders were consulted.

Among the medical and neurological disorders, the majority of studies reported concerned metabolic abnormalities, infectious diseases, and hypoxemic conditions. To address pharmacologically induced cognitive disorders, we consulted recent reviews on alcohol and other drug abuse and dependence, including the neuropsychological effects of abstinence. In terms of prescribed drugs, we reviewed studies of beta-blocking agents and benzodiazepines to provide examples of two commonly prescribed medications that can influence cognitive processes.

References are summarized and presented in tabular form (Table 19–1 and Table 19–2). Particular attention is given to studies with larger sample sizes and those using standardized neuropsychological instruments. Where data permitted, we have subclassified subjects into categories of "demented" and "impaired not demented." This should help define the relative frequency of each "level" of cognitive impairment. In the heading "improvement after treatment" the potential reversibility of cognitive changes is noted (includes improvement following abstinence from substance use).

Common neuropsychological tests used in studies we reviewed include the Wechsler Adult Intelligence Scale—Revised (Wechsler 1981) and one of its subtests, digit span; the Wechsler Memory Scale; the Paced Auditory Serial Addition Test; a subtest from the Halstead-Reitan Neuropsychological Test Battery (Reitan 1979), the Category Test; the Stroop Word Test; the Trail Making Form A and B; and the Paired Associate Learning Test (for descriptions of these tests, see Hartlage et al. 1987). These neuropsychological tests reflect functioning in content areas of verbal-language, attention-immediate recall with auditory stimuli, memory, speed of information processing, abstraction (flexibility of thinking), perceptual-motor abilities, visuomotor skills–parallel processing, and learning, respectively.

In general, in this review we sought citations that described standardized neuropsychological assessment in medical, neurological, and substance use disorders, particularly chronic conditions. Most of the references are from 1987 to 1990. Conditions constituting acute confusional states, such as delirium, are excluded from the search.

Results

Reports addressing the notion of milder neurocognitive disturbance come from three general sources: the literature on alcohol and substance abuse and dependence, the literature on neurological disorders, and the literature on medical disorders with central nervous system complications.

From the standpoint of alcohol use disorders, it has long been recognized that alcoholic persons can experience neuropsychological deficits short of dementia or the Wernicke-Korsakoff syndrome (Grant 1987). These disturbances in learning, recall, abstracting ability, and complex conceptual motor skills often exist in the context of relatively preserved psychometric IQ. It is thought that about 50% of alcoholic persons who have been abstinent for 3–4 weeks have neuropsychological deficit (Grant 1986a). Their impairment can be reliably measured and often is accompanied by supportive laboratory data such as "brain shrinkage" on brain computed tomography and magnetic resonance imaging scans, deficits in cerebral

Table 19–1. Studies involving neuropsychological assessment in medical and neurologic disorders

Author	Study	Subjects	Instruments	Level of cognitive impairment: Demented	Level of cognitive impairment: Impaired not demented	Improvement after treatment	Comments
A. Hypoxemia							
Block et al. 1989	Nocturnal oxygen therapy and snorer's intelligence	17 male heavy snorers, otherwise "normal"; double-blind crossover	WAIS-R; WMS; Rey-Osterrieth Complex Figure; Hooper; Wisconsin Card Sort; Verbal Fluency–using Controlled Oral Word Association Test (FAS version)	None	Implied baseline NP "deficits"	Nocturnal oxygen therapy did not improve NP results	MNCD
Telakivi et al. 1988	Cognitive function in middle-age snorers	46 chronically snoring men ages 41–52 years; 60 age-matched controls	WAIS; WMS; Benton Visual Retention; Trail Making; Clock; Visual Graphic; Symmetry Drawings; others not specified	None	Deficits in delayed recall of logical stories of WMS and spatial orientation of Clock test	Not reported	MNCD
Grant et al. 1987b	NP impairment and hypoxemia	302 COPD patients; mild, moderate, severe hypoxemia; 99 age- and education-matched controls	Average Impairment Rating; WAIS; WMS; Halstead-Reitan Battery; Rennick-Lafayette Repeatable Battery	None	NP "impairment" associated with varying degrees of hypoxemia	Not reported	MNCD
Berry et al. 1986	Nocturnal hypoxia and NP variables	46 male heavy snorers, otherwise healthy; mean age 50 years; mean education 15 years; mean weight/height ratio 2.7; partial correlations controlled for age, weight, and education; no controls	WAIS; WMS; Rey-Osterrieth Complex Figure; Hooper; Wisconsin Card Sort; Verbal Fluency; Finger Tapping	None	Nocturnal index of 4% or more of desaturations reflected significant association with deficits in memory, general intelligence, and expressive verbal fluency	Not reported	MNCD

Findley et al. 1986	Cognitive impairment in obstructive sleep apnea and associated hypoxemia	26 sleep apnea patients; mean age 53 years; mean education 12 years; 17 without hypoxemia, 9 with hypoxemia; no controls	WAIS-R; WMS Trail Making; PASAT; Vigilance and Eye/Hand Coordination test not specified	None	Sleep apnea with hypoxemia > cognitive disturbance than sleep apnea without hypoxemia; hypoxemic condition associated with impaired range in attention, concentration, recall, and complex problem solving	Not reported	MNCD
Heaton et al. 1983	Psychological effects of continuous and nocturnal oxygen therapy in hypoxemic COPD	150 COPD patients; random assignment to continuous and nocturnal oxygen therapy; 53 age- and education-matched controls	WAIS; Halstead-Reitan Battery	None	NP "deficit" in patients with hypoxemic COPD	"Modest improvement" in NP status after 6 months of oxygen therapy, with continuous slightly better than nocturnal	MNCD reversibility
Grant et al. 1982	NP findings in hypoxemic COPD	203 COPD patients; 74 pairs of age-, education-, and social position-matched subjects for comparison and control groups	Halstead-Reitan Battery; WMS; Grooved Pegboard; Halstead Impairment Index; Average Impairment Rating	None	"Cerebral disturbance," particularly abstraction and perceptual motor integration	Not reported	MNCD
B. Autoimmune							
Tarter et al. 1989	NP syndrome in Sjögren's and primary biliary cirrhosis	14 primary biliary cirrhosis female patients; 10 Sjögren's and primary biliary cirrhosis female patients; 10 "normal" female controls	Dominant Signature Time; Shipley IQ; Token; Rey-Osterrieth Copy Score; Trail Making; Finger Tapping; Block Design; Animal Naming; Stroop; Symbol Digit Modality; Digit Span; Grooved Pegboard; Benton Visual Retention	None	"Profound impairment" on NP testing with Sjögren's and primary biliary cirrhosis than primary biliary cirrhosis alone; memory and spatial deficits; cited "intellectual impairments" in Sjögren's	Not reported	MNCD

(continued)

Table 19–1. Studies involving neuropsychological assessment in medical and neurologic disorders *(continued)*

Author	Study	Subjects	Instruments	Level of cognitive impairment: Demented	Level of cognitive impairment: Impaired not demented	Improvement after treatment	Comments
Denburg et al. 1988	NP correlates and serum lymphocytotoxic antibodies in SLE	98 SLE female patients; no controls	WAIS; WMS; Consonant Trigrams; Rey Auditory-Verbal Learning; Rey-Osterrieth; Corsi Block Span; Token; Trail Making; Stroop; Design Fluency; Benton Controlled Word Association; Animal Naming; Finger Tapping; Simplified Hand Preference	None	Cognitive deficits in "anteriorly associated primarily visuospatial functions"; "wide-ranging" cognitive impairment in SLE patients	Not reported	MNCD
Alexander et al. 1988	MRI of cerebral lesions in Sjögren's	38 Sjögren's patients: 16 with active NP findings and mean age of 53 years; 22 without NP findings suggestive of CNS involvement served as controls (mean age of 52 years)	WAIS-R; other tests for memory, attention, concentration, and parietal lobe functions not specified	4 patients with symptoms of dementia	11/16 with "cognitive dysfunction"; 8/16 with "focal neurological deficits"; "subtle" cognitive disturbance noted	Not reported	Dementia, MNCD
Devinsky et al. 1988	Clinical and neuropathologic findings in SLE	50 SLE patients; review of medical records and autopsy reports; no controls	Not reported	2 cases of dementia	About 50% of cases reviewed indicated association between NP and CNS lesions; psychiatric disorders did not particularly address cognitive impairment	Not reported	Dementia, MNCD

Denburg et al. 1987	Cognitive impairment in SLE	86 SLE female patients with mean age of 34.4 years and 12.3 years of education; NP symptom groups of active, inactive, or never; 23 "normal" female controls with mean age of 34.2 years and 11.5 years of education	WAIS; WMS; Rey Auditory Verbal Learning; Rey-Osterrieth; Consonant Trigrams; Trail Making; Stroop; Design Fluency; Controlled Word Association; Animal Naming; Finger Tapping; Handedness	None	"Subclinical CNS involvement"; never NP symptoms group > cognitive impairment than controls; impairment existed in apparently resolved NP symptoms group as in active NP symptoms group reflecting residual CNS involvement	Not reported	MNCD
Sanders et al. 1987	Detection of active terminal complement C5B-9 in cerebrospinal fluid from patients with SLE or Sjögren's	24 Sjögren's patients; 11 SLE patients; no controls	Not reported	None	C5B-9 as possible marker in CNS involvement with "subtle neurologic or neuropsychiatric manifestations" particularly if focal CNS lesion present	Not reported	MNCD
Malinow et al. 1985	NP dysfunction in Sjögren's	16/40 Sjögren's patients received NP testing; no controls	WAIS-R	None	7/16 displayed mild to moderate impairment in attention and concentration	Not reported	MNCD
C. Multiple sclerosis							
Rao et al. 1989a	Correlation of MRI with NP testing in multiple sclerosis	53 multiple sclerosis patients; no controls	WAIS-R; Selective Reminding; 7/24 Spatial Recall; Story Recall; Brown-Peterson Interference; Raven Progressive Matrices; President's; Wisconsin Card Sort; Booklet Category; Stroop; Digit	None	Recent memory and abstract/conceptual reasoning most impaired in multiple sclerosis patients; impaired subgrouping with "relatively substantial cognitive impairment";	Not reported	MNCD

(continued)

Table 19–1. Studies involving neuropsychological assessment in medical and neurologic disorders *(continued)*

Author	Study	Subjects	Instruments	Level of cognitive impairment: Demented	Level of cognitive impairment: Impaired not demented	Improvement after treatment	Comments
			Span; Reaction Time; Sternberg Memory Scanning; Paced Auditory Addition; Boston Naming, Abbreviated; Controlled Oral Word Association; Category Word Generation; Hooper; Judgment of Line Orientation; Facial Recognition; Visual Discrimination; Mini-Mental State Exam		intact subgrouping with "relatively minimal impairment"; abnormal CNS findings on MRI correlated to "cognitive dysfunction"		
Grant et al. 1989	NP impairment in early multiple sclerosis	43 multiple sclerosis patients initially evaluated: 34/43 patients received follow-up after 7 years (median 6 years); 28 age-, sex-, and intelligence-matched controls	WAIS-R; WMS; Trail Making; Brown-Peterson Consonant Trigrams; Kurtzke Expanded Disability Status Scale	None	"Subtle memory deficits" in early stages included encoding, recall, and retrieval; predictive value of Trail Making reflected by Kurtzke disability scale	Not reported	MNCD
Callanan et al. 1989	Cognitive impairment and clinically isolated lesions in multiple sclerosis	48 multiple sclerosis patients with clinically discrete lesions (optic neuritis, brain stem, and spinal cord); 46 physically disabled patients having rheumatic or neurological	National Adult Reading; Schonell Graded Word Reading; WAIS; Recognition Memory for Words; Recognition Memory for Faces; Wisconsin Card Sort; Speed of	None	Cognitive deficit most evident was auditory attention, then abstract thinking; IQ impairment also noted; deficits correlated with abnormal brain MRI findings	Not reported	MNCD

		conditions without CNS involvement serving as one of two age- and sex-matched control groups; 40 "normal" subjects for normative MRI data comparison as other control group	Letter Counting; Auditory Attention (Kaplan); Graded Naming; Jebsen Hand Function; Activities of Daily Living (Haworth and Hollings)				
Nielsen et al. 1989	Cerebral blood flow and cognitive functioning in multiple sclerosis	17 multiple sclerosis patients with 17 age-, sex-, and socioeconomic-matched controls received NP testing; 16/17 multiple sclerosis patients with 16 age-, sex-, and socioeconomic-matched controls received xenon-133 for cerebral blood flow measurements	WAIS-R; Auditory Verbal Learning; Story Recall; Recurring Figures; Visual Gestalt; Symbol Digit Modalities; Trail Making	None	Cognitive slowing with deficits in verbal learning, logical memory, and impaired visuomotor performance	Not reported	MNCD
Rao et al. 1989b	Information processing speed in multiple sclerosis	36 population-based multiple sclerosis patients; 26 age-, education-, and verbal intelligence-matched "normal" controls	Sternberg High Speed Memory Scanning	Nones	Scanning rate indicated "slowing of mental processing" exclusive of motor slowness	Not reported	MNCD
Huber et al. 1987	MRI correlates of dementia in multiple sclerosis	32 multiple sclerosis patients; 12 "normal" controls	WAIS; Mini-Mental State Exam; Diagnostic Criteria for Dementia by Cummings and Benson	28% demented	32% classified as "moderate intellectual impairment"; 38% as "minimal intellectual impairment"; 16% as "no intellectual	Not reported	Dementia, MNCD

(continued)

Table 19–1. Studies involving neuropsychological assessment in medical and neurologic disorders *(continued)*

Authors	Study	Subjects	Instruments	Level of cognitive impairment: Demented	Level of cognitive impairment: Impaired not demented	Improvement after treatment	Comments
					impairment"; memory deficit was most common and early finding		
D. Renal dialysis							
Sprague et al. 1988	Aluminum and neurocognitive dysfunction in chronic dialysis patients	16 chronic dialysis patients; deferoxamine infusion test to monitor body aluminum levels; no controls	Mini-Mental State Exam; Serial Digit Learning; Multilingual Aphasic Exam	None	Impairment in memory without significant difference on dementia test; motor function and memory deficits associated with positive deferoxamine infusion test	Not reported	MNCD
E. Normal pressure hydrocephalus							
Stambrook et al. 1988	NP changes after neurosurgical treatment of normal pressure hydrocephalus	14 normal pressure hydrocephalus patients; mean age 66 years; pre- and postshunt NP testing; no controls	WMS; Mini-Mental State Exam; Finger Tapping; Digit Span; Arithmetic; Trail Making; Aphasia Screening; Spatial Rating	Preshunt NP testing reflected "cognitive symptoms resembling dementia"	None	Postshunt NP testing reflected improvements in memory, attention, arithmetic, concentration, language and communication abilities, and visuomotor skills but not to normal range	Dementia reversibility, MNCD
Mulrow et al. 1987	Clinical findings in normal pressure hydrocephalus	627 dementia cases; retrospective study	Not reported	Dementia as part of gait abnormality and urinary incontinence triad;	None	55% indicate symptom improvement after shunt, with gait abnormality responding better	Dementia reversibility, MNCD

				triad in only 8% of classic normal pressure hydrocephalus		than urinary incontinence better than dementia	
F. Cancer/therapy							
Laaksonen et al. 1988	Dementia-like largely reversible syndrome after cranial irradiation and prolonged interferon treatment	Brief report; single patient; 66-year-old male; 146-week follow-up	WAIS; WMS, Finger Tapping; others not specified	None	"Dementia-like syndrome"	"Dementia-like syndrome" subsided when interferon dose decreased	MNCD reversibility
Laukkanen et al. 1988	Brain irradiation of small cell lung cancer with clinical, CT scan, NP sequelae	94 limited stage small cell lung cancer patients; 12/14 patients alive after 2 years (long-term survivors with mean age of 63.2 years and education of 8.9 grades) received CT, neurologic, oncologic, and NP testing; no controls	WAIS-R; WMS; Benton Visual Retention; Halstead Battery; Trail Making	None of long-term survivors met diagnostic criteria for dementia	Recent memory loss most common cognitive impairment	Not reported	MNCD
Denicoff et al. 1987	NP effects of treatment with interleukin-2 and lymphokine-activated killer cells	44 metastatic cancer patients; age range 22–69 years; longitudinal survey; no controls	Modified Mini-Mental State Exam; Digit Symbol; Road Map Direction Sense; Trail Making	Not specific for dementia diagnosis but noted 22 patients with severe cognitive changes	22 patients with mild to moderate cognitive change rating	Treatment ended prior to discharge with follow-up within 2–4 weeks; 39 patients at follow-up had NP scores return to baseline	Dementia, MNCD reversibility
Adams et al. 1984	NP manifestations of interferon in cancer patients	10 metastatic renal cell cancer patients; age range 36–72 years; follow-up at 1 week and at 1 month of continuous interferon treatment; no controls	WAIS; Trail Making; Bender-Gestalt; Halstead-Reitan Battery; Mental Status Exam not specified	None	"Mild to moderate cognitive" changes with "psychomotor retardation" most noticed	Not reported	MNCD

(continued)

Table 19–1. Studies involving neuropsychological assessment in medical and neurologic disorders *(continued)*

Author	Study	Subjects	Instruments	Level of cognitive impairment: Demented	Level of cognitive impairment: Impaired not demented	Improvement after treatment	Comments
G. HIV infection							
Brunetti et al. 1989	Reversal of brain metabolic abnormalities following treatment of AIDS dementia complex with AZT; a PET-FDG study	3 AIDS dementia complex patients, homosexual males ages 32, 32, and 35; 1 HIV seropositive patient age 11 years with hemophilia	Not reported	3 adult patients with AIDS dementia complex	11-year-old boy with 28-point drop in IQ as compared with prior seroconversion 3 years ago	All subjects reflected cognitive improvement 2 months after treatment, particularly motor functions and memory; 11-year-old boy had return of IQ to "pre-illness level" at 9 months of treatment	Dementia, MNCD reversibility
Dalakas et al. 1989	AIDS and the nervous system	Case report, 32-year-old HIV seropositive homosexual male	Not reported	None	"Psychometric testing revealed mild cognitive dysfunction"	Not reported	MNCD
Perry et al. 1989	NP function in physically asymptomatic HIV seropositive males	20 asymptomatic HIV seropositive homosexual males; age- and education-matched controls of 20 HIV seronegative homosexual males	WAIS-R; Cancellation; Trail Making; PASAT; WMS; California Verbal Learning; Rey-Osterrieth Complex Figure; Boston Naming; Word Production; Shipley Conceptual Quotient; Grooved Pegboard	None	HIV seropositive males had lower scores on 17/20 psychometric measures; correlation of cognitive impairment with lower T_4/T_8 ratios noted; implied "subtle NP impairment" prior to clinical manifestations of cognitive dysfunction or immune suppression	Not reported	MNCD

Schmitt et al. 1988	NP outcome of AZT treatment of patients with AIDS and AIDS-related complex	159 AIDS patients; 122 AIDS-related complex patients; double-blind, placebo-controlled trial of AZT; multicenter (AZT Collaborative Working Group); treatment groups controlled for age, body weight, Karnofsky performance score, symptoms, and mean CD_4^+ at entry into study	Ruff's Two and Seven; WAIS-R; Digit Span; Finger Oscillation; Buschke's Selective Reminding Procedure; Trail Making; Symbol Digit Modalities	None with symptoms of frank AIDS dementia complex	AIDS and AIDS-related complex patient groups with mean NP scores below the standard means at screening	AZT treatment group reflected-improvement in attention, memory, and visuomotor skills; placebo group displayed no change or decline over a 16-week period	MNCD reversibility
Yarchoan et al. 1988	Long-term administration of AZT to patients with AIDS-related neurological disease	3 AIDS patients; 4 AIDS-related complex patients; no controls	WAIS-R; Trail Making; WMS; Kimura's Recurring Figures; Purdue or Grooved Pegboard	3 patients with diagnosis of dementia	3/4 remaining patients had no dementia diagnosis and were not given a cognitive impairment classification	Improvement noted in 3 cases of dementia; all other cases indicated "improvement" but not specific to cognitive impairment	Dementia reversibility, MNCD
Yarchoan et al. 1987	Response of HIV-associated neurological disease to AZT	4 AIDS patients; no controls	WAIS-R; WMS; Kimura's Recurring Figures; Purdue or Grooved Pegboard	3 patients with diagnosis of dementia	1 patient with paraplegia did not have dementia complex	Improvement noted in 3 of 4 cases; 1 patient with paraplegia showed no improvement	Dementia reversibility, MNCD

(continued)

Table 19–1. Studies involving neuropsychological assessment in medical and neurologic disorders *(continued)*

				Level of cognitive impairment			
Author	Study	Subjects	Instruments	Demented	Impaired not demented	Improvement after treatment	Comments
Grant et al. 1987a	Evidence for early CNS involvement in AIDS and other HIV infections: studies with NP testing and MRI	55 homosexual males: 15 Group A (AIDS); 13 Group B (AIDS-related complex); 16 Group C (HIV antibody positive); 11 Group D (HIV antibody negative); age- and education-matched groups	WAIS-R; Category; Trail Making; PASAT; WMS; Symbol-Digit Paired Associate Learning	None	"Atypical and impaired" NP findings reflected in 87% AIDS, 54% AIDS-related complex, 44% HIV-positive, and 9% HIV-negative groupings (common difficulties in speed of processing, learning, remembering, and abstract thinking noted); abnormal MRI findings in 9/13 AIDS and 5/10 AIDS-related complex groupings	Not reported	MNCD
H. Thyroid							
Nystrom et al. 1988	L-thyroxine treatment of women with "subclinical" hypothyroidism	20 subclinical hypothyroid women; double-blind, crossover design; 12-month period; age range 51–73 years	Binglay's Memory; Reaction Time; Thurstone's Identical Forms	None	"Mental lethargy"	Symptom improvement with L-thyroxine	MNCD reversibility
Trzepacz et al. 1988	Psychiatric and NP response to propranolol in Graves' disease	10 Graves' disease patients untreated and newly diagnosed; longitudinal follow-up of hyperthyroid (Stage 1), after 2 weeks propranolol (Stage 2),	WAIS-R; Halstead-Reitan Battery; Categories; Tactual Performance; Finger Tapping; Trail Making; Stroop; Symbol Digit Modalities; Benton Naming; Perceptual Speed; Number Facility	None	NP impairment in memory, concentration, and attention	Propranolol treatment did not reflect improvement in tasks involving attention; after 6 months of antithyroid treatment	MNCD reversibility

		after 6 months antithyroid (Stage 3); no controls				improvement in more difficult memory and attention tasks noted	
Folks 1984	Organic affective disorder and underlying thyrotoxicosis	2 case reports: 23-year-old female with symptoms of depression on referral; 48-year-old female with symptoms of mania on referral	Not reported	None	Both cases presented with "mild cognitive impairment" and implications for an "organic etiology" regarding mood symptoms were noted	"Total remission of symptoms" and "resolution of her manic symptoms" after thyroid treatment and achievement of normal thyroid functions	MNCD reversibility
MacCrimmon et al. 1979	Emotional disturbance and cognitive deficits in hyperthyroidism	19 female hyperthyroid patients; assessments at pretreatment, posttreatment, and euthyroid state; age- and education-matched controls	Competing Voice Messages; Stroop Color-Word; Spokes; Paired Associate Learning; Finger Tapping	None	Pretreatment hyperthyroid condition reflected "subtle disturbance of cognitive functioning," particularly memory, concentration, and attention	Posttreatment assessment (average of 21 days) reflected no significant difference as compared with control group	MNCD reversibility
I. Cardiac							
Barclay et al. 1988	Unrecognized cognitive impairment in cardiac rehabilitation patients	20 cardiac rehabilitation patients; clinically stable without known stroke or dementia; age range 47–85 years; no controls	WAIS-R; Mattis Dementia Rating; Purdue Pegboard; Mental Status Questionnaire; Mini-Mental State Exam; Confrontation Naming	None	40% of subjects displayed "significant memory impairment and disorientation"; 30% had "milder impairment"	Not reported	MNCD

(continued)

Table 19–1. Studies involving neuropsychological assessment in medical and neurologic disorders *(continued)*

Author	Study	Subjects	Instruments	Level of cognitive impairment: Demented	Level of cognitive impairment: Impaired not demented	Improvement after treatment	Comments
Garcia et al. 1984	Underdiagnosis of cognitive impairment in a rehabilitative setting	50 male and 50 female patients; consecutive admissions to a rehabilitation hospital; mean age of 63.4 years; no controls	Mini-Mental State Exam; Cognitive Capacity Screening Examination	None had referral diagnosis of dementia or organic brain syndrome	25% had age-corrected score below 20 on Mini-Mental, which met criteria for "cognitive impairment";15% with cardiac ischemic disease and no stroke had cognitive deficits that were "mild"	Not reported	MNCD
Reich et al. 1983	Unrecognized organic mental disorders in survivors of cardiac arrest	6 case reports	WAIS; WMS	None	4/6 received NP testing only at follow-up; common deficits were in memory and learning of new information; awareness of "subtle cerebral dysfunction" in conditions without focal neurological signs emphasized	Not reported	MNCD
J. Other metabolic disorder							
Basavaraju and Phillips 1989	Cortisol-deficient state: a cause of reversible cognitive impairment and delirium in the elderly	Case report of 79-year-old female; hypopituitarism secondary to postirradiation of pituitary macroadenoma	Mini-Mental State Exam	None	"Severe cognitive impairment" with decreased plasma cortisol level	Prednisone therapy reflected improvement in cognitive functioning	MNCD reversibility

Grabowski and Yeragani 1987	Porphyria and psychosis	Case report of 41-year-old female; diagnosed with acute intermittent porphyria at 26 years old; diagnosed with psychiatric history at 24 years old	WAIS-R	None	NP scores reflected "organic patchy cognitive decline" and "asymmetric cognitive changes"	Not reported	MNCD
Rosselli et al. 1987	Wilson's disease: a reversible dementia	Case report of 30-year-old female, initial medical workup at 17 years old for amenorrhea; unrecognized course of mental and behavioral problems	WAIS; WMS	Implied clinical subcortical dementia with deficits in motor and verbal skills, memory recall, and apathetic personality	None	Improvement of dementia after 7 months of copper chelation with penicillamine	Dementia reversibility, MNCD
Goldstein et al. 1968	Psychiatric and psychometric aspects of Wilson's disease	22 patients with Wilson's disease: 17 patients received psychometric testing, with 13/17 having follow-ups at 16–30 and 63–73 months; no controls	WAIS; WMS; WISC (2 cases); Bender-Gestalt; Shipley-Hartford	None	Implied cognitive deficits based on pretreatment psychometric testing	Treatment with low-copper diet and penicillamine reflected general improvement in all but one mentally retarded patient; improvement most noted in verbal IQ, memory, and concept formation	MNCD reversibility
K. Other chronic infection							
Brooke et al. 1987	Neurosyphilis	Case report, 43-year-old HIV negative homosexual male	Not reported	None	"Intermittent cognitive impairment implied organicity"	Improvement reflecting residual "mild degree of cognitive impairment" after penicillin treatment	MNCD reversibility

(continued)

Table 19–1. Studies involving neuropsychological assessment in medical and neurologic disorders *(continued)*

Author	Study	Subjects	Instruments	Level of cognitive impairment: Demented	Level of cognitive impairment: Impaired not demented	Improvement after treatment	Comments
Weder et al. 1987	Chronic progressive neurological involvement in *Borrelia burgdorferi* infection	5 Lyme disease patients; age range 24–65 years; mean course 2.1 years; no controls	Not reported	None	"Psychointellectual degradation" during chronic progressive course	Symptom improvement after penicillin treatment	MNCD reversibility
L. Intoxicants/pollutants							
Hanninen 1988	Psychological performance profile in occupational intoxications; "reanalyses" of data from epidemiological studies at Institute of Occupational Health in Helsinki	50 patients in carbon disulfide poisoning group; 52 patients in lead poisoning group; 114 patients in organic solvent poisoning group; age range 20–60 years (mean ages 33–44); control (reference) groups matched for age, sex, and occupation	WAIS Similarities; visual reasoning, memory, and visuomotor speed not specified	None	Carbon disulfide poisoning group reflected decrements in "psychomotor" functions; lead exposure results were "rather general"; organic solvent poisoning associated with problems in verbal concept formation during early stage, memory during early and late stages, and visuomotor slowness during late stage	Improvement in cognitive functions with organic solvent poisoning group except short-term memory	MNCD reversibility
Sayers et al. 1987	Effects of carbon dioxide on mental performance	7 males and 3 females exposed to range of inspired CO_2 for 20 minutes; age range 22–26 years; 14 males and 7 females with longer exposure (up to 90–100 minutes)	AB Logic Problems (Baddeley); Digit Span; Longterm Recall (Friedman)	None	At levels greater than 51 Torr of end-tidal pCO_2 "clear detriment in speed of performance of reasoning tests"; only a trend for short-term memory impairment existed at	10-minute lag time for return to baseline functions on breathing room air	MNCD reversibility

		to 6.5% CO_2; age range 20–26 years; all subjects completed study trial as above, and after 7-day interval all received control trial of breathing room air			60 Torr and at inhaled CO_2 of up to 7.5%		
M. Epilepsy							
Homan et al. 1989	Cognitive function and regional cerebral blood flow in partial seizures	47 male and 3 female right-handed patients with known partial seizure; mean age 39.5 years; mean education 12.6 years; antiepileptic drug levels not exceeding toxic range; subjects without clinical signs of toxic side effects; no controls	WAIS-R; Halstead-Reitan Battery WMS (Russell revision)	None	Subjects displayed average intelligence with "mild impairment" on Halstead-Reitan; memory function most impaired, ranging from "mild to severe" in WMS; results supported mild NP dysfunction "without gross structural abnormality"; correlation of NP deficits with decreased perfusion in brain areas, particularly temporal and frontal, noted	Not reported	MNCD

Note. WAIS = Wechsler Adult Intelligence Scale. WMS = Wechsler Memory Scale. NP = neuropsychological. MNCD = mild neurocognitive disorder. COPD = chronic obstructive pulmonary disease. PASAT = Paced Auditory Serial Addition Test. SLE = systemic lupus erythematosus. MRI = magnetic resonance imaging. CNS = central nervous system. C5B-9 = active terminal complement factor. CT = computed tomography. HIV = human immunodeficiency virus. AIDS = acquired immunodeficiency syndrome. AZT = zidovudine. PET-FDG = positron-emission tomography fluorodeoxyglucose. T_4 = helper lymphocytes. T_8 = suppressor lymphocytes. CD_4^+ = cluster determinant 4. WISC = Wechsler Intelligence Scale for Children. CO_2 = carbon dioxide. pCO_2 = alveolar partial pressure of carbon dioxide.

Table 19–2. Studies involving neuropsychological assessment in alcohol and substance use disorders

Author	Study	Subjects	Instruments	Level of cognitive impairment: Demented	Level of cognitive impairment: Impaired not demented	Improvement after treatment	Comments
Sweeney et al. 1989	Assessment of cognitive functioning in polysubstance abusers	200 polysubstance abusers: 2 groups of 100 consecutive admissions to detoxification and rehabilitation program; mean age 33.8 years, 53% males; no controls	WAIS; WAIS-R; WMS; Benton Visual Retention (Form A)	None	NP impairment most notable in functions of memory, motor, and visuospatial; verbal concept formation appears to be relatively preserved as compared with vocabulary	Not reported (all subjects received NP testing within 7 days of admission)	MNCD
Muuronen et al. 1989	Improved drinking habits on brain atrophy and cognitive performance in alcoholic patients; a 5-year follow-up study, Stockholm	52/196 patients satisfied exclusion criteria concerning age, head injury, liver disease, alcohol abuse, and anticonvulsant therapy at baseline; 37/52 satisfied above exclusion criteria and received 5-year follow-up study; 120 age-matched males (random sample) from Stockholm served as control group	SRB (Synonyms, Reasoning, Koh's Block Design); Halstead-Reitan Battery (Category, Tactual Performance, Trail Making A & B, Rhythm, and Finger Tapping); Claeson-Dahl (Verbal Learning and Retention); Graham-Kendall Memory-for-Designs	None	49% of 52 patients had "intellectual impairment" versus 13% of controls; 72% of 52 patients reflected computed tomography findings of brain atrophy versus 16% of controls	Abstinent group (abstinent 1–12 months before follow-up testing or "infrequent drinkers") were 43% of 37 patients and showed significant improvement in visuospatial functions with trends in reasoning and memory; narrowing of 3rd ventricle correlated with cognitive improvement in abstinent group (37% of abstinent group still displayed "intellectual impairment" versus 13% seen in controls)	MNCD reversibility

Varma et al. 1988	Cannabis and cognitive functions; a prospective study	26 heavy users (regular use for 5 years at least 20 times per month and average daily intake equal to 150 mg THC); 26 controls matched for age, education, and occupation; NP testing for heavy users required at least 12-hour abstinent period (monitored by hospitalization)	Pencil Tapping; Reaction Time; Time Perception; Size-Estimation; Trail Making (Form A); Bender-Gestalt; Nahor and Benson; Standard Progressive Matrices; WAIS-R; Bhatia's Short Scale; PGI Memory	None	Heavy users displayed no significant difference in measures of intelligence as compared with controls but did differ by having "lower" scores on recent memory and slower reaction time in perceptual-motor functions	Not reported	MNCD
Guerra et al. 1987	NP performance in opiate addicts after rapid detoxification	65 male and 28 female heroin addicts; mean age 25 years; predetoxification NP testing 2–3 weeks prior to admission; detoxification with clonidine or methadone for 7–10 days; postdetoxification NP testing between 7 and 14 days after admission; 18 male and 13 female controls with mean age of 19 years and matched for education, culture, and demographics	Toulouse-Pieron Cancellation; PMA-F Verbal Fluency; Digit Span; Raven's Progressive Matrices	None	NP scores prior to detoxification were lower than controls in areas of memory, verbal fluency, and attention; in last week prior to testing no significant difference between NP scores of mild (<500 mg consumption) and heavy (>500 mg) opioid addicts	General improvement after detoxification reaching NP scores similar to controls	MNCD reversibility

(continued)

Table 19–2. Studies involving neuropsychological assessment in alcohol and substance use disorders *(continued)*

Author	Study	Subjects	Instruments	Level of cognitive impairment		Improvement after treatment	Comments
				Demented	Impaired not demented		
Grant et al. 1978	Collaborative NP study of polydrug users	276 subjects initial combined groups; 195 subjects follow-up combined groups (polydrug users, psychiatric patients and non-drug-using, nonpsychiatrically ill controls); 8-center collaboration; 151/276 were polydrug users with mean age of 25.5 years and 11.3 years of education; 93/195 polydrug users remained for 3-month follow-up; controls matched for age and education	WAIS; Halstead Battery; Trail Making B; Grooved Pegboard (dominant); Grip-strength (dominant); Aphasia	None	37% of polydrug users had NP impairment on Halstead Battery versus 26% in psychiatrically ill patients and 8% in controls; "perceptuomotor and language-related" skills were common NP deficits in polydrug users; at 3-month follow-up 34% of polydrug users had NP deficits versus 4% in controls, little change in psychiatric group; results implicated "longer-term, slowly reversible" NP deficits with use of central nervous system depressants and opiates	Not reported	MNCD

Note. Refer to Grant 1987 for selected review of alcohol-related studies and to Reed and Grant 1990 for selected review of substance-related studies. WAIS = Wechsler Adult Intelligence Scale. WMS = Wechsler Memory Scale. NP = neuropsychological. MNCD = mild neurocognitive disorder. THC = tetrahydrocannabinol. PGI memory = a clinical test of memory in simple Hindi. PMA-F = F factor of PMA as a measure of verbal fluency.

perfusion and glucose utilization, and electrophysiological changes (Grant 1987). Despite the fact that this syndrome is commonly recognized, it has no place in our current DSM system, since such patients are neither demented nor delirious in the usual sense of the word. It appears that there may also be a slowly reversible mild cognitive disorder among alcoholic persons who remain stably abstinent (Grant et al. 1987a, 1987b).

Research on chronic drug-abusing persons is more fragmentary, but there is good evidence for mild neurocognitive pathology in persons involved in polysubstance abuse (Grant and Reed 1985; Grant et al. 1978; Reed and Grant 1990; Sweeney et al. 1989). In one of the largest studies of its kind, investigators noted that 37% of young persons using more than one substance of abuse had neuropsychological impairment at 3 weeks of detoxification (Grant et al. 1978). The deficiencies were, again, in "higher order" cognitive functions, including abstracting ability and complex perceptual motor skills.

With respect to medical conditions, there is substantial evidence for mild neurobehavioral disorder in persons suffering from chronic obstructive pulmonary disease or sleep apnea who experience chronic or intermittent hypoxemia (Table 19–1, Section A). Neurocognitive disturbances and neuroradiological lesions have also been reported in "autoimmune diseases" such as Sjögren's syndrome and systemic lupus erythematosus (Table 19–1, Section B; Adelman et al. 1986). Furthermore, neurocognitive dysfunction has been associated with thyroid disease (Table 19–1, Section H), vitamin B_{12}-folate deficiency (Hector and Burton 1988; Martin 1988), cardiac rehabilitative condition (Table 19–1, Section I), intoxicants and pollutants (Table 19–1, Section L), and human immunodeficiency virus (HIV) infection (Table 19–1, Section G; Grant and Atkinson 1990; Grant and Heaton 1990).

The treatment of medical conditions can also give rise to mild stable or slowly reversible ("intermediate duration") neurocognitive disorder. For example, many patients receiving beta-blockers for hypertension experience mild to moderate neuropsychological impairment (Blumenthal et al. 1988; Dimsdale et al. 1989; Richardson and Wyke 1988; Shore et al. 1987; Streufert et al. 1989; Wurzelmann et al. 1987). Similarly, patients treated with antiepileptics (Trimble and Thompson 1986) and benzodiazepines (Bergman et al. 1989; Golombok et al. 1988; Kumar et al. 1987; Larson et al. 1987) can experience mild neurocognitive disturbances that can reduce overall intellectual efficiency.

Neurobehavioral deficits are seen in various neurological diseases including neurosyphilis (Brooke et al. 1987), Wilson's disease (Dening and Berriod 1989; Rosselli et al. 1987), Lyme disease (Steere 1989; Weder et al. 1987), porphyria (Grabowski and Yeragani 1987), epilepsy (Homan et al. 1989), normal pressure hydrocephalus (Table 19–1, Section E; Turner and McGeachie 1988), and most prominently in multiple sclerosis (Table 19–1, Section C; Franklin et al. 1988, 1989; Grant 1986b). When considering the early phases of progressive dementing disorders (e.g., Alzheimer's disease, Parkinson's disease, or Huntington's disease), there can also be a prolonged period of mild but definite neurocognitive impairment that has clinical significance, yet fails to reach existing criteria for dementia.

Discussion: Relationship of Proposed Category to Existing Categories

Delirium

The proposed category of mild neurocognitive disorder will differ from delirium in terms of the acuity, severity, and specific features of the presenting phenomena. For example, a severe feature such as "disorganized thinking, as indicated by rambling, irrelevant, or incoherent speech" (American Psychiatric Association 1987, p. 103) would indicate a severity of presentation that exceeds proposed criteria for the mild disorder. Disturbance in consciousness, sleep-wake cycle, and disorientation are other features not embraced by the proposed concept. The rapid evolution of the disorder into a clinically florid phase would be another distinguishing feature between delirium and mild neurocognitive disorder.

Although the differentiation between frank delirium and mild neurocognitive disorder should not be difficult to make, it should be noted that an atypical, slowly evolving delirium might be *preceded* by a period of time in which a patient would satisfy criteria for mild neurobehavioral disorder. In this sense, the proposed category has clinical usefulness in that it may permit early detection of a process before it reaches a more acute and problematic phase. Similarly, persons *recovering* from an episode of delirium may enter a slow recovery period during which they no longer satisfy existing criteria for delirium but continue to have some demonstrable neurocognitive impairment. Recovery from an alcoholic or substance abuse bout, recovery from severe closed head injury, and recovery from a delirium caused by severe metabolic derangement are examples of states that are clinically important, that may reverse gradually with durations of mild neurocognitive impairment lasting weeks to months, but that are currently unclassifiable.

Dementia

Once again, the differentiating features have to do with severity of cognitive disturbance and magnitude of impact on day-to-day functioning. As currently conceived, diagnosis of dementia requires substantial disturbance in memory. The proposed category requires that two neurocognitive areas be affected, but memory does not necessarily have to be one of those. For example, a person might have difficulty in problem solving (abstracting ability) and complex perceptual motor integration without significant impairment in memory. The current concept of dementia also requires "significant" interference with work or usual social activities or relationships with others. Although we believe documented neurocognitive disorder can exist without a clearly documented social-occupational consequence (because occupations are so variable and measurement of work performance can be difficult), we nevertheless propose, in order to avoid inappropriate diagnostic labeling of uncertain cases, to restrict the mild neurocognitive disorder designation to those that manifest at least mild impairment in social or occupational functioning. This impairment must represent a decline from a previous level of functioning.

Other "Organic" Syndromes or Disorders

The proposed category will differ from other "organic" disorders by virtue of the fact that more than one area of neurocognitive functioning must be affected. This will distinguish the proposed category from amnestic syndrome, organic hallucinosis, organic delusional, and mood, personality, and anxiety syndromes.

Developmental Disorders

The key differentiation here is that the predominant disturbance in the developmental disorders is the *acquisition* of cognitive, language, motor, or social skills. In the proposed category of mild neurobehavioral disorders, the key feature is *loss* of previously acquired cognitive capacity.

Recommendations

Proposed Criteria

To address this deficiency in the current DSM nomenclature, we propose the establishment of a new disorder category tentatively entitled, "mild neurocognitive disorder." The criteria proposed are presented in Table 19–3.

By way of comparison, ICD-10 proposes the following criteria for its new category, mild cognitive disorder (F06.7):

> This disorder may precede, accompany, or follow a wide variety of infections and physical disorders, both cerebral and systemic (including HIV infection). Direct neurological evidence of cerebral involvement is not necessarily present, but there may nevertheless be distress and interference with usual activities. The boundaries of this category are still to be firmly established. When associated with a physical disorder from which the patient recovers, mild cognitive disorder does not last for more than a few additional weeks. This diagnosis should not be made if the

condition is clearly attributable to a mental or behavioural disorder classified in any of the remaining blocks in this book. (pp. 64–65)

Diagnostic guidelines

The main feature is a decline in cognitive performance. This may include memory impairment and learning or concentration difficulties. Objective tests usually indicate abnormality. The symptoms are such that a diagnosis of dementia (F00-F03), organic amnesic syndrome (F04), or delirium (F05) cannot be made.

Differential diagnosis

The disorder can be differentiated from postencephalitic syndrome (F07.1) and postconcussional syndrome (F07.2) by its different etiology, more restricted range of generally milder symptoms, and usually shorter duration.

It will be seen that the general approach is similar to that underlying our proposal. However, we believe that our mild neurocognitive disorder criteria are more specific, and therefore should be easier to operationalize in research protocols and field trials.

Table 19–3. Proposed DSM-IV diagnostic criteria for Mild Neurocognitive Disorder

A. The presence of two of the following impairments in cognitive functioning, lasting most of the time for a period of at least 2 weeks (as reported by the individual or a reliable informant):
   (1) memory impairment as identified by a reduced ability to learn or recall information
   (2) disturbance in executive functioning (i.e., planning, organizing, sequencing, abstracting)
   (3) diminished concentration
   (4) slowed thinking
   (5) impairment in language (e.g., comprehension, word finding)

B. Objective evidence of a systemic illness or central nervous system dysfunction from physical examination or laboratory findings (including neuroimaging techniques) that is judged to be etiologically related to the cognitive disturbance.

C. Evidence of an abnormality or decline in performance from neuropsychological testing or quantified cognitive assessment.

D. The cognitive deficits cause a mild impairment in social or occupational functioning and represent a decline from a previous level of functioning.

E. The cognitive disturbance does not meet criteria for any specific Cognitive Impairment Disorder and is not better accounted for by another mental disorder.

References

Adams F, Quesada JR, Gutterman JU: Neuropsychiatric manifestations of human leukocyte interferon therapy in patients with cancer. JAMA 252:938–941, 1984

Adelman DC, Saltiel E, Klinenbert JR: The neuropsychiatric manifestations of systemic lupus erythematosus: an overview. Semin Arthritis Rheum 15:185–199, 1986

Alexander EL, Beall SS, Gordon B, et al: Magnetic resonance imaging of cerebral lesions in patients with the Sjögren syndrome. Ann Intern Med 108:815–823, 1988

American Psychiatric Association: Diagnostic and Statistical Manual of Mental Disorders, 3rd Edition, Revised. Washington, DC, American Psychiatric Association, 1987

Barclay LL, Weiss EM, Mattis S, et al: Unrecognized cognitive impairment in cardiac rehabilitation patients. J Am Geriatr Soc 36:22–28, 1988

Basavaraju N, Phillips SL: Cortisol deficient state: a cause of reversible cognitive impairment and delirium in the elderly. J Am Geriatr Soc 37:49–51, 1989

Bergman H, Borg S, Englebrekston K, et al: Dependence on sedative-hypnotics: neuropsychological impairment, field dependence and clinical course in a 5-year follow-up study. Br J Addict 84:547–553, 1989

Berry DTR, Webb WB, Block AJ, et al: Nocturnal hypoxia and neuropsychological variables. J Clin Exp Neuropsychol 8:229–238, 1986

Block AJ, Hellard DW, Seitzer DA: Nocturnal oxygen therapy does not improve snorers' intelligence. Chest 95:274–278, 1989

Blumenthal JA, Madden DJ, Krantz DS, et al: Short-term behavioral effects of beta-adrenergic addictions in men with mild hypertension. Clin Pharmacol Ther 43:429–435, 1988

Brooke D, Jamie P, Slack R, et al: Neurosyphilis: treatable psychosis. Br J Psychiatry 151:556, 1987

Brunetti A, Berg G, DiChiro G, et al: Reversal of brain metabolic abnormalities following treatment of AIDS dementia complex with 3′-azido-2′,3′-dideoxythymidine (AZT, zidovudine): a PET-FEG study. Clin Sci 30:581–590, 1989

Callanan MM, Logsdail SJ, Ron MA, et al: Cognitive impairment in patients with clinically isolated lesions of the type seen in multiple sclerosis: a psychometric and MRI study, in Mental Disorders and Cognitive Deficits in Multiple Sclerosis. Edited by Jensen K, Knudsen L, Stenager E, et al. London, John Libbey, 1989, pp 63–75

Dalakas M, Wichman A, Sever J: AIDS and the nervous system. JAMA 261:2396–2399, 1989

Denburg SD, Carbotte RM, Denburg JA: Cognitive impairment in systemic lupus erythematosus: a neuropsychological study of individual and group deficits. J Clin Exp Neuropsychol 9:323–339, 1987

Denburg SD, Carbotte RM, Long AA, et al: Neuropsychological correlates of serum lymphocytotoxic antibodies in systemic lupus erythematosus. Brain Behav Immun 2:222–234, 1988

Denicoff KD, Rubinow DR, Papa MZ, et al: The neuropsychiatric effects of treatment with interleukin-2 and lymphokine-activated killer cells. Ann Intern Med 107:293–300, 1987

Dening TR, Berriod GE: Wilson's disease: psychiatric symptoms in 195 cases. Arch Gen Psychiatry 46:1126–1134, 1989

Devinsky O, Petito CK, Alonso DR: Clinical and neuropathological findings in systemic lupus erythematosus: the role of vasculitis, heart emboli, and thrombotic thrombocytopenic purpura. Ann Neurol 23:380–384, 1988

Dickson LR, Ranseen JD: An update on selected organic mental syndromes. Hosp Community Psychiatry 41:290–300, 1990

Dimsdale JE, Newton RP, Joist T: Neuropsychological side effects of beta-blockers. Arch Intern Med 149:514–525, 1989

Findley LJ, Barth JT, Powers DC, et al: Cognitive impairment in patients with obstructive sleep apnea and associated hypoxemia. Chest 90:686–690, 1986

Folks DG: Organic affective disorder and underlying thyrotoxicosis. Psychosomatics 25:243–249, 1984

Franklin GM, Heaton RK, Nelson LM, et al: Correlation of neuropsychological and MRI findings in chronic/progressive multiple sclerosis. Neurology 38:1826–1829, 1988

Franklin GM, Nelson LM, Filley CM, et al: Cognitive loss in multiple sclerosis. Arch Neurol 46:162–167, 1989

Garcia CA, Tweedy JR, Blass JP: Underdiagnosis of cognitive impairment in a rehabilitation setting. J Am Geriatr Soc 32:339–342, 1984

Goldstein NP, Ewert JC, Randall RV, et al: Psychiatric aspects of Wilson's disease (hepatolenticular degeneration): results of psychometric tests during long-term therapy. Am J Psychiatry 124:113–119, 1968

Golinger RC, Fedoroff JP: Characteristics of patients referred to psychiatrists for competency evaluations. Psychosomatics 30:296–299, 1989

Golombok S, Moodley P, Lader M: Cognitive impairment in long-term benzodiazepine users. Psychol Med 18:365–374, 1988

Grabowski J, Yeragani VK: Porphyria and psychosis: a case report. Can J Psychiatry 32:393–394, 1987

Grant I (ed): Neuropsychiatric Correlates of Alcoholism. Washington, DC, American Psychiatric Press, 1986a

Grant I: Neuropsychological and psychiatric disturbances in multiple sclerosis, in Multiple Sclerosis. Edited by McDonald WI, Silberberg DH. London, Butterworth, 1986b, pp 134–152

Grant I: Alcohol and the brain: neuropsychological correlates. J Consult Clin Psychol 55:310–324, 1987

Grant I, Atkinson JH: The evolution of neurobehavioral complications of HIV infection. Psychol Med 20:747–754, 1990

Grant I, Heaton RK: Human immunodeficiency virus-type 1 (HIV-1) and the brain. J Consult Clin Psychol 58:22–30, 1990

Grant I, Reed R: Neuropsychology of alcohol and drug abuse, in Substance Abuse and Psychopathology. Edited by Alterman A. New York, Plenum, 1985, pp 289–341

Grant I, Adams KM, Carlin AS, et al: The collaborative neuropsychological study of polydrug users. Arch Gen Psychiatry 35:1063–1074, 1978

Grant I, Heaton RK, McSweeny AJ, et al: Neuropsychologic findings in hypoxemic chronic obstructive pulmonary disease. Arch Intern Med 142:1470–1476, 1982

Grant I, Atkinson JH, Hesselink JR, et al: Evidence for early central nervous system involvement in the acquired immunodeficiency syndrome (AIDS) and other human immunodeficiency virus (HIV) infections: studies with neuropsychological testing and magnetic resonance imaging. Ann Intern Med 107:828–836, 1987a

Grant I, Prigatano GP, Heaton RK, et al: Progressive neuropsychologic impairment and hypoxemia. Arch Gen Psychiatry 44:999–1006, 1987b

Grant I, McDonald WI, Trimble MR: Neuropsychological impairment in early multiple sclerosis, in Mental Disorders and Cognitive Deficits in Multiple Sclerosis. Edited by Jensen K, Knudsen L, Stenager E, et al. London, John Libbey, 1989, pp 17–26

Guerra D, Sole A, Cami J, et al: Neuropsychological performance in opiate addicts after rapid detoxification. Drug Alcohol Depend 20:261–270, 1987

Hanninen H: The psychological performance profile in occupational intoxications. Neurotoxicol Teratol 10:485–488, 1988

Hartlage LC, Asken MJ, Hornsby JL: Essentials of Neuropsychological Assessment. Springer, NY, 1987

Heaton RK, Pendleton MG: Use of neuropsychological tests to predict adult patients' everyday functioning. J Consult Clin Psychol 49:307–321, 1981

Heaton RK, Grant I, McSweeny AJ, et al: Psychologic effects of continuous and nocturnal oxygen therapy in hypoxemic chronic obstructive pulmonary disease. Arch Intern Med 143:1941–1947, 1983

Hector M, Burton JR: What are the psychiatric manifestations of vitamin B_{12} deficiency? J Am Geriatr Soc 36:1105–1112, 1988

Homan RW, Paulman RG, Devous MD, et al: Cognitive function and regional cerebral blood flow in partial seizures. Arch Neurol 46:964–970, 1989

Huber SJ, Paulson GW, Shuttleworth EC, et al: Magnetic resonance imaging correlates of dementia in multiple sclerosis. Arch Neurol 44:732–736, 1987

Kendler KS: Toward a scientific psychiatric nosology: strengths and limitations. Arch Gen Psychiatry 47:969–973, 1990

Kumar R, Mac DS, Gabrielli WF, et al: Anxiolytics and memory: a comparison of lorazepam and alprazolam. J Clin Psychiatry 48:158–160, 1987

Laaksonen R, Niiranen A, Iivananinen M, et al: Dementia-like largely reversible syndrome after cranial irradiation and prolonged interferon treatment (brief report). Annals of Clinical Research 20:201–203, 1988

Larson EB, Kukull WA, Buchner D, et al: Adverse drug reactions associated with global cognitive impairment in elderly persons. Ann Intern Med 107:169–173, 1987

Laukkanen E, Klonoff H, Allan B, et al: The role of prophylactic brain irradiation in limited stage small cell lung cancer: clinical, neuropsychologic, and CT sequelae. Int J Radiat Oncol Biol Phys 14:1109–1116, 1988

MacCrimmon DJ, Wallace JE, Goldberg WM, et al: Emotional disturbance and cognitive deficits in hyperthyroidism. Psychosom Med 41:331–340, 1979

Malinow KL, Molina R, Gordon B, et al: Neuropsychiatric dysfunction in primary Sjögren's syndrome. Ann Intern Med 103:344–349, 1985

Martin DC: B_{12} and folate deficiency dementia. Clin Geriatr Med 4:841–851, 1988

Mulrow CD, Feussner JR, Williams BC, et al: The value of clinical findings in the detection of normal pressure hydrocephalus. J Gerontol 42:277–279, 1987

Muuronen A, Bergman H, Hindmarsh T, et al: Influence of improved drinking habits on brain atrophy and cognitive performance in alcoholic patients: a five-year follow-up study. Alcoholism: Clinical and Experimental Research 13:137–141, 1989

Nielsen H, Knudsen L, Stenager E, et al: Cerebral blood flow and cognitive functioning in multiple sclerosis, in Mental Disorders and Cognitive Deficits in Multiple Sclerosis. Edited by Jensen K, Knudsen L, Stenager E, et al. London, John Libbey, 1989, pp 89–95

Nystrom E, Caidahl K, Fager G, et al: A double-blind cross-over 12-month study of L-thyroxine treatment of women with "subclinical" hypothyroidism. Clin Endocrinol (Oxf) 29:63–76, 1988

Perry S, Belsky-Barr D, Barr WB, et al: Neuropsychological function in physically asymptomatic, HIV-seropositive men. Journal of Neuropsychiatry 1:296–302, 1989

Rao SM, Leo GJ, Haughton VM, et al: Correlation of magnetic resonance imaging with neuropsychological testing in multiple sclerosis. Neurology 39:161–166, 1989a

Rao SM, St. Aubin-Faubert P, Leo GJ: Information processing speed in patients with multiple sclerosis. J Clin Exp Neuropsychol 11:471–477, 1989b

Reed RJ, Grant I: The long-term neurobehavioral consequences of substance abuse, in Conceptual and Methodological Challenges for Future Research (NIDA Research Monograph No 101). Edited by Spencer J, Boren P. Washington, DC, Department of Health and Human Services, 1990, pp 10–56

Reich P, Regestein QR, Murawski BJ, et al: Unrecognized organic mental disorders in survivors of cardiac arrest. Am J Psychiatry 140:1194–1197, 1983

Reitan RM: Halstead-Reitan Neuropsychological Test Battery. Tucson, AZ, Neuropsychology Laboratory, University of Arizona, 1979

Richardson PJ, Wyke MA: Memory function: effects of different antihypertensive drugs. Drugs 35 (suppl 5):80–85, 1988

Rosselli M, Lorenzana P, Rosselli A, et al: Wilson's disease, a reversible dementia: case report. J Clin Exp Neuropsychol 9:399–406, 1987

Sanders ME, Alexander EL, Koski CL, et al: Detection of activated terminal complement (C5b-9) in cerebrospinal fluid from patients with central nervous system involvement of primary Sjögren's syndrome and of systemic lupus erythematosus. J Immunol 138:2095–2099, 1987

Sayers JA, Smith REA, Holland RL, et al: Effects of carbon dioxide on mental performance. J Appl Physiol 63:25–30, 1987

Schmitt FA, Bigley JW, McKinnis R, et al: Neuropsychological outcome of AZT treatment of patients with AIDS and AIDS-related complex. N Engl J Med 319:1573–1578, 1988

Shore JH, Fraunfelder FT, Meyer SM: Psychiatric side effects from topical ocular timolol, a beta-adrenergic blocker. J Clin Psychopharmacol 7:264–267, 1987

Silver JM, Hales RE, Yudofsky SC: Psychopharmacology of depression in neurologic disorders. J Clin Psychiatry 51 (I, suppl):33–39, 1990

Sprague SM, Corwin HL, Tanner CM, et al: Relationship of aluminum to neurocognitive dysfunction in chronic dialysis patients. Arch Intern Med 148:2169–2172, 1988

Stambrook M, Cardoso E, Hawryluk GA, et al: Neuropsychological changes following the neurosurgical treatment of normal pressure hydrocephalus. Archives of Clinical Neuropsychology 3:323–330, 1988

Steere AC: Medical progress: Lyme disease. N Engl J Med 321:586–596, 1989

Streufert S, DePadova A, McGlynn T, et al: Effects of beta blockade with metoprolol on simple and complex task performance. Health Psychol 8:143–158, 1989

Sweeney JA, Meisel L, Walsh VL, et al: Assessment of cognitive functioning in polysubstance abusers. J Clin Psychol 45:346–350, 1989

Tarter RE, Hays AL, Carra J, et al: Sjögren's syndrome: its contribution to neuropsychiatric syndrome in patients with primary biliary cirrhosis. Dig Dis Sci 34:9–12, 1989

Telakivi T, Kajaste S, Partinen M, et al: Cognitive function in middle-aged snorers and controls: role of excessive daytime somnolence and sleep-related hypoxic events. Sleep 11:454–461, 1988

Trimble MR, Thompson PJ: Neuropsychological aspects of epilepsy, in Neuropsychological Assessment of Neuropsychiatric Disorders. Edited by Grant I, Adams K. Oxford, England, Oxford University Press, 1986, pp 321–346

Trzepacz PT, McCue M, Klein I, et al: Psychiatric and neuropsychological response to propranolol in Graves' disease. Biol Psychiatry 23:678–688, 1988

Turner DA, McGeachie RE: Normal pressure hydrocephalus and dementia—evaluation and treatment. Clin Geriatr Med 4:815–828, 1988

Varma VK, Malhotra AK, Dang R, et al: Cannabis and cognitive functions: a prospective study. Drug Alcohol Depend 21:147–152, 1988

Wechsler D: Wechsler Adult Intelligence Scale—Revised. San Antonio, TX, Psychological Corporation, 1981

Weder B, Wiedersheim P, Matter L, et al: Chronic progressive neurological involvement in *Borrelia burgdorferi* infection. J Neurol 234:40–43, 1987

Wise MG, Taylor SE: Anxiety and mood disorders in medically ill patients. J Clin Psychiatry 51 (suppl):1, 1990

World Health Organization: The ICD-10 Classification of Mental and Behavioural Disorders: Clinical Descriptions and Diagnostic Guidelines. Geneva, World Health Organization, 1992

Wragg RE, Jeste DV: Overview of depression and psychosis in Alzheimer's disease. Am J Psychiatry 146:577–587, 1989

Wurzelmann J, Frishman WH, Aronson M, et al: Neuropsychological effects of antihypertensive drugs. Cardiol Clin 5:689–701, 1987

Yarchoan R, Berg G, Brouwers P, et al: Response of human-immunodeficiency-virus-associated neurological disease to 3′-azido-3′-deoxythymidine. Lancet 1:132–135, 1987

Yarchoan R, Thomas RV, Grafman J, et al: Long-term administration of 3′-azido-2′,3′-dideoxythymidine to patients with AIDS-related neurological disease. Ann Neurol 23S:S82–S87, 1988

Chapter 20

The Proposal for Including Postconcussional Disorder in the Cognitive Disorders Section of DSM-IV

Stephen Brown, M.D.
Igor Grant, M.D.

STATEMENT OF THE ISSUES

It is estimated that two million persons in the United States suffer closed head injuries annually and that 500,000 of these are serious enough to require hospitalization. Although most head injuries resulting in unconsciousness are rated as "mild" (i.e., when first assessed at the site of injury such persons achieve Glasgow Coma Scale [Teasdale and Jennett 1974] scores of 13 or better), it is also now recognized that long-term, perhaps even permanent sequelae frequently complicate even such mild head injuries (Levin et al. 1989). Therefore, postconcussional disorders may represent one of the commonest etiologies of neurobehavioral disorder, especially in younger persons.

Despite increasing recognition of the importance of head injuries in producing changes in thinking, feeling, and behavior, review of the current and proposed DSM taxonomy reveals no adequate location for the signs and symptoms of postconcussional disorder. This constellation does not fit properly under the rubrics of delirium, dementia, or amnestic disorder. Postconcussional disorder does share some features of "secondary disorders due to a general medical condition" as proposed for DSM-IV, for example, proposals involving secondary mood disorder, secondary anxiety disorder, secondary sleep disorder, and secondary personality change. However, as is described below, it would frequently be necessary to code all (plus additional features) to encompass what is typically conceived as postconcussional disorder. There are two other diagnoses that come only slightly closer to describing this syndrome: organic mental disorder not otherwise specified and organic personality syndrome.

Organic mental disorder requires some maladaptive change in social or occupational functioning, and some evidence from physical examination, laboratory tests, or history of "etiology." But this category is very gross and nonspecific. No evidence of cognitive impairment is required. There are few "objective" criteria. Furthermore, by combining a large number of etiologies, it confuses research efforts and makes prognosis, time course, and therapeutic strategies difficult to predict for this diagnosis. Table 20–1 provides a brief outline of DSM-III-R (American Psychiatric Association 1987) criteria for organic personality syndrome. Although these criteria are more specific, once again there is no requirement for cognitive impairment; objective signs are few; and this diagnosis groups together a large variety of etiologies.

Given the scope that the problem head injury presents to society, it seems sensible to propose a specific category, even as has been done for other disorders where the phenomenology and natural course have become better defined (e.g., Alzheimer's disease).

Significance of the Issues

There are serious consequences to the lack of a proper diagnostic category for postconcussional disorder. First, communication among clinicians is made difficult by lack of an adequate diagnostic characterization. Second, research on epidemiology, natural history, phenomenology, and treatment is hampered by use of sometimes imprecise and other times incomplete and contradictory schemata by different groups of authors. Third, the lack of a precise diagnostic framework has perpetuated the myth that many patients, especially those with milder head injuries,

Table 20–1. Abbreviated DSM-III-R diagnostic criteria for Organic Personality Syndrome

1. One of the following:
   - affective instability
   - aggression or rage
   - impaired social judgment
   - apathy and indifference
   - suspiciousness or paranoid ideation
2. Evidence by history, physical examination, or laboratory tests of an etiology.
3. Does not occur as part of Attention-Deficit Hyperactivity Disorder in children.
4. Does not occur uniquely during Delirium, and does not meet criteria for Dementia.

exaggerate their complaints after the fact either because they are "hysterical" or motivated malingerers seeking some sort of compensation. In such instances, the outcome has been stigmatization of patients who are already suffering from a neurobehavioral disorder occasioned by head injury.

Methods

The literature search began through a review of several volumes on closed head injury edited by international authorities (e.g., Brooks 1984; Levin et al. 1982, 1989). Studies cited in these reviews that appeared likely to address the issues were then examined in detail. Additionally, a Medline search covering 1986–1989 identified articles on the definition of concussion and symptom profiles over time. We concentrate on those studies that provide substantial illumination of the main issues (definition, symptomatology, and natural history) without excessive reduplication.

Results

Definition of Concussion

Despite varied approaches, most studies would agree that a concussion has occurred if, after an impact to the head, a person suffers a period of unconsciousness and a period of reduced alertness after emerging from unconsciousness.

Concussion is relatively easy to infer following more severe head injuries characterized by unconsciousness of several hours or more, and posttraumatic confusion and amnesia lasting several days. A greater challenge has been to define sequelae of milder head injuries, typically considered to be those with unconsciousness lasting a few minutes to a few hours, and with Glasgow Coma Scale scores on presentation to a medical team above 12. (The scale is a 15-point clinical rating whose lowest score indicates unresponsiveness and whose upper score [15] indicates normal alertness.) From a public health standpoint, the problem of mild head injury is of great importance, since the majority of head injuries fit into this category (see Table 20–2).

The approaches to defining mild head injury are illustrated by the criteria proposed in several studies selected in Table 20–3. There appears to be a consensus emerging in favor of the criteria developed by a multicenter investigation reported by Levin et al. (1987a, 1987b) (see Table 20–3), which defines mild head injury (concussion) as existing when the period of unconsciousness does not exceed 30 minutes, when the Glasgow Coma Scale score on admission is 13–15 and never falls below 13 on continued observation, and when both clinical neurologic examinations and cranial computed tomography scans (one assumes magnetic resonance imaging could be substituted) are normal.

Symptom Profiles Over Time

The symptoms and complaints of those with postconcussive syndrome have been long known to physicians, with references to "traumatic neurosis" going back at least to H. Oppenheim in 1889. The longer-term sequelae of severe head injuries include poor memory, lack of spontaneity, irritability, restlessness, fatigue, childishness, and emotional lability (Thomsen 1984, 1989). Several studies have also assessed patient-reported symptoms at various intervals after a concussive injury. The results are surprisingly similar even though the time frames varied from 1 month to 3–5 years after concussion. The results from several representative studies are summarized in Table 20–4.

These data, plus the work on more severe head injuries, suggest that three clusters of symptoms occur commonly. There is a *somatic* cluster, which can include headache, fatigue, dizziness (vertigo), and visual or hearing impairments; a *cognitive* cluster, which may include difficulties with concentration and memory; and an *affective* cluster, which may involve irritability, anxiety, and depression, and, in the more severely injured, aspontaneity, lability, childishness, and social isolation (Thomsen 1984, 1989).

Neuropsychological testing has attempted to define the cognitive sequelae more precisely. Data from such studies are important in that they provide more "objective" indicators of persisting postconcussive neurocognitive impairments. Since the presence of cognitive deficits following moderate and severe head injury is considered to be beyond dispute (see Brooks 1984; Levin et al. 1982), our review focused on evidence of persisting neuropsychological impairment following *mild* head injuries.

Most studies we reviewed indicated that neuropsychological deficits could,

Table 20–2. Prevalence of mild head injury

Study	Location	Data (years)	Rate[a]	%[b]
Annegers et al. 1980	Olmstead, MN	1935–1974	149	60
Rimel et al. 1981	North Central, VA	1977–1979	Not given	49
Kraus et al. 1984	San Diego, CA	1981	131	82
Whitman et al. 1984	Chicago area	1979–1980	120–284	80

Note. The importance of "mild head injury" has been quantitated in several populations and epidemiologic studies.
[a]Rate of mild head injury per 100,000. [b]Percentage of all head injury.
Source. Adapted from Kraus and Nourjah 1989.

indeed, be demonstrated. Most commonly, impairments were noted on measures of choice reaction time (Hugenholtz et al. 1988; Jakobsen et al. 1987a; MacFlynn and Montgomery 1984), speeded information and processing (e.g., on Paced Auditory Serial Addition Test [Gronwall 1977]) (Gronwall and Wrightson 1974, 1981), as well as memory and more general neuropsychological functions (Barth et al. 1983).

Although the results of the above studies represent what appears to be an emerging consensus, some disagreements are noted. For example, Gentilini and colleagues (1985) could not distinguish mildly head-injured patients from control subjects on a series of tests that assessed attention, memory, and intelligence. Dikmen and Temkin (1987) cautioned that confounding factors such as alcohol or drug use, prior injuries, and other medical problems may be difficult to sort out from the effects of a mild head injury.

Despite these precautions, the preponderance of evidence favors the conclusion that concussed persons are at risk to develop postconcussional symptoms and

Table 20–3. Examples of criteria for mild head injury

Study	Criteria
Gronwall and Wrightson 1974	Head trauma with posttraumatic amnesia < 24 hours
Minderhoud et al. 1980	Unconscious < 30 minutes and posttraumatic amnesia
Rimel et al. 1981	Cranial trauma with loss of consciousness (20 minutes) and admission GCS score of 13 or better; hospitalization < 48 hours
Barth et al. 1983	Period of unconsciousness not exceeding 20 minutes; GCS score of 13 or more at admission; hospitalization < 48 hours
Edna and Cappelen 1987	One of the following: 1) loss of consciousness following head trauma, 2) a skull fracture, 3) development of an intracranial hematoma
Jakobsen et al. 1987a	A period of complete amnesia no matter how short, but maximum of 24 hours, and caused by a blow to the head
Levin et al. 1987a	Loss of consciousness < 30 minutes; GCS score of 13–15 on hospitalization no decrease of GCS score < 13; normal computed tomography scan; normal neurological examination

Note. A three-center study using the last criteria has gone far in creating a working consensus as to the definition of a concussion (Levin et al. 1987a). Earlier work stressing the importance of the length of the posttraumatic amnesia in assessing severity has been questioned in several studies (Barth et al. 1983; Jakobsen et al. 1987a; Rutherford et al. 1979; Gronwall and Wrightson 1981). GCS = Glasgow Coma Scale.

Table 20–4. Postconcussional symptoms

Study	Symptoms	*n*	%
Jakobsen et al. 1987b[a]	Headache	16	29
	Fatigue	16	29
	Impaired concentration	9	16
	Vertigo	6	11
	Irritability	5	9
Jakobsen et al. 1987b[b]	Headache	8	15
	Fatigue	3	5
	Impaired concentration	5	9
	Vertigo	3	5
	Irritability	1	2
Rutherford et al. 1979[c]	Headache	11	8
	Irritability	7	5
	Anxiety	5	4
	Depression	2	2
	Insomnia	3	2
	Fatigue	3	2
	Loss of concentration	4	3
	Loss of memory	5	4
	Amnesia	2	2
	Diplopia	1	0.8
	Visual defect	3	2
	Hearing defect	2	2
	Dizziness	6	5
	Epilepsy	0	0
	Sensitivity to alcohol	0	0
	Others	1	0.8
Edna and Cappelen 1987[d]	Headache	113	23
	Impaired memory	99	20
	Dizziness	90	19
	Fatigue	89	18
	Irritability (noise and light)	88	18
	Impaired concentration	68	14
	Insomnia	65	13
	Tinnitus	61	13
	Hearing defect	51	11
	Depression	45	9
	Anxiety	37	8
	Double vision	12	2

[a]$N = 55$; symptoms at 1 month. [b]$N = 55$; symptoms at 3 months. [c]$N = 131$; symptoms at 1 year. [d]$N = 485$; symptoms at 3–5 years.

signs. Limited human-pathologic data and animal research also add support to this notion. For example, Oppenheimer (1968) published autopsy results of brain-injured patients. In five patients who suffered mild concussion and died of other causes, he found microglial clusters, evidence of "microscopic destructive foci" that he felt were inflicted on the brain by what were regarded as trivial injuries.

Povlishock and Becker (1983) performed studies of a concussive model in cats, using sham controls. These demonstrated that although the mild concussive injury produced no focal parenchymal hemorrhages, contusions, or lacerations, there was distinct axonal change beginning with intra-axonal peroxidase pooling and leading later to lobulation and then to cloud-like swellings, suggesting axonal separation from distal axonal segments.

Discussion and Recommendations

It is recommended that DSM-IV adopt a diagnostic category entitled "Postconcussional Disorder." Criteria for this disorder are presented in Table 20–5. Criteria A seek to establish that an injury sufficient to cause "commotio cerebri" has taken place. It might be argued that criteria A1 and A2 should be more strict—for example, loss of consciousness for 30 minutes and posttraumatic amnesia lasting

Table 20–5. Proposed DSM-IV diagnostic criteria for Postconcussional Disorder

A. History of head injury that includes at least two of the following:
   1. Loss of consciousness for 5 minutes or more.
   2. Posttraumatic amnesia of 12 hours minimum.
   3. Onset of seizures (posttraumatic epilepsy) within 6 months of head injury.

B. Current symptoms to include (Note: these must be either new symptoms or substantial worsening, if preexisting):
   1. At least the following two cognitive difficulties:
      a. learning or memory (recall)
      b. concentration
   2. At least three of the following affective or vegetative symptoms:
      a. easy fatigability
      b. insomnia or sleep/wake cycle disturbances
      c. headache (substantially worse than before injury)
      d. vertigo/dizziness
      e. irritability and/or aggression on little or no provocation
      f. anxiety, depression, or lability of affect
      g. personality change (examples: social or sexual inappropriateness, child-like behavior)
      h. aspontaneity/apathy

24 hours. In recommending the criteria as we do, we attempt to balance between risking Type 1 error by misdiagnosing momentary, fleeting loss of consciousness with short amnesia (i.e., symptom complexes that might be difficult to diagnose reliably) and risking Type 2 error by missing significant concussive events through excessively restrictive criteria.

We acknowledge that the criteria chosen (greater than 5 minutes loss of consciousness and greater than 12 hours of posttraumatic amnesia) are arbitrary. However, we feel that these criteria, and/or posttraumatic epilepsy, represent good evidence of "commotio cerebri."

Criteria B represent and attempt to look at those effects or vegetative symptoms that are found to be frequent following head injury and that generally occur only following significant head injuries. In addition, we include evidence of cognitive difficulties that are new or have significantly increased.

References

American Psychiatric Association: Diagnostic and Statistical Manual of Mental Disorders, 3rd Edition, Revised. Washington, DC, American Psychiatric Association, 1987

Annegers JF, Grabow JD, Kurland LT, et al: The incidence, causes, and secular trends of head trauma in Olmstead County, Minnesota, 1935–1974. Neurology 30:912–919, 1980

Barth JT, Macciocchi SN, Giordani B, et al: Neuropsychological sequelae of minor head injury. Neurosurgery 13:529–533, 1983

Brooks N (ed): Closed Head Injury: Psychological, Social, and Family Consequences. New York, Oxford University Press, 1984

Dikmen S, Temkin N: Determination of the effects of head injury and recovery in behavioral research, in Neurobehavioral Recovery From Head Injury. Edited by Levin H, Girfman J, Eisenberg H. New York, Oxford University Press, 1987

Edna TH, Cappelen J: Late post-concussional symptoms in traumatic head injury: an analysis of frequency and risk factors. Acta Neurochir (Wien) 86:12–17, 1987

Gentilini M, Nichelli P, Schoenhuber R, et al: Neuropsychological evaluation of mild head injury. J Neurol Neurosurg Psychiatry 48:137–140, 1985

Gronwall D: Paced auditory serial addition task: a measure of recovery from concussion. Percept Mot Skills 44:367–373, 1977

Gronwall D, Wrightson P: Delayed recovery of intellectual function after minor head injury. Lancet 1:605–609, 1974

Gronwall D, Wrightson P: Memory and information processing capacity after closed head injury. J Neurol Neurosurg Psychiatry 44:889–895, 1981

Hugenholtz H, Stuss DT, Stethem LL, et al: How long does it take to recover from a mild concussion? Neurosurgery 5:853–858, 1988

Jakobsen J, Baadsgaard SE, Thomsen P, et al: Prediction of post-concussional sequelae by reaction time test. Acta Neurol Scand 75:341–345, 1987a

Jakobsen J, Thomsen ST, Baadsgaard SE: Sequelae after commotio cerebri. Ugeskr Laeger 149:2198–2200, 1987b

Kraus JF, Nourjah P: The epidemiology of mild head injury, in Mild Head Injury. Edited by Levin HS, Eisenberg HM, Benton AL. New York, Oxford University Press, 1989, pp 8–22

Kraus JF, Black MA, Hessol N, et al: The incidence of acute brain injury and serious impairment in a defined population: Am J Epidemiol 119:186–201, 1984

Levin HS, Benton AL, Grossman RG: Neurobehavioral Consequences of Closed Head Injury. New York, Oxford University Press, 1982

Levin HS, Mattis S, Ruff RM, et al: Neurobehavioral outcome following minor head injury: a three center study. J Neurosurg 66:234–243, 1987a

Levin HS, High WM, Goethe KE, et al: The neurobehavioural rating scale: assessment of the behavioral sequelae of head injury by the clinician. J Neurol Neurosurg Psychiatry 50:183–193, 1987b

Levin HS, Eisenberg HM, Benton AL: Mild Head Injury. New York, Oxford University Press, 1989

MacFlynn G, Montgomery EA: Measurement of reaction time following minor head injury. J Neurol Neurosurg Psychiatry 47:1326–1331, 1984

Minderhoud JM, Bouleins MM, Huizenga J, et al: Treatment of minor head injuries. Clin Neurol Neurosurg 82:127–140, 1980

Oppenheim H: Die Traumatischen Neurosen. Berlin, Germany, Hirschwald, 1889

Oppenheimer D: Microscopic lesions in the brain following head injury. J Neurol Neurosurg Psychiatry 31:299–306, 1968

Povlishock J, Becker D: Axonal change in minor head injury. J Neuropathol Exp Neurol 22:225–242, 1983

Rimel RW, Girodani B, Barth JT, et al: Disability caused by minor head injury. Neurosurgery 9:221–228, 1981

Rutherford W, Merret J, McDonald JR: Symptoms at one year following concussion from minor head injuries. Injury 10:225–230, 1979

Teasdale G, Jennett B: Assessment of coma and impairment of consciousness: a practical scale. Lancet 2:81–84, 1974

Thomsen IV: Late outcome of very severe head trauma: a ten-fifteen year second followup. J Neurol Neurosurg Psychiatry 47:260–268, 1984

Thomsen IV: Do young patients have worse outcomes after severe blunt head trauma? Brain Inj 3:157–162, 1989

Whitman S, Coonley-Hoganson R, Desai BT: Comparative head trauma experience in two socioeconomically different Chicago area communities: a population study. Am J Epidemiol 119:570–580, 1984

Chapter 21

Should Aging-Associated Memory Decline Be Included in DSM-IV?

Eric D. Caine, M.D.

Statement of the Issues

Researchers and clinicians who work with geriatric patient populations have recommended the development of a new diagnostic entity, "aging-associated memory impairment." In this review, I examine whether developing such a classification is warranted in light of available research data.

To decide whether aging-associated memory impairment, or a related diagnostic construct, should be included in DSM-IV, several specific issues relating to reliability and validity were considered. Who complains of memory impairment? What are the primary factors contributing to the process of complaint? Are subjective complaints related to objective deficits? Are aging-related decrements stable, or are they prodromal to a further progressive (pathological) cognitive decline? Does the aging-associated memory impairment construct, as currently defined, suitably describe a clinical syndrome or disorder that has pathological, therapeutic, or prognostic significance?

This chapter was supported, in part, by Public Health Service Grant MH40381 to the University of Rochester National Institute of Mental Health Clinical Research Center for the Study of Psychopathology of the Elderly. The unpublished data shared by Drs. Susan Bassett, Joy Taylor, Enid Light, and Kenneth Davis were especially helpful. Drs. Thomas Crook, Steven Ferris, Mary Ganguli, Glenn Larrabee, Barry Lebowitz, Paul Newhouse, Barry Reisberg, Jerome Yesavage, and Steven Zarit provided valuable critiques and comments regarding the early drafts of this review. Janet Werkheiser assisted with the Geriatric Diagnosis Workshop and manuscript preparation. Wendy Davis, M.Ed., has given valued support through the American Psychiatric Association's Office of Research.

Significance of the Issues

As part of the process leading to the development of DSM-IV, the National Institute of Mental Health (NIMH) and the University of Rochester-NIMH Clinical Research Center for the Study of Psychopathology of the Elderly convened a Geriatric Diagnosis Workshop, along with the American Psychiatric Association, to consider which psychiatric disorders, syndromes, or symptoms might be specifically related to the process of aging. During this May 1989 meeting, Dr. J. Yesavage recommended the inclusion of a new diagnostic entity, aging-associated memory impairment. This proposal was a direct result of nearly a decade's work, and the product of three NIMH/industry cosponsored workshops to consider memory dysfunction among nondemented elderly, and reflected as well the enthusiastic support of the Council on Aging of the American Psychiatric Association. It was intended to underscore the frequent finding that aging-related intellectual deficits can prove distressing for many elderly.

The concept of aging-associated memory impairment has roots in both the cognitive psychology and medical literatures. The former has been well developed over the past 30 years, with reliable and repeated documentation of robust declines in memory efficiency during the last decades of life (Craik 1977; Craik and McDowd 1987). However, ample data indicate that aging-associated cognitive alterations go well beyond memory, including general intelligence, visuospatial processing, abstraction and set maintenance, and language processing (Albert 1988). Kral (1958, 1962) introduced the term *benign senescent forgetfulness* (as opposed to malignant forgetfulness) to describe the memory complaints of the retirement home residents he studied. This term has been repeated often in the medical literature and has become a generally accepted notion among many clinicians. However, close evaluation of Kral's work revealed that he never objectively distinguished between his "normal" and his "benign" patient groups. He never evaluated a healthy elderly comparison population, rather examining nursing home residents or patients housed chronically in psychiatric hospitals. Moreover, many of his "benign" subjects showed evidence suggestive of significant neurological disease (Bamford and Caine 1988).

As proposed by Crook and colleagues (1986), the specific criteria for aging-associated memory impairment include 1) persons at least 50 years of age; 2) a gradual onset of memory dysfunction in daily life activities (e.g., misplacing objects or difficulty remembering names); 3) subjective complaints substantiated by psychometric evidence of memory failure, as measured by performance at least one standard deviation below the mean established for young adults on a well-standardized test of secondary or recent memory (e.g., logical memory or paired associates subtests of the Wechsler Memory Scale [Wechsler 1987]); 4) intact global intellectual function; and 5) absence of dementia (e.g., score ≥ 24 on the Mini-Mental State Exam [Folstein et al. 1975]). Persons would be excluded if they had a definable disorder that might account for their condition (including psychiatric disturbances). In effect, these criteria include healthy elderly, as long as each potential patient *complains* of cognitive dysfunction.

Methods

The initial review was based on the product of a literature search dealing with amnestic disorders, producing more than 300 papers that were published between 1984 and late 1989. With the exception of two articles, this search was remarkably unproductive regarding citations that might help consider aging-associated memory impairment as a putative entity. Thus other sources of information were examined. The experimental psychology literature regarding aging-related cognitive changes was a central focus. Although this literature was useful for background consideration, it did not specifically pertain to diagnostic, therapeutic, pathological, or prognostic issues. Thus little from that area has been cited. There has been a growing interest among cognitive psychologists in "metamemory," and some of that work pertained to the questions at hand. The term *metamemory* captures two concepts, comprising self-perceptions regarding one's memory capability as well as one's beliefs about how memory abilities relate to a variety of processes, such as aging or memory rehearsal. In addition, epidemiological data were provided by Bassett and Folstein (in press) of Johns Hopkins University, Baltimore, Maryland. Unpublished descriptive findings were shared by J. Taylor and J. Tinklenberg of Stanford University, California, and E. Light of NIMH (who analyzed test results collected initially by T. Crook). In a similar vein, K. Davis of Mt. Sinai Medical Center, New York, provided unpublished information regarding the follow-up of control subjects.

Results

Who Complains?

The available data suggest that complaining subjects are not representative of the elderly population at large. Bassett and Folstein (in press) and O'Connor and colleagues (1990) find that memory complaint is common in randomly assessed elderly populations and that it increases with increasing age and decreasing education. Affective symptoms are associated with increasing subjective memory complaints among presumably healthy subjects who are not syndromically depressed (O'Connor et al. 1990), although subjective complaints are not apparently related in these sample populations to cognitive performances measured by the Mini-Mental State Exam. Taylor and colleagues (1992) and Light (1988) described self-selected subject samples who were "competent intellectually" (J. L. Taylor, personal communication, June 26, 1989). Typically these were college-educated volunteers, from high socioeconomic groups, who had concerns regarding memory functioning. They had responded to newspaper advertisements or other solicitations for individuals who might be concerned regarding problems with memory functioning.

What Are the Primary Contributing Factors?

Two broadly defined factors seem to contribute to the aging-associated memory impairment phenomenon. One has been touched on in the metamemory literature and reflects the apparent beliefs of subjects about how memory changes with aging. This has been cited in the work of Herrmann (1982), as well as many others. In addition, ample literature is now available to indicate that memory complaints and metamemory perceptions are most closely tied to the affective status of the subject (Bolla et al. 1991; Light 1988; Niederehe and Yoder 1989; O'Connor et al. 1990; Popkin et al. 1982).

Are Subjective Complaints Related to Objective Deficits?

There are virtually no available data to suggest that there is a powerful correlation between subjective appraisal and objective performance (Bolla et al. 1991; Herrmann 1982; Light 1988; Niederehe and Yoder 1989; O'Connor et al. 1990; Popkin et al. 1982). It has been suggested in the past that a failure to show such a correlation may be a reflection of the use of experimental or laboratory measures of memory, as opposed to "ecologically valid" everyday measures of memory. However, Light (1988) failed to show a robust correlation between everyday measures and subjective complaints. (Indeed, the movement to everyday memory measures has been based, in part, on the notion of ecological validity, but it remains to be demonstrated whether these measures are more useful than either the experimental or clinical measures employed previously. Experimental measures may have the utility of clearly defining discrete, easily altered independent variables, which are useful for research purposes. No doubt, they are far removed [in terms of face validity] from the complaints that patients present, but it may not be wise to discard them until we show that everyday memory measures are, in fact, more utilitarian.)

Are Aging-Related Decrements Stable, or Are They Prodromal to a Further Progressive (Pathological) Cognitive Decline?

There are relatively few follow-up studies of elderly control subjects with an eye to detecting the onset of dementia. Taylor and colleagues (1992) followed 30 of 43 subjects for 4 years; although evidence of a very slow decline in memory performance was apparent for the group as a whole, largely accounted for by older participants, only one subject developed signs of dementia (J. L. Taylor, personal communication, October 9, 1992). Davis and colleagues (K. L. Davis, personal communication, November 13, 1989) monitored 52 control subjects for at least 1 year, and 38 of them for 2 years. There was no indication that there is a worsening in cognitive performance with aging over this period of the control subjects, a situation that contrasts rather dramatically with the Alzheimer's patients who quite clearly worsen with time.

Larrabee and colleagues (1986) assessed their cohort of patients after 1 year, having defined a subgroup who had particularly poor cognitive function, and found no deterioration in any of the members when they were reevaluated 1 year later. Similarly, Reisberg and colleagues (1986) prospectively followed patients with Alzheimer's disease and comparison subjects, rating them with the Global Deterioration Scale (GDS) (Reisberg et al. 1982), a scale ranging from "normal" (GDS 1) to "late dementia" (GDS 7). Of the 72 subjects who were at a stage less than GDS 4 on entry, 62 showed no progression, 5 deteriorated significantly, and 3 improved (the latter were among the GDS 3 patients). Of those who declined, 2 were from the GDS 2 group, and 3 were from the GDS 3 group.

Katzman and colleagues (1989) followed 434 apparently healthy volunteers, ages 75–85 years, for a 5-year period. Of these, 56 (12.9%) developed dementing disorders (most having Alzheimer's disease) during that time. The major predictor of development of dementia of the Alzheimer type was the mental status score on entry into the study. Among the 254 (58.5%) patients who made 0–2 errors on a 33-item mental status test, the rate of developing dementia of the Alzheimer type was 0.6% per year; 73 (16.8%) of the original sample made 5–8 errors on the test, and among these 12% per year developed Alzheimer's disease. Katzman and colleagues concluded that it may be possible in the future to identify those 80-year-old patients who are at a low risk for developing dementia of the Alzheimer type and a smaller group that has a very substantial risk.

Does the Aging-Associated Memory Impairment Construct, as Currently Defined, Suitably Describe a Clinical Syndrome or Disorder That Has Pathological, Therapeutic, or Prognostic Significance?

As originally proposed, the diagnostic criteria for aging-associated memory impairment are ultimately dependent on the presence of subjective complaints. Given the relatively poor correlation between memory complaints (or self-assessed memory functioning) and objective indices of performance, the use of this criterion is most tenuous. As the proposed objective cutoff (one standard deviation below the mean for young age groups) may be overinclusive, a clinician could be faced with a very large group of elderly patients who have no uniquely identifying feature beyond their complaint. Perceived deficits are culturally variable and, in this instance, unrelated to any other definable disorder.

On the other hand, it is also evident that there are potentially identifiable subjects within the elderly population who have cognitive decrements that are separable or definable relative to age-comparable peers, and who might either have a decline that is prodromal to progressive dementia or a form of "exaggerated" age-related cognitive decline. It is also important to emphasize that the cognitive impairment experienced as part of normal aging is not restricted to memory, and thus any future nomenclature will have to account for multifunctional deficits.

Discussion and Recommendations

Utilizing a diagnostic label implies the definition of a syndrome that we connect with a pathological disease process. Diagnosis conveys in a shorthand fashion what is known regarding symptoms, signs, and clinical history. It is utilitarian in nature and most helpful when specifying prognosis and pointing toward treatment intervention.

Normal aging-related cognitive declines occur on a continuum of performance, ranging from near the higher performance levels encountered among young individuals to deficits that are suggestive of dementia of the Alzheimer type. It may be very difficult to establish an arbitrary or numerical level where a disease state should be proclaimed. We typically associate diagnosis with dysfunction, and functional impairment may be a useful parameter for defining those age-related conditions that might be called "disorders." Subjective complaint has proven unreliable; indeed, subjective complaint is not consistently related to performance in diagnosed dementing or amnestic populations. However, the cognitive decline that exceeds the decrement of age-matched peers may be the precursor of a more severe, progressive disorder. The data of Reisberg and colleagues (1986) and Katzman and colleagues (1989) suggest that these patients require close monitoring, even when a diagnosis of dementia is not yet warranted.

Thus two major points emerge. First, changes in intellect that are related to age are readily demonstrable, but do not lead to the picture of the dementia that is the hallmark of progressive neurodegenerative disease. In contrast, elderly patients who show subtle but significant cognitive impairment relative to age- and education-matched peers may be at increased risk of developing a dementing disorder, with mild but definable deficits reflecting the earliest measurable manifestations of a beginning decline.

Second, given the needs of clinicians to reassure healthy elderly that they are not suffering early dementia of the Alzheimer type, a designation in DSM-IV remains a laudable goal. In light of the inadequacies of aging-associated memory impairment as a diagnostic label, a more appropriate designation might be known as "aging-associated cognitive decline." Aging-associated cognitive decline would be listed among conditions that are not attributable to a mental disorder, but are a focus of attention or treatment (called V Codes in DSM-III-R [American Psychiatric Association 1987], and Z Codes during DSM-IV planning). Aging-associated cognitive decline is intended to capture the robust, objectively identified, age-related decrement in cognitive processing abilities, including an array of intellectual functions; these are not so severe as to impair personal or vocational functioning significantly. Individuals who experience this condition note occasional problems remembering names or appointments, may experience some greater difficulty solving complex problems, and often develop compensatory strategies to deal with these symptomatic but not impairing difficulties. The exact standards for defining the limits of aging-associated cognitive decline are not immediately clear, as there might be substantial debate regarding how much performance decrement relative to young control subjects is necessary to qualify, and to what extent education and socioeconomic status affect the expression of these problems. Despite robust performance changes on neuropsychological testing, aging-associated cognitive decline is not the harbinger of serious illness or reduced longevity. However, evaluation of possible contributing medical and primary psychiatric disturbances would remain an important aspect of initial clinical assessment.

Thus cognitive decline in the elderly can be considered dimensionally or hierarchically, involving aging-associated cognitive decline, mild cognitive impairment, and dementia. One would establish aging-associated cognitive decline based on the presence of a reported cognitive decline, the absence of significant overall functional decrement, and performance on standardized neuropsychological tests that place the patient within the normal range of similarly age- and education-matched peers. As compared with aging-associated memory impairment, a criterion involving subjective complaint is unnecessary. Those patients who demonstrate mild cognitive deficits (relative to aged peers), and related mild functional impairment, could be classified as having "cognitive impairment disorder, not otherwise specified" (a category that will include "mild cognitive impairment"). Such a diagnosis would be established by a history indicative of intellectual decline; evidence of interference in higher-order vocational, social, and interpersonal tasks; and objective demonstration of cognitive impairment on one or more cognitive parameters. However, both the cognitive deficits and the functional impairments remain relatively mild and not impairing enough to qualify for a diagnosis of dementia. This category can be particularly appropriate for individuals where the progressive nature of the disorder remains to be clarified, or a definitive diagnosis of dementia of the Alzheimer type seems unwarranted. Consideration of this diagnosis should trigger an extensive neuropsychiatric evaluation to determine whether a specific disorder is causing its appearance.

The third level of this diagnostic hierarchy would involve the designation of dementia. In comparison to mild cognitive impairment, a greater degree of cognitive dysfunction would require the use of the dementia label. Although DSM-III-R makes no attempt at gradation, this is a common practice clinically, where mild disorders are not yet diagnosed confidently. It is worthwhile to maintain this distinction in our classification, especially as some patients do not progress to a full-blown syndrome.

It seems desirable to avoid the designation "impairment" when describing the cognitive changes that occur in the healthy elderly, and inappropriate to use a psychiatric diagnostic (disease) label for a condition that is not associated with a negative long-term outcome or significant functional interference. Having a V Code (or Z Code) for "Aging-Associated Cognitive Decline" provides recognition of this robust phenomenon and allows for the use of an accepted term when reassuring individuals that they do not have Alzheimer's disease, as well as providing a descriptive label for those individuals who might benefit from memory-cognitive enhancement through behavioral or (in the future) pharmacological intervention.

References

Albert MS: Cognitive function, in Geriatric Neuropsychology. Edited by Albert MS, Moss MB. New York, Guilford, 1988, pp 33–53

American Psychiatric Association: Diagnostic and Statistical Manual of Mental Disorders, 3rd Edition, Revised. Washington, DC, American Psychiatric Association, 1987

Bamford KA, Caine ED: Does "benign senescent forgetfulness" exist?, in Treatment Considerations for Alzheimer's Disease and Related Dementing Illnesses, Clinics in Geriatric Medicine, Vol 4. Edited by Maletta GJ. Philadelphia, PA, WB Saunders, 1988, pp 897–916

Bassett SS, Folstein MF: Memory complaint, memory performance and psychiatric diagnosis: a community study. J Geriatr Psychiatry Neurol (in press)

Bolla KI, Lindgren KN, Bonaccorsy C, et al: Memory complaints in older adults: fact or fiction? Arch Neurol 48:61–64, 1991

Craik FIM: Age differences in human memory, in Handbook of the Psychology of Aging. Edited by Birren JE, Schaie KW. New York, Van Nostrand Reinhold, 1977

Craik FIM, McDowd J: Age differences in recall and recognition. J Exp Psychol [Learn Mem Cogn] 13:474–479, 1987

Crook T, Bartus RT, Ferris SH, et al: Age-associated memory impairment: proposed diagnostic criteria and measures of clinical change—report of a National Institute of Mental Health work group. Developmental Neuropsychology 2:261–276, 1986

Folstein MF, Folstein SE, McHugh PR: Mini-Mental State: a practical method for grading the cognitive state of patients for the clinician. J Psychiatr Res 12:189–198, 1975

Herrmann DJ: Know thy memory: the use of questionnaires to assess and study memory. Psychol Bull 92:434–452, 1982

Katzman R, Aronson M, Fuld P, et al: Development of dementing illness in an 80-year-old volunteer cohort. Ann Neurol 25:317–324, 1989

Kral VA: Neuro-psychiatric observations in an old peoples home. J Gerontol 13:169–176, 1958

Kral VA: Senescent forgetfulness: benign and malignant. Can Med Assoc J 86:257–260, 1962

Larrabee GJ, Levin HS, High WM: Senescent forgetfulness: a quantitative study. Dev Neuropsychol 2:373–385, 1986

Light E: The relationship of subjective memory, affective status and performance on simulated everyday memory tasks across the adult lifespan. Unpublished doctoral dissertation, University of Maryland, College Park, 1988

Niederehe G, Yoder C: Metamemory perceptions in depressions of young and older adults. J Nerv Ment Dis 177:4–14, 1989

O'Connor DW, Pollitt PA, Roth M, et al: Memory complaints and impairment in normal, depressed and demented elderly people identified in a community survey. Arch Gen Psychiatry 47:224–227, 1990

Popkin SJ, Gallagher D, Thompson LW, et al: Memory complaint and performance in normal and depressed older adults. Exp Aging Res 8:141–145, 1982

Reisberg B, Ferris SH, de Leon MJ, et al: The Global Deterioration Scale for assessment of primary degenerative dementia. Am J Psychiatry 139:1136–1139, 1982

Reisberg B, Ferris SH, Shulman E, et al: Longitudinal course of normal aging and progressive dementia of the Alzheimer's type: a prospective study of 106 subjects over a 3.6 year mean interval. Prog Neuropsychopharmacol Biol Psychiatry 10:571–578, 1986

Taylor JL, Miller TP, Tinklenberg JR: Correlates of memory decline: a 4-year longitudinal study of older adults with memory complaints. Psychol Aging 7:185–193, 1992

Wechsler D: Wechsler Memory Scale—Revised. San Antonio, TX, Psychological Corporation, 1987

Section III

Schizophrenia and Other Psychotic Disorders

Contents

Section III
Schizophrenia and Other Psychotic Disorders

Introduction to Section III

Schizophrenia and Other Psychotic Disorders

Nancy Andreasen, M.D., Ph.D.

The issues confronted by the Work Group charged with responsibility for schizophrenia and other psychotic disorders are complex and difficult. Unlike many other disorders under the purview of DSM, the concept of schizophrenia has a long history that has been informed by a variety of competing perceptions and definitions. The boundaries of the concept have shifted over time, and modest variations exist internationally, depending on whether particular nations adhere to attitudes that are predominantly Kraepelinian (Kraepelin 1919/1971), Bleulerian (Bleuler 1911/1950), Schneiderian (Schneider 1959), or eclectic. Paradoxically, controversy about the nature and definition of schizophrenia and other psychoses is created, not by an absence of research and data, but rather by a wealth of information. The complexity and diversity of the issues mirror the complexity and diversity of the disease itself. Until we understand schizophrenia and other major psychoses at the pathophysiological and etiological level, we are not likely to achieve firm consensus on what they are or how they should be defined and delineated.

As adumbrated in detail in subsequent chapters in the Sourcebook, the Work Group grappled with five major issues: 1) the characteristic symptoms of schizophrenia as presented in criterion A, 2) the breadth versus narrowness of the category of schizophrenia, 3) the relationship of schizophrenia to brief psychoses, 4) the subtypes of schizophrenia, and 5) the relationship of nonpsychotic conditions to the schizophrenia spectrum.

Because of the large research data bases already in existence, combined with the clinical importance of schizophrenia, the Work Group responsible for this disorder and related conditions achieved a consensus that might be referred to as "progressive conservatism." That is, they agreed that changes would be made only when a preponderance of evidence indicated that the advantages of change outweighed the disadvantages. A large body of research is already in existence that uses DSM-III (American Psychiatric Association 1980) or DSM-III-R (American Psychiatric Association 1987) criteria. Because of the inconvenience and confusion that could be produced through major changes, the Work Group concurred that it would be important to maintain as much continuity as possible between DSM-III-R and DSM-IV. On the other hand, other factors also impinged to inform the identification of issues and their subsequent resolution. These forces included the impending arrival of ICD-10 (World Health Organization 1992), recognition that the presentation of psychotic conditions in DSM-III-R might be unduly complex and difficult to learn, and a variety of problems with the reliability of particular symptoms. The consensus toward progressive conservatism led to an agreement that, as far as possible, decisions about changes would be guided by the basic principles that caseness should be changed as little as possible, but that changes could be made if they were informed by an adequate data base and if they improved consonance with ICD-10, user friendliness, or reliability.

Characteristic Symptoms

Prior to the development of DSM-III, three different algorithms were available to provide objective methods for the diagnoses of schizophrenia: the DIAGNO system of the Present State Examination (PSE) (Wing et al. 1974), the Washington University criteria (Feighner et al. 1972), and the Research Diagnostic Criteria (RDC) (Spitzer et al. 1978). DIAGNO emphasized a cross-sectional approach, asking interviewers to focus on symptoms present during the past month. If a characteristic constellation of symptoms was present, a certain diagnosis of schizophrenia was made; the constellation of symptoms emphasized Schneiderian first-rank symptoms. The Washington University criteria stressed that symptoms must be present for at least 6 months, enumerated a mixture of characteristic symptoms ranging from flat affect through hallucinations, and included manifestations of social dysfunction within the criteria. The RDC required 1 week of characteristic symptoms (which were a mixture of first-rank symptoms, other types of delusions and hallucinations, and some "negative symptoms" such as affective flattening), and further subdivided schizophrenia into acute, subacute, subchronic, and chronic on the basis of duration.

The DSM-III-R criteria were developed within this environment and represented a compromise between these three competing methods. DSM-III required 1 week of "active symptoms" and an overall duration of 6 months. For the first time, the concept of prodromal and residual symptoms was introduced; these symptoms contributed to the overall duration criterion. DSM-III-R retained these concepts, with some modest modifications.

The overall net effect of DSM-III and DSM-III-R was to reduce the boundaries of the concept of schizophrenia to a relatively narrow construct and to require the presence of psychotic symptoms for the diagnosis of schizophrenia. This was a clear break with prior American traditions, which had been heavily influenced by Bleulerian concepts, which involved a broader construct and based the diagnosis primarily on nonpsychotic or "negative" symptoms.

The first task of the Work Group was to evaluate the characteristic symptoms of schizophrenia, as presented in criterion A. Three different issues were noted: the complexity of the algorithm, the possible unreliability of the concept of "bizarreness," and the emerging importance of negative symptoms.

Issues concerning the complexity of the algorithm are enumerated in Chapter 22 by Andreasen and Flaum. Briefly, a variety of problems were noted, including redundance, logical inconsistencies, selection of symptoms with low base rates or poor reliability, and excessive complexity. The MacArthur data reanalyses confirmed some of these concerns, and field trials were mandated to collect additional information. Overall, the Work Group agreed that, if supporting evidence was provided by the field trials that caseness would not be changed significantly, it would be desirable to simplify the DSM-III-R algorithm, which was a compromise position between PSE, RDC, and Washington University criteria.

The concept of bizarre delusions was a second issue. The concept of bizarre delusions had undergone a gradual metamorphosis from the PSE to DSM-III and DSM-III-R. The PSE construct relied heavily on Schneiderian symptoms; if present, Schneiderian symptoms mandated a diagnosis of schizophrenia. DSM-III originally included the same concept; as DSM-III was being written, however, a series of reports appeared in the literature indicating that Schneiderian first-rank symptoms were not pathognomonic of schizophrenia. In this context, Schneiderian symptoms were de-emphasized in DSM-III, and more generic terms were used to refer to delusions and hallucination. When DSM-III-R was written, a new concept was added to the definition of bizarre delusions. The DSM-III definition indicated that such delusions would be "impossible," whereas the DSM-III-R definition indicated that they would be "implausible." The latter definition represented an effort to invoke Jasperian concepts of "nonunderstandability." A variety of concerns were raised in Work Group discussions that the translation from Schneiderian to Jasperian concepts had introduced some blurring and that clinicians might not understand what was meant by the concept of bizarre. Several studies were completed during the DSM-IV developmental process, some of which confirmed this concern and some of which did not. This issue is also discussed in the Andreasen review and was deferred to the field trials for definitive resolution.

The third issue concerning characteristic symptoms involved the role of negative symptoms in the diagnosis of schizophrenia. Negative symptoms have a rich tradition, reaching back to Bleuler and Kraepelin, both of whom saw as central to the concept symptoms such as loss of drive, loss of ability to experience pleasure, loss of the capacity to speak fluently, or loss of emotional tone. In addition to their historical importance, negative symptoms were also recognized as important in producing severe morbidity among patients with schizophrenia. Finally, a literature has been amassed, indicating that they may have predictive validity, as reviewed in Chapter 23 by McGlashan and Fenton. These symptoms had been minimized in DSM-III and DSM-III-R because of a concern that they were not reliable. During the 1980s, however, a substantial literature accumulated that indicated that the symptoms could be rated reliably if clearly defined. In this context, the Work Group felt that the reintroduction of negative symptoms to a more important role in the diagnosis of schizophrenia should be considered and that a move in this direction had good evidentiary support.

Breadth Versus Narrowness of the Concept of Schizophrenia

The concept of schizophrenia, as defined by DSM-III and DSM-III-R, constituted a significant narrowing. These changes are summarized in Chapters 22, 24, and 28. Many patients who would previously have been diagnosed as having schizophrenia, schizoaffective type, or even as having schizophrenia were reclassified in DSM-III and DSM-III-R as having affective or mood disorders. Essentially, the DSM conceptualization gave primacy to the presence of affective symptoms over psychotic symptoms, for reasons that made good clinical sense. Nevertheless, this changed the American construct of schizophrenia so that it became the narrowest in the world. ICD, on the other hand, retains a broader concept of schizophrenia, including both schizoaffective disorder (relatively broadly defined) and schizotypal disorder within the overall construct of schizophrenia. Consequently, the Work Group was obliged to review the boundaries between schizophrenia, schizoaffective disorder, and affective disorder. The conclusions of this review are summarized in Chapter 28 by Kendler. Basically, Kendler suggests that it is worthwhile to retain the relatively narrow construct of schizophrenia.

A second boundary issue is related to the boundary between schizophrenia and delusional disorder. The DSM-III construct had a relatively "fuzzy boundary," which was clarified by DSM-III-R. The DSM-III-R definition introduced additional defining criteria by clarifying the concept of bizarreness and also including other markers of "paranoia vera" such as preserved affect and good social functioning. These issues were also reviewed in Chapter 28 by Kendler, with a recommendation that the DSM-III-R construct be retained.

Relationship to Brief Psychoses

The ICD-10 construct is based heavily on the PSE tradition. It defines schizophrenia cross-sectionally, requiring the presence of 1 month of characteristic symptoms; among the characteristic symptoms, emphasis is placed on Schneiderian first-rank symptoms. This construct is quite different from the concepts that evolved from the RDC and the Washington University criteria into the DSM-III and DSM-III-R construct, which requires 6 months of symptoms overall, but only 1 week of "active symptoms" (i.e., psychotic symptoms of various types). The Work Group was required, therefore, to review existing literature that was available to support a distinction based on 1 week versus 1 month versus 6 months of symptoms and to evaluate which types of symptoms must be present during those various time periods. This review is provided in Chapter 24 by Keith and Matthews. As they indicate, the evidence to support each of these various positions is not definitive. Various conclusions can be reached. Reviewing the evidence, the Work Group suggested that 1 month of "active symptoms" be considered for DSM-IV to provide consistency with ICD; on the other hand, they also suggested that an overall duration of 6 months be retained to provide continuity with DSM-III and DSM-III-R.

The 6-month duration criterion is closely related to the concept of prodromal and residual symptoms. These symptoms were a new construct introduced by DSM-III and were supported by a relatively small data base. The Work Group concluded that a review of the data base accumulated since DSM-III was appropriate. As reviewed in Chapter 24 by Keith and Matthews, however, only modest evidence has been accrued since 1980 when DSM-III was published. In this context, the field trials were felt to be particularly important, and the field trial studies were designed to collect additional information about prodromal and residual symptoms (e.g., whether they can be assessed reliably).

Subtypes of Schizophrenia

Bleuler (1911/1950) elected to subtitle his book on dementia praecox: "or the Group of Schizophrenias." Since the 19th century, clinicians and investigators have concurred that the concept of schizophrenia probably refers to a heterogeneous group of conditions. Further, most clinicians and investigators concur that the disorder(s) is both phenomenologically and etiologically heterogeneous. In recognition of this heterogeneity, a variety of subtypes have been defined. McGlashan and Fenton (Chapter 25) consider the classical subtypes of schizophrenia. The traditional subtypes have included paranoid, hebephrenic, undifferentiated, catatonic, and simple. The DSM system opted for a relatively traditional approach to subtyping. Nevertheless, the Work Group felt that a review of approaches to subtyping was appropriate in the context of developing DSM-IV. The suggestion by Crow (1980) and others that a new system of subtyping, based on positive versus negative symptoms, should be introduced, was considered worthy of evaluation. The results of this literature review are summarized in Chapter 23 by McGlashan and Fenton. The conclusions reached were that the traditional subtypes performed reasonably well, although far from perfectly.

In Chapter 26, McGlashan considers late-onset schizophrenia.

Relationship of Nonpsychotic Conditions to the Schizophrenia Spectrum

DSM-III and DSM-III-R have tended to group the mood disorders under a single category and to include milder forms of mood or affective disorders in the overall category. In an effort to narrow the construct of schizophrenia, however, milder forms were either excluded altogether (i.e., simple schizophrenia) or moved to other sections (i.e., schizotypal personality). The Work Group concluded that it was important to review this issue. The topic of schizotypal personality was reviewed by Siever and colleagues (1991); simple schizophrenia is considered in Chapter 25 by McGlashan and Fenton. Although the evidence is far from conclusive, the consensus appears to be to retain schizotypal disorder within the Personality Disorders section. The concept of simple schizophrenia may be recommended for inclusion in an appendix to DSM-IV.

In Chapter 27, Siris discusses secondary depression in schizophrenia.

Trait Markers

A variety of trait markers have been proposed for schizophrenia. This issue is considered in Chapter 29 by Szymanski, Kane, and Lieberman.

Summary and Conclusions

The Work Group charged with responsibility for schizophrenia and other psychotic disorders faced a variety of weighty decisions. Many of these were addressed through the literature reviews that follow. Others have been deferred until additional evidence was amassed from the field trials. The field trials have focused in particular on issues pertaining to caseness, duration criteria, prodromal and residual symptoms, and bizarre delusions. Clear areas of agreement, based on committee consensus and literature reviews, included the importance of maintaining continuity with DSM, the desirability of creating consistency with ICD, the value of retaining caseness and doing as little "tinkering" as possible, the value of improving clarity and "user friendliness," and the importance of negative symptoms. The final criteria chosen for DSM-IV will reflect this consensus, as modulated by evidence gleaned from the field trials.

References

American Psychiatric Association: Diagnostic and Statistical Manual of Mental Disorders, 3rd Edition. Washington, DC, American Psychiatric Association, 1980

American Psychiatric Association: Diagnostic and Statistical Manual of Mental Disorders, 3rd Edition, Revised. Washington, DC, American Psychiatric Association, 1987

Bleuler E: Dementia Praecox or the Group of Schizophrenias (1911). Translated by Zinkin J. New York, International Universities Press, 1950

Crow TJ: Molecular pathology of schizophrenia: more than one disease process? BMJ 12:66–68, 1980

Feighner JP, Robins E, Guze SB, et al: Diagnostic criteria for use in psychiatric research. Arch Gen Psychiatry 26:57–63, 1972

Kraepelin E: Dementia Praecox and Paraphrenia (1919). Translated by Barclay RM. Edited by Robertson GM. New York, RE Krieger, 1971

Schneider K: Clinical Psychopathology. Translated by Hamilton MW. New York, Grune & Stratton, 1959

Siever LJ, Bernstein DP, Silverman JM: Schizotypal personality disorder: a review of its current status. Journal of Personality Disorders 5:178–193, 1991

Spitzer RL, Endicott J, Robins E: Research Diagnostic Criteria: rationale and reliability. Arch Gen Psychiatry 35:773–782, 1978

Wing JK, Cooper JE, Sartorius N: The Measurement and Classification of Psychiatric Symptoms. New York, Cambridge University Press, 1974

World Health Organization: The ICD-10 Classification of Mental and Behavioural Disorders: Clinical Descriptions and Diagnostic Guidelines. Geneva, World Health Organization, 1992

Chapter 22

Characteristic Symptoms of Schizophrenia

Nancy Andreasen, M.D., Ph.D.
Michael Flaum, M.D.

Statement of the Issues

An evaluation of the characteristic symptoms used to define schizophrenia has raised a variety of issues. These include the following:

1. Should the characteristic symptoms, in conjunction with the duration criterion, be revised to make the definition of schizophrenia in DSM-III-R (American Psychiatric Association 1987) more similar to the definition in ICD-10 (World Health Organization 1992)?
2. Are the symptoms used to define schizophrenia in criterion A appropriately supported by an empirical data base, which demonstrates adequate reliability, a high enough base rate to provide face validity, and specificity?
3. Have the criteria used to define schizophrenia become excessively complex, making it difficult for them to serve the basic clinical, research, and teaching functions that are fundamental in the diagnostic process?
4. Given the research and clinical interest in negative symptoms, should they be given more prominence among the defining features of schizophrenia?

This research was supported in part by NIMH Grants MH31593, MH40856, and MHCRC 43271; the Nellie Ball Trust Fund, Iowa State Bank and Trust Company, Trustee; and a Research Scientist Award, MH00625. This chapter was revised and adapted from an article originally published in Andreasen N: "Schizophrenia and Related Disorders in DSM-IV: Editor's Introduction." *Schizophrenia Bulletin* 17:27–49, 1991.

Significance of the Issues

Consonance With ICD-10

DSM-III-R and ICD-10 differ in several important ways. ICD specifies a much shorter duration (1 month), requires that the characteristic symptoms listed in the ICD equivalent of criterion A be present for 1 month, and does not include the concept of prodromal or residual symptoms. The listing of characteristic symptoms stresses Schneiderian concepts much more prominently than does DSM-III-R; any one from a list of four is sufficient to make the diagnosis. There are major differences in the definition of terms. Criterion A1D of ICD ("persistent delusions of other kinds that are culturally inappropriate and completely impossible" (World Health Organization 1992, p. 87) is comparable to the "bizarre delusions" (p. 194) criterion of DSM-III-R, but the examples provided in the two systems indicate that they are conceptually far apart; DSM-III-R lists Schneiderian-like symptoms, whereas ICD lists "religious or political identity, or superhuman powers and abilities" (World Health Organization 1992, p. 87).

Very little data are available at present to indicate the effects of DSM-III-R on the diagnostic boundaries defined by DSM-III (American Psychiatric Association 1980), but the existing evidence indicates that DSM-III-R has further narrowed the concept of schizophrenia by requiring that, if delusions are the only positive symptom present, they must be bizarre (Fenton et al. 1988). Criterion B, if interpreted to require impairment in role function, will further narrow the definition. The ICD definition has not been in use as yet, although it is closely similar to the Present State Examination CATEGO system (Wing et al. 1974), since it depends heavily on requiring the presence of positive symptoms during the past month. This system has been shown to be broader than DSM.

Thus, the major difference between ICD and DSM is that the ICD criteria probably embody a broader concept of schizophrenia than do the DSM criteria. Further, ICD contains the category of simple schizophrenia, which is defined on the basis of negative symptoms alone and specifically excludes cases characterized by prominent positive symptoms. This further broadens the conceptual definition of schizophrenia in ICD. ICD also gives explicit recognition to the importance of negative symptoms by mentioning them in criterion A2H, although negative symptoms alone are not sufficient to make a diagnosis of schizophrenia. (This appears to introduce some inconsistency in the system, since simple schizophrenia is a subtype of schizophrenia.)

The problems of consonance with ICD raise the following questions. Should the duration criterion be modified? Should the concept of prodromal or residual symptoms be abandoned? Should Schneiderian symptoms be given more prominence? Should negative symptoms be given more prominence? Should the overall concept of schizophrenia be broadened?

The Value of an Empirical Base

The DSM-III-R criteria were developed by slow accretions and modifications of previous methods for diagnosing schizophrenia. Because of a concern about excessive breadth and poor reliability, Bleulerian approaches were abandoned in the development of the Washington University criteria, which is also referred to as Feighner's criteria (Feighner et al. 1972), and subsequently the Research Diagnostic Criteria (RDC) (Spitzer et al. 1978), which jointly formed the basis for DSM-III. The items selected for DSM-III, and subsequently for DSM-III-R, were not subjected to a systematic empirical examination of their reliability, base rate, or discriminating power. The need to develop DSM-IV, combined with the current existence of a variety of data sets consisting of patients who have been previously diagnosed as having schizophrenia, may provide an opportunity to develop diagnostic criteria using modern biometric methods, thereby leading to criteria that will be more efficient, have better coverage, and be more scientifically valid.

Excessive Complexity

Despite attempts to simplify, DSM-III-R criteria remain very complex. To make a diagnosis of schizophrenia, clinicians must assess the presence or absence of a total of at least 12 different signs and symptoms: delusions, prominent hallucinations, incoherence, loosening of associations, catatonic behavior, flat affect, inappropriate affect, nonaffective verbal hallucinations, voices commenting, voices conversing, bizarre delusions, and thought broadcasting. They must remember which symptoms permit the diagnosis to reach criterion level when only one is present, and when two are required. They must make distinctions among delusions and hallucinations as to whether they are Schneiderian or non-Schneiderian, bizarre or "nonbizarre," and mood congruent or mood incongruent. They must employ some concepts that are often poorly understood, such as thought broadcasting. Further, clinicians must be aware of and assess a list of 9 prodromal symptoms in addition to the 12 symptoms in criterion A. Finally, the new definition of bizarre delusions, which occupies a crucial role in DSM-III-R since it provides a major component of the distinction between schizophrenia and delusional disorder, may be problematic (Flaum et al. 1991). A relatively more subjective definition has replaced a more objective one (implausible, as opposed to impossible); the major differences between the DSM-III-R examples (Schneiderian symptoms) and ICD-10 examples (religious or political identity, superhuman powers) illustrate how different concepts of implausibility may be. Several studies have noted problems with the criteria for schizophrenia that reflect this apparent lack of user-friendliness (Jampala et al. 1988; Lipkowitz and Idupuganti 1985).

Coverage of Negative Symptoms

Historically, negative symptoms have formed the conceptual core of schizophrenia. Both Kraepelin and Bleuler agreed that these were the defining features of this disorder. Kraepelin (1904) stated:

> The complete loss of mental activity and of interest in particular, and the failure of every impulse to energy, are such characteristic and fundamental indications that they give a very definite stamp to the condition in both cases. Together with the weakness of judgment, they are invariable and permanent fundamental features of dementia praecox, accompanying the whole evolution of the disease. Compared with these, all other disturbances, however prominent they may be in individual cases, must be regarded as merely transitory, and therefore not absolutely diagnostic, features. This holds good, for instance, of delusions and hallucinations, which are very frequently present, but may be developed in very different degrees or be altogether absent, or disappear, without the fundamental features of the disease or its course and issue being in any way affected. (pp. 26–27)

Bleuler (1911/1950) stated:

> Certain symptoms of schizophrenia are present in every case and at every period of the illness even though, as with every other disease symptom, they must have attained a certain degree of intensity before they can be recognized with any certainty. For example, the peculiar association disturbance is always present, but not each and every aspect of it. Sometimes the anomalies of association may manifest themselves in "blocking" or in the splitting of ideas; at other times in different schizophrenic symptoms. As far as we know, the fundamental symptoms are characteristic of schizophrenia, while the accessory symptoms may also appear in other types of illness. (p. 13)

With the de-emphasis on Bleulerian symptoms embodied in the Washington University criteria, RDC, and DSM-III, the study of negative symptoms was minimized during the 1970s to early 1980s. However, a resurgence of interest in negative symptoms has occurred, and a substantial empirical research literature has been amassed. The DSM-III-R criteria require the presence of positive symptoms but do not require any negative symptoms at all. Thus the historical concept of schizophrenia has been substantially changed. As described in more detail below, this was done primarily to pursue the goal of improved reliability.

Methods

This literature review was based on both a Medline search and a historical review. The Medline search involved entering the terms *schizophrenia/nosology, schizophrenia/phenomenology, schizophrenia/symptoms, schizophrenia/negative symptoms,* and *schizophrenia/positive symptoms,* obtaining a listing of all references that ran back to 1960. This yielded a total of 580 references. Unfortunately, since DSM-III is not a key word available through Medline, this could not be used to assist in either identifying or sifting references. These references were screened to identify those studies containing information that would be specifically useful to the issues and problems described below, reducing the list to about 250. In addition, it was also considered important to review major seminal contributions occurring before 1960, since the diagnosis of schizophrenia has been in existence for more than 100 years and since this disorder has been the subject of intensive empirical research during most of that time period. The size and breadth of this research literature precluded conducting a Medline search during that entire interval (as well as the time limitations of Medline itself), but seminal contributions were identified by selecting very frequently referenced articles or books from the references identified via the Medline search. Analyses of data sets, prepared for MacArthur analyses, were provided by N. C. Andreasen (unpublished data, 1988), M. F. Green and K. H. Nuechterlein (unpublished data, 1988), G. Haas (unpublished data, 1990), and J. Lieberman (unpublished data, 1989).

Results

Historical Data

The definition and criteria of schizophrenia in DSM-III-R cannot be understood without examining the historical background that led to the development of the definition in DSM-III, since only minor changes were made between DSM-III and DSM-III-R, whereas the differences between DSM-II (American Psychiatric Association 1968) and DSM-III were major.

The definition of schizophrenia in DSM-III represented a sharp break with decades of American and European nosological tradition. Prior to DSM-III, most American psychiatrists used a relatively broad definition of schizophrenia based largely on the Bleulerian four A's: associations, affect, autism, and ambivalence. At its broadest, the boundaries of the concept of schizophrenia included Kasanin's (1933) schizoaffective disorder, Hoch and Polatin's (1949) pseudoneurotic schizophrenia, and good prognosis schizophrenia (Stephens et al. 1966; Vaillant 1964), as well as nonpsychotic variants such as simple and latent schizophrenia (Bleuler 1911/1950). With a few swift strokes of the nosological scalpel, many of these forms of traditional schizophrenia were dissected away and included in other categories: psychosis not elsewhere classified (schizoaffective, schizophreniform, and paranoid disorders), affective disorders (mood incongruent manic and major depressive disorders), and even personality disorders (schizotypal personality disorder). The resulting concept of schizophrenia that emerged in DSM-III has been repeatedly shown to be among the narrowest in existence in the world (Endicott et al. 1982; Helzer et al. 1981; Klein 1982; Loranger 1990; McGlashan 1984: Moller et al. 1989; Stephens et al. 1982).

The decision to reduce the concept of schizophrenia to its "bare bones" was to a large extent based on the empirical evidence available at the time DSM-III was being developed. During the late 1960s and early 1970s, several important cross-national studies of schizophrenia were conducted: the International Pilot Study of Schizophrenia (IPSS) (World Health Organization 1973), and the United States-United Kingdom study (Cooper et al. 1972; Kendell et al. 1971). Both of these studies suggested that American psychiatrists used a much broader definition of schizophrenia than their colleagues in other parts of the world. Specifically, American psychiatrists often tended to see schizophrenia in patients their international colleagues viewed as manic-depressive.

A second important conceptual development during the 1970s, which exerted a major influence on the DSM-III concept of schizophrenia, was an increased emphasis on improving the reliability of diagnosis and the evaluation of symptoms. Several influential studies presented critiques of the reliability of diagnosis (Beck et al. 1962; Kreitman et al. 1961; Sandifer et al. 1964, 1968; Spitzer and Fleiss 1974). The critiques led in turn to an interest in identifying symptoms that were more "objective," such as delusions and hallucinations, and could therefore be defined more reliably; delusions and hallucinations are essentially all-or-none phenomena and are sharply delimited from normal experience. Bleulerian symptoms, on the other hand, were seen as relatively softer, since they tend to be on a continuum with normality. British psychiatrists, such as Frank Fish (1962) and John Wing (Wing 1970; Wing et al. 1974), stressed the importance of empirical approaches to phenomenology, in addition to emphasizing the importance of German approaches. The Schneiderian school, which proposed the pathognomonic nature of "first-rank symptoms," assumed great importance during the 1970s (Mellor 1970; Schneider 1959, 1974). These symptoms were given prominence in standard interviewing instruments such as the Present State Examination (Wing et al. 1974) or the Schedule for Affective Disorders and Schizophrenia (SADS) (Endicott and Spitzer 1978), which have formed the basis for most research on schizophrenia during the past two decades (Wing 1970). A final influential contribution during the 1970s was an emphasis on using course of illness, in addition to cross-sectional symptoms, as a way of improving the reliability and validity of the diagnosis of schizophrenia; the influential Washington University criteria required a duration of symptoms of at least 6 months before a diagnosis of schizophrenia could be given. A large number of studies were conducted that indicated these criteria to have strong predictive validity (Bland and Orn 1979; Guze et al. 1983; Helzer et al. 1981, 1983; Loyd and Tsuang 1985; Moller et al. 1989; Tsuang et al. 1979).

These influences all impinged on the DSM-III definition of schizophrenia. The new schizophrenia in DSM-III was defined as a disorder lasting at least 6 months, including both prodromal and residual periods, which was characterized primarily by delusions and hallucinations during the active period of illness. The description of characteristic symptoms placed great emphasis on Schneiderian first-rank symptoms.

Relatively minor modifications were made in the DSM-III criteria as DSM-III-R was being developed. The changes and their rationale have been reviewed by Kendler and colleagues (1989). Because the criteria were seen as too complex, an effort was made to simplify them based on both historical tradition and research findings. Negative symptoms were given more emphasis by increasing the relative weighting of flattened and inappropriate affect. In an effort to recognize that bizarreness may be culturally dependent, bizarre delusions were redefined. A definition seeking to reflect Jasperian concepts of "nonunderstandability" (i.e., involving a phenomenon that the person's culture would regard as totally implausible) replaced the previous more objective definition ("content is patently absurd and has no possible basis in fact" [American Psychiatric Association 1980, p. 188]), and a listing of four Schneiderian symptoms (delusions of being controlled, thought broadcasting, thought insertion, or thought withdrawal) was replaced by examples of one Schneiderian symptom (thought broadcasting) and one symptom similar to Schneiderian delusions of control (being controlled by a dead person). In DSM-III-R, the major distinction between schizophrenia and delusional disorder turns on this definition of bizarre delusions, since delusional disorder is defined in terms of the presence of nonbizarre delusions. A 1-week duration criterion was added for the group of symptoms appearing in criterion A. Criterion B, which specified deterioration in functioning in DSM-III, was rewritten to broaden it. Overall, the net effect of these changes appears to be a further narrowing of the definition of schizophrenia in DSM-III-R.

The publication of DSM-IV will coincide with the publication of ICD-10. Several factors make it desirable that the DSM-IV definitions approximate those of ICD-10 as closely as possible. Improving international communication is one important pressure. The research community that studies schizophrenia is truly international, and it is important that investigators be able to conduct cross-national attempts to validate one another's findings. The disparate findings concerning D_2 receptors measured with positron-emission tomography scanning highlights the problems that may arise when different constructs of schizophrenia are applied, since the Swedish sample represented a more acute, younger, floridly psychotic sample, whereas the Hopkins sample was older and more chronic (Andreasen et al. 1988). A second major pressure arises from the fact that American diagnoses must be coded using the ICD system for administrative and clinical purposes; consequently, it is important that the American definitions corresponding to the ICD-10 codes be as close to the ICD-10 definition as possible, so that maximal diagnostic precision and clarity will be achieved.

The ICD-10 system for defining schizophrenia and related disorders is quite different from the American system. All conditions within the schizophrenia-psychotic spectrum are grouped together under the major heading "Schizophrenia, Schizotypal, and Delusional Disorders" (the F20 group). The definition of schizophrenia requires a duration of only 1 month (in contrast to the 6-month duration criterion of DSM-III-R). Positive symptoms of psychosis, and particularly Schneiderian symptoms, are given even more prominence than in DSM-III-R. Negative symptoms are given somewhat more prominence as well, in that they are mentioned specifically and can be used to diagnose schizophrenia if present in conjunction with relatively mild thought disorder (e.g., irrelevant speech). Simple schizophrenia, a purely negative form of schizophrenia, is included as one of the subtypes in ICD-10. The definition of schizoaffective disorder is markedly different from DSM-III-R in that it takes a predominantly cross-sectional approach and requires the simultaneous presence and approximate balance of psychotic and mood symptoms; consequently, many patients classified as mood incongruent manic or major depressive disorder (and probably even some classified as mood congruent) will be classified as schizoaffective disorder in ICD-10.

Conceptual Principles

Most of the early attempts to develop diagnostic criteria depended on common sense and clinical experience in judging the number and type of characteristic symptoms that should be used to select criteria. Once criteria have been selected in this manner, their reliability and predictive validity can then be assessed. This strategy is quite appropriate when nosological systems are in a young developmental period and when very little empirical data are available concerning the frequency and severity of defining or characteristic symptoms. It was used for the development of the Washington University criteria, permitting many subsequent efforts to assess their reliability and validity, providing the foundation on which DSM-III and DSM-III-R were built.

All this previous work has important implications for the formulation of criteria for DSM-IV.

The development of a variety of structured interviews and rating scales, which have been applied to a large number of data sets, may make it possible, however, to employ even more empirical, data-based, biometric approaches to the development of criteria for schizophrenia for DSM-IV (Frances et al. 1989). The reliability of most characteristic symptoms of schizophrenia has been improved through the development of structured interviews such as the SADS, the Diagnostic Interview Schedule (Robins et al. 1981), the Structured Clinical Interview for DSM-III (Spitzer and Williams 1984), and the Comprehensive Assessment of Symptoms and History (CASH) (Andreasen 1985). The base rate of the symptoms of schizophrenia have been, or are being, evaluated in large groups of patients at various stages of the illness. Once a group of patients has been identified who are considered to have schizophrenia according to some acceptable definition (e.g., that used in the RDC, DSM-III, or DSM-III-R), biometric approaches such as discriminant function analysis can be applied to identify which symptoms are more powerful in achieving that classification efficiently (Pfohl and Andreasen 1978).

Several basic biometric principles guide the selection of symptoms that should be selected to be included in diagnostic criteria. One characteristic that is widely agreed on is that the symptoms must have adequate reliability; a kappa of 0.5 or 0.6 is usually considered to be acceptable, but a kappa of 0.7 or greater is preferable. Other things being equal, symptoms that have demonstrated high rates of reliability are more desirable, and ideally this high rate of reliability should be demonstrated in more acute and more chronic samples and in a relatively large number of diagnostic settings.

A second desirable characteristic is an adequate base rate. If a particular symptom or sign (e.g., thought withdrawal) is pathognomonic of schizophrenia but occurs very infrequently, then that symptom is very useful diagnostically when it occurs, but it should probably not be incorporated as a criterion symptom in a standard nomenclature. No specific minimal base rate has been agreed on at this point, but common sense suggests that a sign or symptom probably should not be included if its base rate is less than 10%–15%. Criteria should be limited to those symptoms that occur relatively frequently, and an ideal rate would probably be greater than 30% or 40%.

In addition to evaluating the performance characteristics of the specific items used in diagnostic criteria, the overall purposes of diagnostic criteria themselves should also be considered. Diagnostic criteria serve two basic purposes: 1) gatekeeping (as efficiently as possible) and 2) describing and educating.

To achieve the gatekeeping function, the criteria should emphasize the inclusion of a minimal number of symptoms that will help clinicians and researchers classify patients, including those who "belong" within the syndromal construct and excluding those who do not. The major purpose of the gatekeeping function is simply to classify. Ideally, to achieve this function, the list of symptoms used to define the disorder should be as parsimonious as possible; in fact, if a clustering of only two or three symptoms (or even one) were pathognomonic of the disorder, only a very short list would be necessary. The gatekeeping rationale was behind Bleuler's emphasis on thought disorder as a pathognomonic symptom, or Schneider's emphasis on first-rank symptoms. Cloninger and colleagues' (1985) work with the clinic 500 sample exemplifies the use of modern biometric approaches to identify criteria useful for gatekeeping; a stepwise discriminant function analysis or other such multivariate techniques can assist in identifying the shortest list of symptoms possible to achieve classification.

A second function of criteria is to provide a comprehensive description of the disorder and to educate clinicians, residents, and medical students about its characteristic symptoms. The DSM-III or DSM-III-R criteria have been widely used as teaching tools for residents and medical students. Thus trainees acquire their concepts of the characteristic symptoms of each of the disorders from the criteria themselves. This means that the criteria used to define schizophrenia should be selected to convey its full clinical flavor.

In general, the existing DSM-III-R criteria tend to provide a compromise between these two purposes, which are potentially at cross purposes with one another. The gatekeeping function is best served by a very short list of symptoms; the descriptive and educational function is best served by a long and comprehensive list. Ideally, as we revise the criteria to serve both of these functions, we should be striving toward simultaneously identifying the list of symptoms that will assist in efficient classification, but that will also provide a comprehensive description of the disorder that captures its full clinical flavor.

Selection of criteria for DSM-IV will inevitably be influenced by two major controversies that have previously been addressed in the development of DSM-III and DSM-III-R: polythetic versus monothetic and broad versus narrow.

Polythetic versus monothetic. Kraepelin's (1904, 1919/1971) concept of schizophrenia was polythetic, although he clearly considered negative or deficit symptoms to be more important clinically. Bleuler (1911/1950) introduced the concept of pathognomonic symptoms and derived an essentially monothetic construct in that he said that thought disorder was pathognomonic of schizophrenia. The search for a pathognomonic symptom was further extended by Kurt Schneider (1959), who selected a completely different type of symptom as pathognomonic; that is, Schneider selected particular forms of positive symptoms as his pathognomonic markers of the disorder. The Washington University criteria represented a polythetic construct. The RDC, deriving from the Schneiderian thinking that informed the Present State Examination and the work of Wing and colleagues (1974), emphasized Schneiderian first-rank symptoms (Spitzer et al. 1975). This emphasis was carried over to DSM-III, although with some modifications and corrections as evidence emerged that Schneiderian first-rank symptoms were not in fact pathognomonic. The DSM-III-R system can be regarded as either polythetic or monothetic, depending on what one considers to be a primal element. DSM-III-R is monothetic in that it requires that all patients with schizophrenia have some type of positive symptom of psychosis. It is polythetic in that the positive symptoms may be variable and may include delusions, or hallucinations, or positive formal thought disorder.

Broad versus narrow. As the above historical review indicates, the boundaries of schizophrenia have expanded and contracted over the years. Kraepelin's original definition of the disorder was relatively narrow, but this concept was broadened by Bleuler. The concept continued to be steadily broadened by psychoanalysts throughout the world (but particularly in the United States), peaking in the 1950s, at which point substantially more than 1% of patients seen by psychiatrists were diagnosed as having schizophrenia, at least in some sections of the United States (Cooper et al. 1972). This was impressively demonstrated by Kuriansky and colleagues (1974), who found that more than 80% of psychiatric admissions to a New York hospital during the early 1950s received a clinical diagnosis of schizophrenia, as opposed to less than 40% at the same hospital a decade earlier. Rediagnosis by research psychiatrists revealed no differences between the patient groups.

The Washington University criteria, RDC, and DSM-III represented an attempt to "correct" this excessive breadth of the definition. The narrowing was done in two ways: one involved the introduction of the 6-month duration criteria, and the other was to emphasize florid or positive symptoms of psychosis and to de-emphasize deficit, Bleulerian, or negative symptoms of psychosis. The DSM-III-R criteria include only positive symptoms, plus catatonia and abnormalities of affect; the criteria are essentially written so that some form of positive psychotic symptoms (delusions, hallucinations, or positive formal thought disorder) is required to make the diagnosis. The ICD-10 criteria are narrower in that they stress the importance of Schneiderian symptoms, but broader in that they also recognize negative symptoms, have a shorter duration criterion, include simple schizophrenia, and operationally are likely to include a larger number of patients within the overall category of schizophrenia.

The structure of DSM-III-R criteria. The DSM-III-R criteria represent an attempt to modify and correct the DSM-III criteria further. The overall structure consists of six criteria. Criterion A specifies the characteristic symptoms. Criterion B requires deterioration in functioning. Criterion C defines the boundary between schizophrenia, schizoaffective disorder, and mood disorder. Criterion D specifies the duration of the disturbance and also includes a list of prodromal and residual symptoms that may be present before or after the characteristic symptoms listed in criterion A and can be used to demonstrate that psychopathology has been present during the entire 6-month period that symptoms are required. Criterion E rules out organic factors that may have initiated or maintained the disturbance. Criterion F defines the boundary between schizophrenia and autism. In this review, I focus primarily on criterion A, with some discussion of criterion B and criterion D.

Criterion A of DSM-III consisted of a relatively complex list that placed considerable emphasis on positive symptoms of psychosis and especially Schneiderian symptoms. The DSM-III-R criteria require any one of three defining features to be present.

Criterion A1 is polythetic. Essentially, it requires any two of five different symptoms. This list includes delusions, prominent hallucinations (defined on the basis of duration rather than severity), several forms of formal thought disorder (incoherence or marked loosening of associations), catatonic behavior, and abnormalities in affect (either flat or grossly inappropriate). Criterion A2 indicates that the diagnosis can be made on the basis of delusions alone if they are present in an "extreme" form. In DSM-III, the definitional emphasis was on Schneiderian symptoms. In DSM-III-R, the emphasis was changed to "bizarre delusions," which are defined as "involving a phenomenon that the person's culture would regard as totally implausible" (p. 194) and exemplified by a Schneiderian symptom (thought broadcasting) and a modification of the Schneiderian concept of delusions of control ("being controlled by a dead person").

Criterion A3 permits the diagnosis of schizophrenia to be made only in the presence of hallucinations, if these are sufficiently severe; the "rate limiting" item in this instance is auditory hallucinations that are relatively persistent and nonaffective in content or that involve one of two Schneiderian symptoms (voices commenting or voices conversing).

Criterion B requires that some type of deterioration in functioning has occurred. This was stated relatively explicitly in DSM-III (deterioration from a previous level of functioning in such areas as work, social relations, and self-care). DSM-III-R elaborates this further:

> During the course of the disturbance, functioning in such areas as work, social relations, and self-care is markedly below the highest level achieved before the onset of the disturbance (or, when the onset is in childhood or adolescence, failure to achieve expected level of social development). (p. 194)

This modification was meant to assist in identifying deterioration in those cases where the actual age at onset is difficult to identify due to the presence of poor premorbid functioning. Since the concept of "deterioration in functioning" is no longer stated in the criterion, however, it may be subject to misinterpretation. Because the criterion now begins with "during the course of the disturbance," students and residents often interpret it to mean that chronic impairment in functioning is required and that schizophrenia cannot be diagnosed in individuals who are able to work, have relatively normal social relationships, or care for themselves.

The prodromal or residual symptoms, listed in criterion D, include a list of nine signs and symptoms. These have been reordered between DSM-III and DSM-III-R, and one additional symptom has been added (marked lack of initiative, interests, or energy) to provide more recognition of the importance of negative symptoms. Some of these are redundant with criterion A (blunted or inappropriate affect) or criterion B (marked impairment in role functioning as wage earner, student, or homemaker). The list mixes mild positive and mild negative symptoms somewhat randomly, and sometimes it mixes both positive and negative signs within a single item (digressive, vague, overelaborate, or circumstantial speech, or poverty of speech, or poverty of content of speech). Two of these symptoms are required during the prodromal or residual phase, and the prodromal phase is defined somewhat differently from criterion B ("a clear deterioration in functioning before the active phase of the disturbance" [American Psychiatric Association 1987, p. 194]). The list is similar, but not identical, to the nine symptoms used to define schizotypal personality. Some items are nearly identical (e.g., odd beliefs, unusual perceptual experiences, odd or eccentric behavior); some items appear in one list but not the other (impairment in role functioning among prodromal symptoms, suspiciousness or paranoid ideation among schizotypal symptoms).

Empirical Data

Narrowness of definition and consonance with ICD. A number of studies have established that DSM-III criteria provide a relatively narrow definition of schizophrenia, as compared with several other systems that enjoy wide usage. Six such studies are summarized in Table 22–1 (Coryell and Zimmerman 1987; Endicott et al. 1982; Helzer et al. 1981; Klein 1982; McGlashan 1984; Stephens et al. 1982). The results of these studies indicate that the Washington University and DSM-III criteria appear to yield the narrowest definitions, whereas the others such as RDC, the IPSS 12-Point Flexible System (Carpenter et al. 1973b), and the New Haven Schizophrenia Index (Astrachan et al. 1972) have somewhat broader definitions. Thus it seems clear that DSM-III substantially reduced the boundaries of schizophrenia. The study by Klein appears to indicate that basing the diagnosis on the presence of first-rank symptoms actually broadens the definition beyond DSM-III.

Table 22–1. Breadth of definitions of schizophrenia, in percentages

Diagnostic system	Helzer et al. 1981 ($N = 125$)[a]	Stephens et al. 1982 ($N = 283$)[b]	Endicott et al. 1982 ($N = 168$)[c]	Klein 1982 ($N = 46$)[d]	McGlashan 1984 ($N = 400$)[c]	Coryell and Zimmerman 1987 ($N = 97$)[a]
DSM-III	15	37	11	28	29	37
Research Diagnostic Criteria (probable and definite)	22	46	18	33	30	22
Feighner	14	38	7	24	24	20
New Haven	—	88	26	—	46	—
Flexible (≥5 points)	—	53	13	63	—	—
Taylor-Abrams	—	66	4	26	—	—
Presence of first-rank symptoms	—	37	—	56	—	—
DSM-I[e]	—	83	—	—	—	—
CATEGO (all schizophrenia groups)	42	—	—	—	—	—

[a]All patients had psychotic symptoms but the sample was not limited to schizophrenia. [b]All patients had a hospital diagnosis of either schizophrenic, schizoaffective, or paranoid state. [c]The patient sample was diagnostically heterogeneous. [d]All patients had a DSM-II hospital diagnosis of schizophrenia. [e]American Psychiatric Association 1952.

A comparative study by Fenton and colleagues (1988) indicated that DSM-III-R has further narrowed the definition of schizophrenia, principally by requiring that delusions, if the only positive psychotic feature present, be bizarre. Inevitably, no studies exist that compare DSM-III-R criteria against ICD-10, making this a primary issue for the upcoming field trials.

Does the increased narrowness of DSM-III produce gains in predictive validity? This literature review identified four studies that addressed this question, all of which involved the patient samples listed in Table 22–1. Helzer and colleagues (1981) found that the DSM-III and Washington University criteria for schizophrenia were more strongly predictive of chronicity and social decline than RDC and CATEGO. Although the authors initially speculated that this was probably attributable to the 6-month duration criterion alone, a later study revealed that nontemporal symptom factors also appeared to play an important role (Helzer et al. 1983). Endicott and colleagues (1986) found that although there was up to an eightfold difference in diagnostic rates among the criteria systems compared, they all performed similarly but poorly in predicting indices of short-term outcome. McGlashan (1984) also found the predictive validity to be roughly equivalent between the four systems evaluated in that sample (DSM-III, RDC, Washington University, and New Haven), but found that each demonstrated reasonably good diagnostic stability and prediction of long-term outcome. Coryell and Zimmerman (1987) evaluated diagnostic validity in terms of short-term outcome and familial aggregation and concluded that of the three criteria for schizophrenia that were tested (DSM-III, RDC, and Washington University), each appeared to be validated by these measures, and there were no significant differences between them. Thus, although the empirical evidence is far from conclusive, there appears to be some support for the predictive validity of the more stringent criteria such as DSM-III, but the evidence also suggests that the broader RDC definition may also have equal predictive validity.

First-rank symptoms. Another important issue raised by ICD is the importance of first-rank symptoms. As shown in Table 22–2, Koehler and colleagues (1977) compared the frequency with which these symptoms were rated in four different studies: one done in Germany by the authors, one done in England by Mellor (1970), one done of an American sample by Carpenter and colleagues (1973a), and one of an international sample by Carpenter and Strauss (1974). The base rate of any single Schneiderian symptom is relatively low and tends to vary somewhat unnervingly from one center to another. The figures presented in Table 22–2 are based only on Schneider-positive schizophrenic patients, whereas Table 22–3 shows the overall prevalence of at least one first-rank symptom in all patients with a diagnosis of schizophrenia. Again, the number varies significantly, ranging from a low of 28% to a high of 72%.

A related problem is the specificity of first-rank symptoms. When first-rank symptoms were originally introduced to English-speaking psychiatrists, they were touted as being highly specific. If they were present, a diagnosis of schizophrenia was virtually certain. This view was widely accepted during the late 1960s and early

Table 22–2. Frequency distribution of 10 first-rank symptoms in Schneider-positive schizophrenic patients

First-rank symptom	Germany (Koehler et al. 1977) (*N* = 69)	England (Mellor 1970) (*N* = 173)	United States (Carpenter et al. 1973a) (*N* = 53)	International (Carpenter and Strauss 1974) (*N* = 354)
Audible thoughts	1.5	11.6	20	28
Voices arguing	7.2	13.3	—	22
Voices commenting	24.6	13.3	—	10
Thought broadcasting	27.5	21.4	33	26
Thought insertion	17.4	19.7	20	23
Thought withdrawal	24.6	9.8	15	25
"Made" affect, feelings, or impulses	1.5	9.3	11	16
"Made" volition	20.3	9.2	28	29
Somatic passivity	37.7	11.6	17	—
Delusional perception	55.1	6.4	—	—

Source. Adapted from Koehler et al. 1977.

Table 22–3. Prevalence of first-rank symptoms in schizophrenia

Study	Number with schizophrenia	Percentage with first-rank symptoms
Case record		
Huber 1967	195	72
Taylor 1972	78	28
Abrams and Taylor 1973	71	34
Prospective		
Mellor 1970	166	72
Carpenter et al. 1973a	103	51
Carpenter and Strauss 1974	811	57

Source. Adapted from Koehler et al. 1977.

1970s, but in the mid-1970s, a series of studies began to question the specificity of first-rank symptoms. Table 22–4 summarizes three such studies, two of them done by Taylor and Abrams (1973, 1975) and a third by Carpenter and Strauss (1974). These studies suggest that first-rank symptoms occur in a substantial number of patients suffering from affective illness, indicating that they are in fact nonspecific and not pathognomonic of schizophrenia.

In summary, although including first-rank symptoms may be appropriate based on their historical importance, limitations regarding their reliability, base rates, and specificity suggest that they should not be given undue prominence or treated as the major criterion symptoms that are pathognomonic of the disorder.

Empirical data concerning reliability and base rates. Since the original development of DSM-III, a substantial empirical data base has been amassed concerning the reliability of the symptoms used in criterion A, as well as the reliability of a variety of other symptoms that might be included in DSM-IV.

The reliability of the specific symptoms used in DSM-III or DSM-III-R is one important empirical issue. If the symptoms are not sufficiently reliable, they probably should not be included. Table 22–5 presents reliability data from three different studies using two different instruments and two different sets of diagnostic criteria. The earlier Andreasen and colleagues (1982) study involved a variety of patients, as well as interviewers from a variety of backgrounds, who rated patients evaluated on videotape. The Endicott and colleagues (1982) study also examined a diagnostically heterogeneous sample of larger size and applied DSM-III criteria. Although the data for other criteria are not presented in this particular table, in general higher reliability was achieved when interviewers used the SADS to make diagnoses with RDC than when they applied DSM-III criteria. The reliability data collected for symptoms using the CASH tended to show the highest reliability for the various symptoms.

Negative symptoms tended to be minimized in diagnostic criteria in the era that followed the articulation of the Washington University criteria. The primary

Table 22–4. Specificity of first-rank symptoms

Study	Sample	Percentage with first-rank symptoms
Taylor and Abrams 1975	Manic: 53	8
Taylor and Abrams 1973	Manic: 52	12
Carpenter and Strauss 1974	Manic: 66	23
	Depressive: 119	16

reason was that investigators suspected that these symptoms would have poor reliability. With the development of more objective definitions of negative symptoms, such as are embodied in scales such as the Scale for the Assessment of Negative Symptoms (Andreasen 1983), it became evident that adequate reliability could be achieved for negative symptoms. Reliability coefficients of negative symptoms in five different cultural settings are summarized in Table 22–6 (N. C. Andreasen, unpublished data, 1986; Humbert et al. 1986; Moscarelli et al. 1987; Ohta et al. 1984; Phillips 1987). As this table indicates, objective definitions lead to good-to-excellent reliability of most negative symptoms. Global ratings are consistently above 0.6 in all studies. Data concerning positive symptoms, as assessed by the Scale for the Assessment of Positive Symptoms (Andreasen 1984), are also summarized. In general, the reliability coefficients for positive symptoms shown in Table 22–6 are higher than those reported in earlier studies. The reason for this is unclear, but it may reflect the possibility that reliability is improved by more detailed definitions and the use of extensive descriptions and examples.

As the concept of bizarre delusions assumed a pivotal role in DSM-III-R, the reliability with which the bizarre versus nonbizarre distinction could be made became important. Kendler and colleagues (1983) reported that of the five dimen-

Table 22–5. Reliability of DSM-III or DSM-III-R symptoms of schizophrenia

Symptoms	Andreasen et al. 1982 (SADS-RDC)[a]	Endicott et al. 1982 (SADS-DSM-III)[b]	Andreasen et al. in press (CASH)[a]
Delusions	.86	.59	.76
Hallucinations	.92	—	.93
Incoherence	.70	.57	.79
Loosening of associations	.57	.47	.70
Catatonic behavior	—	—	—
Flat affect	.70	.13	.80
Inappropriate affect	.62	—	.61
Nonaffective verbal hallucinations	.61	.47	—
Voices commenting	.84	—	.98
Voices conversing	—	—	.82
Thought broadcasting	.34	.48	.97
Bizarre delusions	.75[c]	.29[c]	.44
Mood incongruent delusions	.47	—	—

Note. SADS = Schedule for Affective Disorders and Schizophrenia. RDC = Research Diagnostic Criteria. CASH = Comprehensive Assessment of Symptoms and History.
[a]Intraclass *r*. [b]K coefficient. [c]Definition differs from DSM-III-R.

sions of delusional experience he examined (conviction, extension, bizarreness, disorganization, and pressure), bizarreness had the lowest reliability (weighted kappa = .30). Flaum and colleagues (1991) conducted a study to address this question specifically and found a similarly low reliability estimate (kappa of 0.31) using the DSM-III-R wording. This suggests that the concept either be reduced in importance in DSM-IV or that the definition and examples of what is meant by bizarre be more clearly stipulated.

There is very little empirical evidence regarding the reliability of assessing prodromal and residual symptoms. During the process of revising DSM-III, it was suggested that prodromal and residual symptoms be dropped from the criteria, largely because of concerns that the severity and duration of these symptoms could not be reliably assessed (Kendler et al. 1989). At the time, only one study had addressed this issue (Endicott et al. 1982), and it was therefore decided to hold off on such a change and reconsider the suggestion during the DSM-IV process. Unfortunately, this review did not identify any subsequently published reports that provide reliability data for prodromal and residual symptoms. In the Endicott study, the interrater reliability was found to be poor for three of the prodromal symptoms (kappa < 0.15 for vague speech, unusual perceptions and flat affect), moderate for three others (kappa = 0.5–0.6 for social isolation, impaired role

Table 22–6. Interrater reliability of negative and positive symptoms in different cultural settings, intraclass *r*

Symptoms	Iowa (Andreasen 1986)[a]	Italy (Moscarelli et al. 1987)	Spain (Humbert et al. 1986)	Japan (Ohta et al. 1984)	China (Phillips 1987)
Negative symptoms (global ratings)					
Alogia	.65	.69	.95	.63	.99
Affective flattening	.85	.69	.84	.72	.90
Avolition-apathy	.94	.75	.86	.75	.82
Anhedonia-asociality	.90	.73	.77	.73	.86
Inattentiveness	.88	.66	.89	.79	.83
Positive symptoms (global ratings)					
Hallucinations	.96	.86	.93	—	.84
Delusions	.96	.88	.90	—	.42
Bizarre behavior	.90	.83	.88	—	.99
Positive formal thought disorder	.93	.82	.99	—	.94

[a]Unpublished data.

functioning, and odd thinking), and good for two symptoms (kappa = 0.73 for peculiar behavior and impairment in hygiene). A study of the reliability of prodromal and residual symptoms was conducted in the context of a large reliability study of the CASH (Andreasen et al., in press). The results are shown in Table 22–7 and demonstrate that when the ratings are made jointly (interrater design), the agreement between two raters is reasonably good for both prodromal and residual symptoms. However, a more stringent test of reliability, and one that more closely approximates clinical reality, is one in which two raters evaluate the symptoms on the basis of independent interviews (test-retest design). This design yielded a consistently low level of agreement for all prodromal symptoms. Further, the ability to assess the onset and duration of these symptoms (which is critical, given their role in the criteria) may also prove to be problematic. No data that address this specifically could be identified, and therefore this issue will be explored in the upcoming field trials.

Criterion B was substantially rewritten between DSM-III and DSM-III-R. This rewriting may have introduced a major change that may substantially narrow the definition of schizophrenia in DSM-III-R. No reliability data are available concerning the "deterioration criteria" in either DSM-III or DSM-III-R. It would clearly be worthwhile to collect some data concerning the reliability of this judgment. This will also be done in the field trials.

The base rate of symptoms is another important empirical issue. Table 22–8 summarizes the base rates for the signs and symptoms used to diagnose schizophrenia in DSM-III-R (the criterion A symptoms), as assessed in two Iowa samples. In general, the base rates of most DSM symptoms are acceptably high. The base rates

Table 22–7. Interrater and test-retest reliability of DSM-III prodromal and residual symptoms

	Interrater intraclass r		Test-retest intraclass r	
Symptoms	Prodromal	Residual	Prodromal	Residual
Social isolation	0.63	1.00	0.00	0.63
Impairment in work or school	0.73	0.17	0.36	0.81
Peculiar behavior	0.62	0.00	0.34	0.00
Impairment in personal hygiene	0.79	1.00	0.25	1.00
Blunted or inappropriate affect	0.71	0.57	0.52	0.75
Odd speech (e.g., digressive, vague)	0.91	0.84	0.21	0.41
Odd beliefs, magical thinking, etc.	1.00	1.00	0.33	1.00
Unusual perceptual experiences	0.79	0.65	0.00	0.47
Mean	*0.77*	*0.65*	*0.25*	*0.63*

of three symptoms—incoherence, marked loosening of associations, and thought broadcasting—may, however, be marginal.

Empirical data concerning the relevance of negative symptoms. As the above historical and conceptual review has indicated, negative symptoms have traditionally been considered a prominent component of schizophrenia, and possibly as the core or fundamental symptoms of the disorder. DSM introduced a radical change by requiring the presence of positive symptoms to make the diagnosis of schizophrenia. One important aspect of DSM-IV is an evaluation as to whether there is a sufficient data base to support giving negative symptoms more prominence. If they are given more prominence, then an important related issue is the way in which this prominence should be achieved. Several alternatives are possible. One is to add more negative symptoms to the list required to make the diagnosis. A second is to use the positive and negative dimensions as a method for subtyping schizophrenia. A third is to reintroduce the concept of a purely negative form of schizophrenia, usually referred to as simple schizophrenia, characterized by the presence of severe negative symptoms in the absence of delusions and hallucinations.

In this chapter, we cover only the first issue. The subjects of subtyping and simple schizophrenia are presented in other literature reviews for DSM-IV.

Table 22–8. DSM-III-R symptoms: base rates in two Iowa samples

Symptoms	1985 (*N* = 111)	1988 (*N* = 55)
Delusions	85	89
Prominent hallucinations	50	35
Incoherence	7	0
Marked loosening of associations	17	19
Catatonic behavior	—	15
Affective flattening	88	86
Inappropriate affect	50	37
Bizarre delusions	—	—
Thought broadcasting	14	22
Auditory hallucinations	70	56
Voices commenting	33	30
Voices conversing	31	23

Note. Base rates are based on a rating of ≥2 ("mild but definitely present") coded for this item on the Scale for the Assessment of Negative Symptoms (SANS) or the Scale for the Assessment of Positive Symptoms (SAPS). Symptoms specified in the criteria as "prominent" or "marked" are equated with SANS/SAPS ratings of 4 (marked) or 5 (severe).

During the past decade, interest in negative symptoms has increased substantially. Although Hughlings-Jackson (1931), Strauss and colleagues (1974), Wing and colleagues (1974), and others had also stressed their importance, the publication of Crow's article in the *British Medical Journal* in 1980, proposing a two-syndrome hypothesis of schizophrenia based on positive and negative dimensions, was a seminal piece of research. There is now a very large research literature examining the reliability, internal consistency, and predictive validity of negative symptoms. Much of this research is summarized in two overview book chapters: Barnes and Liddle (1990) have evaluated the evidence for the validity of negative symptoms; Marks and Luchins (1990) have examined the relationship between brain imaging findings and positive and negative symptoms.

Briefly, both these reviews support the importance of the construct of negative symptoms. Negative symptoms have been very consistently found to be reliable, if they are adequately defined (Andreasen 1982; Kay et al. 1987; Krawiecka et al. 1977; Lewine et al. 1983; Overall and Gorham 1962). They have also been found to be internally consistent and highly correlated with one another, suggesting that they in some sense represent a valid construct (Andreasen and Olsen 1982; Bilder et al. 1985; Liddle 1987). They have also been shown to be associated with a number of independent validators in a variety of studies, including cognitive impairment (Andreasen et al. 1990; Bilder et al. 1985; Cornblatt et al. 1985; Johnstone et al. 1978; Liddle 1987), a differential treatment response (Angrist et al. 1980; Brier et al. 1987; Singh et al. 1987; Van Kammen and Boronow 1988), and poor outcome (Carpenter et al. 1978; Johnstone et al. 1979; Pogue-Geile and Harrow 1984, 1985). Negative symptoms also tend to be quite stable over time (Biehl et al. 1989; Johnstone et al. 1986; Pfohl and Winokur 1983; Pogue-Geile and Harrow 1985). They are also correlated with motor abnormalities (Barnes 1988; Jeste et al. 1984; Owens and Johnstone 1980; Waddington et al. 1987).

Among external validators, the relationship between negative symptoms and evidence of structural brain abnormality has been most widely studied. As reviewed by Marks and Luchins (1990), a total of 18 studies have shown a direct relationship between neuroanatomical abnormalities and positive or negative symptoms; two more showed an indirect relationship. On the other hand, five studies showed no relationships, and three showed a relationship in the direction opposite to the one usually hypothesized (i.e., an association of ventricular enlargement with positive symptoms rather than negative symptoms).

Thus a substantial body of literature appears to support the importance of negative symptoms in schizophrenia. In fact, at present the literature supporting their stability and validity is stronger than the literature that can be marshaled in support of the stability and validity of first-rank symptoms or even positive symptoms generally. This evidence seems to suggest that it would be appropriate to consider giving negative symptoms a more prominent position within DSM-IV.

Discussion and Recommendations

Several conclusions appear to emerge from this overview that suggest future directions and potential options.

First, the DSM and ICD definitions of schizophrenia are currently very different. This difference lies primarily in two areas. ICD places more emphasis on first-rank symptoms than does DSM, and it requires a shorter duration. Simply put, the ICD definition describes a disorder characterized by relatively short periods of severe psychosis, whereas the DSM definition places less emphasis on persistent psychotic symptoms but greater emphasis on chronicity. No analyzed data are currently available that will permit us to determine whether American psychiatrists diagnose and treat patients who have prominent positive symptoms that persist for at least a month. It is noteworthy, however, that the feasibility of establishing a 1-month period of psychotic symptoms is only relevant in first-admission patients. Patients with established chronicity are likely to be diagnosed the same by both systems.

This situation presents several options. One option is to adopt an approach similar to ICD and to require only 1 month of symptoms, reducing the emphasis on prodromal and residual symptoms. This approach would have the benefit of reducing dependence on prodromal and residual symptoms, which at this stage do not have any adequacy of reliability documented or their base rate assessed. A second option is to require 1 month of "positive symptoms," as does ICD, but to remain reasonably consonant with DSM-III-R by requiring a 6-month duration for both positive and negative symptoms; this option has the advantages of striking a compromise between the two systems and reducing the emphasis on potentially unreliable prodromal and residual symptoms: its major disadvantage is that it is new and untested. The above literature review suggests that it would be difficult to adopt the ICD definition in toto, however, because of the heavy emphasis on Schneiderian first-rank symptoms; the review suggests that these symptoms do not have adequate specificity to make them the primary defining features of schizophrenia, nor do they have an adequate base rate (or perhaps adequate reliability).

Second, more use can be made of modern biometric approaches to developing diagnostic criteria. Such approaches are based on identifying symptoms with established reliability and a high enough base rate to provide adequate coverage of the symptoms observed in schizophrenia. There are now a reasonably large number of data sets consisting of both chronic and first-episode patients. An additional large data set is being amassed in the field trials. These data sets can be used to develop a more data-based and empirical approach to developing diagnostic criteria. This approach will require data sets comprised of both schizophrenic patients and patients with other major illnesses (e.g., manic disorder, severe depression). Discriminant analyses can be used to identify the symptoms most useful in classifying patients. The discriminant analyses can be compared across independently collected samples. As these analyses are done, consideration should be given to the possibility that different criteria may be necessary for first-episode patients and for more chronic patients. This represents a "bootstrapping" approach to the development of criteria. That is, alternative sets of criteria can be written that appear to have desirable characteristics, such as simplicity and adequate coverage. If these criteria are equally good in classifying patients previously diagnosed as having schizophrenia by DSM-III or DSM-III-R, and excluding patients with other diagnoses, then their improved simplicity and coverage suggest that they would be better alternatives. This type of biometric approach will be applied to field trial data and to analysis of data sets made available through MacArthur Foundation Funding.

Third, negative symptoms have long been recognized to be very important symptoms of schizophrenia, and possibly the most fundamental symptoms. Although they have been minimized in DSM-III and DSM-III-R, their historical importance and the resurgence of research studies suggesting their internal consistency and validity suggest that they should be given more prominence in DSM-IV. Several types of criteria can be written that would increase the emphasis on negative symptoms. One approach might be to have two listings of symptoms, both of which would be required; one list would consist of positive symptoms (e.g., delusions, hallucinations, positive formal thought disorder), and the other would consist of negative symptoms (e.g., affective blunting, alogia, avolition, anhedonia). Another alternative would be to couch criterion B, the "deterioration in functioning criterion," in terms of negative symptoms. Yet a third alternative would be to refurbish the list of prodromal symptoms so that they are subdivided into positive and negative, and thereby to stress the concept that mild negative symptoms may occur as either a prodrome or a residual state in patients who have transient episodes of more severe positive symptoms. The first approach is probably the best, based on empirical data concerning the poor reliability of prodromal-residual symptoms.

Fourth, DSM-III and DSM-III-R have substantially narrowed the definition of schizophrenia. DSM-III-R appears to be even narrower than DSM-III. Since the ICD definition may lead to a broader classification net, and since consonance with ICD is an important goal, the possibility of broadening the criteria must at least be considered. The importance of negative symptoms and the possibility that there is in fact a relatively pure negative form of schizophrenia (e.g., simple schizophrenia) also suggest that broadening the concept could be desirable.

Several options are possible. One option is to maintain the existing definition and continue to have a narrow definition of schizophrenia. If this decision is selected, then any modifications in the criteria will strive toward maintaining the inclusion of the same patients as were classified within schizophrenia by DSM-III or DSM-III-R. This approach has the advantage of being the most conservative, in the sense that it would not produce any sharp breaks with existing practice, but has the disadvantage of making the American system different from ICD and possibly in employing a concept contrary to the overall historical concept of the disorder.

A second alternative would be to broaden the definition. If this approach were chosen, the most logical direction to take would be to adopt a definition similar to ICD. This approach would rely primarily on reducing the duration criteria. A third approach would involve broadening the coverage of symptoms so that negative systems are given more prominence and so that the diagnosis of schizophrenia can be made in patients who have a "pure negative" syndrome. Either of these later two alternatives has the disadvantage of producing a break with existing practices and would be much less conservative than the first option discussed above.

The field trials will play an important role in making the final assessment of these various options. They will assist in the collection of reliability data on some important issues, such as prodromal and residual symptoms and bizarre delusions. They will also provide information concerning the effects of changing the duration criterion (1 month versus 6 months) on "caseness." In addition, they will provide important information concerning the feasibility of using a 1-month duration criterion for positive symptoms in an American clinical setting. At present, six American sites are involved in the field trials, as well as two international sites. Emphasis has been placed on obtaining regional and ethnic diversity. Thus the field trials will yield useful information concerning the application of criteria and the frequency of symptoms in cross-cultural settings. After the data are collected, information concerning reliability and base rates will be summarized. In addition, biometric approaches to generating classification algorithms will be explored.

Although important, field trial data will not be treated as definitive. All judgments concerning various options will be made based on three lines of evidence: literature reviews, MacArthur analyses, and field trials. Final decisions will attempt to strike a reasonable balance between maintaining tradition and continuity and developing improvements that improve reliability, educational description, and user friendliness.

References

Abrams R, Taylor M: First-rank symptoms, severity of illness, and treatment response in schizophrenia. Compr Psychiatry 14:353–355, 1973

American Psychiatric Association: Diagnostic and Statistical Manual: Mental Disorders. Washington, DC, American Psychiatric Association, 1952

American Psychiatric Association: Diagnostic and Statistical Manual of Mental Disorders, 2nd Edition. Washington, DC, American Psychiatric Association, 1968

American Psychiatric Association: Diagnostic and Statistical Manual of Mental Disorders, 3rd Edition. Washington, DC, American Psychiatric Association, 1980

American Psychiatric Association: Diagnostic and Statistical Manual of Mental Disorders, 3rd Edition, Revised. Washington, DC, American Psychiatric Association, 1987

Andreasen NC: Negative symptoms in schizophrenia: definition and reliability. Arch Gen Psychiatry 39:784–788, 1982

Andreasen NC: The Scale for the Assessment of Negative Symptoms (SANS). Iowa City, IA, The University of Iowa, 1983

Andreasen NC: The Scale for the Assessment of Positive Symptoms (SAPS). Iowa City, IA, The University of Iowa, 1984

Andreasen NC: The Comprehensive Assessment of Symptoms and History (CASH). Iowa City, IA, The University of Iowa, 1985

Andreasen NC, Olsen S: Negative vs positive schizophrenia: definition and validation. Arch Gen Psychiatry 39:789–793, 1982

Andreasen NC, Mcdonald-Scott P, Grove WM, et al: Assessment of reliability in multicenter collaborative research with a videotape approach. Am J Psychiatry 139:876–882, 1982

Andreasen NC, Carson R, Diksic M, et al: Workshop on schizophrenia, PET, and D_2 receptors in the human neostriatum. Schizophr Bull 14:471–484, 1988

Andreasen NC, Flaum M, Swayze VW, et al: Positive and negative symptoms in schizophrenia: a critical reappraisal. Arch Gen Psychiatry 47:615–621, 1990

Andreasen NC, Flaum M, Arndt S: The Comprehensive Assessment of Symptoms and History (CASH): an instrument for assessing psychopathology and diagnosis. Arch Gen Psychiatry (in press)

Angrist B, Rotrosen J, Gershon S: Differential effects of amphetamine and neuroleptics on negative vs positive symptoms in schizophrenia. Psychopharmacology 72:17–19, 1980

Astrachan BM, Harrow M, Adler D, et al: The checklist for the diagnosis of schizophrenia. Br J Psychiatry 121:529–539, 1972

Barnes TR: Tardive dyskinesia: risk factors, pathophysiology, and treatment, in Recent Advances in Clinical Psychiatry, No 6. Edited by Granville-Grossman K. Edinburgh, Churchill Livingstone, 1988

Barnes TR, Liddle P: Evidence for the validity of negative symptoms, in Modern Problems of Pharmacopsychiatry, Vol 24: Positive and Negative Symptoms and Syndromes. Edited by Andreasen NC. Basel, Switzerland, Karger, 1990, pp 43–72

Beck AT, Ward CH, Mendelson M: Reliability of psychiatric diagnosis, II: a study of consistency of clinical judgements and ratings. Am J Psychiatry 119:351–357, 1962

Biehl H, Maurer K, Juang E, et al: The WHO psychological impairments rating schedule (WHO/PIRS), II: impairments in schizophrenics in cross-sectional and longitudinal perspective: the Mannheim experience in two independent samples. Br J Psychiatry 155 (suppl 7):71–77, 1989

Bilder RM, Mukherjee S, Rieder RO, et al: Symptomatic and neuropsychological components of defect states. Schizophr Bull 11:409–419, 1985

Bland RC, Orn H: Schizophrenia: diagnostic criteria and outcome. Br J Psychiatry 134:34–38, 1979

Bleuler E: Dementia Praecox or the Group of Schizophrenias (1911). Translated by Zinkin J. New York, International Universities Press, 1950

Brier A, Wolkowitz OM, Doran AR, et al: Neuroleptic responsivity of negative and positive symptoms in schizophrenia. Am J Psychiatry 144:1549–1555, 1987

Carpenter WT, Strauss JS: Cross-cultural evaluation of Schneider's first-rank symptoms of schizophrenia: a report from the International Pilot Study of Schizophrenia. Am J Psychiatry 131:682–687, 1974

Carpenter WT, Strauss JS, Muleh S: Are there pathognomonic symptoms in schizophrenia? an empiric investigation of Schneider's first-rank symptoms. Arch Gen Psychiatry 28:847–852, 1973a

Carpenter WT, Strauss JS, Bartko JJ: Flexible system for the diagnosis of schizophrenia: report from the World Health Organization International Pilot Study of Schizophrenia. Science 182:1275–1278, 1973b

Carpenter WT, Bartko JJ, Strauss JS, et al: Signs and symptoms as predictors of outcome: a report from the International Pilot Study of Schizophrenia. Am J Psychiatry 135:940–944, 1978

Cloninger R, Martin RL, Guze SB, et al: Diagnosis and prognosis in schizophrenia. Arch Gen Psychiatry 42:15–25, 1985

Cooper JE, Kendell RE, Gurland BJ, et al: Psychiatric diagnosis in New York and London (Institute of Psychiatry, Maudsley Monograph Series No 20). London, Oxford University Press, 1972

Cornblatt BA, Lenzenweger MF, Dworkin RH, et al: Positive and negative schizophrenic symptoms: attention and information processing. Schizophr Bull 11:397–407, 1985

Coryell W, Zimmerman M: Progress in the classification of functional psychoses. Am J Psychiatry 144:1471–1473, 1987

Crow TJ: Molecular pathology of schizophrenia: more than one disease process? BMJ 280:66–68, 1980

Endicott J, Spitzer RL: A diagnostic interview: the Schedule for Affective Disorders and Schizophrenia. Arch Gen Psychiatry 35:837–844, 1978

Endicott J, Nee J, Fleiss J, et al: Diagnostic criteria for schizophrenia: reliabilities and agreement between systems. Arch Gen Psychiatry 39:884–889, 1982

Endicott J, Nee J, Cohen J, et al: Diagnosis of schizophrenia: prediction of short term outcome. Arch Gen Psychiatry 43:13–19, 1986

Feighner JP, Robins E, Guze SB, et al: Diagnostic criteria for use in psychiatric research. Arch Gen Psychiatry 26:57–63, 1972

Fenton WS, McGlashan TH, Heinssen RK: A comparison of DSM-III and DSM-III-R schizophrenia. Am J Psychiatry 145:1446–1449, 1988

Fish FJ: Schizophrenia. Bristol, England, John Wright 1962

Flaum M, Arndt S, Andreasen NC: Reliability of bizarre delusions. Compr Psychiatry 32:59–65, 1991

Frances AJ, Widiger TA, Pincus HA: The development of DSM-IV. Arch Gen Psychiatry 46:373–375, 1989

Guze SB, Cloninger R, Martin RL, et al: A follow-up in a family study of schizophrenia. Arch Gen Psychiatry 40:1273–1276, 1983

Helzer JR, Brockington IF, Kendell RE: Predictive validity of DSM-III and Feighner definitions of schizophrenia. Arch Gen Psychiatry 38:791–797, 1981

Helzer JE, Kendell RE, Brockington IF: Contribution of the six-month criterion to the predictive validity of the DSM-III definition of schizophrenia. Arch Gen Psychiatry 40:1277–1280, 1983

Hoch P, Polatin P: Pseudoneurotic forms of schizophrenia. Psychiatr Q 23:248–276, 1949

Huber G: Symptomwandel der Psychosen und Pharmakopsychiatrie, in Pharmakopsychiatrie und Psychopathologie. Edited by Kranz H, Heinrich K. Stuttgart, West Germany, Thieme, 1967

Hughlings-Jackson J: Selected Writings. Edited by Taylor J. London, Hodder & Stoughton, 1931

Humbert M, Salvador L, Segui J, et al: Estudio interfiabilidad version espanola evaluacion de sintomas positivos y negativos. Rev Departmento Psiquiatria Facultad de Medicine, University of Barcelona 13:28–36, 1986

Jampala VC, Sierles FS, Taylor MA: The use of DSM-III in the United States: a case of not going by the book. Compr Psychiatry 29:39–47, 1988

Jeste DV, Karson CN, Iager A, et al: Association of abnormal involuntary movements and negative symptoms. Psychopharmacol Bull 20:380–381, 1984

Johnstone EC, Crow TJ, Frith CD, et al: The dementia of dementia praecox. Acta Psychiatr Scand 57:305–325, 1978

Johnstone EC, Frith CD, Gold A, et al: The outcome of severe acute schizophrenic illnesses after one year. Br J Psychiatry 134:28–33, 1979

Johnstone EC, Owens DG, Frith CD, et al: Relative stability of positive and negative features in chronic schizophrenia. Br J Psychiatry 150:60–64, 1986

Kasanin J: The acute schizoaffective psychosis. Am J Psychiatry 90:97–126, 1933

Kay SR, Fizbein A, Opler LA: The Positive and Negative Syndrome Scale (PANSS) for schizophrenia. Schizophr Bull 13:261–267, 1987

Kendell RE, Cooper JE, Gourlay AG: Diagnostic criteria of American and British psychiatrists. Arch Gen Psychiatry 25:123–130, 1971

Kendler KS, Glazer WM, Morgenstern H: Dimensions of delusional experience. Am J Psychiatry 140:466–469, 1983

Kendler KS, Spitzer RL, Williams JBL: Psychotic disorders in DSM-III-R. Am J Psychiatry 146:953–962, 1989

Klein D: Relation between current diagnostic criteria for schizophrenia and the dimensions of premorbid adjustment, paranoid symptomatology, and chronicity. J Abnorm Psychol 91:319–325, 1982

Koehler K, Guth W, Grimm G: First-rank symptoms of schizophrenia in Schneider-oriented German centers. Arch Gen Psychiatry 34:810–813, 1977

Kraepelin E: Lectures on Clinical Psychiatry. Translated and edited by Johnstone T. New York, Hafner, 1904

Kraepelin E: Dementia Praecox and Paraphrenia (1919). Translated by Barclay RM. Edited by Robertson GM. New York, RE Krieger, 1971

Krawiecka M, Goldberg D, Vaughan MA: Standardized psychiatric assessment for rating chronic patients. Acta Psychiatr Scand 55:299–308, 1977

Kreitman N, Sainsbur P, Morrissey J: The reliability of psychiatric assessment: an analysis. Journal of Mental Science 107:887–908, 1961

Kuriansky JB, Deming WE, Gurland BJ: On trends in the diagnosis of schizophrenia. Am J Psychiatry 131:402–408, 1974

Lewine RR, Fogg M, Meltzer HY: Assessment of negative and positive symptoms in schizophrenia. Schizophr Bull 9:368–376, 1983

Liddle PF: The symptoms of chronic schizophrenia: a reexamination of the positive-negative dichotomy. Br J Psychiatry 151:145–151, 1987

Lipkowitz M, Idupuganti S: Diagnosing schizophrenia in 1982: the effect of DSM-III. Am J Psychiatry 142:634–637, 1985

Loranger AW: The impact of DSM-III on diagnostic practice in a university hospital: a comparison of DSM-II and DSM-III in 10,914 patients. Arch Gen Psychiatry 47:672–675, 1990

Loyd DW, Tsuang MT: Duration criteria and long-term outcome in affective disorder and schizophrenia. J Affective Disord 9:35–39, 1985

Marks RC, Luchins DJ: Relationship between brain imaging findings in schizophrenia and psychopathology: a review of the literature relating to positive and negative symptoms, in Modern Problems of Pharmacopsychiatry, Vol 24: Positive and Negative Symptoms and Syndromes. Edited by Andreasen NC. Basel, Switzerland, Karger, 1990, pp 89–123

McGlashan TH: Testing four diagnostic systems for schizophrenia. Arch Gen Psychiatry 41:141–144, 1984

Mellor CS: First-rank symptoms of schizophrenia. Br J Psychiatry 117:15–23, 1970

Moller HJ, Hohschramm M, Cording-Tommel C, et al: The classification of functional psychoses and its implications for prognosis. Br J Psychiatry 154:467–472, 1989

Moscarelli M, Maffei C, Cesana BM: An international prospective on assessment of negative and positive symptoms in schizophrenia. Am J Psychiatry 144:1595–1598, 1987

Ohta T, Okazaki Y, Anzai N: Reliability of the Japanese version of the Scale for the Assessment of Negative Symptoms (SANS). Japanese Journal of Psychiatry 13:999–1010, 1984

Overall JE, Gorham D: Brief Psychiatric Rating Scale. Psychol Rep 10:799–812, 1962

Owens DG, Johnstone EC: The disabilities of chronic schizophrenia: their nature and the factors contributing to their development. Br J Psychiatry 136:384–395, 1980

Pfohl B, Andreasen NC: Development of classification systems in psychiatry. Compr Psychiatry 19:197–207, 1978

Pfohl B, Winokur G: The micropsychopathology of hebephrenic/catatonic schizophrenia. J Nerv Ment Dis 171:296–300, 1983

Phillips M: Scale for the Assessment of Negative Symptoms and Scale for the Assessment of Positive Symptoms, Chinese Version. Shashi, Hubei, People's Republic of China, National Center for Psychiatric Training, Shashi Psychiatric Hospital, 1987

Pogue-Geile MF, Harrow M: Negative and positive symptoms in schizophrenia and depression: a follow-up. Schizophr Bull 10:371–387, 1984

Pogue-Geile MF, Harrow M: Negative symptoms in schizophrenia: their longitudinal course and prognostic importance. Schizophr Bull 11:427–439, 1985

Robins LN, Helzer JE, Croughan J, et al: National Institute of Mental Health Diagnostic Interview Schedule: its history, characteristics, and validity. Arch Gen Psychiatry 38:381–389, 1981

Sandifer MG, Petus G, Quad ED: A study of psychiatric diagnosis. J Nerv Ment Dis 139:350–356, 1964

Sandifer MG, Hordern A, Timbury GC, et al: Psychiatric diagnosis: a comparative study in North Carolina, London, and Glasgow. Br J Psychiatry 114:1–9, 1968

Schneider K: Clinical Psychopathology. Translated by Hamilton MW. New York, Grune & Stratton, 1959

Schneider K: Primary and secondary symptoms in schizophrenia, in Themes and Variations in European Psychiatry. Edited by Hirsch SR, Shepherd M. Bristol, England, John Wright, 1974, pp 40–46

Singh MM, Kay SR, Opler LA: Anticholinergic-neuroleptic antagonism in terms of positive and negative symptoms of schizophrenia: implications for psychobiological subtyping. Psychol Med 17:39–48, 1987

Spitzer RL, Fleiss JL: A reanalysis of the reliability of psychiatric diagnosis. Br J Psychiatry 125:341–347, 1974

Spitzer RL, Williams JBW: Structured Clinical Interview for DSM-III (SCID). New York, New York State Psychiatric Institute, 1984

Spitzer RL, Endicott J, Robbins E: Research Diagnostic Criteria. New York, Biometrics Research Division, New York State Psychiatric Institute, 1975

Spitzer RL, Endicott J, Robins E: Research Diagnostic Criteria: rationale and reliability. Arch Gen Psychiatry 35:773–782, 1978

Stephens JH, Astrup C, Mangrum J: Prognostic factors in recovered and deteriorated schizophrenics. Am J Psychiatry 122:1116–1121, 1966

Stephens JH, Astrup C, Carpenter WT, et al: A comparison of nine systems to diagnosis of schizophrenia. Psychiatry Res 6:127–143, 1982

Strauss J, Carpenter WT, Bartko J: The diagnosis and understanding of schizophrenia, III: speculations on the processes that underlie schizophrenia symptoms and signs. Schizophr Bull 1:61–69, 1974

Taylor M: Schneiderian first-rank symptoms and clinical prognostic features in schizophrenia. Arch Gen Psychiatry 26:64–67, 1972

Taylor MA, Abrams R: The phenomenology of mania: a new look at some old patients. Arch Gen Psychiatry 29:520–522, 1973

Taylor MA, Abrams R: Acute mania: clinical and genetic study of responders and non-responders to treatments. Arch Gen Psychiatry 32:863–865, 1975

Tsuang MT, Woolson RF, Fleming JA: Longterm outcome of major psychoses, I: schizophrenia and affective disorders compared with psychiatrically symptom-free surgical conditions. Arch Gen Psychiatry 36:1295–1301, 1979

Vaillant GE: Prospective prediction of schizophrenic remission. Arch Gen Psychiatry 11:509–518, 1964

Van Kammen DP, Boronow JJ: Dextro-amphetamine diminishes negative symptoms in schizophrenia. Int Clin Psychopharmacol 3:111–121, 1988

Waddington JL, Youseff HA, Dolphin C, et al: Cognitive dysfunction, negative symptoms, and tardive dyskinesia in schizophrenia: their association in relation to topography of involuntary movements and criterion of their abnormality. Arch Gen Psychiatry 44:907–912, 1987

Wing JK: A standard form of psychiatric Present State Examination and a method for standardizing the classification of symptoms, in Psychiatric Epidemiology: An International Symposium. Edited by Hare EH, Wing JK. London, Oxford University Press, 1970, pp 93–108

Wing JK, Cooper JE, Sartorius N: The Measurement and Classification of Psychiatric Symptoms. New York, Cambridge University Press, 1974

World Health Organization: The International Pilot Study of Schizophrenia. Geneva, World Health Organization, 1973

World Health Organization: The ICD-10 Classification of Mental and Behavioural Disorders: Clinical Descriptions and Diagnostic Guidelines. Geneva, World Health Organization, 1992

Chapter 23

The Positive-Negative Distinction in Schizophrenia: Review of Natural History Validators

Thomas H. McGlashan, M.D.
Wayne S. Fenton, M.D.

Statement of the Issues

The issue broadly addressed by this review concerns the natural history validity of negative or deficit symptoms in schizophrenia and whether they deserve a place among the core defining features of the disorder.

Significance of the Issues

In the past decade, the distinction between positive and negative symptoms in schizophrenia has captured the attention of researchers and clinicians alike. Perhaps, in retrospect, the revitalized focus on this perspective was long overdue, fueled by frustrations with the vast heterogeneity of schizophrenia and by disenchantments with the preexisting (classic) subtyping schema. Furthermore, developing diagnostic systems of the past generation leaned heavily on the more reliable positive symptoms to define schizophrenia, an emphasis that many considered psychometrically sound but scientifically suspect. Eschewing negative symptoms or deficit psychopathologies, some postulated, weakens construct validity by ignoring processes that have been considered central to schizophrenia for almost 100 years. The recent reliable operationalization of negative phenomenologies, however, rendered empirical study of these issues within the purview of many investigators, and a literal explosion of investigative effort ensued. We attempt here to review only a segment of this effort, that dealing with the natural history validators of the positive-negative distinction. Other validating criteria such as neuroimaging, neurochemistry, or neuropsychological testing, although no less important, have been reviewed elsewhere (Andreasen 1990). We focus here on the longitudinal clinical perspective—that is, how the person and the disease present and interact over a significant proportion of the life span.

Brief History of the Positive-Negative Distinction

The distinction between positive and negative schizophrenia is ubiquitous historically, and no single person can lay claim to its original formulation. In the 19th century, Hughlings-Jackson (1931) used the terms *negative symptoms* and *positive symptoms* to describe insanity and speculated that the former came from disease-induced loss of higher mental functioning and the latter from release phenomena secondary to this loss of higher control. The distinction was present in the thinking of our nosologic forefathers of the 20th century. Kraepelin (1919/1971) described "two principle disorders that characterize the malady [dementia praecox] . . . a weakening of those emotional activities which permanently form the mainspring of volition and . . . the loss of the inner unity of activities of intellect, emotion, and volition" (pp. 74–75). Bleuler (1911/1950) had a similar negative-positive dichotomy in mind with his fundamental versus accessory symptoms. The former involved loss of function (e.g., of attention, volition, affective responsiveness, association) and was always present. The latter involved an aberration of function (e.g., hallucinations, delusions, catatonia) and was present only during severe relapse.

This distinction was carried through the 20th century in one form or another. In fact, the most anecdotal but telling validation of the positive-negative distinction comes from the degree to which it has entered—and saturated—our everyday clinical language. Schizophrenia has almost always been described in terms of a bipolarity, the valence of which suggests today's positive-negative distinction. The following dichotomies from Sass (1989) are illustrative: acute (+) versus chronic (–), reactive (+) versus process (–), secondary (+) versus primary (–), accessory (+) versus fundamental (–), active (+) versus residual (–), florid (+) versus quiescent (–), and productive (+) versus deficient (–).

The first explicit hypothesis that these phenomenologies represented distinct pathophysiologies within schizophrenia came from Strauss and colleagues (1974). This notion was elaborated soon after by Crow (1980), who postulated two syndromes and psychopathological processes in schizophrenia. Type I schizophrenia had mainly positive symptoms, good premorbid functioning, acute onsets, neuroleptic responsive symptoms, and better long-term course and outcome without intellectual deterioration. Type II schizophrenia had mainly negative symptoms, poor premorbid functioning, insidious onset, drug-resistant symptoms, and poorer long-term course and outcome with intellectual deterioration or dementia. Crow (1985) later added behavioral deterioration and abnormal involuntary movements to Type II. Type I was postulated to reflect reversible hyperdopaminergic activity in a normal brain and Type II to reflect irreversible neuronal loss in a structurally abnormal brain.

Crow's (1980) powerfully heuristic hypothesis catalyzed a chain reaction of research, once systems for operationalizing positive and negative phenomenologies became available, first from Britain (Krawiecka et al. 1977) and then from America (Andreasen 1982). The 1980s witnessed the appearance of literally hundreds of articles on the topic, studying virtually every class of validation, including clinical phenomenology, laboratory findings, family history, treatment responsiveness, long-term course, and outcome. Many of these investigations have already become the subject of reviews (Barnes and Liddle 1990; Kay and Opler 1987; Marks and Luchins 1990; Pickar et al. 1990; Pogue-Geile and Zubin 1988; Walker and Lewine 1988).

Definitions and Reliability of Positive and Negative Symptoms

Many systems have been devised to define positive and negative symptoms. The following have been used most frequently over the past decade: 1) the Manchester Scale (Hyde 1989; Krawiecka et al. 1977) and Crow's (1985) modification of this scale; 2) the Positive and Negative Symptom Scale (PANSS) (Kay et al. 1989); 3) the Scale for the Assessment of Negative Symptoms (SANS) (Andreasen and Olsen 1982); 4) the Scale for the Assessment of Positive Symptoms (SAPS) (Andreasen and Olsen 1982); 5) the Rating Scale for Emotional Blunting (Abrams and Taylor 1978); 6) the Deficit and Non-deficit categorization (Carpenter et al. 1988); and 7) scales devised by Lewine and colleagues (1983) and by Pogue-Geile and Harrow (1984).

Which symptoms are considered positive or negative varies across these systems. *All* systems include flat affect and poverty of speech among the negative symptoms and hallucinations and delusions among the positive symptoms. Most systems regard anhedonia, apathy, and avolition or abulia as negative symptoms when they are included. Thought disorder, bizarre behavior, and inappropriate affect, on the other hand, are classified as positive or negative with variability. Kulhara and colleagues (1986), Liddle (1987a, 1987b), and Liddle and colleagues (1989) suggested they constitute a third factor that is orthogonal to the positive-negative distinction. Lewine and Sommers (1985) asserted that inappropriate affect and poverty of content of speech (a form of thought disorder) fit better in a separate domain reflecting a loss of higher integrative capacity. Fenton and McGlashan (1991) found thought disorder and bizarre behavior, in contrast to hallucinations and delusions, to correlate with negative symptoms and with poorer premorbid functioning. On the other hand, thought disorder and bizarre behavior were unlike negative symptoms but like positive symptoms in being unrelated to a variety of measures of long-term outcome. Therefore, it appears that these domains of psychopathology stand in ambiguous relation to the positive-negative distinction. Nevertheless they are occasionally included in the definitions used in the studies reviewed and as such this may confound the interpretation of results in ways that are difficult to specify since comparisons are almost always made between samples defined by groups of symptoms (e.g., by composite scores).

Operationalizing the assessment of negative symptoms has had a positive effect on reliability. All of the scales specified above have generated levels of interrater reliability in the acceptable range. For example, the intraclass correlations for the SANS and SAPS symptom complex global ratings ranged between .70 and .88 (Andreasen 1982), and the interrater Pearson correlations for the negative symptom items of the PANSS averaged .85 (Kay et al. 1989). A more complete comparison of these assessment systems vis-à-vis reliability and other psychometric parameters is the subject of another communication (Fenton and McGlashan 1991). For now, suffice it to say negative symptoms can be rated with as much reliability as positive symptoms. Whether they actually were rated reliably in the studies cited here is another matter. Reliability of assessment was tested and reported in only about one of five of the investigations reviewed. Clearly, there is room for improvement.

Methods

This review is limited to the set of "natural history" validators (Robins and Guze 1970)—that is, those variables that can be elaborated at the clinical phenomenological level (Table 23–1). Approximately 200 potentially relevant articles from the

Table 23–1. Natural history validators

■ Demography Age Sex Marital status ■ Premorbid functioning Social/sexual Education/work IQ	■ Illness loading Family history of mental illness Twin concordance Age at onset Established chronicity at baseline Neurological abnormalities ■ Relationship between positive and negative symptoms ■ Course of positive and negative symptoms ■ Prognosis and outcome

English psychiatric and psychological literature of the past 15 years were collected with the aide of computer searches using key words such as *positive, negative, deficit, Type I/II, anhedonia, apathy, flat* or *blunted affect, asociality, avolition, alogia,* and *poverty of speech.*

The methodological standards applied were modestly rigorous. Selected were studies of schizophrenia that characterized diagnosis and the positive-negative or deficit-nondeficit typology using current operational criteria. Also included were studies in which these parameters could be translated easily into these constructs. Reliability testing was not required for inclusion; had it been this review would be remarkably brief. Studies without tests of significance were excluded as were studies with sample sizes that were probably too small for meaningful results (e.g., populations or comparison groups of less than 12 subjects).

Results

Tables 23–2 through 23–5 summarize the findings across a variety of natural history parameters. The number of citations supporting a particular finding or direction

Table 23–2. Positive and negative symptom literature: demography and premorbid functions

Parameter	Finding	Number of citations
Demography		
Age differences	Negative patients older	1
	Nonsignificant	11
Gender differences	Male patients more negative	9
	Male patients less negative	1
	Nonsignificant	13
Marital status	Negative patients more single	1
	Nonsignificant	7
Premorbid functioning		
Social/sexual function	Poorer in negative patients	7
	Poorer in negative male patients	2
	Better in acute negative patients	1
Education	Lower in negative patients	10
	Lower in negative male patients	2
	Higher in negative female patients	1
	Nonsignificant	6
Work	Inferior in negative patients	7
Intelligence	Lower in negative patients	7
	Lower in negative male patients	1

Table 23–3. Positive and negative symptom literature: illness morbid characteristics

Parameter	Finding	Number of citations
Family history of mental illness	Positive linkage of schizophrenia with negative symptoms	1
	No linkage of schizophrenia	4
	Positive linkage of negative symptoms with affective disorder absence	2
Age at first hospitalization	More negative in early cases	3
	More negative in later cases	3
	Nonsignificant	11
Chronicity[a]	More hospitalizations in positive patients	2
	Longer duration in negative patients	3
	Nonsignificant	17
Neurological abnormalities	Abnormal motor movements[b] and negative symptoms associated	10
	Soft neurological signs and negative symptoms	1
	Parietal sensory signs and negative symptoms	1
	Tardive dyskinesia: correlation with negative symptoms	11
	Tardive dyskinesia: no correlation with negative symptoms	3

[a]Number and length of prior hospitalizations, total length of illness.
[b]Choreiform, athetoid, dyskinetic, synchrony.

Table 23–4. Positive and negative symptom literature: manifest illness characteristics

Parameter	Finding	Number of citations
Linkage between positive and negative symptoms	Negative correlation	2
	Positive correlation	3
	Nonsignificant	21
Course of positive and negative symptoms	Negative symptoms unstable in early acute cases	4
	Negative symptoms stable in early acute cases	3
	Negative symptoms stable in subacute cases	3
	Negative symptoms stable in subchronic and chronic cases	9
	Negative symptoms increase with time	7

Table 23–5. Positive and negative symptom literature: prognosis and outcome

Parameter	Finding	Number of citations
Short-term outcome (0–2 years)	Poorer outcome in negative patients	2
	Better outcome in negative patients	3
Medium-term outcome (3–5 years)	Poorer outcome in negative patients	4
	Poorer outcome in high negative and high positive symptom patients	2
	Poorer outcome (hospitalization) in high positive patients	1
Long-term outcome (6–22 years)	Poorer outcome in medicated patients with high positive and negative symptoms	1
	Poorer outcome in high positive and negative patients	1
	Poorer outcome in negative patients	3

is tabulated in the right margin and provides a rough estimate of the direction, if any, of the empirical data. In the interest of space, constituent references are not elaborated but can be found in the original publication (McGlashan and Fenton 1992). In the tables, the phrase "more negative" means negative symptoms or subtype cohorts that are higher in number or greater in severity.

Summary of Empirical Findings

The natural history validators of the positive-negative distinction may be summarized as follows.

Demographically, age does not discriminate between patients with predominantly negative symptomatology and patients with predominantly positive symptomatology. Neither does marital status, but this is a poor measure because of its low frequency in schizophrenia generally. Where gender differences exist, they associate negative symptoms with male patients in the vast majority of instances.

Premorbid distinctions are more striking. Negative or deficit symptom schizophrenic patients consistently have a history of inferior premorbid social-sexual functioning, lower educational level, and compromised work capacity. IQ data are preliminary but suggest an association between negative symptoms and lower intelligence, either premorbidly or early in the morbid process.

Illness loading parameters present a less dramatic picture. Family history studies are sparse and equivocal. Twin concordance studies suggest a greater genetic loading with negative symptoms, but more data are needed. Age at onset and established chronicity at baseline fail to discriminate, perhaps because of measurement and sampling bias; that is, these variables are measured relative to hospitalization. Age at onset is not defined as the age when symptoms first appear, but the age at which symptoms become disruptive enough to require institutionalization. It is possible that negative symptoms begin significantly earlier than positive symptoms but never get the patient into enough trouble to be recorded. Thus the failure to find distinctions here may be a false negative. The robust correlation between negative symptoms and abnormal voluntary and involuntary movements is the most striking finding in this realm of parameters. It strongly suggests that negative symptomatology is linked with psychopathological processes different from those associated with positive symptoms.

Studies of the intercorrelations among positive and negative symptoms uphold their content validity and overwhelmingly suggest they are independent or semi-independent processes in schizophrenia.

The course of positive and negative symptoms in schizophrenia is variable, depending on phase of disorder. In first or early episodes, positive symptoms are frequent; negative symptoms are infrequent; and both types are unstable, fluctuating, and usually treatment responsive. In subacute-subchronic stages of the illness, negative symptoms increase in prevalence, are at least as common as positive symptoms, and fluctuate less. In the latter stages of the illness, negative symptoms are quite stable and usually dominate the clinical picture. The different character and course of negative symptoms in early versus mid- to later-phases of schizophrenia strongly suggest they may be generated by different underlying mechanisms.

Such a distinction is further upheld by the findings on prognosis and outcome. Negative symptoms have a polymorphous prognostic potential early in the disorder and do not become consistently prognostic until well after the acute and/or initial phases. Negative symptoms are then consistent predictors of poor medium-term and longer-term outcome, more so than positive symptoms, which can also be predictive at times in a similar direction.

Discussion

The prototypic negative symptom or deficit schizophrenic patient is a single male. He has problems socializing through adolescence and does not date. He is not among the better students and works sporadically or not at all. He is physically uncoordinated and evinces other motor abnormalities that add to an aura of weirdness. During the illness, his positive and negative symptoms fluctuate a fair amount at first, but negative symptoms and poor functioning dominate the picture over time. The process is chronic and disabling, requiring some form of institutional or community asylum for a lifetime. Other elements to this prototypic picture are less established and more speculative: a higher familial-genetic loading for schizophrenia and perhaps for negative symptoms, earlier onset of illness, and more rapid establishment of chronicity.

The literature does not, however, uniformly support such a singular or prototypic portrait. The variability of findings among studies probably stems from both methodological inconsistencies and heterogeneity in the nature of negative symptoms themselves. As noted, the definition of what constitutes a negative symptom or syndrome varies across studies and assessment schemes. Some phenomenologies such as flat affect and poverty of speech are commonly identified as negative. Others such as inappropriate affect and poverty of content of speech are sometimes classified as negative and sometimes as positive and sometimes regarded as indeterminant and dropped altogether. Furthermore, the stringency with which phenomenologies achieve the status of a particular category also varies among studies. In many, a negative symptom is defined on the basis of a single cross-sectional observation. In others, consistency across longitudinal windows of observation of varying length (e.g., up to 1 year) is required. Thus one possible source of the difference in the relationships of negative symptoms to validating criteria may be the definition of negative symptoms used. Finally, even given comparable definitions, the reliability with which they are applied undoubtedly varies across studies. The impact of this, however, is hard to estimate given that so few investigations test for or report interrater reliability.

Another source of variability in findings probably derives from the likelihood that negative symptoms, in themselves, are pleomorphic. The natural history data outline at least three negative symptom phases or syndromes that may be quite distinct or that may signal qualitatively different underlying processes at work. The first is associated with compromised premorbid functioning and suggests a link between negative symptoms and the vulnerability(ies) to schizophrenia. In severe cases, like the negative symptom-laden children of schizophrenic mothers described by Fish (1987), the deficits linked to such vulnerability may not be progressive but rather may be in place more or less from birth. The second negative or deficit process is associated with the acute and/or florid states of schizophrenia. Here negative symptoms are like positive symptoms, rapidly forming and rapidly receding, responsive to environmental pressures and treatment interventions. A theory by Tandon and Greden (1989), for example, postulates that negative symptoms result from cholinergic hyperactivation, which is a protective response to positive symptom-generating dopaminergic hyperactivity. The third negative or deficit process is associated with manifest illness chronicity. Here negative symptoms are more dominant, persistent, intervention resistant, and functionally disabling; they may reflect the structural abnormalities of Crow's (1980, 1985) Type

II hypothesis or the deteriorating process that Kraepelin (1919/1971) originally postulated as central to dementia praecox.

As noted by Carpenter and colleagues (1988), negative symptoms can arise from many sources: drugs, depression, institutionalization, demoralization, and a variety of positive symptoms (e.g., paranoid anxieties leading to muteness). A distinction is made between negative symptoms that are secondary to these antecedent (causal) sources and negative symptoms that are primary or core to the disorder. This distinction is useful as long as "primary" is not assumed to be "unitary." As seen above, the natural history literature may outline at least three forms of primary negative symptoms (i.e., negative or deficit processes that form a necessary if not sufficient condition for the development of schizophrenia). These are 1) negative or deficit processes linked to vulnerability (perhaps genetic), 2) processes akin to those that generate positive symptoms (perhaps biochemical), and 3) processes linked to deterioration (perhaps structural or developmental). All are important, but which process can claim to be primary etiologically has yet to be explicated.

Despite our ignorance concerning etiology, however, we now possess abundant knowledge concerning the manifest behavior (i.e., the natural history of negative symptoms in schizophrenia). They are frequent; they can be assessed accurately; and they have a profound influence on the life-long variances of schizophrenia.

Recommendations

Negative symptoms have rightfully recaptured the interest of clinicians and researchers, and their importance needs to be recaptured in our diagnostic nosology and nomenclature. DSM-III (American Psychiatric Association 1980) and DSM-III-R (American Psychiatric Association 1987) de-emphasized them to prodromal-residual symptoms because of questionable reliability, specificity, and validity. The issue of reliability appears to have been resolved, and, as reviewed in this chapter, the literature on natural history provides overwhelming support of validity. Specificity, especially the distinction between negative symptoms in schizophrenia versus depression, remains an issue. Nevertheless, whether or not negative symptoms are found in other disorders, they are a common and important component of schizophrenia. That much is clear and that much is sufficient to justify changes in the DSM-IV criteria for schizophrenia.

Among all the assessment systems reviewed here, flat affect and poverty of speech were considered to be negative symptoms. Accordingly, we suggest that flat affect and poverty of speech become one of the defining criteria A alongside delusions, hallucinations, thought disorder, and disorganized behavior. The negative symptoms of avolition, apathy, anhedonia, and asociality could also perhaps be added, or they could be listed among the prodromal-residual cluster where, in fact, some of them currently reside. The exact number and their precise placement in the criteria set are issues for current debate and future investigation. As a defining class, however, we feel negative symptoms have met the test of validity with respect to data concerning natural history of disorder.

References

Abrams R, Taylor MA: A rating scale for emotional blunting. Am J Psychiatry 135:226–229, 1978

American Psychiatric Association: Diagnostic and Statistical Manual of Mental Disorders, 3rd Edition. Washington, DC, American Psychiatric Association, 1980

American Psychiatric Association: Diagnostic and Statistical Manual of Mental Disorders, 3rd Edition, Revised. Washington, DC, American Psychiatric Association, 1987

Andreasen NC: Negative symptoms in schizophrenia: definition and reliability. Arch Gen Psychiatry 39:784–788, 1982

Andreasen NC (ed): Schizophrenia: Positive and Negative Symptoms and Syndromes. Basel, Switzerland, Karger, 1990

Andreasen NC, Olsen S: Negative vs positive schizophrenia: definition and validation. Arch Gen Psychiatry 39:789–794, 1982

Barnes TRE, Liddle PF: Evidence for the validity of negative symptoms, in Schizophrenia: Positive and Negative Symptoms and Syndromes. Edited by Andreasen NC. Basel, Switzerland, Karger, 1990, pp 43–72

Bleuler E: Dementia Praecox or the Group of Schizophrenias (1911). Translated by Zinkin J. New York, International Universities Press, 1950

Carpenter WT, Heinrichs DW, Wagman AMI: Deficit and nondeficit forms of schizophrenia: the concept. Am J Psychiatry 145:578–583, 1988

Crow TJ: Molecular pathology of schizophrenia: more than one disease process? Br Med J 12:66–68, 1980

Crow TJ: The two-syndrome concept: origins and current status. Schizophr Bull 11:471–486, 1985

Fenton WS, McGlashan TH: Natural history of schizophrenia subtypes II: positive and negative symptoms and long-term course. Arch Gen Psychiatry 48:978–986, 1991

Fish B: Infant predictors of the longitudinal course of schizophrenic development. Schizophr Bull 13:395–409, 1987

Hughlings-Jackson HJ: Selected Writings. Edited by Taylor J. London, Hodder & Stoughton, 1931

Hyde CE: The Manchester Scale: a standardised psychiatric assessment for rating chronic psychotic patients. Br J Psychiatry 155 (suppl 7):45–48, 1989

Kay SR, Opler LA: The positive-negative dimension in schizophrenia: its validity and significance. Psychiatric Developments 2:79–103, 1987

Kay SR, Opler LA, Lindenmayer J-P: The positive and negative syndrome scale (PANSS): rationale and standardisation. Br J Psychiatry 155 (suppl 7):59–65, 1989

Kraepelin E: Dementia Praecox and Paraphrenia (1919). Translated by Barclay RM. Edited by Robertson GM. New York, RE Krieger, 1971

Krawiecka M, Goldberg D, Vaughan M: A standardized psychiatric assessment scale for rating chronic psychotic patients. Acta Psychiatr Scand 55:299–308, 1977

Kulhara P, Kota SK, Joseph S: Positive and negative subtypes of schizophrenia: a study from India. Acta Psychiatr Scand 74:353–359, 1986

Lewine RJ, Sommers AA: Clinical definition of negative symptoms as a reflection of theory and methodology, in Controversies in Schizophrenia: Changes and Constancies. Edited by Alpert M. New York, Guilford, 1985, pp 267–279

Lewine R, Fogg L, Meltzer H: The development of scales for the assessment of positive and negative symptoms in schizophrenia. Schizophr Bull 9:368–376, 1983

Liddle PF: Schizophrenic syndromes, cognitive performance, and neurological dysfunction. Psychol Med 17:49–57, 1987a

Liddle PF: The symptoms of chronic schizophrenia: a re-examination of the positive-negative dichotomy. Br J Psychiatry 151:145–151, 1987b

Liddle PF, Barnes TRE, Morris D, et al: Three syndromes in chronic schizophrenia. Br J Psychiatry 155 (suppl 7):119–122, 1989

Marks RC, Luchins DJ: Relationship between brain imaging findings in schizophrenia and psychopathology: a review of the literature relating to positive and negative symptoms, in Schizophrenia: Positive and Negative Symptoms and Syndromes. Edited by Andreasen NC. Basel, Karger, 1990, pp 89–123

McGlashan TH, Fenton WS: The positive/negative distinction in schizophrenia: review of natural history validators. Arch Gen Psychiatry 49:63–72, 1992

Pickar D, Litman RE, Konicki PE, et al: Neurochemical and neural mechanisms of positive and negative symptoms in schizophrenia, in Schizophrenia: Positive and Negative Symptoms and Syndromes. Edited by Andreasen NC. Basel, Karger, 1990, pp 124–151

Pogue-Geile MF, Harrow M: Negative and positive symptoms in schizophrenia and depression: a follow-up. Schizophr Bull 10:371–387, 1984

Pogue-Geile MF, Zubin J: Negative symptomatology and schizophrenia: a conceptual and empirical review. International Journal of Mental Health 16:3–45, 1988

Robins E, Guze SB: Establishment of diagnostic validity in psychiatric illness: its application to schizophrenia. Am J Psychiatry 126:983–987, 1970

Sass H: The historical evolution of the concept of negative symptoms in schizophrenia. Br J Psychiatry 155 (suppl 7):26–31, 1989

Strauss J, Carpenter WT, Bartko J: The diagnosis and understanding of schizophrenia, III: speculations on the processes that underlie schizophrenic symptoms and signs. Schizophr Bull 1:61–69, 1974

Tandon R, Greden JF: Cholinergic hyperactivity and negative schizophrenic symptoms: a model of cholinergic/dopaminergic interactions in schizophrenia. Arch Gen Psychiatry 46:745–753, 1989

Walker E, Lewine RJ: The positive/negative symptom distinction in schizophrenia: validity and etiological relevance. Schizophr Res 1:315–328, 1988

Chapter 24

The Diagnosis of Schizophrenia: A Review of Onset and Duration Issues

Samuel J. Keith, M.D.
Susan M. Matthews, M.D.

Overview

One of the essential considerations for the diagnosis of schizophrenia has been how to capture the time-honored concept of its tendency toward chronicity. That schizophrenia is an illness that tends to have a lifelong course or to spawn problems that are long lasting fits nearly everyone's picture of the clinical condition. Diagnosticians have struggled, however, with how to characterize chronicity. The problem becomes particularly pointed with the scientific necessity of developing reliable criteria as was done with DSM-III (American Psychiatric Association 1980) and DSM-III-R (American Psychiatric Association 1987). In these diagnostic systems, specific and quantifiable periods of time were selected for various symptom durations to characterize illness and to accomplish the goal of reliability. However, no sooner had the time interval and the symptom requirements been selected, when critics of the selection process suggested that perhaps these were either not the right time periods or not the right symptoms. To review in general terms, DSM-III and DSM-III-R required a relatively brief duration of psychotic symptoms (1 week, or less if successfully treated), with the remaining duration requirement composed of either persistent psychotic symptoms *or* prodrome or residual symptoms (less than 6 months for schizophreniform or greater than 6 months for schizophrenia diagnosis).

Two forces have come together that have made a reexamination of these issues significant. First, internal to the DSM-III-R revision toward DSM-IV has been a discussion of the following:

1. Could prodromal symptoms be reliably identified and dated?
2. Was "1 week or less if successfully treated" a sufficient duration to establish the relevance of psychotic symptomatology for a diagnosis potentially as stigmatizing as schizophrenia?
3. Was 6 months the optimal time duration for separating schizophreniform illness from schizophrenia?

Second, the ICD-9 (World Health Organization 1978) to ICD-10 (World Health Organization 1988) process of revision independently made several major distinctions in establishing criteria for the diagnosis of schizophrenia that were potentially incompatible with DSM-III-R:

1. Although acknowledging that prodromal symptoms were a part of the clinical syndrome of schizophrenia, because of reliability of assessment issues, they would not be used in ICD-10.
2. To meet the criteria for schizophrenia, psychotic symptoms must have occurred over the period of 1 month during which they were present most of the time.
3. For those clinical cases where psychotic symptomatology did not last 1 month, a wide variety of brief psychotic syndromes were described with emphases on the presence or absence of characteristic schizophrenic symptoms or the relative lability of symptoms. The ICD-10 was silent on the issue of 6 months.

In the three sections of this chapter, we review each of these issues and bring what data are available to bear on these topics. It should be noted that no studies were designed to address these issues absolutely and directly, and therefore much of the data relevant to these topics were extrapolated from other types of research projects.

Prodrome and Residual Symptoms

Statement of the Issues

The concept of schizophrenia or schizophreniform illness having a gradual onset or insidious course is one that has always been a part of the illnesses. What has conflicted contemporary psychiatry are issues of how best to capture and characterize this clinically accepted phenomenon. With residual symptoms, there has been relatively less debate, because for the most part these symptoms are collected prospectively following psychotic symptomatology—a phenomenon that will color many aspects of the patient's future life as well as the confidence with which residual symptoms are assessed. With prodrome, however, we are usually in the position of having to assess potentially "low-grade" symptoms retrospectively—inescapable for reasons of efficiency and acceptable because of the place of retrospective data in the history of psychiatry and medicine in general. Critical, then, becomes the characterization of the components of prodrome in terms of their reliability and duration.

Significance of the Issues

The role of prodromal and residual phases of schizophrenia and schizophreniform illnesses characterizes a significant difference between ICD-10 and DSM-III-R. The ICD-10 recognizes that the prodrome exists, but has chosen not to include its characterization or duration into the diagnostic criteria. The ICD-10 stated:

> Viewed retrospectively it may be clear that a prodromal phase in which symptoms and behavior, such as loss of interest in work, social activities and personal appearance and hygiene, together with generalized anxiety and mild degrees of depression and preoccupation may precede the onset of psychotic symptoms by weeks or months. Because of the difficulty in timing onset, the one month duration criterion applies only to specific symptoms listed above and not to any prodromal nonpsychotic phase. (World Health Organization 1988, p. 60)

By this system, they have confined the issue of retrospective data collection to 1 month only and limited criteria to those that are clearly definable and hence most reliable. There is no reference to treatment response; negative symptoms are included only to a limited extent; and residual symptoms are restricted to these limited negative symptoms:

> clearly defined delusions and hallucinations are not always present, particularly in chronic conditions. The diagnosis will then often depend on establishing the presence of "negative" symptoms such as:
>
> . . . blunting or incongruity of emotional responses, increasing apathy, paucity of speech; and
>
> . . . breaks or interpolations in the train of thought. Although these various deficits are equally characteristic of schizophrenia, depression or neuroleptic drugs can sometimes produce a very similar clinical picture. (World Health Organization 1988, p. 60)

Other than the above statement regarding neuroleptic-induced negative symptoms, ICD-10 essentially ignores treatment response except to note that, "conditions meeting such symptomatic requirements but of a duration less than one month (whether treated or not) should be diagnosed . . . as acute schizophrenia-like psychotic disorder (F23.2) and reclassified as schizophrenia if the symptoms persist for longer periods [1 month] of time" (World Health Organization 1988, p. 60).

In practical terms, this difference between the two diagnostic systems is highlighted with the first-episode patient. For DSM, the characteristic psychotic symptoms in this patient may assume somewhat less significance in terms of duration, with the only requirement being that symptoms be present for 1 week (or less if symptom successfully treated) at some point. The remainder of the criteria for diagnosis for the first-episode patient is dependent on the accurate assessment of the presence of prodrome. If the symptoms that brought the patient to psychiatric attention are of relatively recent onset, a diagnosis of schizophreniform (provisional) is made with a 6-month time clock started. After the 6-month time period has elapsed, if either psychotic or residual symptoms persist, a diagnosis of schizophrenia is made.

If, however, there has been an insidious onset, and the presence of characteristic symptoms is established, then the diagnosis hinges on an accurate, retrospective dating of prodromal symptoms for up to 6 months in the past. Further, if the highest degree of difficulty in diagnosis lies with the first-episode patient, then the focus of a discussion of "6 months" becomes in actuality the utility, reliability, and implication of prodrome as defined in DSM, because *after* 6 months of manifest illness (either active psychotic symptoms or residual symptoms as assessed prospectively), the diagnosis becomes considerably easier regardless of the system used.

The current controversy is consistent with enduring debate in the scientific literature on the importance of prodrome. Over the past 25 years, leaders in schizophrenia research (e.g., Bleuler 1978; Wing 1988; Wynne 1988) have held strong opinions on the clinical importance of this issue.

Methods

There has been considerable discussion in the literature over what constitutes a prodromal symptom. Currently it is reasonably accurate to say that prodrome has become a heterogeneous group of behaviors related in a temporal manner to the onset of psychosis. The reader is referred to DSM-III-R (pp. 194–195) for a full listing of the criteria.

For the purposes of this review, we have elected to examine the reliability of date of onset and prodromal symptoms of both sets of variables. We also discuss conceptual problems that arise from combining these two types of symptoms into a single entity of prodrome.

Gradually emerging psychosis. For gradually emerging "prepsychotic" symptoms, in older literature we relied extensively on the seminal review by Docherty and colleagues (1978). For the most part, the reviewed studies provide a clinical descriptive account of prodromal symptoms from retrospective reports. Most, however, take the form of clinical vignettes and, although rich in clinical material, they provide little methodological rigor. From 1980 to date, we have attempted to review all articles in which premorbid or prodromal symptoms were studied. We preferred those that looked at the phenomenon prospectively, but this required examining relapse rather than original prodromal symptoms for obvious logistical reasons. We have included the retrospective study of the Herz group (Herz and Melville 1980) because of its major impact on the clinical field.

Early morbid patterns of withdrawal or negative symptoms. For the assessment of reliability and duration of early morbid patterns of withdrawal or negative symptoms, we examined the premorbid adjustment literature, focusing on four major reviews of this field (W. T. Carpenter, J. S. Strauss, A. E. Pulver, et al.: Prediction of outcome in schizophrenia, IV: eleven-year follow-up of the Washington IPSS cohort, unpublished manuscript, 1987; Fenton and McGlashan 1987; Stephens 1978; Vaillant 1964a, 1964b). Again, it should be noted that these studies were examining retrospectively the premorbid adjustment of already manifest cases of schizophrenia and, because of the extensive span of time, were utilizing varying editions of DSM. However, because the issue of assessment of these early morbid signs is clinically a retrospective decision in most cases, this point is less critical.

Results

Gradually emerging psychosis. In 1980, Herz and Melville published a retrospective study of prodromal symptoms as they occurred in relapse. Of relevance to our review are both the frequency and duration findings of the report.

The reported rank order of symptoms that appeared or worsened in at least 50% of schizophrenic patients prior to hospitalization is listed in Table 24–1.

In the same report, family members and patients at another site (Atlanta, Georgia) were interviewed concerning these signs and, although not perfect, the rank-order correlation of frequency of symptoms was quite good ($r = .78$, $P < .001$), giving some indication that these prodromal symptoms can be reliably assessed over the short term. It is interesting, however, that the symptoms that showed the greatest disagreement were those of a more prepsychotic nature—talking in a nonsensical way and hearing voices and seeing things. In terms of duration of symptoms, approximately 50% of patients had prodromal symptoms for less than 1 month prior to hospitalization.

As noted in Subotnik and Neuchterlein's (1988) article, there have now been four prospective studies of prodromal prepsychotic symptoms: Herz and colleagues (1982), Heinrichs and Carpenter (1985), Marder and colleagues (1984), and their own (1988). This group of studies includes only those patients who are at risk for relapse, as the prospective identification of first-episode patients is not yet possible.

Herz and colleagues (1982) reported that "typical symptoms were sleep disturbances, agitation, anxiety, anger, social anxiety . . . and all were reversed with medication. . . . Episodes lasted an average of 1.4 weeks" (p. 920). Clearly, in terms of prodromal symptoms that are identified early, active treatment will reverse their course.

Heinrichs and Carpenter (1985) listed the following "common prodromal symptoms" in order of their frequency: hallucinations; suspiciousness; change in sleep; anxiety; cognitive inefficiency; anger-hostility; somatic symptoms or delusions; thought disorder; disruptive, inappropriate behavior; and depression.

Marder and colleagues (1984) conducted a study, again examining relapse, in which they found the paranoia and depression factors from the Brief Psychiatric Rating Scale (BPRS) (Overall and Gorham 1962) and the psychoticism factor from the Hopkins Symptom Checklist—90 (Derogatis et al. 1974) were the most discriminating factors. Further they reported that "anxiety, depression and interpersonal sensitivity increase earlier than did BPRS thought disorder" (p. 46).

The final prospective study of relapse (Subotnik and Neuchterlein 1988) included patients in early phases of schizophrenia with their first psychotic episode occurring not longer than 2 years before study contact. Several interesting comparisons were done in this study using the patient as his or her own control (the "within-patient comparison") and with patients who did not relapse (the "between-patients comparison"). Symptomatology was compared during the 6 weeks prior to relapse with periods that did not precede relapse using factors from the BPRS. For the within-patient comparison, increases were reported for thought disturbance and anxiety-depression. Subtle changes were detected in unusual

Table 24–1. Rank order of symptoms

Symptom	%	Symptom	%
Tense and nervous	80.4	Preoccupied	59.6
Eating less	71.7	Seeing friends less	59.6
Trouble concentrating	69.6	Feeling laughed at	59.6
Trouble sleeping	67.4	Loss of interest	56.5
Enjoy things less	65.2	More religious thinking	54.3
Restlessness	63.0	Feeling bad for no reason	54.3
Can't remember things	63.0	Feeling too excited	52.2
Depression	60.9	Hear voices/see things	50.0

thought content and hallucinations. Less change was found for depression, somatic concern, and guilt. The between-patient comparison found increases in hostility and grandiosity. Small increases were reported for strange thought content and unusual perceptual experiences. Subotnik and Neuchterlein's conclusions from the differences found in comparing "within" to "between" patient groups were that those patients with hostility and grandiosity were at higher risk for relapse in general, but that these symptoms did not predict imminent relapse as a prodromal symptom. Further, they, like Marder and colleagues (1984), found that the odd thought content increased quite late (2–4 weeks) prior to relapse.

Early morbid pattern of emotional withdrawal and negative symptoms. In general, the early morbid patterns of schizophrenia are a reflection of more enduring characteristics than the subthreshold psychotic symptoms discussed above.

The premorbid adjustment literature provides us with a description of the difficulty working in this area. As several studies have shown, the categorical presence or absence of a symptom can be assessed reliably (Fenton and McGlashan 1987; Stephens 1978; Vaillant 1964a, 1964b), but the timing of onset is uncertain. Further, each of these studies concluded that the predictive value of its scale in either a positive or negative direction is a dimensional phenomenon that makes the total score a better predictor than any single predictor.

Discussion

It is clear that there is a period of time prior to the onset of psychosis that includes symptoms other than those listed under A in DSM-III-R (p. 194). Lieberman and colleagues (1992) demonstrated this with a sample of first-break patients. They found

- Age at first psychiatric symptoms: 21.3
- Age at first psychotic symptoms: 23.3
- Age at first treatment: 23

The implication of this is that there was a year of psychiatric symptoms before the patient was seen in treatment, and slightly more than a year before the onset of psychotic symptoms. The diagnostic problem caused by the assessment of prodrome then is not hypothetical.

Gradually emerging psychosis. In general, the above studies indicate that prodromal symptoms of gradually emerging psychosis (remembering these are for relapse—how relevant this is to first episode is difficult to estimate) can be reliably rated (Herz and Melville 1980). Further, prospective studies are able to validate the relevance and proximity of prodromal symptoms to onset of psychotic symptoms. What is equally important to note, however, is that prodromal symptoms appear quite proximate to relapse (1–2 months) and do not seem to extend to 6 months.

Early morbid pattern of emotional withdrawal and negative symptoms. The problems noted above are clear: the presence as determined by a composite score is reliable, but the actual dating of their onset remains elusive.

General. Although it becomes clear that the symptoms of prodrome can be reasonably assessed in terms of presence or absence, there are two substantial problems. First is the conceptual problem created by combining prepsychotic symptoms (e.g., markedly peculiar behavior, odd beliefs, unusual perceptual experiences) with "negative-like symptoms" (e.g., marked social isolation, blunted or inappropriate affect, marked lack of initiative) (Andreasen 1982). It seems logical that these symptoms may come from entirely different domains of psychopathology. The clinical implications of the onset of psychosis are different for patients who have had long-standing negative or negative-like symptoms as compared with patients who have not or whose psychosis began relatively recently (e.g., 2 months) with prepsychotic symptoms only.

Second, possibly stemming from the above, is that the prepsychotic symptoms, although easier to date for onset, occur relatively closer to the beginning of frank psychotic symptoms than 6 months; and the negative-like symptoms, which are longer in duration, are quite difficult to date in terms of onset.

Duration of Psychotic Symptoms

Statement of the Issues

The purpose of this review is to examine the difference between two potential duration periods for psychotic symptoms—1 week or 1 month—to meet criteria for schizophrenia. The need for considering these two time intervals has been caused by the proposed criteria for ICD-10, emphasizing 1 month of psychotic symptoms.

ICD-10 proposed that "psychotic" symptoms "should have been clearly present for most of the time during a period of one month or more" (World Health Organization 1988, p. 60). It further specified:

> Viewed retrospectively it may be clear that a prodromal phase in which symptoms and behavior, such as loss of interest in work, social activities and personal appearance and hygiene, together with generalized anxiety and mild degrees of depression and preoccupation may precede the onset of psychotic symptoms by weeks or months. *Because of the difficulty in timing onset,* the one month duration

> criterion applies only to specific symptoms listed above and not to any prodromal nonpsychotic phase. (World Health Organization 1988, p. 60, italics added)

As noted earlier, ICD-10 defined the issue of retrospective data collection to refer to 1 month only. Other than the above statement regarding neuroleptic-induced negative symptoms, ICD-10 essentially ignores treatment response except to note that "conditions meeting such symptomatic requirements but of a duration less than one month (whether treated or not) should be diagnosed . . . as acute schizophrenia-like psychotic disorder (F23.2) and reclassified as schizophrenia if the symptoms persist for longer periods [1 month] of time" (World Health Organization 1988, p. 60).

The DSM-III-R criteria require a 6-month duration of illness for the diagnosis of schizophrenia. However, in terms of psychotic symptoms (criteria A), it requires only 1 week and even that has a proviso. The exact criteria requires 1 week (or less if symptoms have been successfully treated) of psychotic symptoms; the remaining 5 months and 3 weeks may be composed of either prodromal or residual symptoms.

Significance of the Issues

The significance of duration becomes quite apparent particularly with initial-onset patients. DSM-III-R criteria imply that characteristic psychotic symptoms *may* be "successfully treated" in less than 1 week, or in any event that 1 week of psychotic symptoms is sufficient to meet the diagnosis of schizophrenia. If this is correct, many patients who would be classified as having schizophrenia under DSM-III-R criteria would not meet ICD-10 criteria and would fall into the ICD-10 category of acute schizophrenia-like psychotic disorder. For the well-established case of schizophrenia (long course of psychotic symptoms with progressive deterioration), meeting either criteria for the diagnosis is not difficult because symptoms will have been present for enough time to satisfy either diagnostic system.

We have attempted to determine the origins of the 1-month time period as a tradition of diagnosis. There would appear to be only limited data addressing this point, most which are not distinctly set up to address the difference between one week and one month of symptomatology. From a traditional standpoint, the British development of the Present State Examination (PSE) (Wing et al. 1974), which has used a 1-month time frame, appears to have relied on clinical judgment in this determination. We were able trace this origin back to the following passages from Wing and colleagues:

> The time period covered is one month before the interview. During the development stage, periods of three months and one week were tried out, as was a purely

> "present state" interview. The last of these alternatives [present state interview] was least satisfactory since the time of most intense subjective experience of the symptoms was often a week or two before interview; that is, before the patient had contacted the service. Similarly, one week was often too short a period. On the other hand, many patients found it difficult to cover a period as long as three months without constant reminders. One month appeared to be a comfortable period to keep in mind. No doubt for special purposes a shorter or longer period would need to be specified (if examinations were to be conducted at weekly intervals for example) but the schedule itself is written in terms of one month. . . .
>
> It should be noted that the effect of limiting the period covered to four weeks is to exclude from consideration certain traits which can only be assessed on the basis of a much larger knowledge of the subject's attitudes, behaviour and reactions. Thus personality disorders and mental retardation, for example, could not be evaluated on the basis of only four weeks in the subject's life. The PSE schedule is not intended to cover such conditions. (pp. 13–14)

Although it seems reasonable to assume that most persons who would be diagnosed as having schizophrenia by ICD-10 would meet criteria for either schizophrenia or schizophreniform in DSM-III-R, the reverse is not true in that those people who had more than 1 week, but less than 4 weeks of psychotic symptoms, would meet DSM-III-R but not ICD-10 standards. The major group of concern would be those who respond to treatment within this 1- to 4-week period.

Methods

Our literature review found no studies that were designed to evaluate the question of whether 1 week (or less if successfully treated) or 1 month of psychotic symptoms was a "better" length of time. Ideally, the study of such a question would require consideration of the following:

1. All patients who presented with psychotic symptomatology for the first time would be diagnosed by both DSM-III-R and ICD-10.
2. Symptom rating scales would be conducted daily to establish both duration and the ICD-10 requirement that these symptoms be present "most of the time."
3. Longitudinal follow-up would be conducted to determine whether those who recovered early differed in clinical course from those whose symptoms persisted for 1 month.
4. Genetic and eventually biological studies of the two groups from item 3 above would be undertaken to evaluate genetic or biological validation of the dichotomy.

Because the ideal study was not available, we turned to other types of studies within which were partial answers to the duration issue. The body of literature that we found most helpful, therefore, in examining the 1 week-1 month issue came from clinical trials studies. It was our expectation that the clinical trials would provide information about the likelihood of symptom remission within the first month of treatment and would therefore provide information on the magnitude of the impact of a criterion change from 1 week to 1 month. It should be remembered, however, that these studies selected patients based on a diagnosis of schizophrenia made from DSM of varying versions. As a result, even in relatively acute onset patients, some degree of use of prodrome may have been considered.

Specifically, what we were interested in was the time it takes for psychotic symptoms, once observed and treated, to be considered no longer present. Because in most of these studies the date of onset of symptoms is not stated, we were forced to date onset from when the patient first came to the study (or treatment) and to ask how long it took from this point for the symptoms to remit. This is far from an exact methodology for determining a 1 week-1 month difference.

We therefore chose representative studies from several methodological perspectives (clinical and biological) to examine these issues. There are, no doubt, many other studies that would bear on this early phase of treatment response, but the clinical trial studies noted above provided examples of relevant data and the inferential limitations of the data. It is the limitations that restrict the review to only a limited number of reports. A complete literature review of all clinical trials would not have been fruitful because they were not designed to address our questions. Our inclusion criteria required the study of patients with relatively acute onset of psychotic symptoms who were in their initial episode or whose relapse was observed under research conditions, as well as data collected during the first month of symptomatology. These criteria greatly reduced the literature available. The studies that were selected had the following characteristics.

First, the studies involve patients already diagnosed as schizophrenic through some system of classification and therefore did not include patients presenting with psychotic symptomatology for the first time. It seems to us that the use of hospitalized patients as a starting point would skew the sample toward the most severely ill and therefore the group least likely to recover in the 1- to 4-week time period. In fact, many of those who might fall into this rapid recovery group might avoid psychiatric hospitalization altogether.

Second, the patients were at varying points in the course of their illness and so most probably had had well over a month of symptoms prior to the treatment study.

Third, the results for the most part were reported as group means and thus would not reflect individual outlying patients who might have had mild symptoms or none at all in the time period being assessed. It was these patients who were particularly important in establishing the impact of a 1 week versus 1 month difference in symptom duration.

The following section includes relevant data from two ongoing studies. Again, these studies were not designed to answer the 1 week-1 month question, but they do provide relevant data on this topic.

Results

Literature review. From the early studies of phenothiazine treatment of acute schizophrenia (Cole et al. 1964), it has generally been assumed that treatment response in the first month of treatment is striking. In that original study of more than 400 patients, 60% were first admissions; 50% were first-episode patients with a mean symptom duration of 2.6 months. It is important to recall that diagnostic criteria were not up to DSM-III standards and reflect a broader group of patients than would ever enter a study today. The results indicate that at 6 weeks, approximately 50% of the sample had almost no symptoms, but that auditory hallucinations were one of the symptoms that changed least compared with such symptoms as agitation and tension.

As noted by Baldessarini (1980), the length of time for resolution of psychotic symptoms is considerably longer from a clinical standpoint than we might have previously thought. He concluded that, for as long as 6 weeks, psychotic symptoms are still responding to antipsychotic medication and that the early responses are mainly from the sedative quality of the drug and not from its antipsychotic property.

In a study designed to test the correlation of plasma homovanillic acid levels (a dopamine metabolite) with clinical change, Pickar and colleagues (1986) provided support for Baldessarini's (1980) clinical observations in finding that a 6-week period of time is required to reach clinical improvement. The study was obviously not designed to test a 1-week versus 1-month duration of psychotic symptoms, although it would lend some support for symptoms still persisting at 4–6 weeks.

Kay and Singh (1989) reported on a study from pooled data on 62 schizophrenic patients treated over an extensive period of time at the Bronx Veterans Administration Hospital in New York. The patients were "mainly in the acute or subacute phase of illness" (p. 712) for as long as 5 years of illness. During a drug-free baseline period, Kay and Singh reported good stability of both positive and negative symptoms. Their next outcome point was after 3–4 months of neuroleptic treatment, at which time they found 51.5% improvement in positive symptoms.

Johnstone and colleagues (1978) conducted a double-blind trial of an alpha-isomer of flupenthixol (a dopamine blocker) and beta-flupenthixol (a nondopamine receptor blocker) on 45 acute schizophrenic patients who had developed PSE symptoms of schizophrenia within the past month. For our needs, the important issue is whether symptoms significantly improved in either group over the 4-week trial. Total scores improved for the dopamine blocker by a magnitude of about 70%, but of even more importance is that hallucinations and incoherence fell to almost zero. Negative symptoms changed relatively little, and delusions were in an intermediate position of some change.

Breier and colleagues (1987) conducted a study of neuroleptic withdrawal, followed by neuroleptic treatment in 19 young "patients meeting DSM-III criteria for schizophrenia" (p. 1550) to determine the responsiveness of negative symptoms to neuroleptics. In addition to finding that negative symptoms that occur in conjunction with positive symptoms on neuroleptic withdrawal are responsive to reinstitution of the neuroleptic, the study provided a view of symptom evolution and neuroleptic responsiveness over a 4-week period. On neuroleptic withdrawal, positive and negative symptoms increased approximately 25%, with a peak at 3 weeks. On neuroleptic reinstitution, a 25% decline was seen—within 2 weeks for positive symptoms and over 4 weeks for negative symptoms.

It does appear, then, that there is clinical improvement over the first 4 weeks of treatment. Data from the National Institute of Mental Health (1983) Treatment Strategies in Schizophrenia (TSS) Cooperative Agreement Program below clearly show that this early improvement is significant in predicting early outcome results.

Relevant data. The TSS is an ongoing study examining the treatment outcome of various dosing strategies in interaction with family management strategies. For the preliminary data analysis, the TSS study identified variables collected during the stabilization period that could predict likelihood of stabilization; demographic characteristics, diagnosis, psychopathology, social adjustment, treatment history, and assignment to applied or supportive family treatment. Each of these variables is utilized as the dependent measure in analyses (categorical or linear) that also allow the examination of three-way categorization of "stabilization status" (entered double-blind study, nonstabilized, noncooperative), the five sites, and the interaction of site and stabilization status. Table 24–2 presents the severity of psychopathology at the first evaluation period approximately 1 month after hospitalization (Hargreaves et al. 1990). It is important to note several features:

1. Positive symptoms from the BPRS after 1 month are now in the mild-moderate range, and their decline predicts the likelihood of stabilization at a later time.
2. Negative symptoms—either BPRS or the Scale for the Assessment of Negative Symptoms (Andreasen and Olsen 1982)—changed relatively little and did not predict early outcome.
3. For our purposes, the results are subject to all the criticisms described above.

In a prospective study of the psychobiology of first-episode schizophrenic patients (Lieberman et al. 1992), preliminary data on 57 patients showed the majority (78%) received a diagnosis of schizophrenia and the remaining patients were diagnosed as schizoaffective-manic (7%) and schizoaffective-depressive (14%).

The course of illness also provides us with some interesting data:

- Age at study entrance: 23.9 years
- Age at first psychiatric symptoms: 21.3 years
- Age at first psychotic symptoms: 23.3 years
- Age at first treatment: 23 years

This study seems to come as close as we are likely to get to answering our question based on clinical trials. It should be noted, however, that there is approximately a year and a half from the onset of "psychotic symptoms" to the entrance into this research project. Although this may be as good as we can hope for in any research project, it still does not provide information on the first month of psychotic symptoms. It appears, however, that there will indeed be diagnosis

Table 24–2. Treatment strategies in schizophrenia study stabilization analyses: mean severity of psychopathology during stabilization

	Stabilization status				
	Entered double-blind	**Non-stabilized**	**Non-cooperation**	*F*	*P*
Time from admission to baseline evaluations (days)	38.2	34.4	35.4	0.35	NS[a]
BPRS factors *n*	132	40	22		
Anxiety-depression	2.2	2.4	2.9	4.97	.008[b]
Anergia	2.0	2.1	2.4	2.55	NS
Thought disturbance	2.3	3.0	2.5	4.64	.01[a]
Activation	1.5	1.6	1.8	2.89	.05
Hostile-suspicious	1.9	2.2	2.7	7.52	.0007
Severity of illness	4.0	4.6	4.4	7.32	.0009[a]
SANS global ratings *n*	93	32	13		
Affective flattening	2.4	2.4	2.6	0.06	NS
Alogia	1.8	1.9	1.8	0.04	NS
Avolition/apathy	2.4	2.8	2.7	1.48	NS
Anhedonia	2.5	2.8	2.7	0.83	NS
Attention	2.0	2.2	2.2	0.11	NS[a]

Note. NS = not significant. BPRS = Brief Psychiatric Rating Scale. SANS = Schedule for the Assessment of Negative Symptoms.
[a]Site main effect significant.
[b]Site by stabilization status interaction and site main effect significant.

questions for treating clinicians as patients apparently do seek treatment at the time of or even slightly prior to the onset of psychotic symptoms. Whether there is an absolute need to have a diagnosis at this point is questionable, but certainly diagnostic (classification) uncertainty would occur.

Regarding the time course for stabilization and for positive and negative symptoms, Lieberman's (personal communication, 1990) preliminary findings show that there is a small group of patients (10%–15%) who would respond in the first 4 weeks of treatment. However, the time course above should be borne in mind—these are people who on average have had psychotic symptoms for more than a year. Whether there is a small group with onset in the last week is not known. It is interesting to note as well that the investigators have defined a rapid response group but that 11 weeks is the cutoff point.

Discussion

It is our assessment that the data needed to resolve completely the issue of 1 week versus 1 month are not available. It appears likely, however, that if the prepsychotic prodromal symptoms are included, and for most cases even if they are not, very few psychotic episodes last less than 1 month; those that do, we know almost nothing about. Still, altering the current DSM criteria to 1 month would create several logistic and scientific problems that need to be considered.

First, most ongoing studies in the United States are based on the 1 week criterion, and a change would require a rediagnosis of entire research samples.

Second, for a select group of patients (e.g., acute onset, first break), there would be a 1-month delay in establishing a diagnosis of schizophrenia. Either the entrance into a variety of protocols would be delayed, or, if they are entered, some patients might later have to be dropped for not meeting criteria. Further, a month in the prevailing current rapid discharge zeitgeist (average length of stay approximately 14 days, although in the TSS study the range was 22.8–52.1 days) would mean that the waiting period necessary to establish a diagnosis might exceed the observation period available.

Third, not altering DSM-IV to meet international diagnostic criteria will leave us with an idiosyncratic national system, making international collaboration and interpretation of results impossible.

Six-Month Duration Criterion

Statement of the Issues

The purpose of this review is to examine the appropriateness of the 6-month criterion for diagnosing schizophrenia. The original pressure for a thorough review of this area has been somewhat overtaken by the decision by ICD-10 to use 1 month of psychotic symptoms as the duration criterion and to eliminate prodromal and residual symptoms as contributing to duration.

As mentioned earlier, DSM-III-R criteria require a 6-month duration of illness for the diagnosis of schizophrenia. This duration may, however, be composed of 1 week (or less if successfully treated) of psychotic symptoms and, for the remaining 5 months and 3 weeks, be composed of either prodromal or residual symptoms. It is not difficult for the well-established case of schizophrenia (long course of psychotic symptoms with progressive deterioration) to meet this diagnostic criteria. It becomes problematic, however, with the patient's first presentation to a clinician. The questions for meeting criteria have become whether symptoms should be assessed prospectively or retrospectively, what symptoms count, and how long they need to be present.

Significance of the Issues

We feel a discussion of the 6-month criterion is still merited because even if DSM-IV were to accept the ICD-10 1-month duration, it would still be possible to nest a 6-month category within this framework—for example, by defining a more chronic condition of schizophrenia that requires persistent symptomatology of some kind (positive, negative, residual).

The central rationale for having this review thus becomes a reconsideration of the idea that over a single day (5 months, 29 days versus 6 months), a diagnosis should change from schizophreniform (not even a part of the schizophrenia section of DSM-III-R) to schizophrenia. It is an idea that many find intellectually unsatisfying.

At first it must be decided whether a pattern of onset of illness should be a significant factor in establishing a diagnosis. At this point in the history of medicine, little argument will be found over this issue, both from a practical standpoint (this is frequently when the patient is first seen) and from a scientific one (the early evolution of symptoms may contribute to diagnosis and prognosis). But once this has been decided, the various means of characterizing the early course of illness must be considered. Many writers have noted that the current diagnosis of schizophrenia with its requirement of 6 months of symptoms skews toward chronicity of outcome (Kendell 1988; Wynne 1988). In general, at issue is that the current criterion potentially establishes a tautology—the longer one has an illness, the more likely one is to have it for a long time. Or as McGlashan (1988) noted, there is the "Heisenberg Uncertainty Principle" of predicting outcome in schizophrenia—"the entity you are measuring moves simply by virtue of how you define it" (p. 533).

Ultimately, of course, the validity of a 6-month duration depends on how it *defines* or *contributes* to the form of illness by predicting outcome or genetic or biological homogeneity. Treatment response may also help to define illness (e.g., lithium with bipolar disorder), but in a less exact manner due to the broad spectrum of response with some treatments (e.g., aspirin and fever, neuroleptics and psychosis) and individual response differences (host factors).

As validating features become an increasingly significant companion to reliability of diagnostic criteria in psychiatry, the interaction of validity and reliability assumes greater importance. Critical in establishing the validity of a diagnosis is the reliability of the information used in making it. Factors that increase reliability of data are prospective collection and marked or discreet differences between a symptom and normal range of behavior. Factors that decrease reliability of data are retrospective collection and similarity between a symptom and normal range of behavior. Lying between these two would be combinations of them—prospective collection and similarity between a symptom and normal range of behavior and retrospective collection and marked or discreet differences between a symptom and normal range of behavior. A secondary factor relevant to retrospectively collected data is how retrospective (length of time) and how exact the dating must be.

The 6-month criterion for prodromal symptoms, which are defined as a "clear deterioration in functioning before the active phase of the disturbance" (American Psychiatric Association 1987, p. 194), appears to be an attempt to define specifically what has often been called with less specificity "insidious onset." For example, in Helzer and colleagues' (1983) article, which has often been cited as the benchmark study for the 6-month criterion, the authors accepted the premise that "it seems more appropriate to view the six month criterion as insidious onset rather than established chronicity" (p. 1280). What seems unfortunate in this process is that in creating an appearance of exactness by giving an actual time frame, we may actually be losing a potentially valuable concept of pattern of onset in the debate over whether 6 months is the exactly correct time period. A further problem is created by assigning a 6-month criterion to equal insidious onset—duration of symptoms or prodrome at initial presentation may well be more dependent on sociocultural differences in help seeking than on the disorder itself (Lin et al. 1978).

It appears, however, that there is value to longitudinal criteria, and indeed the studies below provide us with ample support for that. The question remains, however: how should it be used?

Methods

We examined the literature on longitudinal studies that used varying lengths of illness either to predict outcome or to examine familial aggregation based on varying lengths of illness. Relatively few studies were actually designed to provide information directly on this point, and even those that purportedly were designed for this purpose may have fallen victim to the circularity noted below.

Results

Several comprehensive reviews have clearly demonstrated that the addition of longitudinal criteria to the cross-sectional psychotic symptoms of schizophrenia add predictive validity to the diagnosis (Angst 1988; Harding 1988; McGlashan 1988). Others have pointed out that creation of a tautological validity (the longer a person has a disorder, the more likely one is to continue with it) is a clear risk of this approach (Fenton and McGlashan 1987; Strauss and Carpenter 1979). Again, it may be important to restate that for well-established courses of illness, the differential diagnosis of schizophrenia may not be as difficult, and therefore the pattern of illness (e.g., well-established chronicity) is highly relevant. Even here, however, we are faced with several excellent studies that amply demonstrate the heterogeneity of outcome of schizophrenia after many years of established illness (Ciompi 1980; Harding et al. 1987a, 1987b; McGlashan 1984a, 1984b, 1987). The problem of examining longitudinal outcome in a cross-sectional approach is that the cutoff point has a high degree of likelihood of establishing its own validity because the more chronic group, those lying at and beyond the cutoff point, will include those for whom established outcome (usually negative) is more homogeneous. Those who are in the stage of illness before the cutoff point will be a mixed group, some of whom will indeed progress on to a chronic course, and some of whom may recover. Even extending this logic further, one could move the cutoff point, but what would we learn from this?

A similar problem also exists in determining duration of illness as it did in determining duration of prodrome. For example, are there differences between someone whose "criterion A" symptoms remain for 6 months and someone who has a lower level of symptoms (residual and prodrome are the same) "post-psychotic" or someone whose symptoms following the acute episode are mainly negative or "negative-like."

Only one study that we were able to identify examined this latter point, and it did so only indirectly (Beiser et al. 1988). As we noted earlier, one way of looking at the 6-month criterion would be to examine schizophreniform versus schizophrenia diagnoses. Beiser and colleagues studied 29 subjects with schizophreniform disorder and found that 8 (28%) recovered and 18 (62%) went on to be diagnosed as schizophrenic at the 9-month follow-up. Three patients (10%) were rediagnosed as having affective disorder. In their conclusions, Beiser and colleagues noted that the schizophreniform patients who did not recover resembled the first-episode schizophrenic patients in outcome measures, emphasizing the point made by Lin and colleagues (1978) earlier that help seeking may bring some people in before 6 months have elapsed. They then went on to examine predictors for the recovered or "true" schizophreniform category, noting that the recovered group, when compared with the nonrecovered group, was characterized by better premorbid functioning (88%), less restricted affect (75%), and generally better rapport with the interviewer (87%). Although these may be important factors in prognosis, and they indeed reached statistical significance, whether they create a diagnostically separate group is questionable. Their data suggest that on these same variables—good premorbid adjustment, less restricted affect, and good rapport—the nonrecovered schizophreniform patients (NR SZF) and the schizophrenic patients (SZ) had appreciable representation as follows:

- Good premorbid adjustment: NR SZF 17%, SZ 25%
- Less restricted affect: NR SZF 44%, SZ 44%
- Good rapport: NR SZF 63%, SZ 69%

It is also useful to note that the inverse of these variables (poor premorbid, restricted affect, and poor rapport) would all fall in the negative or negative-like symptom category. Further, from this study, we can suggest that the 6-month period may be important if a patient *recovers* in that time frame. This should be contrasted, however, with how long a patient had had the illness when first seen.

The remainder of the studies examined the relevance of duration of illness on presentation and whether this type of longitudinal approach added to the validity of the diagnosis. Helzer and colleagues (1981) (also see critique by Fenton 1982) found support for the 6-month criterion being predictive of outcome in differentiating schizophrenia from schizophreniform disorder. Helzer and colleagues' (1983) elegantly designed study established that those who had been ill less than 6 months had a better outcome than those who had been ill 6 months or more. Obviously, however, not all those who had been ill less than 6 months had good outcomes, otherwise there would never have been a group with more than 6 months of illness! What this demonstrates is that for defining poor outcome, an illness duration of 6 months or more defines a group with worse outcomes than those with a duration of less than 6 months. For defining good outcome, the inverse is also true—duration of less than 6 months captures a group whose outcome is better than those with a duration of more than 6 months.

We return now to the question regarding moving the cutoff point. Regardless of the movement of the cutting point, as long as the group "past the cutoff point" contains all patients beyond it, such patients will have a significantly poorer outcome on tests of between-group differences. The longer one extends the cutoff point, the *more* homogeneous will be the poor outcome in the group past the cutoff point. A general assumption has been that if one extended the cutoff point to 7 months, 1 year, 2 years, or 10 years, one would find a level of increasing homogeneity of poor outcome in the group past the cutoff point at the expense of increasing the heterogeneity of the group before the cutoff point.

In a meta-analysis review of outcome studies, McGlashan (1988) suggested that the chronicity threshold may be from 6 months to 1 year. He based this conclusion on the difference in outcome found among the three studies of patients with short-term illness—the Massachusetts Mental Health study (Vaillant 1964a, 1964b), the Phipps Clinic study (Stephens 1970, 1978; Stephens and Astrup 1963, 1965), and the Alberta study (Bland et al. 1976)—and the Iowa 500 (Tsuang et al. 1979, 1980). He concluded:

> The outcome of the Iowa 500 cohort was decidedly worse than the other cohorts [above] and all of the Iowa 500 patients had been manifestly ill for more than 6 months, as required by the Feighner criteria, or for more than one year (85%), but not much longer. (p. 529)

Studies that followed chronicity further indicate still worse outcomes as chronicity gets longer (G. Gardos, J. O. Cole, R. A. LaBrie: A twelve-year follow-up study of 124 chronic hospitalized schizophrenics, I: current psychosocial adjustment, unpublished manuscript, 1982; Gardos et al. 1982; McGlashan 1984a, 1984b, 1987), with the single exception being the Vermont State Hospital Followup (Harding et al. 1987a, 1987b). However, the process appears to plateau by 5 years, as exemplified by the lack of change between the 5- and 11-year follow-up in the Washington International Pilot Study of Schizophrenia (Carpenter et al., unpublished manuscript, 1987).

Carpenter and colleagues (unpublished manuscript, 1987) concluded that cross-sectional data alone offer little predictive validity in terms of heterogeneity of outcome. Helzer and colleagues' (1983) examination of 121 patients with functional psychosis demonstrated clearly how the combination of 6 months of illness when combined with DSM-III symptoms added to the prediction of outcome, but because he did not test other lengths of duration, we do not have a test of a minimum or maximum threshold period.

Coryell and Tsuang (1982) provided us with just such an analysis for a relatively short-term follow-up: 3.1 year average. They looked at six different time periods: 2 weeks to 1 month; 1 month to 6 months; 6 months to 1 year; 1 year to 2 years; 2 years to 5 years; and more than 5 years. Only 1 month or less symptomatology predicted a significantly better outcome than the next time duration group. In comparing the 1–6 months category, statistically significant differences were not found until the category was compared with the more than 5 years group. In their 40-year follow-up group, Coryell and Tsuang found that no duration threshold "recommended itself over any other" (p. 68). In the comparisons between schizophreniform and schizophrenia over four outcome domains—marital, occupational, mental, and residential—statistical differences were found only for the marital status category, although small trends were present favoring schizophreniform patients in the latter three. Although this study is quite persuasive, one must still realize that the duration criterion was established at index admission and is subject to the help-seeking differences confound mentioned earlier.

In a follow-up of the United States/United Kingdom cohort at an average of 6.5 years after the index admission, Helzer and colleagues (1981) reported that there were no differences found between those patients with schizophrenia and those with schizophreniform diagnoses on the following symptom scales: passivity, auditory hallucinations, delusions, persecution, and defect state. Only manic symptoms of all those measured showed a significant difference. On general outcome measures, percentage of time in hospital, and combined social status score and outcome regression score there were significant differences favoring the schizophreniform group. This would appear to be in contrast to Coryell and Tsuang (1982), but the variables of hospitalization, social status, and outcome regression scores were probably influenced by sample selection as well as by psychopathology (see McGlashan 1988 for a discussion of sample selection and outcome variables). At a minimum, the psychopathology findings support the Iowa study. Further potentially influencing the samples were the small numbers of subjects involved (19 with schizophrenia; 7 with schizophreniform disorder).

Discussion

There can be relatively little question that duration of symptoms will predict outcome, but the question remains as to whether it does so more than the inherent tautology would predict. As we noted earlier, a diagnosis that uses duration as a criterion, particularly one that goes beyond the necessity of establishing "true presence" of symptoms (in our case not just a "puff of madness" or as the French system refers to it—bouffee delirante), is going to be subject to that criticism. We would like to suggest that a certain time period, therefore, certainly needs to be a part of any system just to ensure that a symptom is present. Beyond that, however, it would seem to us that it may well be the negative or "negative-like" symptoms, whether existing prior to the onset of psychosis or developing in the postpsychotic period (and likewise their absence in either of these periods) that may be what clinicians, researchers, and nosologists would find more useful.

Recommendations

Prodrome and Residual Symptoms

Whether to use prodrome and residual symptoms at all is the first decision point. Our recommendation takes into consideration that ICD-10 will not be using these symptoms in its diagnostic criteria. For DSM to include them as part of the diagnostic classification will leave us with a conflicting nosology. We would therefore prefer to recommend their use to characterize, not classify.

If prodrome and residual symptoms are to be kept, one additional possibility would be to subdivide them into two subtypes (or three if role functioning is separated) of positive and negative character. These symptoms would then potentially account for the additional 5 months of symptomatology required to reach a diagnosis (as is the case for DSM-III-R). Further, the presence or absence of negative-like or frank negative symptoms could be used as a characterizing or subtyping variable either preceding or following the onset of the characteristic criterion A symptoms.

Duration of Psychotic Symptoms

It is difficult to make a recommendation as of this writing, and no solution will be universally satisfactory. The impact on the research community in the United States either of changing or of having an idiosyncratic national diagnostic system by not changing does not suggest much in the way of a compromise position. At this point it may, however, be the better of the two choices to adopt the 1 month of psychotic symptoms as a base requirement for entering the schizophrenia spectrum. Whether to then extend a category from 1 month to 6 months and call it schizophreniform, and to call what extends beyond 6 months schizophrenia, will require a judgment on whether there are data to support this dichotomization. At least this way, the schizophreniform and schizophrenia categories will nest within what the ICD-10 is labeling schizophrenia.

Six-Month Duration Criteria

Although we feel that the 6-month criterion suffers from less support than we would like, the established use of this time period in at least American psychiatry may make its retention useful. Subdividing schizophrenia into 1-month and 6-month segments would still permit it to be "nested" within the ICD-10 system. We would again like to call for additional research on this topic in an effort to use duration to characterize schizophrenia, not classify it.

With each of these topics, the current review represents a data base in evolution. The forthcoming field trials will examine many of these issues and permit the final decisions on them to be increasingly well informed.

References

American Psychiatric Association: Diagnostic and Statistical Manual of Mental Disorders, 3rd Edition. Washington, DC, American Psychiatric Association, 1980

American Psychiatric Association: Diagnostic and Statistical Manual of Mental Disorders, 3rd Edition, Revised. Washington, DC, American Psychiatric Association, 1987

Andreasen NC: Negative symptoms in schizophrenia: definition and reliability. Arch Gen Psychiatry 39:784–788, 1982

Andreasen NC, Olsen S: Negative v positive schizophrenia: definition and validation. Arch Gen Psychiatry 39:789–794, 1982

Angst J: European long-term follow-up studies of schizophrenia. Schizophr Bull 14:501–513, 1988

Baldessarini RJ: Drugs and the treatment of psychiatric disorders, in The Pharmacologic Basis of Therapeutics. Edited by Gilman AG, Goodman LS, Gilman A. New York, Macmillan, 1980, pp 391–447

Beiser M, Fleming JAE, Iacono WG, et al: Refining the diagnosis of schizophreniform disorder. Am J Psychiatry 145:695–700, 1988

Bland RC, Parker JH, Orn, H: Prognosis in schizophrenia: a ten-year follow-up of first admissions. Arch Gen Psychiatry 33:949–954, 1976

Bleuler M: The Schizophrenic Disorders: Long-Term Patient and Family Studies. Translated by Clemens S. New Haven, CT, Yale University Press, 1978

Breier A, Wolkowitz OM, Doran AR, et al: Neuroleptic responsivity of negative and positive symptoms in schizophrenia. Am J Psychiatry 144:1549–1555, 1987

Ciompi L: Catamnestic long-term study on the course of life and aging of schizophrenics. Schizophr Bull 6:606–618, 1980

Cole JO, Klerman GL, Goldberg SC: Phenothiazine treatment in acute schizophrenia. Arch Gen Psychiatry 10:246–261, 1964

Coryell WC, Tsuang MT: DSM-III schizophreniform disorder: comparisons with schizophrenia and affective disorder. Arch Gen Psychiatry 39:66–69, 1982

Derogatis LR, Lipman RS, Rickels K, et al: The Hopkins Symptom Checklist (HSCL): a self-report symptom inventory. Behav Sci 19:1–15, 1974

Docherty JP, Van Kammen DP, Siris SG, et al: Stages of onset of schizophrenic psychosis. Am J Psychiatry 135:420–426, 1978

Fenton WS: Definition of schizophrenia. Arch Gen Psychiatry 39:357, 1982

Fenton W, McGlashan T: Prognostic scale for chronic schizophrenia. Schizophr Bull 13:277–286, 1987

Gardos G, Cole JO, LaBrie RA: A twelve-year follow-up study of chronic schizophrenics. Hosp Community Psychiatry 33:983–984, 1982

Harding CM: Course types in schizophrenia: an analysis of European and American studies. Schizophr Bull 14:633–643, 1988

Harding CM, Brooks GW, Ashikaga T, et al: The Vermont longitudinal study of persons with severe mental illness, I: methodology, study sample, and overall status 32 years later. Am J Psychiatry 144:718–726, 1987a

Harding CM, Brooks GW, Ashikaga T, et al: The Vermont longitudinal study of persons with severe mental illness, II: long-term outcome of subjects who retrospectively met DSM-III criteria for schizophrenia. Am J Psychiatry 144:727–735, 1987b

Hargreaves WA, Kane JM, Ninan PT, et al: The Treatment Strategies in Schizophrenia Collaborative Study Group: demographic characteristics, treatment history, presenting psychopathology and early course in schizophrenia. Psychopharmacol Bull 25:340–343, 1990

Heinrichs DW, Carpenter WT: Prospective study of prodromal symptoms in schizophrenic relapse. Am J Psychiatry 142:371–373, 1985

Helzer JE, Brockington IF, Kendell RE: Predictive validity of DSM-III and Feighner definitions of schizophrenia: a comparison with research diagnostic criteria and CATEGO. Arch Gen Psychiatry 38:791–797, 1981

Helzer JE, Kendell RE, Brockington IF: Contributions of the six-month criterion to the predictive validity of the DSM-III definition of schizophrenia. Arch Gen Psychiatry 40:1277–1280, 1983

Herz MI, Melville C: Relapse in schizophrenia. Am J Psychiatry 137:801–807, 1980

Herz MI, Szymanski MV, Simon JC: Intermittent medication of stable schizophrenic outpatients: an alternative to maintenance medication. Am J Psychiatry 139:918–922, 1982

Johnstone EC, Crow TJ, Frith CD: Mechanism of the antipsychotic effect in the treatment of acute schizophrenia. Lancet 1:848–851, 1978

Kay SR, Singh MM: The positive-negative distinction in drug-free schizophrenic patients. Arch Gen Psychiatry 46:711–717, 1989

Kendell RE: Long-term follow-up studies: a commentary. Schizophr Bull 14:663–667, 1988

Lieberman JA, Alvir J, Woerner M, et al: Prospective study of psychobiology in first episode schizophrenia at Hillside Hospital. Schizophr Bull 18:351–371, 1992

Lin T, Tardiff K, Donetz G, et al: Ethnicity and patterns of help-seeking. Cult Med Psychiatry 2:3–13, 1978

Marder SR, Van Putten T, Mintz J, et al: Maintenance therapy in schizophrenia: new findings, in Drug Maintenance Strategies in Schizophrenia. Edited by Kane JM. Washington, DC, American Psychiatric Press, 1984

McGlashan TH: The Chestnut Lodge follow-up study, I: follow-up methodology and study sample. Arch Gen Psychiatry 41:573–585, 1984a

McGlashan TH: The Chestnut Lodge follow-up study, II: long-term outcome of schizophrenia and affective disorders. Arch Gen Psychiatry 41:586–601, 1984b

McGlashan TH: Late onset improvement in chronic schizophrenia: characteristics and prediction, in Schizophrenia and Aging. Edited by Miller NE, Cohen GD. New York, Guilford, 1987, pp 61–73

McGlashan TH: A selective review of recent North American long-term follow-up studies of schizophrenia. Schizophr Bull 14:515–542, 1988

National Institute of Mental Health: Request for Applications: Treatment Strategies in Schizophrenia Cooperative Agreement Program. Rockville, MD, Department of Health and Human Services, 1983

Overall JE, Gorham DR: The Brief Psychiatric Rating Scale. Psychol Rep 10:799–812, 1962

Pickar D, Labarca R, Doran AR, et al: Longitudinal measurement of plasma homovanillic acid levels in schizophrenic patients. Arch Gen Psychiatry 43:669–676, 1986

Stephens JH: Long-term course and prognosis in schizophrenia. Seminars in Psychiatry 2:464–485, 1970

Stephens JH: Long-term prognosis and follow-up in schizophrenia. Schizophr Bull 4:25–47, 1978

Stephens JH, Astrup C: Prognosis in "process" and "non-process" schizophrenia. Am J Psychiatry 119:945–953, 1963

Stephens JH, Astrup C: Treatment of outcome in "process" and "nonprocess" schizophrenics treated by "A" and "B" types of therapists. J Nerv Ment Dis 140:449–456, 1965

Strauss JS, Carpenter WT: The prognosis of schizophrenia, in Disorders of the Schizophrenia Syndrome. Edited by Bellack L. New York, Basic Books, 1979, pp 472–491

Subotnik KL, Neuchterlein KH: Prodromal signs and symptoms of schizophrenic relapse. J Abnorm Psychol 97:405–412, 1988

Tsuang MT, Woolson RF, Fleming JA: Long-term outcome of major psychoses, I: schizophrenia and affective disorders compared with psychiatrically symptom-free surgical conditions. Arch Gen Psychiatry 39:1295–1301, 1979

Tsuang MT, Woolson RF, Fleming JA: Premature deaths in schizophrenia and affective disorders: an analysis of survival curves and variables affecting the shortened survival. Arch Gen Psychiatry 37:979–983, 1980

Vaillant GE: An historical review of the remitting schizophrenias. J Nerv Ment Dis 138:48–56, 1964a

Vaillant GE: Prospective prediction of schizophrenic remission. Arch Gen Psychiatry 11:509–518, 1964b

Wing J: Comments on the long-term outcome of schizophrenia. Schizophr Bull 14:669–673, 1988

Wing JK, Cooper JE, Sartorius N: The Measurement and Classification of Psychiatric Symptoms. New York, Cambridge University Press, 1974

World Health Organization: Manual of the International Classification of Diseases, Injuries, and Causes of Death, 9th Revision. Geneva, World Health Organization, 1978

World Health Organization: Manual of the International Classification of Diseases, 10th Revision. Geneva, World Health Organization, 1988

Wynne LC: The natural histories of schizophrenic processes. Schizophr Bull 14:653–659, 1988

Chapter 25

Classical Subtypes for Schizophrenia

Thomas H. McGlashan, M.D.
Wayne S. Fenton, M.D.

Statement of the Issues

Subtyping attempts to deal with the vast heterogeneity of schizophrenia; however, without sufficient evidence for validity and clinical utility, there is little reason for retaining the subtype construct. This is the primary question of this review. If there is reason to keep the classical subtypes of schizophrenia in DSM-IV, the second question focuses on whether to retain some or all of the subtypes, and the third question addresses the need to change any of the current defining criteria.

Significance of the Issues

The subtypes of schizophrenia have a rich tradition within clinical psychiatry (Black and Boffeli 1989; Kendler and Tsuang 1981; Morrison 1974; Wender 1963). The "classical" subtypes are so named because they relate back to Kraepelin and Bleuler, the two fathers of psychopathologic nosology. This tradition defined several subcategories of the schizophrenic disorder: latent, simple, catatonic, paranoid, hebephrenic, undifferentiated, and residual. Over the years the list has undergone several changes; only the latter five are retained in DSM-III-R (American Psychiatric Association 1987).

The 1970s brought major challenges to the concept of subtypes in general and to the classical subtypes of schizophrenia in particular. They were criticized as being temporally unstable, phenomenologically nonspecific, and of questionable validity (Carpenter and Stephens 1979; Guggenheim and Babigian 1974; Hay and Forrest 1972; Katz et al. 1964; Munoz et al. 1972; Van der Velde 1976). Their communicative value, or descriptive validity, also came under question (Carpenter and Strauss 1979; Carpenter et al. 1976).

DSM-III (American Psychiatric Association 1980) dropped simple schizophrenia and reformulated latent schizophrenia as schizotypal personality disorder on Axis II. The other classical subtypes were retained, however, despite the questions about their validity. DSM-III-R maintained the same subtype categories, but significantly altered the criteria for the paranoid, disorganized, and undifferentiated subtypes. The paranoid criteria were modeled after those of Tsuang and Winokur (1974), and specific exclusion criteria were added to the disorganized and undifferentiated subtypes, thus creating a functional hierarchy among the subtype group (Kendler et al. 1989).

In this review we focus on paranoid, undifferentiated, and disorganized (hebephrenic) schizophrenias and their validity and criteria; on catatonic schizophrenia and its criteria; and on simple schizophrenia and whether to return it to official nosology and with what criteria.

Methods

A search was conducted of the English psychiatric and psychological literatures using the Social Science Citation Index, Psychological Abstracts, and MEDLARS computer data bases. The search keyed in on literature from the last decade when DSM-III criteria were extant. Review articles covering the classical subtype literature up to and encompassing the last decade were also included. Relevant presentations from major psychiatric meetings were added where relevant, as were relevant data from an ongoing study of schizophrenic subtypes at the authors' institution (Fenton and McGlashan 1991a, 1991b).

Specifically selected were studies that compared the classical subtypes with each other or with their nonclassical counterparts (e.g., paranoid versus nonparanoid). Investigations were excluded if they did not use operationalized criteria in constructing study groups or failed to subject their findings to statistical tests of significance.

Many of the studies found tested the DSM-III subtype criteria. However, *no* study was located that tested the DSM-III-R subtype criteria. Other subtype sets and criteria that were studied included Research Diagnostic Criteria (RDC) (Spitzer et al. 1977), ICD-9 (World Health Organization 1978), and Tsuang-Winokur (1974) criteria. Simple schizophrenia is not included in DSM-III and DSM-III-R and has no criteria. Latent schizophrenia is reformulated on Axis II as schizotypal personality disorder, and will not be considered further here.

Results and Discussion

Paranoid, Undifferentiated, and Disorganized Subtypes

Most of the results are organized and summarized by validating dimensions into Tables 25–1 through 25–5. We provide minimal elaboration in the text.

Table 25–1: Familial and Genetic Studies

Five studies and one review are relevant to the familial-genetic realm of validation. The study by Kendler and colleagues (1985) arose from and updated an earlier study by Winokur and colleagues (1974). Most reports focus on the paranoid-nonparanoid dichotomy, and all of the studies rely on the rating of records. Two major questions are addressed: 1) the relative risk of schizophrenia among family members across schizophrenic proband subtypes, and 2) the concordance of subtype among schizophrenic family members with identified schizophrenic probands.

With regard to the first question, Kendler and Davis (1981) suggested that the genetic loading for schizophrenia is higher in nonparanoid schizophrenic subtypes. The studies by McGuffin and colleagues (1984) and Jorgensen and colleagues (1987) uphold this assertion, but the study by Kendler and colleagues (1988) does not. Overall, there appears to be modest evidence suggesting a different genetic composition between paranoid and nonparanoid schizophrenia, but more data are clearly needed. Fenton and McGlashan (1991a, 1991b) found a higher loading of general psychopathology in the families of hebephrenic patients, but the records on which this is based are unable to be more diagnostically specific.

With regard to the second question, Kendler and Davis (1981) suggested that paranoid schizophrenia runs in families to a moderate degree. High tendencies for subtype concordance across the paranoid-nonparanoid distinction were recorded by McGuffin and colleagues (1984) and by Kendler and Adler (1984). Jorgensen and colleagues (1987) and Kendler and colleagues (1988), on the other hand, found no familial factor specific to subtype. The evidence that subtype breeds true within families, therefore, is suggestive but even more equivocal than the evidence supporting question 1.

Table 25–2: Subtype Stability Studies

Four investigations are relevant to the issue of subtype stability over time. Parnas and colleagues (1988) documented a high degree of stability in the paranoid-nonparanoid distinction over 6 years among female schizophrenic patients. Studying hebephrenic and catatonic schizophrenic patients, on the other hand, Pfohl and Winokur (1983) recorded a persistent tendency toward subtype nonspecificity with time (increase in undifferentiated and residual types). The studies by Kendler and

Table 25–1. Familial and genetic studies

Study	Kendler and Davis 1981	McGuffin et al. 1984	Kendler and Adler 1984	Jorgensen et al. 1987	Kendler et al. 1988	Fenton and McGlashan 1991a, 1991b
Sample	Review of genetic studies up to 1980	Maudsley Twin Registry	Margit Zehnder's case report of pairs of psychotic siblings	Copenhagen High Risk; mothers with schizophrenia and offspring	Iowa 500 and non-500	Chestnut Lodge follow-up schizophrenic cohort
Country	—	England	Switzerland	Denmark	United States	United States
N	—	60 probands	30 sibling pairs	108 mothers with DSM-III schizophrenia; 175 offspring	Approximately 250 schizophrenic probands; 723 first-degree relatives	187 probands, unknown number of relatives
Schizophrenia diagnosis	—	Blind consensus of 6 clinicians	DSM-III	DSM-III and ICD-8	DSM-III, RDC, ICD-9, T-W	Mostly DSM-III
Subtype diagnosis	Paranoid	T-W paranoid	DSM-III paranoid; ICD-9 paranoid; T-W paranoid	ICD-8 paranoid	DSM-III paranoid, hebephrenic, catatonic, undifferentiated; T-W paranoid, hebephrenic, undifferentiated; ICD-9 paranoid, hebephrenic, catatonic; RDC paranoid, hebephrenic, catatonic, undifferentiated	Hebephrenic (T-W), paranoid (DSM-III and T-W), undifferentiated (DSM-III-R)

Comparison group	Nonparanoid	T-W hebephrenic and undifferentiated	Nonparanoid	Nonparanoid	DSM-III paranoid, hebephrenic, catatonic, undifferentiated; T-W paranoid, hebephrenic, undifferentiated; ICD-9 paranoid, hebephrenic, catatonic; RDC paranoid, hebephrenic, catatonic, undifferentiated	Hebephrenic (T-W), paranoid (DSM-III and T-W), undifferentiated (DSM-III-R)
Method	—	Blind rating of clinical abstract	Blind reevaluation of case reports (entire course of illness)	Rediagnosis of hospital records (mothers)	Rescoring hospital records (probands) and interview records (relatives)	Rescoring hospital records (probands and relatives)
Reliability	—	Kappa	Not reported	Not reported	Kappa for hospital records; ? for interview records	Kappa
Result measure	Risk of schizophrenia in first-degree relatives of paranoid vs. nonparanoid probands Risk of paranoid schizophrenia in schizophrenic relatives of paranoid schizophrenic probands	Probandwise risk pairs; Subtype concordance pairs	Concordance of paranoid/nonparanoid across subtype of schizophrenia pairs	Risk of schizophrenia in offspring Subtype concordance across generations	Risk of schizophrenia & schizophrenia spectrum in relatives across generations Proband-relative subtype concordance	Risk of schizophrenia, affective disorder, mental hospitalization in relatives, across subtype

(continued)

Table 25–1. Familial and genetic studies *(continued)*

Study	Kendler and Davis 1981	McGuffin et al. 1984	Kendler and Adler 1984	Jorgensen et al. 1987	Kendler et al. 1988	Fenton and McGlashan 1991a, 1991b
Results	Lower risk in 8/9 family studies & 2/3 twin studies Higher risk in 4/9 studies; no difference in 5/9; higher concordance in 3/3 twin studies	Risk: paranoid MZ: 40% DZ: 7% nonparanoid MZ: 62% DZ: 15% Concordance MZ: 13/15 DZ: 3/3	ICD-9 $P = .04$ DSM-III $P = .56$ T-W NS	Risk: Higher (29%) for nonparanoid mothers than for paranoid schizophrenic mothers (5%) Concordance paranoid offspring and paranoid mother: 33% nonparanoid offspring and paranoid mother: 50%	NS NS	NS increase in schizophrenia and affective disorder in relatives of hebephrenic probands; significant increase in hospitalization for any mental disorder in relatives of hebephrenic probands
Conclusions	Suggests genetic loading for schizophrenia higher in non-paranoid schizophrenia Suggests paranoid schizophrenia runs in families to a moderate degree	Paranoid is less familial for schizophrenia High tendency for subtype concordance	Supports subtype concordance and broader definition of paranoid	Genetic loading for schizophrenia higher in non-paranoid schizophrenia Subtype does not breed true	Familial factors similar across subtype No familial factor specific to subtype	Loading for general and severe psychopathology higher in hebephrenic schizophrenia

Note. T-W = Tsuang-Winokur 1974 criteria. MZ = monozygotic. DZ = dizygotic. NS = not significant.

Table 25–2. Studies of subtype stability

Study	Pfohl and Winokur 1983	Kendler et al. 1985	Parnas et al. 1988	Fenton and McGlashan 1991a, 1991b
Sample	Iowa 500	Iowa 500	Copenhagen High Risk	Chestnut Lodge follow-up schizophrenic cohort
Country	United States	United States	Denmark	United States
N	52 predrug	139	64	125 patients with sufficient early course data
Schizophrenia diagnosis	Feighner criteria	Feighner criteria	DSM-III-R	Mostly DSM-III
Subtype diagnosis	Hebephrenic/catatonic	RDC paranoid, undifferentiated, hebephrenic; DSM-III paranoid, undifferentiated, hebephrenic; ICD paranoid, hebephrenic; T-W paranoid, undifferentiated, hebephrenic	ICD-9 paranoid/nonparanoid	Hebephrenic (T-W), paranoid (DSM-III and T-W), undifferentiated (DSM-III-R)
Method	Chart review of symptoms over 25 years	Blind rating of index record; blind rating of follow-up records; follow-up = 25 years	Review of index and follow-up records; blind and independent; follow-up = 6 ± 2 years	Review of hospital records prior to and including index hospitalizations
Reliability	Not reported	Kappa for index, ? for follow-up	Not reported	Kappa

(continued)

Table 25–2. Studies of subtype stability *(continued)*

Study	Pfohl and Winokur 1983	Kendler et al. 1985	Parnas et al. 1988	Fenton and McGlashan 1991a, 1991b
Results	Time brings: decrease in hallucinations/delusions; increase in avolition, flat affect, disorientation, impaired social interest	Three samples: A = all patients; B = A minus residual schizophrenia & latent schizophrenia at follow-up; C = only patients with specific subtype at index and follow-up (paranoid, hebephrenic)	6-year rehospitalization: Index / paranoid / nonparanoid paranoid: 48, 3 nonparanoid: 2, 14 $P \leq .0001$	Subtype diagnosis at first hospitalization and index admission 4.5 years later (average) First admission: # (%) Index admission: # (%) / paranoid 61 (49) / hebephrenic 12 (10) / undifferentiated 52 (42) paranoid 45 (36): 38 (62), 0, 7 (13) hebephrenic 22 (18): 5 (8), 8 (67), 9 (17) undifferentiated 58 (46): 18 (30), 4 (33), 36 (69) kappa = 0.44
Conclusions	Time brings increase in nonspecific subtypes	Subtype stability modest in A & B, considerable in C; stability best for paranoid, modest for hebephrenic, absent for undifferentiated; time brings increase in nonspecific subtypes (undifferentiated, latent, residual); specific subtypes evolve into nonspecific but rarely into each other	Paranoid/nonparanoid subtype highly stable	Subtype stability modest; 66% retain same subtype; rank order of stability (most to least): paranoid, hebephrenic, undifferentiated; time brings increase in hebephrenic and undifferentiated subtypes

Note. T-W = Tsuang-Winokur 1974 criteria.

colleagues (1985) and Fenton and McGlashan (1991a, 1991b) perhaps integrate these disparate findings. They too noted that time generates an increase in the number of nonspecific subtypes of schizophrenia. Subtype stability, therefore, is modest at best when looking at total samples. However, when specific subtypes can be identified at both index and follow-up, they tend to be relatively stable—the paranoid subtype to a considerable degree, the hebephrenic subtype to some degree, and the undifferentiated subtype to the least degree.

Table 25–3: Outcome Studies

Two outcome studies are relevant. The first is by Kendler and colleagues (1984) on the Iowa 500 sample of schizophrenic patients defined by the Washington University criteria (Feighner et al. 1972). There are no studies of outcome prior to 1980 using operationalized criteria except Tsuang and Winokur (1974). This study has been updated by the one cited here. The 1984 study of the Iowa 500 presents data about both short-term (2.5 years) and long-term (24 years) outcome of three classical subtypes (paranoid, hebephrenic, and undifferentiated). The data indicate that paranoid and nonparanoid schizophrenic patients are different by short-term and long-term outcome and that these differences increase with follow-up length. Outcome fails, however, to differentiate the hebephrenic and undifferentiated subgroups.

The paranoid-nonparanoid differences are greatest using the Tsuang-Winokur criteria because this set selects patients with better prognoses (older onset, no family history of schizophrenia, married, or working premorbidly), and without comorbid schizophrenic psychopathology from other domains (prominent thought disorder, affective disorganization, bizarre behavior, motor abnormalities). The latter exclusion criterion appears to contribute the most to the differences in predictive validity among the four definitions of the paranoid subtype. For this reason, such an exclusion criterion was incorporated into the DSM-III-R definition of paranoid schizophrenia.

The Fenton and McGlashan (1991a, 1991b) study of the Chestnut Lodge follow-up schizophrenic cohort indicated that the hebephrenic patients are significantly inferior to the paranoid and undifferentiated subtypes on most long-term outcome dimensions. A narrowly defined paranoid subtype (i.e., one without any blunted affect or thought disorder) scores a significantly better outcome than hebephrenic or undifferentiated, thus replicating Kendler and colleagues (1984).

Table 25–4: Neurological and Neuropsychological Studies

It is clear from the three studies in Table 25–4 that there are little data from neurology or from neuropsychological testing that support (with any stringency) the validity of subtyping schizophrenia according to DSM-III. More data are

Table 25–3. Outcome studies

Study	Kendler et al. 1984	Fenton and McGlashan 1991a, 1991b
Sample	Iowa 500	Chestnut Lodge follow-up schizophrenic cohort
Country	United States	United States
N	187	162 patients with follow-up
Schizophrenia diagnosis	Feighner criteria	Mostly DSM-III
Subtype diagnosis	RDC paranoid, undifferentiated, disorganized hebephrenic; T-W paranoid, hebephrenic, undetermined-undifferentiated; DSM-III paranoid, undifferentiated, disorganized hebephrenic; ICD-9 paranoid, hebephrenic	Hebephrenic (T-W), paranoid (DSM-III and T-W), undifferentiated (DSM-III-R)
Method	Blind rating of index admission records	Blind interview of subjects and/or significant others
Reliability	Kappa	Kappa and intraclass correlation
Outcome	**Short-term**: 2.5 years; Hospital record; Improved yes/no **Long-term**: 24 years; Interview; Improved yes/no for 3 dimensions	Long-term 19 years (average); 5-point ratings on 35 outcome dimensions
Results	Paranoid short-term outcome better than hebephrenic for T-W; paranoid long-term outcome better than hebephrenic for all 4 systems on most dimensions; paranoid outcome better than undifferentiated for T-W and DSM for some dimensions	Undifferentiated better than hebephrenic on most dimensions; paranoid better than undifferentiated for narrowly defined paranoid subtype (*no* blunted affect or thought disorder) paranoid better than hebephrenic on most dimensions
Conclusions	By short- and long-term outcome, paranoid and nonparanoid are different; the differences increase with time; outcome does not differentiate hebephrenic and undifferentiated	Outcome differentiates hebephrenic from paranoid and undifferentiated and narrowly defined paranoid from hebephrenic and undifferentiated

Note. T-W = Tsuang-Winokur 1974 criteria.

Table 25–4. Neurological and neuropsychological studies

Study	Manschreck and Ames 1984	Langell et al. 1987	Bornstein et al. 1989
Sample	Inpatients	Veterans Administration inpatients	Outpatients
Country	United States	United States	United States
N	See below	See below	See below
Schizophrenia diagnosis	DSM-III	DSM-III	DSM-III
Subtype diagnosis	DSM-III paranoid ($N = 19$) undifferentiated ($N = 21$) hebephrenic ($N = 13$) affective disorder ($N = 21$) nonpsychiatric control ($N = 20$)	DSM-III paranoid ($N = 45$) undifferentiated ($N = 45$) nonpsychiatric control ($N = 45$)	DSM-III paranoid ($N = 28$) nonparanoid (undifferentiated, hebephrenic) ($N = 27$) schizoaffective ($N = 18$) nonpsychiatric control ($N = 52$)
Method	Neurological evaluation	Neuropsychological battery (nonblind)	Neuropsychological battery
Reliability	Not tested for this sample	None	?
Results	Neurological abnormal features indistinguishable among subtypes	Paranoid schizophrenic patients performed better on tests of complex motor function, concentration, and processing of complex information	Nonparanoid schizophrenic patients performed the worst on neuropsychiatric summary score; however, results may relate more to symptom level than to subtype
Conclusions	No relationship between subtype and neurological abnormalities	Potential relationship between subtype and neuropsychological abnormalities	Equivocal relationship between subtype and neuropsychological abnormalities

needed from this realm before any definitive trend is likely to be apprehended.

Table 25–5: Biological Studies

Two reviews and one study address biological differences associated with schizophrenic subtypes, meaning the paranoid-nonparanoid breakdown almost exclusively. The results overall are highly equivocal and are not compelling enough one way or the other to inform nosologic judgments at this time.

Other Studies

Age at onset. As cited in Zigler and Glick (1984), three studies found that paranoid schizophrenic patients are older at first psychiatric admission (Gift et al. 1981; Winokur et al. 1974; Zigler and Levine 1981). Gruenberg and colleagues (1985) applied the four sets of subtype criteria to the Iowa 500 sample (see Table 25–3). They find age at onset to be significantly discriminating between the paranoid, undifferentiated, and hebephrenic subtypes, with the paranoid patients being oldest and the hebephrenic patients being the youngest. This distinction holds up no matter which of the four systems are used. With the Chestnut Lodge follow-up sample of schizophrenic patients, Fenton and McGlashan (1991a, 1991b) found the paranoid subtype to have a significantly older age at onset than the hebephrenic and undifferentiated subtypes. By age at onset, therefore, the paranoid, undifferentiated, and hebephrenic subgroups appear to be valid and distinct.

Social competence. Zigler and Glick's (1984) review also cited three studies asserting that paranoid schizophrenic patients "typically" obtain higher social competence scores than nonparanoid schizophrenic patients (Cantor et al. 1980; Zigler et al. 1976, 1977). It is not clear if they are referring to social competence as a premorbid, comorbid, or postmorbid (outcome) measure. Concurrent ratings of social competence do not distinguish paranoid from nonparanoid subtypes in a sample of acutely ill inpatients and in a sample of remitted outpatients (Dobson and Neufeld 1987). Better premorbid social contacts, marital status, and instrumental capacities do characterize the paranoid subtype in the Chestnut Lodge cohort (Fenton and McGlashan 1991a, 1991b).

Perinatal insult. Wilcox and Nasrallah (1987) found that a history of perinatal distress (prolonged labor and/or instrument delivery) is significantly more common in the medical histories of 30 paranoid schizophrenic inpatients compared with the histories of 60 nonparanoid schizophrenic inpatients matched for sex, age, race, and social status ($P < .0005$). DSM-III criteria are applied in an unspecified manner without any report of reliability. Family history of schizophrenia is negatively correlated with perinatal distress ($r = .41$, $P < .05$). Fenton and McGlashan

Table 25–5. Biological studies

Study	Zureick and Meltzer 1988	Ko et al. 1988	McGuffin and Sturt 1986
Topic	MAO activity	Plasma MHPG	Human leukocyte
Sample	Review of 9 studies (1977–1984)	Drug-free chronic schizophrenic inpatients (NIH)	Review of 9 studies (1976–1984)
Country	—	United States	—
N	Meta-analysis of 165 paranoid, 152 nonparanoid, 985 nonpsychiatric controls	14	—
Schizophrenia diagnosis	—	RDC	—
Subtype diagnosis	—	DSM-III paranoid, undifferentiated, nonpsychiatric controls	—
Method	Meta-analysis	Blood samples	—
Reliability	—	None	—
Result measure	Platelet MAO activity	Plasma MHPG	HLA
Results	Paranoid schizophrenic patients had MAO activity lower than 61% of nonparanoid patients and 79% of control subjects; effect size (% decrease in MAO activity to control): paranoid 30%, nonparanoid 24%	Paranoid schizophrenic patients had nonsignificant trend toward higher levels than nonparanoid schizophrenic patients	7/9 studies show an association between paranoid schizophrenia and HLA A9, although strength of association low (relative risk of A9 positive individual = 1.6)
Conclusions	Equivocal relationship between paranoid/nonparanoid status and MAO activity	Equivocal to no relationship between paranoid/undifferentiated status and plasma MHPG	Equivocal relationship of paranoid schizophrenia to HLA genetic marker

Note. MAO = monoamine oxidase. MHPG = 3-methoxy-4-hydroxyphenylglycol. NIH = National Institutes of Health. HLA = human lymphocyte antigens.

(1991a, 1991b) found a nonsignificant trend in the opposite direction (i.e., more frequent birth and neonatal trauma in the hebephrenic and undifferentiated subtypes).

Seasons of birth. Hsieh and colleagues (1987) examined the seasonal rate of birth in 472 schizophrenic inpatients subdivided by gender and paranoid-nonparanoid subtype. Patients carried an ICD-9 clinical discharge diagnosis of schizophrenia and a clinical subtype diagnosis of paranoid schizophrenia or nonparanoid schizophrenia (simple, hebephrenic, catatonic, residual, undifferentiated). Seasonal variation was not significant for the group as a whole or for the group broken down by gender. By season quartiles (January-March, April-June, July-September, October-December), however, there was a significant increase in births for the male paranoid schizophrenic patients for the first quartile.

This study partially replicates that by Nasrallah and McCalley-Whitters (1984), who found no seasonality of birth in a group of 577 chronic schizophrenic patients. However, a breakdown of the sample by gender and paranoid-nonparanoid status demonstrates that winter-month births includes an increase in the number of paranoid males and nonparanoid females.

Other validating parameters. Fenton and McGlashan (1991a, 1991b) reported that the paranoid subtype patients have a more acute onset of disorder and display an illness that is relatively field dependent (i.e., sensitive to life events and more intermittent [versus continuous] in its course).

Andreasen and Grove (1986) found that a measure of loose associations significantly discriminated RDC hebephrenic patients (more) from paranoid patients (less).

Other studies of paranoid-nonparanoid differences include investigations of facial movements (Pitman et al. 1987) and perceptual processing (Wells and Leventhal 1984). Neither study has more than 10 subjects in any comparison group. No conclusions can be drawn on such preliminary findings.

Zigler and Glick (1984) summarized other differences in behavior between paranoid and nonparanoid schizophrenic patients. From this literature, paranoid schizophrenic patients are superior on such parameters as distractibility, capacity to process complex information, ability to shift concept, boundary articulation, reaction time, perceptual closure, and so on. The reader is referred to Zigler and Glick's review for details. Overall, this body of work suggests that the paranoid schizophrenic subtype is healthier and better functioning than the nonparanoid schizophrenic subtype, findings that dovetail with their better outcome over time (Kendler et al. 1984).

Reliability and Comprehensiveness

Gruenberg and colleagues (1985) tested the reliability and concordance of the four subtyping systems used in their studies. All four systems are reliable using unweighted kappas. The DSM-III and RDC systems are the most concordant, and the Tsuang-Winokur and ICD-9 systems the least concordant. The number of patients assigned to paranoid and hebephrenic subtypes is lowest for the Tsuang-Winokur system and highest for the ICD-9 system. The number of patients assigned to the undifferentiated subtype is highest for the Tsuang-Winokur system and lowest for the ICD-9 system. DSM-III and RDC are intermediate on these measures of comprehensiveness.

Fenton and McGlashan (1991a, 1991b) found the RDC, DSM-III, ICD-9, and Tsuang-Winokur criteria reliable for the paranoid-nonparanoid distinction. Furthermore, hebephrenic and undifferentiated patients can be reliably ascertained using ICD-9 and Tsuang-Winokur, but not RDC or DSM-III.

Summary of the Data

The data concerning three of the classical subtypes (paranoid, hebephrenic, undifferentiated) may be summarized as follows. There appears to be a modest distinction genetically between paranoid and nonparanoid schizophrenia, the latter being more familial than the former. The evidence is more equivocal for subtype concordance. Premorbid functioning is usually superior in the paranoid subtype. Across all studies, age at onset clearly separates the three subtypes. The early character of illness course is also different among the three subtypes, with that of the paranoid patients being acute, intermittent, distinct, and reactive; that of the hebephrenic patients being insidious, continuous, and distinct but nonreactive; and that of the undifferentiated patients being insidious, continuous, nonreactive, and poorly distinguished from the patient's premorbid character. Over time the paranoid and hebephrenic subtypes retain some phenomenologic sameness, but often evolve into less specific groups (undifferentiated, residual). Long-term outcome data provide robust validation for the distinctiveness of the paranoid subtype on the one hand (Kendler et al. 1985), and the hebephrenic and undifferentiated subtypes on the other (Fenton and McGlashan 1991a, 1991b).

Catatonic Schizophrenia

Precious little literature exists to inform or guide considerations about catatonic schizophrenia. Although statements that the subtype is extinct may be premature, the number of times it has been cited (or sighted) has dropped dramatically, especially in samples from Western industrialized cultures. Only one reference was found to catatonic schizophrenia: a study by Chandrasena (1986) describing 35 hospitalized International Pilot Study of Schizophrenia (World Health Organization 1973) catatonic schizophrenic patients from Sri Lanka. The study found the most common "catatonic" symptoms to be mutism, stupor, mannerisms, stereotypies, and negativism.

Where catatonia does exist, its specificity to schizophrenia has come under scrutiny. For example, Abrams and Taylor (1976) found that only 4 of 55 patients exhibiting one or more signs of catatonia satisfied their research criteria for schizophrenia. More than two-thirds of them satisfied their research criteria for affective disorder, usually mania. Furthermore, cases have been described of acutely developing catatonic symptoms in young adults that are nonresponsive to neuroleptic treatments but highly responsive to electroconvulsive treatment (Max Fink, M.D., personal communication to Allen Frances, M.D., December 20, 1989). Thus, in terms of at least one validating criterion (i.e., treatment response), catatonia may not be specific to the schizophrenic spectrum.

Simple Schizophrenia

Black and Boffeli (1989) reviewed the history of simple schizophrenia and asserted that if the disorder exists, it is characterized by a quietly impoverished psychological life without active phases or symptoms. It is a relatively pure form of negative or deficit schizophrenia. The disorder is generally seen outside an institution, with most of those afflicted able to function marginally. The most frequently described symptoms include insidious onset (usually in adolescence), shallow or blunted affect, and avolition and deteriorating course.

A second article (Levit 1977) reported a Russian study conducted at the Institute of Psychiatry in Moscow. Two hundred cases, mostly first hospitalizations, with predominant symptoms of sluggishness, apathy, and passivity were followed up approximately 20 years after admission. All subjects presented with sluggish schizophrenia. There were three gross outcome trajectories: one group improved, one group evolved into other typical schizophrenia subtypes, and one group remained sluggish and deteriorated. This group seems to fit the classical description of simple schizophrenia. The author was struck with the changing picture of the simple form to other forms of psychosis and concluded that the classical simple form was often the initial stage in the development of the schizophrenic process.

Recommendations

Paranoid, Undifferentiated, and Disorganized Subtypes

Unlike the skeptical studies of the 1970s, the studies of the last decade lend overall support to the validity of these classical subtypes. This goes especially for the paranoid subtype and, albeit with less force, for the disorganized and undifferentiated subtypes. All these should be retained in DSM-IV. Furthermore, the data lend support to several changes in specific criteria that have already been incorporated into DSM-III-R. First, a definition of paranoid schizophrenia that excludes patients with significant thought disorder or affective deterioration appears to have the greatest predictive validity. Second, disorganized patients may show some paranoid symptoms but, in contrast, disorganized symptoms are exclusion criteria for paranoid subtype. In this respect, DSM-III-R effectively organizes the major subtypes hierarchically. Third, undifferentiated schizophrenia is only a subtype of exclusion. Defined in this way, the undifferentiated category appears to lie on a midpoint of severity between the paranoid and disorganized (hebephrenic) types.

Table 25–6 lists the proposed DSM-IV subtypes of schizophrenia and their criteria. The paranoid subtype is retained with identical criteria from DSM-III-R. These derive from the Tsuang-Winokur paranoid subtype criteria, which demonstrate robust antecedent and predictive validity. The disorganized (hebe-

Table 25–6. Proposed DSM-IV diagnostic criteria for Paranoid, Disorganized, Undifferentiated, and Residual Subtypes of Schizophrenia

Paranoid

A type of schizophrenia in which there are:

A. Preoccupation with one or more systematized delusions or with frequent auditory hallucinations related to a single theme.

B. *None* of the following: incoherence, marked loosening of associations, flat or grossly inappropriate affect, catatonic behavior, grossly disorganized behavior

Disorganized (hebephrenic)

A type of schizophrenia in which the following are met:

A. Incoherence or marked loosening of associations

B. Flat or inappropriate affect

C. Grossly bizarre or disorganized behavior

D. Does not meet the criteria for Catatonic Type

Undifferentiated

A type of schizophrenia in which there are:

A. Prominent delusions, hallucinations, incoherence, or grossly disorganized behavior

B. Does not meet the criteria for Catatonic, Paranoid, or Disorganized Type

Residual

A type of schizophrenia in which there are:

A. Absence of prominent delusions, hallucinations, incoherence, marked loosening of associations, or grossly disorganized behavior

B. Continuing evidence of the disturbance, as indicated by two or more of the following: any residual symptoms listed in criterion B of DSM-IV Schizophrenia, or blunted, flat affect, or poverty of speech

phrenic) subtype is also retained, but with modified criteria that are somewhat more stringent than DSM-III-R. Fenton and McGlashan (1991a, 1991b) required the presence of three domains in their definition of disorganized (hebephrenic): disorganized thought and flat or inappropriate affect and bizarre or disorganized behavior. These criteria defined a subgroup with a distinct profile on many longitudinal parameters. The undifferentiated subtype is retained with DSM-III-R criteria. As in DSM-III-R, it is a diagnosis of exclusion. With these criteria it is hypothesized that the likelihood of overlap between the undifferentiated and disorganized subtypes will be reduced.

The residual subtype is retained. The format of the criteria is essentially the same as in DSM-III-R, but the details here depend on the specific proposed DSM-IV criteria for schizophrenia. Basically, criterion 1 notes the absence of positive symptoms, and criterion 2 notes the presence of negative symptomatology.

Catatonic Schizophrenia

Although it is clear that catatonia may not be specific to schizophrenia, it can still characterize a subtype of schizophrenia. As a symptom complex, it is like paranoia and can describe patients with mania, depression, or delusional disorder as well as schizophrenia. As such the subtypes should be retained, but catatonic symptoms should be dropped from the defining criterion A for schizophrenia to guard against misdiagnosing affective or other forms of catatonia as schizophrenia.

The DSM-III-R criteria for the catatonic subtype perseverate on the term *catatonic* (e.g., catatonic stupor, catatonic negativism, catatonic rigidity, catatonic excitement, and catatonic posturing). A less redundant and potentially more comprehensive set of criteria is suggested in Table 25–7.

Simple Schizophrenia

Black and Boffeli (1989) favored restoring simple schizophrenia as a category because

> 1) there are historic precedents for the disorder; 2) there is evidence for its genetic relationship to core schizophrenia; 3) simple and core schizophrenia are similar descriptively and clinically; and 4) research emphasizing the schizophrenic spectrum would benefit from an operational definition of simple schizophrenia. (p. 1272)

We agree. However, to avoid its pejorative association with the politically volatile Soviet classification of "sluggish schizophrenia," it should be labeled Simple Deteriorative Disorder and categorized under Psychotic Disorders Not Otherwise Specified.

Two variations in criteria are suggested (Table 25–8). The first is isomorphic

Table 25–7. Proposed DSM-IV diagnostic criteria for Catatonic Schizophrenia

A type of schizophrenia with the following clinical features

A. At least one of the following:

1. Catalepsy/stupor: marked decrease in reactivity to the environment and/or reduction in spontaneous movements and activity
2. Extreme negativism: apparently motiveless resistance to all instructions and/or maintenance of a rigid posture against efforts to be moved
3. Extreme agitation: excessive motor activity, apparently purposeless and not influenced by external stimuli
4. Extreme suggestibility/compliance: automatic obedience or waxy flexibility in which externally imposed body postures are maintained indefinitely.

and/or

B. At least three of the following:

1. Stereotypes
2. Mannerisms or grimacing
3. Posturing or the assumption of inappropriate/bizarre postures
4. Echo phenomena (echolalia, echopraxia)
5. Mutism
6. Staring

Table 25–8. Proposed DSM-IV diagnostic criteria for Simple Schizophrenia

Simple Deterioration Disorder (Simple Schizophrenia) Version 1

All of the following:

A. Never demonstrated 1 month of active phase psychotic symptoms (criterion A of DSM-IV Schizophrenia)

B. Current absence of prominent delusions, hallucinations, incoherence, marked loosening of associations, or grossly disorganized behavior

C. Evidence of disturbance as indicated by two or more of the following: any residual symptom listed in criterion B of DSM-IV Schizophrenia or blunted, flat affect, of poverty of speech

D. Continuous signs of disturbance for at least 6 months

E. Deterioration of functioning (same as criterion D of DSM-IV Schizophrenia)

F. Schizophrenia, Schizoaffective Disorder, and Mood Disorder with Psychotic Features have been ruled out (same as criterion E of DSM-IV Schizophrenia)

G. Organic disorder exclusion (same as criterion F of DSM-IV Schizophrenia)

Simple Deterioration Disorder (Simple Schizophrenia) Version 2

All of the following:

A. Meets criteria for Axis II Schizotypal Personality Disorder

B. Deterioration of functioning (criterion D of DSM-IV Schizophrenia)

C. Continuous signs of disturbance for at least 6 months

D. Schizophrenia, Schizoaffective Disorder, and Mood Disorder with Psychotic Features have been ruled out (same as criterion E of DSM-IV Schizophrenia)

E. Organic disorder exclusion (same as criterion F of DSM-IV Schizophrenia) with the residual subtype of schizophrenia minus criterion A for schizophrenia. The second is isomorphic with Schizotypal Personality Disorder plus the criterion of deterioration in functioning.

References

Abrams R, Taylor MA: Catatonia: a prospective clinical study. Arch Gen Psychiatry 33:579–581, 1976

American Psychiatric Association: Diagnostic and Statistical Manual of Mental Disorders, 3rd Edition. Washington, DC, American Psychiatric Association, 1980

American Psychiatric Association: Diagnostic and Statistical Manual of Mental Disorders, 3rd Edition, Revised, Washington, DC, American Psychiatric Association, 1987

Andreasen NC, Grove WM: Thought, language, and communication in schizophrenia: diagnosis and prognosis. Schizophr Bull 12:348–359, 1986

Black D, Boffeli T: Simple schizophrenia: past, present, and future. Am J Psychiatry 146:1267–1273, 1989

Bornstein RA, Nasrallah, HA, Coffman JA, et al: Neuropsychological deficit in subtypes of schizophrenia. Paper presented at International Congress on Schizophrenia Research, San Diego, CA, May 1989

Cantor N, Smith E, French R, et al: Psychiatric diagnosis as prototype categorization. J Abnorm Psychol 89:181–193, 1980

Carpenter WT, Stephens JH: An attempted integration of information relevant to schizophrenia subtypes. Schizophr Bull 5:490–506, 1979

Carpenter WT, Strauss JS: Diagnostic issues in schizophrenia, in Disorders of the Schizophrenic Syndrome. Edited by Bellak L. New York, Basic Books, 1979

Carpenter WT, Bartko JJ, Langsner CA et al: Another view of schizophrenia subtypes: a report from the International Pilot Study of Schizophrenia. Arch Gen Psychiatry 33:508–516, 1976

Chandrasena R: Catatonic schizophrenia: an international comparative study. Can J Psychiatry 31:249–252, 1986

Dobson DJG, Neufeld RWJ: Association of social competence with episodic vs remitted status in paranoid and nonparanoid schizophrenia. Canadian Journal of Behavioral Science 19:67–73, 1987

Feighner JP, Robins E, Guze SB, et al: Diagnostic criteria for use in psychiatric research. Arch Gen Psychiatry 26:57–63, 1972

Fenton WS, McGlashan TH: Natural history of schizophrenia subtypes, I: longitudinal study of paranoid, hebephrenic, and undifferentiated schizophrenia. Arch Gen Psychiatry 48:969–977, 1991a

Fenton WS, McGlashan TH: Natural history of schizophrenia subtypes, II: positive and negative symptoms and long-term course. Arch Gen Psychiatry 48:978–986, 1991b

Gift T, Strauss JS, Harder DW, et al: Established chronicity of psychotic symptoms in first-admission schizophrenic patients. Am J Psychiatry 138:779–784, 1981

Gruenberg AM, Kendler KS, Tsuang MT: Reliability and concordance in the subtyping of schizophrenia. Am J Psychiatry 142:1355–1358, 1985

Guggenheim FG, Babigian HM: Diagnostic consistency in catatonic schizophrenia. Schizophr Bull 11:103–198, 1974

Hay AJ, Forrest AD: The diagnosis of schizophrenia and paranoid psychosis: an attempt at clarification. Br J Med Psychol 45:233–241, 1972

Hsieh HH, Khan MH, Atwal SS, et al: Seasons of birth and subtypes of schizophrenia. Acta Psychiatr Scand 75:373–376, 1987

Jorgensen A, Teasdale TW, Parnas J, et al: The Copenhagen High-Risk Project: the diagnosis of maternal schizophrenia and its relation to offspring diagnosis. Br J Psychiatry 151:753–757, 1987

Katz MM, Cole JO, Lowert HA: Non-specificity of diagnosis of paranoid schizophrenia. Arch Gen Psychiatry 11:197–202, 1964

Kendler KS, Adler D: The pattern of illness in pairs of psychotic siblings. Am J Psychiatry 141:509–513, 1984

Kendler KS, Davis KL: The genetics and biochemistry of paranoid schizophrenia and other paranoid psychoses. Schizophr Bull 7:689–709, 1981

Kendler KS, Tsuang MT: Nosology of paranoid schizophrenia and other paranoid psychoses. Schizophr Bull 7:594–609, 1981

Kendler KS, Gruenberg AM, Tsuang MT: Outcome of schizophrenic subtypes defined by four diagnostic systems. Arch Gen Psychiatry 41:149–154, 1984

Kendler KS, Gruenberg AM, Tsuang MT: Subtype stability in schizophrenia. Am J Psychiatry 142:827–832, 1985

Kendler KS, Gruenberg AM, Tsuang MT: A family study of the subtypes of schizophrenia. Am J Psychiatry 145:57–62, 1988

Kendler KS, Spitzer RL, Williams JBW: Psychotic disorders in DSM-III-R. Am J Psychiatry 146:953–962, 1989

Ko GN, Jimerson DC, Wyatt RJ, et al: Plasma 3-methoxy-4-hydroxyphenylglycol changes associated with clinical state and schizophrenic subtype. Arch Gen Psychiatry 45:842–846, 1988

Langell ME, Purisch AD, Golden CJ: Neuropsychological differences between paranoid and nonparanoid schizophrenics on the Luria-Nebraska Battery. International Journal of Clinical Neuropsychology 9:88–95, 1987

Levit VG: Simple form of schizophrenia: what did it turn out to be? in New Dimensions in Psychiatry: A World View, Vol 2. Edited by Arieti S, Chrzanowski G. New York, Wiley, 1977, pp 378–403

Manschreck TC, Ames D: Neurologic features and psychopathology in schizophrenic disorders. Biol Psychiatry 19:703–719, 1984

McGuffin P, Sturt E: Genetic markers in schizophrenia. Hum Hered 36:65–88, 1986

McGuffin P, Farmer AE, Gottesman II, et al: Twin concordance for operationally defined schizophrenia. Arch Gen Psychiatry 41:541–545, 1984

Morrison JR: Changes in subtype diagnosis of schizophrenia: 1920–1966. Am J Psychiatry 136:674–677, 1974

Munoz RA, Kulak G, Marten S, et al: Simple and hebephrenic schizophrenia: a follow-up study, in Life History Research in Psychopathology, Vol 2. Edited by Roff M, Robbins LN, Pollack M. Minneapolis, University of Minnesota Press, 1972, pp 228–235

Nasrallah HA, McCalley-Whitters M: Seasonality of birth in subtypes of chronic schizophrenia. Acta Psychiatr Scand 69:292–295, 1984

Parnas J, Jorgensen A, Teasdale TW, et al: Temporal course of symptoms and social functioning in relapsing schizophrenics. Compr Psychiatry 29:361–371, 1988

Pfohl B, Winokur G: The micropsychopathology of hebephrenic/catatonic schizophrenia. J Nerv Ment Dis 171:296–300, 1983

Pitman RK, Kolb B, Orr SP, et al: Ethological study of facial behavior in nonparanoid and paranoid schizophrenic patients. Am J Psychiatry 144:99–102, 1987

Spitzer RL, Endicott J, Robins E: Research Diagnostic Criteria (RDC) For a Selected Group of Functional Disorders, 3rd Edition. New York, New York State Psychiatric Institute, Biometrics Research, 1977

Tsuang MT, Winokur G: Criteria for subtyping schizophrenia: clinical differentiation of hebephrenic and paranoid schizophrenia. Arch Gen Psychiatry 31:43–47, 1974

Van der Velde CD: Variability in schizophrenia: indication of a regulatory disease. Arch Gen Psychiatry 33:489–496, 1976

Wells DS, Leventhal D: Perceptual grouping in schizophrenia: replication of Place and Gilmore. J Abnorm Psychol 93:231–234, 1984

Wender PH: Dementia praecox, the development of the concept. Am J Psychiatry 120:1143–1151, 1963

Wilcox JA, Nasrallah HA: Perinatal insult as a risk factor in paranoid and nonparanoid schizophrenia. Psychopathology 20:285–287, 1987

Winokur G, Morrison J, Clancy J, et al: Iowa 500: the clinical and genetic distribution of hebephrenic and paranoid schizophrenia. J Nerv Ment Dis 159:12–19, 1974

World Health Organization: The International Pilot Study of Schizophrenia. Geneva, World Health Organization, 1973

World Health Organization: Mental Disorders: Glossary and Guide to Their Classification in Accordance with the 9th Revision of the International Classification of Diseases. Geneva, World Health Organization, 1978

Zigler E, Glick M: Paranoid schizophrenia: an unorthodox view. Am J Orthopsychiatry 54:43–70, 1984

Zigler E, Levine J: Age on first hospitalization of schizophrenics: a developmental approach. J Abnorm Psychol 90:458–467, 1981

Zigler E, Levine J, Zigler B: The relation between premorbid competence and paranoid-nonparanoid status in schizophrenia: a methodological and theoretical critique. Psychol Bull 83:303–313, 1976

Zigler E, Levine J, Zigler B: Premorbid social competence and paranoid-nonparanoid status in female schizophrenics. J Nerv Ment Dis 164:333–339, 1977

Zureick JL, Meltzer HY: Platelet MAO activity in hallucinating and paranoid schizophrenics: a review and meta-analysis. Biol Psychiatry 24:63–78, 1988

Chapter 26

Late-Onset Schizophrenia

Thomas H. McGlashan, M.D.

Statement and Significance of the Issues

In response to clinical feedback and opinion, the DSM-III (American Psychiatric Association 1980) age limit of 45 for schizophrenia was eliminated in DSM-III-R (American Psychiatric Association 1987). The first question of this review, therefore, addresses the validity of this move. If late-onset schizophrenia appears legitimate, the second question addresses its subtype status, and the third question concerns any needed changes in criteria.

Results

Harris and Jeste (1988) reviewed the literature on late-onset schizophrenia: more than 30 publications, mostly European, from between 1913 and 1986. This includes volumes from geriatric psychiatry and foreign language articles. It appears to be a very comprehensive review. It is also sophisticated in its methodological critique of the included studies.

The following data could be gleaned from the literature.

- Incidence and prevalence. Schizophrenia after age 40 is far from rare, although the studies do not allow a decent estimate at this time. The order of magnitude is approximately 10%.
- Gender. Late-onset schizophrenia has a high female-to-male ratio, and this does not appear to be secondary to differences in longevity.
- Family pedigree. The prevalence of schizophrenia in first-degree relatives is greater than that found in the general population but less than the prevalence of schizophrenia in first-degree relatives in early-onset probands.
- Symptoms. Symptoms in late-onset schizophrenia are similar to those in early-onset schizophrenia, especially the paranoid type.

- Course. The course is more or less chronic, with a poor prognosis.
- Premorbid. Premorbidity may consist of schizoid or paranoid traits.
- Biology. There appears to be a higher than normal prevalence in auditory and visual sensory deficits. Magnetic resonance imaging suggests there is a subgroup with structural abnormalities.
- Differential diagnosis. It is especially important to rule out major affective disorder, organic brain syndrome, delusional disorder, and schizophrenia before age 45 years.
- Treatment. There is frequent symptomatic improvement with neuroleptics.

Harris and Jeste (1988) concluded that late-onset schizophrenia is no less valid than early-onset schizophrenia. Whether it represents a subtype of schizophrenia is unclear.

Harris and colleagues (1988) examined five cases of late-onset schizophrenia, four men and one woman. The predominant symptomatology consisted of bizarre delusions, usually persecutory, and auditory hallucinations. It is clear that the patients are functioning quite well up until age 45, that they have a marked deterioration in functioning with onset, and that organic etiologic factors are satisfactorily ruled out. The authors made the point that late-onset schizophrenia is a clinically diagnosable entity.

Jeste and colleagues (1988b) studied the face validity and descriptive validity of late-onset schizophrenia. Their study consists of two investigations.

In the first study, they compare late-onset schizophrenia across four centers: 1) the University of California at San Diego (UCSD); 2) the University of California at Los Angeles; 3) Johns Hopkins in Baltimore, Maryland; and 4) Douglas Hospital in Montreal. The inclusion criteria for this collaborative study (which is ongoing) are from DSM-III-R. Stringent exclusion criteria are used at UCSD. They insist on adequate information, including independent historical corroboration, usually from a family member. They also are careful to rule out organic brain syndrome, mood disorder, substance abuse, institutionalization, and schizophrenia with onset prior to age 45. In this report each center has approximately 10 subjects. The cases are similar in the following ways: 1) most are married; 2) sensory deficits are not common (6 of 36 patients); 3) the most frequent symptoms are delusions (often bizarre) followed by hallucinations; 4) loose associations and inappropriate affect are uncommon; 5) the Mini-Mental Status Exam (Folstein et al. 1975) scores are 26–28 (scores ≤ 24 being equivalent to dementia); 6) the course is chronic; and 7) the type is paranoid.

In the second study, they compare late-onset schizophrenia (N = 10) with early-onset schizophrenia (N= 15) from UCSD. The following similarities between groups are noted: 1) the duration is 7–9 years; 2) sensory deficits are rare; 3) there is a high frequency of bizarre delusions and hallucinations; 4) the subtype is paranoid; and 5) the course is chronic. The following differences are noted: 1) those with younger-onset schizophrenia have a greater prevalence of loose associations and inappropriate affect; and 2) they are single compared with those with late-onset schizophrenia, most of whom are married. The early and late onsets are roughly equivalent in prevalence of positive symptomatology, but the early onsets present with definitely more negative symptoms.

Jeste and colleagues (1988a) wrote a summary article for a comprehensive text. It includes most of the points covered in Jeste and colleagues (1988b). Additional points include that, premorbidly, patients with late-onset schizophrenia tend to have fairly adequate occupational and social adjustment until the beginning of middle life. They noted that the most common brain abnormality (on magnetic resonance imaging) is nonspecific subcortical white matter changes. Overall, they asserted that late-onset schizophrenia is clinically characterized by 1) female predominance; 2) paranoid symptomatology (paranoid delusions most common, auditory hallucinations second); 3) a chronic course; 4) symptomatic improvement with low-dose neuroleptics; 5) premorbid schizoid and paranoid personality types that are, nevertheless, not too severe because premorbid occupational and social functioning are relatively intact; and 6) a positive family history of schizophrenia that is frequently *lacking*.

Pearlson and Rabins (1988) reviewed the literature on risk factors for development of schizophrenia and affective disorders in late life. They listed the risk factors for late-onset schizophrenia as 1) a genetic predisposition; 2) premorbid schizotypal personality disorder or paranoid personality disorder; 3) increasing social isolation with age (leading to the prominent symptom of suspiciousness); 4) advancing visual, auditory, and sensory defects (leading to frequent misinterpretations of the environment); 5) menopause and other hormonal problems for women (leading to an excess of dopamine D_2 receptors); and 6) nonspecific brain atrophy (leading to a variety of cognitive problems).

Pearlson and colleagues (G. Pearlson, L. Creger, P. V. Rabins, et al., Late life onset schizophrenia, unpublished manuscript, 1989) conducted a chart review study of selected patients. A single rater examined all of the charts. No reliability data are available.

Three groups were constructed: 54 late-onset schizophrenia patients; 22 elderly, early-onset patients matched for current age; and 54 young, early-onset patients matched for gender and socioeconomic status. Compared with the control groups, the patients with late-onset schizophrenia have the following characteristics.

- Description. Of the patients, 87% are female, and 93% are married. Furthermore, 78% of the married females have children.

- Symptoms. Patients with late-onset schizophrenia have more visual, tactile, and olfactory hallucinations as well as hallucinations in more senses than either control group. Patients with late-onset schizophrenia have more persecutory delusions but less thought disorder and less affective blunting. Both thought disorder and affective blunting decrease significantly with age. There are no significant differences in the frequency of catatonia or first-rank symptoms.
- Premorbid. Patients with late-onset schizophrenia have more premorbid schizoid personalities and more auditory and visual impairments. They also tend to be living alone. Family history of schizophrenia does not discriminate.
- Treatment response. A significantly higher percentage of the group with late-onset schizophrenia have a complete remission with neuroleptics.
- Predictors. Thought disorder and schizoid personality disorder have a negative effect on treatment response.

Discussion and Recommendations

Diagnostic Category

Is there schizophrenia of late onset? Yes. The above reviews and prospective survey strongly suggest that late-onset schizophrenia is a valid entity. It appears DSM-III-R was correct in eliminating the age limit of 45.

Subtype Status

Late-onset schizophrenia has some interesting differences from early-onset schizophrenia, although it is unknown how robust they will turn out to be since the data are very new, preliminary, and based on a relatively small number of patients. The following features currently characterize late-onset schizophrenia and may be incorporated in a textual description.

- Symptoms. Can overlap with those of early-onset schizophrenia but tend more in direction of bizarre paranoid delusions and hallucinations, especially auditory. Thought disorder, inappropriate affect, and negative symptoms are uncommon.
- Course. Chronic, although patients are often quite responsive symptomatically to low-dose neuroleptics.
- Premorbid. High frequency of schizoid, schizotypal, and paranoid personality disorder. On the other hand, most patients are or have been married, and their premorbid instrumental capacity is high.
- Prevalence. Not really known but not rare. Estimated at 10% of cases of schizophrenia.

- Sex ratio. Many more females than males.
- Family history of schizophrenia. Frequently lacking.
- Biological risk factors. Sensory deficits with aging have an undetermined association with late-onset schizophrenia and may not be as common as initially thought.
- Differential diagnosis. Affective disorder, organic brain syndromes, and delusional disorder.

Criteria

P. V. Rabins and D. V. Jeste (personal communication, 1989) feel there is a difficulty with the "deteriorating of functioning" criterion for older people. The criterion requires deterioration from the "highest level" of functioning. However, in geriatric populations that develop late-onset schizophrenia, premorbid general level of functioning can already be quite compromised. They suggest that a caveat be incorporated somehow in the criterion much like that which exists for childhood onset schizophrenia.

References

American Psychiatric Association: Diagnostic and Statistical Manual of Mental Disorders, 3rd Edition. Washington, DC, American Psychiatric Association, 1980

American Psychiatric Association: Diagnostic and Statistical Manual of Mental Disorders, 3rd Edition, Revised. Washington, DC, American Psychiatric Association, 1987

Folstein MF, Folstein SE, McHugh PR: Mini-Mental State: a practical method for grading the cognitive state of patients for the clinician. J Psychiatr Res 12:189–198, 1975

Harris MJ, Jeste D: Late onset schizophrenia: an overview. Schizophr Bull 14:39–55, 1988

Harris MJ, Cullum CM, Jeste DB: Clinical presentation of late onset schizophrenia. J Clin Psychiatry 49:356–360, 1988

Jeste DB, Harris MJ, Zweifach M: Late onset schizophrenia, in Psychiatry. Edited by Michels R. Philadelphia, PA, JB Lippincott, 1988a

Jeste DB, Harris MJ, Pearlson GD, et al: Late onset schizophrenia: studying clinical validity. Psychiatr Clin North Am 11:1–13, 1988b

Pearlson G, Rabins P: The late onset psychoses: possible risk factors. Psychiatr Clin North Am 11:15–32, 1988

Chapter 27

Secondary Depression in Schizophrenia

Samuel G. Siris, M.D.

Statement of the Issues

Inasmuch as ICD-10 (World Health Organization 1992) will include a diagnostic category of Post-Schizophrenic Depression, is it valid and worthwhile for DSM-IV to include such a category?

Significance of the Issues

Since the initial descriptions of schizophrenia, it has been recognized that a variety of depression-like symptoms may precede, accompany, or follow the flagrant manifestations of psychosis in these patients (Berrios and Bulbena 1987). These symptoms have consistently presented diagnostic problems, even when their consideration has been confined to the epoch following the resolution (complete or partial) of flagrant psychotic symptomatology. DSM-III-R (American Psychiatric Association 1987) has dealt with this situation by suggesting consideration of the additional diagnosis of Depressive Disorder Not Otherwise Specified (NOS) or Bipolar Disorder NOS when episodes of marked mood disturbance are confined to the residual phase of schizophrenia. The critique has been advanced, however, that this approach offers no more than limited assistance to clinicians faced with crucial treatment decisions (Bartels and Drake 1988), and the need has been articulated for a clearly defined, criteria-based diagnosis of secondary depression in schizophrenia (Becker et al. 1985).

ICD-10 proposes to introduce specific criteria for the definition of secondary

This work was supported, in part, by Grants MH34309 and DA05039.

depression in schizophrenia. For such a diagnosis to be warranted, however, there needs to be demonstration of the existence of a corresponding definable syndrome, and evidence that the definition of such a syndrome would represent a meaningful and helpful clinical entity.

Methods

The literature was reviewed by means of a Medline computer search of the topic of depression as coexisting with schizophrenia, augmented by the author's personal files. Papers were selected for emphasis on the basis of the clarity of the diagnostic criteria employed. Review of psychopharmacologic trials was limited to double-blind, placebo-controlled studies.

Results

Observations Supporting the Existence of a Definable Secondary Depression Syndrome in Schizophrenia

Numerous studies have been published over the years describing a state in the course of patients with schizophrenia that bears phenotypic resemblance to the syndrome of depression (Abuzzahab and Zimmerman 1982; Barnes et al. 1989; Carney and Sheffield 1973; Donlon et al. 1976; Falloon et al. 1978; Floru et al. 1975; Guze et al. 1983; Hirsch et al. 1989; Hogarty and Munetz 1984; House et al. 1987; Johnson 1973, 1981b, 1988; Knights et al. 1979; Leff et al. 1988; Mandel et al. 1982; Martin et al. 1985; McGlashan and Carpenter 1976a; Moller and von Zerssen 1982; Munro et al. 1984; Planansky and Johnston 1980; Roy 1980, 1981, 1986; Siris et al. 1981; Stern et al. 1972; Summers et al. 1983; Van Putten and May 1978; Weissman et al. 1977; Winokur 1972). These studies vary in a number of respects. A wide diversity of diagnostic criteria are employed; different "postpsychotic intervals" are examined (some studies are simply cross-sectional in nature); and various definitions of a depression-like state are employed (some categorical, others dimensional). Yet all of these published studies find a meaningful incidence of some sort of depression-like state among schizophrenic patients who are no longer flagrantly psychotic. Indeed, the very diversity of these studies gives them the strength of generalizability. The rates of reported depression, of course, varied widely with the different intervals and definitions examined, ranging from as few as 7% to as many as 70% of cases. The rate of 25%, as culled from the early literature by McGlashan and Carpenter (1976b), would seem a fair approximation of a modal rate estimate.

One of the important critiques of the "true" existence of secondary depression of schizophrenia concerns the question of whether or not it might be a neuroleptic-induced phenomenon. Some descriptions, particularly in the earlier psychopharmacology literature, raised a serious question of whether this might indeed be the case (Ananth and Ghadirian 1980; Carney and Sheffield 1976; DeAlarcon and Carney 1969; Floru et al. 1975; Galdi 1983; Galdi et al. 1981; Johnson 1981a). More recently, however, the weight of evidence has seemed to come down against this being an explanation that could account for all or nearly all the cases of secondary depression in schizophrenia.

This evidence stems mostly from three types of studies. In the first type, acutely psychotic patients are followed for evidence of depression-like symptomatology throughout the course of their acute treatment with neuroleptic medication (Alfredsson et al. 1984; Donlon et al. 1976; Green et al. 1990; Hirsch et al. 1989; House et al. 1987; Knights and Hirsch 1981; Leff et al. 1988; Moller and von Zerssen 1982; Shanfield et al. 1970; Strian et al. 1982; Szymanski et al. 1983). The studies found that considerable depression-like symptomatology exists at the height of the psychotic episodes (although it may not be obvious due to the more florid psychotic symptomatology). During the course of neuroleptic treatment, not only does the psychotic symptomatology subside, but the depression-like symptomatology also generally diminishes, although perhaps at a slower rate. This is contrary to what would be expected if the depression-like symptoms were to be caused by the neuroleptic medication.

The second type of relevant study examines neuroleptic-treated schizophrenic patients being compared with patients not treated with neuroleptics (Hirsch et al. 1973, 1989; Hogarty and Munetz 1984; Wistedt and Palmstierna 1983). In these studies, as much or more depression-like symptomatology is found among patients not treated with neuroleptics as among neuroleptic-treated patients. Additionally, one retrospective study that examined chronic schizophrenic patients from the era before neuroleptics found a high incidence of depression-like symptomatology (Planansky and Johnston 1980).

The third category of relevant study compared schizophrenic patients with depression and those without depression. These studies found that neuroleptic doses were not higher in schizophrenic patients with depression (Barnes et al. 1989; Berrios and Bulbena 1987; Roy 1984; Roy et al. 1983) and that there was no relationship between the extent of depression and neuroleptic dosage (Siris et al. 1988a), plasma neuroleptic level (Siris et al. 1988a), or cerebrospinal fluid neuroleptic concentration (Alfredsson et al. 1984).

Two neuroleptic side effects deserve careful consideration in this context, however. One is the syndrome of neuroleptic-induced akinesia (Rifkin et al. 1975, 1978; Van Putten and May 1978), which may be subtle yet devastating. Patients with this side effect lack spontaneity and fail to initiate or sustain activities properly. The resultant anergic and anhedonic state can very closely resemble depressive symptomatology (Martin et al. 1985; Siris 1987), a distinction that may be rendered even more difficult because the akinesia syndrome can occur with insidious onset (Van Putten and May 1978) and without other concomitant extrapyramidal symptomatology (Siris 1987; Van Putten and May 1978) and can be accompanied by blue mood (Siris 1987; Van Putten and May 1978). The other neuroleptic-induced syndrome easily mistaken for depression is akathisia (Martin et al. 1985; Van Putten 1974, 1975). Akathisia is often accompanied by intense dysphoria and has been associated with suicide (Drake and Ehrlich 1985; Shear et al. 1983; Van Putten and Marder 1987). Prominent restlessness makes blatant cases of akathisia obvious, but more subtle cases can present difficult diagnostic problems.

Comparisons of Schizophrenic Patients With Versus Without Secondary Depressions

A crucial validator of the utility of making a diagnostic distinction between schizophrenia with and without secondary depression concerns whether or not making this distinction helps us know anything else of value about the patient. A number of studies have been conducted comparing schizophrenic patients who do versus do not manifest a pattern of secondary depression-like symptomatology (Barnes et al. 1989; Berrios and Bulbena 1987; Glazer et al. 1981; Mandel et al. 1982; McGlashan and Carpenter 1976a; Munro et al. 1984; Roy 1981; Roy et al. 1983). Although these studies differ widely in terms of diagnostic strategies and the definition of secondary depression in schizophrenia, each finds various differences between the secondary depression and nondepression groups in terms of historical and demographic information, prognosis, biological attributes, and treatment response. Specifically, patients with secondary depressions were found to have a more impaired level of social functioning (Glazer et al. 1981; McGlashan and Carpenter 1976a; Roy et al. 1983), to be more likely to be rehospitalized (Berrios and Bulbena 1987; Mandel et al. 1982), to be more likely to have suffered early parental loss (Roy 1980, 1981; Roy et al. 1983), to have more previous episodes of depression and past suicide attempts (Roy et al. 1983), to have more previous hospitalizations (Mandel et al. 1982; Roy et al. 1983), and to have more auditory hallucinations (Barnes et al. 1989; Berrios and Bulbena 1987).

Perhaps the most crucial question is the relationship, if any, between the occurrence of secondary depression in schizophrenia and overall prognosis. In terms of this issue, the literature is somewhat divided. The earlier writings, which have been well-reviewed (Goplerud and Depue 1979; McGlashan and Carpenter 1976b), tend to favor the notion that depression-like symptomatology in schizophrenia represents a positive prognostic indicator. A problem with many of these papers, however, is that clear distinctions are not made between depressive symptomatology that occurs prior to or concomitant with the flagrant psychosis and depressive symptomatology that follows its resolution. More recent chart reviews also wrestle with the same dilemma (McGlashan 1986). A further problem is that most of the early studies preceded the advent of modern operationalized diagnostic criteria, so that at least some of the patients who eventually had favorable outcomes might now have been considered to be suffering from affective or schizoaffective disorders.

A number of more recent studies have generated evidence that specifically postpsychotic depressive symptomatology may be associated with unfavorable prognostic significance (Bartels and Drake 1988; Becker 1988; Becker et al. 1985). Patients manifesting secondary depression in schizophrenia have been found to be significantly more likely to experience a relapse into psychosis (Falloon et al. 1978; Mandel et al. 1982), an observation that appears to be separable from the depression-like symptomatology that frequently occurs as an early stage in the process of psychotic decompensation in schizophrenia (Docherty et al. 1978; Herz 1985; Herz and Melville 1980; Wistedt and Palmstierna 1983). In terms of their unfavorable implications, these reports are conceptually consistent with the findings of correlations between a postpsychotic depressive state in schizophrenia and poor premorbid adjustment, schizoid and neurotic traits, insidious onset of the first and index psychotic episodes (Moller and von Zerssen 1986), and histories of more early parental loss (Roy 1980, 1981; Roy et al. 1983).

Another blatantly unfavorable outcome in schizophrenia is suicide, the means by which approximately 10% of schizophrenic lives terminate (Drake et al. 1984; Roy 1986). More schizophrenic suicides have been observed to have histories of depressive episodes, or to have shown depression-like symptomatology at their last contact, than suitable control groups (Roy 1982). Suicide in schizophrenia may correlate specifically with hopelessness and the more psychological aspects of depression in these patients, rather than with more vegetative features (Drake and Cotton 1986). Furthermore, significantly more depression-like symptomatology has been observed in schizophrenic patients who attempt suicide (Prasad 1986; Prasad and Kumar 1988), and significantly more schizophrenic patients who have attempted suicide have been found to have histories of depressive episodes (Roy 1986; Roy et al. 1984). Suicidal ideation has also been found more frequently in those schizophrenic patients who have other depression-like symptomatology (Barnes et al. 1989).

Studies of biological features potentially differentiating schizophrenic patients with secondary depressions from those without have included studies of the dexamethasone suppression test, the thyrotropin-releasing hormone test, and studies of platelet monoamine oxidase activity. Results of the dexamethasone suppression test have been mixed, with both a relationship of nonsuppression to depression (Coppen et al. 1983; Munro et al. 1984) and no such relationship being reported (Siris et al. 1984; Whiteford et al. 1988). The one reported series to investigate the thyrotropin-releasing hormone test in schizophrenic patients with secondary depressions found comparable rates among these patients to a control group of primary depressed patients matched for age and gender (Siris et al. 1989b). Higher levels of platelet monoamine oxidase activity were found in patients with schizophrenia-related depressions, compared with both nonschizophrenic control subjects and nondepressed schizophrenic patients (Schildkraut et al. 1978, 1980).

From an alternative biological perspective, some evidence has accumulated that schizophrenic patients who develop secondary depressions may be distinguished in terms of their genetic predispositions. Schizophrenic patients with unipolar depressed first-degree relatives have been found to be significantly more likely to have a depression-like syndrome develop following the resolution of a psychotic episode (Kendler and Hays 1983), and neuroleptics have been specifically associated with the emergence of depression-like symptomatology in schizophrenic patients who have depressed relatives (Galdi et al. 1981). In the latter study, this "pharmacogenetic depression" seemed to be associated with the development of extrapyramidal effects (i.e., akinesia). On the other hand, two other studies have specifically found no differences in the rates of primary affective disorders among the relatives of schizophrenic patients with and without intercurrent episodes of depression (Berrios and Bulbena 1987; Guze et al. 1983). The risk of a Type II error in these relatively small *N* (70 and 44, respectively) negative studies, however, is greater than the risk of a Type I error in the reported positive studies.

Treatment Studies

A number of treatment studies have been undertaken to investigate the utility of adjunctive antidepressant medication in schizophrenia with secondary depression. Since antidepressant medication has generally been found to be without value in the acute treatment of schizophrenic patients who do not manifest secondary depression-like symptomatology (Siris et al. 1978), or who manifest their depressive symptomatology only in the context of a flagrant psychotic episode (Kramer et al. 1989), the finding of antidepressant efficacy in the context of secondary (i.e., postpsychotic) depression would constitute practical evidence that the identification of such a syndrome has clinical utility.

Nine double-blind studies of adjunctive antidepressant medications added to the neuroleptic regimen of schizophrenic patients with secondary depression-like symptomatology have been reported (Siris 1990). Four of these show an advantage to the addition of the antidepressant; five found no such advantage. The methodology of the negative studies, however, makes their interpretation difficult. In one, the dose of antidepressant may have been too low (Waehrens and Gerlach 1980); in another, the antidepressant dose may have been too high (Johnson 1981b); in one, a different neuroleptic was used for those patients who received the antidepressant than for the patients who did not (Becker 1983); and in the final two, the issue is unclear as to whether or not the patients were flagrantly psychotic at the time of the study (Dufresne et al. 1988; Kurland and Nagaraju 1981). In each of these final two studies, there is also the question of adequacy of antidepressant dosage and treatment duration.

The three acute treatment studies that have shown a benefit to adjunctive antidepressant medication in stabilized schizophrenic patients with secondary depressions, who are not flagrantly psychotic, do not suffer these same methodological drawbacks. Two of these showed modest amounts of clinical improvement, generally in the dimension of depression-like symptomatology (Prusoff et al. 1979; Singh et al. 1978). The final positive acute treatment study found substantial improvement in both depressive symptoms and the depression syndrome (Siris et al. 1987). In this study, patients had been identified as having a full depression syndrome before the start of the trial, and this was the only study in which a rigorous attempt had been made before the trial to rule out the confound of neuroleptic-induced akinesia. Additionally, there has been one trial suggesting the benefit of maintenance adjunctive antidepressant treatment in schizophrenic patients with secondary depression (Siris et al. 1989a). Finally, in one small double-blind study, 6 of 11 medication-free depressed schizophrenic patients showed improvement in response to the addition of lithium (Van Kammen et al. 1980). Otherwise, lithium has not been studied in the context of secondary depression in schizophrenia.

In summary, then, although the issue is not conclusively established, there is some degree of evidence that adjunctive tricyclic-type antidepressants may be useful for at least a subset of secondarily depressed schizophrenic patients, and that secondarily depressed schizophrenic patients may therefore be a category worthy of distinguishing for purposes of psychopharmacologic intervention.

Differential Diagnosis

Various conditions occurring in the course of schizophrenia can present with symptomatology consistent with the picture of secondary depression.

The first differential diagnosis consists of medical conditions, alcoholism, substance abuse, and other organic causes of depression that can occur during the course of schizophrenia (Bartels and Drake 1988). Next to be considered are neuroleptic-induced akinesia and akathisia, which have been referred to earlier. Also, with regard to neuroleptic medications, there is the controversial topic, as detailed earlier, about whether or not these medications can produce an iatrogenic state of "true" depression.

The next differential diagnosis for a secondary depression syndrome in schizophrenia is "prepsychotic" depressive symptomatology. The frequent occurrence of various depression-like symptoms, if not a full depression-like syndrome, during the course of decompensation into psychosis has been well described in schizophrenia (Docherty et al. 1978; Herz 1985; Herz and Melville 1980; Wistedt and Palmstierna 1983). In this case a relatively brief period of watchful waiting would be sufficient for the condition to declare its true identity. A second condition detectable by watchful waiting is the situational disappointment reaction (Siris et al. 1986). A more difficult differential diagnosis for secondary depression in schizophrenia, which is not distinguishable by watchful waiting, is the syndrome of chronic discouragement known as demoralization (Frank 1973; Klein 1974).

The negative symptom syndrome of schizophrenia has prominent features of anergia and anhedonia, as well as a flattening of affect (Andreasen and Olsen 1982; Carpenter et al. 1985; Crow 1980; Pogue-Geile and Zubin 1988; Strauss et al. 1974). With such features, it can easily be mistaken for depression, especially in schizophrenic individuals who do not always express their affect in typical ways. Indeed, the negative symptom syndrome has been described as overlapping phenomenologically, if not conceptually, with the postpsychotic depression syndrome of schizophrenia (Martin et al. 1985; Prosser et al. 1987; Siris et al. 1988b). The deficit syndrome of schizophrenia is another concept related to the negative symptom syndrome, and, by extension, then also related to the secondary depression syndrome (Carpenter et al. 1988). An additional syndrome that has been described in schizophrenia—related to the negative symptom and deficit concepts—and that can easily be confused with secondary depression is a state of psychic blankness maintained adaptively for aims that are psychodynamically defensive in nature (McGlashan 1982).

Discussion and Recommendations

Arguing for the inclusion of the state of secondary depression in schizophrenia is the large bulk of evidence that it exists as a definable clinical state, that it may have prognostic and therapeutic implications, and that it may have distinct associations with other clinical phenomena and demographic characteristics. Arguing against the inclusion of secondary depression in schizophrenia as a DSM-IV diagnosis is the difficulty involved in its differential diagnosis.

On balance, the secondary depression syndrome in schizophrenia appears to be important, and the only way to learn more about it and deal with it is to identify it. Even if our initial boundaries for identifying the syndrome are not perfect, they provide a place to begin—to learn more about the syndrome, its proper boundaries, its correct amount of overlap (or lack of it) with other syndromes, and its correct role in our understanding of the clinical phenomenology we encounter. For that reason, it seems logical to follow the lead of ICD-10 and include a category of secondary depression in schizophrenia in the DSM-IV. For the sake of scientific uniformity, DSM-IV might adopt the criteria proposed for inclusion in ICD-10 as Post-Schizophrenia Depression.

One problem with the adoption of the ICD-10 criteria is its requirement for a flagrant episode of schizophrenic illness to have occurred within the past 12 months. The literature reviewed earlier does not substantiate this arbitrarily timed cutoff. One perhaps should therefore consider eliminating the arbitrary 12-month limitation and simply confirm that the patient has had a schizophrenic illness meeting the general criteria for schizophrenia "at some time in the past." The literature suggests that this change would work quite well, as long as the second ICD-10 criterion—"some schizophrenic symptoms are still present" (World Health Organization 1992, p. 93)—is preserved.

References

Abuzzahab FS, Zimmerman RL: Psychopharmacological correlates of post-psychotic depression: a double-blind investigation of haloperidol vs thiothixene in outpatient schizophrenia. J Clin Psychiatry 43:105–110, 1982

Alfredsson G, Harnryd C, Wiesel F-A: Effects of sulpiride and chlorpromazine on depressive symptoms in schizophrenic patients: relationship to drug concentrations. Psychopharmacology (Berlin) 84:237–241, 1984

American Psychiatric Association: Diagnostic and Statistical Manual of Mental Disorders, 3rd Edition, Revised. Washington, DC, American Psychiatric Association, 1987

Ananth J, Ghadirian AM: Drug-induced mood disorders. International Pharmacopsychiatry 15:59–73, 1980

Andreasen NC, Olsen S: Negative vs positive schizophrenia: definition and validation. Arch Gen Psychiatry 39:789–794, 1982

Barnes TR, Curson DA, Liddle PF, et al: The nature and prevalence of depression in chronic schizophrenic in-patients. Br J Psychiatry 154:486–491, 1989

Bartels SJ, Drake RE: Depressive symptoms in schizophrenia: comprehensive differential diagnosis. Compr Psychiatry 29:467–483, 1988

Becker RE: Implications of the efficacy of thiothixene and a chlorpromazine-imipramine combination for depression in schizophrenia. Am J Psychiatry 140:208–211, 1983

Becker RE: Depression in schizophrenia. Hosp Community Psychiatry 39:1269–1275, 1988

Becker RE, Singh MM, Meisler N, et al: Clinical significance, evaluation, and management of secondary depression in schizophrenia. J Clin Psychiatry 46 [11, sec 2]:26–32, 1985

Berrios GE, Bulbena A: Post psychotic depression: the Fulbourn cohort. Acta Psychiatr Scand 76:89–93, 1987

Carney MWP, Sheffield BF: The long-term maintenance treatment of schizophrenic outpatients with depot fluphenthixol. Curr Med Res Opin 1:423–426, 1973

Carney MWP, Sheffield BF: Comparison of antipsychotic depot injections in the maintenance treatment of schizophrenia. Br J Psychiatry 129:476–481, 1976

Carpenter WT Jr, Heinrichs DW, Alphs LD: Treatment of negative symptoms. Schizophr Bull 11:440–452, 1985

Carpenter WT Jr, Heinrichs DW, Wagman AMI: Deficit and nondeficit forms of schizophrenia: the concept. Am J Psychiatry 145:578–583, 1988

Coppen A, Abou-saleh M, Milln P, et al: Dexamethasone suppression test in depression and other psychiatric illness. Br J Psychiatry 142:498–504, 1983

Crow TJ: Molecular pathology of schizophrenia: more than one disease process? BMJ 280:66–68, 1980

DeAlarcon R, Carney MWP: Severe depressive mood changes following slow-release intramuscular fluphenazine injection. BMJ 3:564–567, 1969

Docherty JP, Van Kammen DP, Siris SG, et al: Stages of onset of schizophrenic psychosis. Am J Psychiatry 135:420–426, 1978

Donlon PT, Rada RT, Arora KK: Depression and the reintegration phase of acute schizophrenia. Am J Psychiatry 133:1265–1268, 1976

Drake RE, Cotton PG: Depression, hopelessness and suicide in chronic schizophrenia. Br J Psychiatry 148:554–559, 1986

Drake RE, Ehrlich J: Suicide attempts associated with akathisia. Am J Psychiatry 142:499–501, 1985

Drake RE, Gates C, Cotton PG, et al: Suicide among schizophrenics: who is at risk? J Nerv Ment Dis 172:613–617, 1984

Dufresne RL, Kass DJ, Becker RE: Bupropion and thiothixene versus placebo and thiothixene in the treatment of depression in schizophrenia. Drug Development Research 12:259–266, 1988

Falloon I, Watt DC, Shepherd M: A comparative controlled trial of pimozide and fluphenazine decanoate in the continuation therapy of schizophrenia. Psychol Med 8:59–70, 1978

Floru L, Heinrich K, Wittek F: The problem of post-psychotic schizophrenic depressions and their pharmacological induction. International Pharmacopsychiatry 10:230–239, 1975

Frank JD: Persuasion and Healing. Baltimore, MD, Johns Hopkins University Press, 1973

Galdi J: The causality of depression in schizophrenia. Br J Psychiatry 142:621–625, 1983

Galdi J, Rieder RO, Silber D, et al: Genetic factors in the response to neuroleptics in schizophrenia: a pharmacogenetic study. Psychol Med 11:713–728, 1981

Glazer W, Prusoff B, John K, et al: Depression and social adjustment among chronic schizophrenic outpatients. J Nerv Ment Dis 169:712–717, 1981

Goplerud E, Depue RA: Affective symptoms, schizophrenia, and the conceptual ambiguity of postpsychotic depression. Schizophr Bull 5:554–559, 1979

Green MF, Nuechterlein KH, Ventura J, et al: The temporal relationship between depressive and psychotic symptoms in recent-onset schizophrenia. Am J Psychiatry 147:179–182, 1990

Guze SB, Cloninger CR, Martin RL, et al: A follow-up and family study of schizophrenia. Arch Gen Psychiatry 40:1273–1276, 1983

Herz M: Prodromal symptoms and prevention of relapse in schizophrenia. J Clin Psychiatry 46 [11, sec 2]:22–25, 1985

Herz M, Melville C: Relapse in schizophrenia. Am J Psychiatry 137:801–805, 1980

Hirsch SR, Gaind R, Rohde PD, et al: Outpatient maintenance of chronic schizophrenic patients with long-acting fluphenazine: double-blind placebo trial. BMJ 1:633–637, 1973

Hirsch SR, Jolley AG, Barnes TRE, et al: Dysphoric and depressive symptoms in chronic schizophrenia. Schizophr Res 2:259–264, 1989

Hogarty GE, Munetz MR: Pharmacogenic depression among outpatient schizophrenic patients: a failure to substantiate. J Clin Psychopharmacol 4:17–24, 1984

House A, Bostock L, Cooper J: Depressive syndromes in the year following onset of a first schizophrenic illness. Br J Psychiatry 151:773–779, 1987

Johnson DAW: The side-effects of fluphenazine decanoate. Br J Psychiatry 123:519–522, 1973

Johnson DAW: Depressions in schizophrenia: some observations on prevalence, etiology, and treatment. Acta Psychiatr Scand 63 (suppl 291):137–144, 1981a

Johnson DAW: Studies of depressive symptoms in schizophrenia. Br J Psychiatry 139:89–101, 1981b

Johnson DAW: The significance of depression in the prediction of relapse in chronic schizophrenia. Br J Psychiatry 152:320–323, 1988

Kendler KS, Hays P: Schizophrenia subdivided by the family history of affective disorder: a comparison of symptomatology and course of illness. Arch Gen Psychiatry 40:951–955, 1983

Klein DF: Endogenomorphic depression: a conceptual and terminological revision. Arch Gen Psychiatry 31:447–454, 1974

Knights A, Hirsch SR: "Revealed" depression and drug treatment for schizophrenia. Arch Gen Psychiatry 38:806–811, 1981

Knights A, Okasha MS, Salih MA, et al: Depressive and extrapyramidal symptoms and clinical effects: a trial of fluphenazine versus flupenthixol in maintenance of schizophrenic out-patients. Br J Psychiatry 135:515–523, 1979

Kramer MS, Vogel WH, DiJohnson C, et al: Antidepressants in "depressed" schizophrenic inpatients: a controlled trial. Arch Gen Psychiatry 46:922–928, 1989

Kurland AA, Nagaraju A: Viloxazine and the depressed schizophrenic: methodological issues. J Clin Pharmacol 21:37–41, 1981

Leff J, Tress K, Edwards B: The clinical course of depressive symptoms in schizophrenia. Schizophr Res 1:25–30, 1988

Mandel MR, Severe JB, Schooler NR, et al: Development and prediction of postpsychotic depression in neuroleptic-treated schizophrenics. Arch Gen Psychiatry 39:197–203, 1982

Martin RL, Cloninger RC, Guze SB, et al: Frequency and differential diagnosis of depressive syndromes in schizophrenia. J Clin Psychiatry 46 [11, sec 2]:9–13, 1985

McGlashan TH: Aphanisis: the syndrome of pseudodepression in chronic schizophrenia. Schizophr Bull 8:118–134, 1982

McGlashan TH: The prediction of outcome in chronic schizophrenia, IV: the Chestnut Lodge follow-up study. Arch Gen Psychiatry 43:167–176, 1986

McGlashan TH, Carpenter WT Jr: An investigation of the postpsychotic depressive syndrome. Am J Psychiatry 133:14–19, 1976a

McGlashan TH, Carpenter WT Jr: Postpsychotic depression in schizophrenia. Arch Gen Psychiatry 33:231–239, 1976b

Moller HJ, von Zerssen D: Depressive states occurring during the neuroleptic treatment of schizophrenia. Schizophr Bull 8:109–117, 1982

Moller HJ, von Zerssen D: Depression in schizophrenia, in Handbook of Studies on Schizophrenia. Edited by Burrows RK, Norman LA, Rubinstein M. New York, Elsevier, 1986

Munro JG, Hardiker TM, Leonard DP: The dexamethasone depression test in residual schizophrenia with depression. Am J Psychiatry 141:250–252, 1984

Planansky K, Johnston R: Psychotropic drugs and depressive syndrome in schizophrenia. Psychiatr Q 52:214–221, 1980

Pogue-Geile MF, Zubin J: Negative symptomatology and schizophrenia: a conceptual and empirical review. International Journal of Mental Health 16:3–45, 1988

Prasad AJ: Attempted suicide in hospitalized schizophrenics. Acta Psychiatr Scand 74:42–42, 1986

Prasad AJ, Kumar N: Suicidal behavior in hospitalized schizophrenics. Suicide Life Threat Behav 18:265–269, 1988

Prosser ES, Csernansky JG, Kaplan J, et al: Depression, parkinsonian symptoms, and negative symptoms in schizophrenics treated with neuroleptics. J Nerv Ment Dis 175:100–105, 1987

Prusoff BA, Williams DH, Weissman MM, et al: Treatment of secondary depression in schizophrenia. Arch Gen Psychiatry 36:569–575, 1979

Rifkin A, Quitkin F, Klein DF: Akinesia: a poorly recognized drug-induced extrapyramidal behavioral disorder. Arch Gen Psychiatry 32:672–674, 1975

Rifkin A, Quitkin F, Kane J, et al: Are prophylactic antiparkinsonian drugs necessary? a controlled study of procyclidine withdrawal. Arch Gen Psychiatry 35:483–489, 1978

Roy A: Depression in chronic paranoid schizophrenia. Br J Psychiatry 137:138–139, 1980

Roy A: Depression in the course of chronic undifferentiated schizophrenia. Arch Gen Psychiatry 38:296–297, 1981

Roy A: Suicide in chronic schizophrenia. Br J Psychiatry 141:171–177, 1982

Roy A: Do neuroleptics cause depression? Biol Psychiatry 19:777–781, 1984

Roy A: Depression, attempted suicide, and suicide in patients with chronic schizophrenia. Psychiatr Clin North Am 9:193–206, 1986

Roy A, Thompson R, Kennedy S: Depression in chronic schizophrenia. Br J Psychiatry 142:465–470, 1983

Roy A, Mazonson A, Pickar D: Attempted suicide in chronic schizophrenia. Br J Psychiatry 144:303–306, 1984

Schildkraut JJ, Orsulak PJ, Schatzberg AF, et al: Elevated platelet MAO activity in schizophrenia-related depressive disorders. Am J Psychiatry 135:110–112, 1978

Schildkraut JJ, Orsulak PJ, Schatzberg AF, et al: Platelet monoamine oxidase activity in subgroups of schizophrenic disorders. Schizophr Bull 6:220–225, 1980

Shanfield S, Tucker G, Harrow M, et al: The schizophrenic patient and depressive symptomatology. J Nerv Ment Dis 151:203–210, 1970

Shear K, Frances A, Weiden P: Suicide associated with akathisia and depot fluphenazine treatment. J Clin Psychopharmacol 3:235–236, 1983

Singh AN, Saxena B, Nelson HL: A controlled clinical study of trazodone in chronic schizophrenic patients with pronounced depressive symptomatology. Current Therapeutics Research 23:485–501, 1978

Siris SG: Akinesia and post-psychotic depression: a difficult differential diagnosis. J Clin Psychiatry 48:240–243, 1987

Siris SG: Pharmacological treatment of depression in schizophrenia, in Depression in Schizophrenia. Edited by DeLisi LE. Washington, DC, American Psychiatric Press, 1990, pp 141–162

Siris SG, Van Kammen DP, Docherty JP: Use of antidepressant drugs in schizophrenia. Arch Gen Psychiatry 35:1368–1377, 1978

Siris SG, Harmon GK, Endicott J: Postpsychotic depressive symptoms in hospitalized schizophrenic patients. Arch Gen Psychiatry 38:1122–1123, 1981

Siris SG, Rifkin A, Reardon GT, et al: The dexamethasone suppression test in patients with post-psychotic depressions. Biol Psychiatry 19:1351–1356, 1984

Siris SG, Rifkin A, Reardon GT, et al: Stability of the post-psychotic depression syndrome. J Clin Psychiatry 47:86–88, 1986

Siris SG, Morgan V, Fagerstrom R, et al: Adjunctive imipramine in the treatment of post-psychotic depression: a controlled trial. Arch Gen Psychiatry 44:533–539, 1987

Siris SG, Strahan A, Mandeli J, et al: Fluphenazine decanoate dose and severity of depression in patients with post-psychotic depression. Schizophr Res 1:31–35, 1988a

Siris SG, Adan F, Cohen M, et al: Post-psychotic depression and negative symptoms: an investigation of syndromal overlap. Am J Psychiatry 145:1532–1537, 1988b

Siris SG, Cutler J, Owen K, et al: Adjunctive imipramine maintenance in schizophrenic patients with remitted post-psychotic depressions. Am J Psychiatry 146:1495–1497, 1989a

Siris SG, Strahan A, Frechen K, et al: Thyroid-releasing hormone test in schizophrenic patients with post-psychotic depressions. Paper presented at the annual meeting of the American College of Neuropsychopharmacology, Washington, DC, December 13, 1989b

Stern MJ, Pillsbury JA, Sonnenberg SM: Postpsychotic depression in schizophrenics. Compr Psychiatry 13:591–598, 1972

Strauss JS, Carpenter WT Jr, Bartko JJ: The diagnosis and understanding of schizophrenia, III: speculations on the processes that underlie schizophrenic symptoms and signs. Schizophr Bull 11:61–75, 1974

Strian F, Heger R, Klicpera C: The time structure of depressive mood in schizophrenic patients. Acta Psychiatr Scand 65:66–73, 1982

Summers F, Harrow M, Westermeyer J: Neurotic symptoms in the postacute phase of schizophrenia. J Nerv Ment Dis 171:216–221, 1983

Szymanski HV, Simon J, Gutterman N: Recovery from schizophrenic psychosis. Am J Psychiatry 140:335–338, 1983

Van Kammen DP, Alexander PE, Bunney WE Jr: Lithium treatment in post-psychotic depression. Br J Psychiatry 136:479–485, 1980

Van Putten T: Why do schizophrenic patients refuse to take their drugs? Arch Gen Psychiatry 31:67–72, 1974

Van Putten T: The many faces of akathisia. Compr Psychiatry 16:43–47, 1975

Van Putten T, Marder SR: Behavioral toxicity of antipsychotic drugs. J Clin Psychiatry 48 [9, suppl]:13–19, 1987

Van Putten T, May PRA: "Akinetic depression" in schizophrenia. Arch Gen Psychiatry 35:1101–1107, 1978

Waehrens J, Gerlach J: Antidepressant drugs in anergic schizophrenia: a double-blind cross-over study with maprotiline and placebo. Acta Psychiatr Scand 61:438–444, 1980

Weissman MM, Pottenger M, Kleber H, et al: Symptom patterns in primary and secondary depression: a comparison of primary depressives with depressed opiate addicts, alcoholics, and schizophrenics. Arch Gen Psychiatry 34:854–862, 1977

Whiteford HA, Riney SJ, Savala RA, et al: Dexamethasone nonsuppression in chronic schizophrenia. Acta Psychiatr Scand 77:58–62, 1988

Winokur G: Family history studies, VIII: secondary depression is alive and well, and. . . . Diseases of the Nervous System 33:94–99, 1972

Wistedt B, Palmstierna T: Depressive symptoms in chronic schizophrenic patients after withdrawal of long-acting neuroleptics. J Clin Psychiatry 44:369–371, 1983

World Health Organization: The ICD-10 Classification of Mental and Behavioural Disorders: Clinical Descriptions and Diagnostic Guidelines. Geneva, World Health Organization, 1992

Chapter 28

The Nosologic Validity of Mood-Incongruent Psychotic Affective Illness

Kenneth H. Kendler, M.D.

STATEMENT AND SIGNIFICANCE OF THE ISSUES

One of the most important changes in DSM-III (American Psychiatric Association 1980) was the widening of the diagnostic concept of affective illness to include patients with mood-incongruent psychotic (MICP) symptoms. Such patients, who had been considered schizoaffective or schizophrenic in many other diagnostic systems, present with both a full affective syndrome (manic or depressive) and delusions or hallucinations the content of which is unrelated to grandiose or depressive themes (e.g., persecutory delusions not connected to "deserved punishment") and which is often bizarre and schizophrenia-like (e.g., thought insertion, delusions of control). To meet criteria for affective illness in DSM-III, these MICP symptoms must be restricted to periods when the patient is displaying a full affective syndrome. The purpose of this chapter is to review empirical evidence regarding the validity of the concept of mood-incongruent psychotic affective illness (MICPAI).

From a historical perspective, it is possible to articulate three hypotheses regarding the proper nosologic assignment of cases of affective illness with MICP symptoms.

Hypothesis 1

As advocated by Kraepelin (1921) and Lewis (1934, 1936), and as articulated in the DSM-III and DSM-III-R (American Psychiatric Association 1987) criteria,

This chapter is adapted from Kendler, *Archives of General Psychiatry* 48(April, 4):362–369, copyright 1991, American Medical Association, with permission.

MICPAI should be considered a form of affective illness. Within this viewpoint, it is useful to articulate two "subhypotheses." Subhypothesis 1A, as suggested by Pope and Lipinski (1978), is that these cases should all be considered to have affective illness and that they *will not* form a valid subtype because they will not be found to differ meaningfully, on any validating criteria, from cases with more typical affective illness. Subhypothesis 1B, as articulated by DSM-III and DSM-III-R, suggests that such cases should be considered as a subtype of affective illness. That is, using validating criteria, they will be found to resemble most closely cases with typical affective illness, but also to have some meaningful differences from them.

Hypothesis 2

As in the Research Diagnostic Criteria (RDC) (Spitzer et al. 1978), these cases should be considered as a form of schizoaffective disorder, which is in turn separable from both schizophrenia and affective disorder. That is, using validating criteria, cases of MICPAI should differ substantially from both schizophrenia and typical affective illness and should most closely resemble cases of schizoaffective disorder (e.g., as defined by DSM-III-R).

Hypothesis 3

As advocated by Bleuler (1924), and as articulated in DSM-I (American Psychiatric Association 1952) and DSM-II (American Psychiatric Association 1968), cases of MICPAI should be considered as a subtype of schizophrenia. That is, using validating criteria, they will be found to resemble most closely typical cases of schizophrenia.

Methods

An article was included in this review if it met the following criteria:

1. Data were reported on the diagnostic category of MICPAI using either DSM-III criteria *or* RDC for mainly affective schizoaffective disorder or using criteria that were described in sufficient detail to establish that they were approximately equal to these criteria.
2. One or more systematic comparison groups were used, including at least one of the following: for DSM-III criteria—schizophrenia, schizoaffective disorder, mood-congruent psychotic (MCP) affective illness or nonpsychotic affective illness; and for RDC—schizophrenia, mainly schizophrenic schizoaffective disorder, MCP affective illness or nonpsychotic affective illness.
3. The measurement of one or more potential validators in the various diagnostic groups.

4. Data were presented or described so as to make possible a statistical statement regarding the comparison of the validators in the various diagnostic groups.

Although not precisely identical, RDC for mainly affective schizoaffective disorder are close to the DSM-III criteria for MICPAI. Given the sparsity of data in this diagnostic area, the decision was made for this review to assume that RDC mainly affective schizoaffective disorder is an adequate "proxy" for MICPAI. Therefore, for the purposes of this report, patients meeting RDC for schizoaffective disorder, mainly affective type, will be termed MICPAI.

Utilizing diagnostic validators, I focus in this review on evaluating the three hypotheses regarding the proper nosologic position of MICPAI outlined above. Space precluded presenting the details of the results or methodology of each study. Tables are used to present most data; the text is reserved for summary and interpretation.

Results

Antecedent Validators

Family History

Table 28–1 summarizes the results of six studies that report the risk or prevalence of affective illness and/or schizophrenia in relatives of MICPAI patients and one or more relevant comparison groups (Abrams and Taylor 1983; Baron et al. 1982; Coryell and Zimmerman 1987; Coryell et al. 1982, 1985; Rosenthal et al. 1980). In addition, a seventh study of psychotic depression (Coryell and Zimmerman 1988) found "the risk of various illnesses among first-degree relatives failed to distinguish mood-congruent from mood-incongruent groups" (p. 25).

Hypothesis 1. The results of these studies are broadly consistent with this hypothesis. Relatives of individuals with MICPAI, like relatives of individuals with more typical affective illness, tend to have high rates of affective illness and low rates of schizophrenia in their relatives. The results, however, are more consistent with subhypothesis 1B than subhypothesis 1A as two studies (Coryell et al. 1982, 1985) produced four significant results showing lower rates for affective illness or higher rates for schizophrenia in relatives of patients with MICPAI versus more typical affective illness.

Hypothesis 2. Only one study reported findings relevant to this hypothesis (Baron et al. 1982). Those results, showing that relatives of MICPAI probands had

Table 28–1. Studies reporting risk of affective illness or schizophrenia in relatives of patients with mood-incongruent psychotic affective illness

Study	Polarity	Morbid risk for affective illness					Morbid risk for schizophrenia				
		NPAI	MCPAI	MICPAI	SA	SCH	NPAI	MCPAI	MICPAI	SA	SCH
Rosenthal et al. 1980[a]	B	24.8[b]		24.6	—	—	—	—	—	—	—
Coryell et al. 1982	U	13.3[c]	12.8	8.2	—	5.8	0.2[c]	0.8	1.6	—	2.8
Baron et al. 1982[a]	U,B	25.6[b]		28.1	10.9[c]	5.1[c]	0.3[b]		0	4.1	7.4[c]
Abrams and Taylor 1983	U	12.9	—	19.3	—	6.8[c]	0	—	0	—	1.6
Coryell et al. 1985[d]	U	27.0[c]	29.7[c]	16.3	—	—	0.4	0.9	1.8	—	—
Coryell and Zimmerman 1987[e]	U	—	21.9	22.2	—	12.5[c]	—	—	—	—	—

Note. NPAI = nonpsychotic affective illness. MCPAI = mood-congruent psychotic affective illness. MICPAI = mood-incongruent psychotic affective illness. SA = schizoaffective disorder. SCH = schizophrenia. U = unipolar illness only. B = bipolar illness only. U,B = both unipolar and bipolar illness.

[a]Research Diagnostic Criteria diagnoses. Presents results for nonpsychotic and mood-congruent psychotic patients only.

[b]These values placed in between NPAI and MCPAI because diagnoses are not sufficiently distinguished.

[c]$P < .05$ from MICPAI.

[d]Life-time prevalence.

[e]Risk only for Major Depression.

substantially higher rates of affective illness and lower rates of schizophrenia than relatives of schizoaffective probands, were not supportive of this hypothesis.

Hypothesis 3. The available studies provide consistent evidence *against* this hypothesis; compared with relatives of schizophrenic patients, relatives of MICPAI probands have higher rates of affective illness and lower rates of schizophrenia.

Demographics

Table 28–2 summarizes the results from seven studies that presented information on sex ratio and/or age at onset for MICPAI and one or more relevant comparison groups (Abrams and Taylor 1983; Breslau and Meltzer 1988; Coryell and Zimmerman 1988; Coryell et al. 1982, 1985; Rosenthal et al. 1980; Winokur et al. 1990). In addition, four studies were found that examined marital status in patients with MICPAI (Coryell and Zimmerman 1988; Coryell et al. 1982, 1985, 1986). Three studies compared the marital status of MCP and MICP depressed patients. Two found that MICP patients were more likely to be single (Coryell et al. 1982, 1985) (one statistically significant and one not), whereas one found MICP patients to be nonsignificantly less likely to be single (Coryell et al. 1986). One study found that patients with MICPAI were significantly less likely to be single than schizoaffective patients (Coryell and Zimmerman 1988).

Hypothesis 1. Regarding sex ratio, the results are consistent with this hypothesis; particularly, depression with MICP features appears to share with more typical depressions a substantial female preponderance. Data on marital status are sufficiently inconsistent as to be uninformative. However, the results regarding age at onset are not fully consistent with subhypothesis 1A. In all six reported comparisons, age at onset was earlier in MICPAI than in either nonpsychotic or MCP affective illness, and in four of these the difference was statistically significant.

Hypothesis 2. Only one study reported relevant information (Coryell and Zimmerman 1988). This study found that patients with MICP depression, compared with those with schizoaffective depressed type, are more likely to be female and to have a later age at onset and are significantly less likely to be single. These results argue weakly against the validity of hypothesis 2.

Hypothesis 3. Only one study (Abrams and Taylor 1983) reported relevant information, which was not consistent with this hypothesis. Compared with patients with MICPAI, patients with schizophrenia were significantly less likely to be female and had a significantly earlier age at onset.

Table 28–2. Studies reporting demographic characteristics of mood-incongruent psychotic affective illness

Study	Polarity	Female (%)					Mean age at onset (years)				
		NPAI	MCPAI	MICPAI	SA	SCH	NPAI	MCPAI	MICPAI	SA	SCH
Rosenthal et al. 1980[a]	B	—	59[b]	52	—	—	—	29[b,d]	24	—	—
Coryell et al. 1982	U	—	[c]	[c]	—	—	—	47[d]	29	—	—
Abrams and Taylor 1983	U	86	—	77	—	42[d]	34[d]	—	29	—	25[d]
Coryell et al. 1985	U	57	66	78	—	—	—	—	—	—	—
Coryell and Zimmerman 1988[a]	U	—	—	67	57	—	—	—	32	25	—
Breslau and Meltzer 1988[a]	U	—	64	65	—	—	—	26	25	—	—
Winokur et al. 1990	U,B										
Depression		64	68	73	—	—	37[d]	32	31	—	—
Mania		57	50	53	—	—	31	33	25	—	—

Note. NPAI = nonpsychotic affective illness. MCPAI = mood-congruent psychotic affective illness. MICPAI = mood-incongruent psychotic affective illness. SA = schizoaffective disorder. SCH = schizophrenia. B = bipolar illness only. U = unipolar illness only. U,B = both unipolar and bipolar illness.

[a]Research Diagnostic Criteria diagnoses.

[b]Mixed nonpsychotic and mood-congruent psychotic cases.

[c]Reported only as not significantly different.

[d]$P < .05$ from MICPAI.

Concurrent Validators

Clinical Variables

Only clinical variables that are unrelated to the diagnostic criteria used to select patients can be useful as diagnostic validators. Four reports were found that examined "depressive" or "melancholic" symptoms in MICP depressed patients versus more typical depressive patients. Coryell and colleagues (1985) compared the severity of 17 depressive symptoms in MCP versus MICP depressed patients and found that they differed significantly on five of them: guilt, negative evaluations of self, weight loss, fatigue, and dysphoria. For all five, the symptoms of the MICP patients were less severe than those of MCP patients. Two articles compared the proportion of patients with MCP versus MICP depression who met DSM-III criteria for melancholia (Caroff et al. 1983; Coryell et al. 1986), and both found melancholia to be significantly more common in MCP than in MICP depressed patients. Breslau and Meltzer (1988) compared the severity of 13 key depressive symptoms in patients with MCP and MICP depression. MCP depressed patients had higher scores on 9 of the 13 symptoms, but none of the differences were statistically significant.

Of the four studies, three produced results clearly inconsistent with subhypothesis 1A; the other had weak trends in the same direction. There is probably a meaningful difference in the severity of melancholic symptoms in depressed patients with MICP versus MCP symptoms.

Biologic Variables

The only potential biologic validator that was presented in more than one report was the dexamethasone suppression test (DST), which was reported on in MICP depressed patients and one or more relevant comparison groups in seven publications (Ayuso-Gutierrez et al. 1985; Caroff et al. 1983; Coryell et al. 1986; Katona and Roth 1985; Maj 1986; Sauer et al. 1984; Winokur et al. 1990). Although the specific method of assessment of suppression (e.g., dose of dexamethasone, timing of sampling, criteria for escape) varied across studies, the same method was always applied to each comparison group within each study. Six of these reports provide raw numbers and a total of 97 cases of MICP depression, of which 44 (45%) were defined as having escaped suppression.

Hypothesis 1. Six studies compared the rates of escape from DST in nonpsychotic versus MICP depressed patients (Ayuso-Gutierrez et al. 1985; Caroff et al. 1983; Katona and Roth 1985; Maj 1986; Sauer et al. 1984; Winokur et al. 1990). In one study (Sauer et al. 1984), a significant difference was found (higher rates of escape in the MICP patients); in the remaining five studies, the rates of escape were not significantly different (higher in MICP patients in two studies, higher in non-psychotic patients in three studies). Four studies compared the rates of escape from DST in MCP and MICP depressed patients (Ayuso-Gutierrez et al. 1985; Caroff et al. 1983; Coryell et al. 1986; Winokur et al. 1990). In two studies, the MCP patients had significantly higher rates of escape; in the other two reports, the rates were not significantly different (higher in MCP patients in one study and in MICP patients in the other). In summary, the DST results broadly support the validity of hypothesis 1. Patients with MICP depression appear to have elevated rates of DST escape broadly similar to that found with other forms of major depression. However, the results could be interpreted as modest evidence against subhypothesis 1A, as MICP cases probably have lower rates of DST escape than affective disorder cases with more typical psychotic features.

Hypothesis 2. Only one study examined this hypothesis (Maj 1986), reporting identical rates of DST escape in patients with MICP depression and schizoaffective disorder, depressed type. These results provide weak evidence in favor of this hypothesis.

Hypothesis 3. Two studies found substantially lower rates of DST escape in schizophrenic patients versus MICP depressed patients (Katona and Roth 1985; Sauer et al. 1984), and this difference was statistically significant in one of the reports. These results provide evidence against the validity of hypothesis 3.

Predictive Validators

Treatment Response

Three reports were found that examined response to electroconvulsive therapy (ECT) in MICPAI and one or more relevant comparison groups. Minter and Mandel (1979) reported that the rate of good response to ECT in MICP depression (80%) was very similar to that of patients with MCP depression (83%). Coryell and colleagues (1982) found the response to ECT similar among MCP patients (48% recovered at discharge) and MICP patients (52% recovered at discharge). Winokur and colleagues (1990) found a similar rate of "marked improvement" with ECT in depressed patients without psychosis (59%), with MCP (56%), and with MICP (70%).

Three reports examined the response to lithium prophylaxis in MICPAI and relevant comparison groups (Maj 1988; Maj et al. 1985; Rosenthal et al. 1980). Rosenthal and colleagues found no substantial difference in response to lithium over 2 years in MICP bipolar patients versus a mixed group of MCP and non-psychotic bipolar patients. By contrast, examining only depressed patients, Maj and colleagues found that, compared with MICP patients (19% good response), both MCP and nonpsychotic patients had a better response to lithium (39% and 58%, respectively), and the difference between the MICP and nonpsychotic patients was statistically significant. In another study of patients with mixed polarity, Maj, using RDC, found that the response rate to lithium was nonsignificantly greater in MICPAI (64%) than in schizoaffective patients (30%). Surprisingly, we were unable to locate two reports that examined response to tricyclic antidepressants or antipsychotic drugs in MICPAI and one or more relevant comparison groups.

Interpretation of these results is problematic. The response to ECT, which appears to be the same in MICP and more typical depression, supports the validity of hypothesis 1, and particularly subhypothesis 1A. However, the fact that the prophylactic response to lithium may be poorer in MICP patients argues against the validity of hypothesis 1. The better response to lithium in MICP versus schizoaffective illness argues, weakly, against hypothesis 2.

Outcome

Fourteen studies were found that provided outcome information on patients with MICPAI and one or more relevant comparison groups (Abrams and Taylor 1983; Brockington et al. 1982, 1983; Coryell and Tsuang 1985; Coryell and Zimmerman 1987, 1988; Coryell et al. 1982, 1986, 1990a, 1990b; M. Harrow, personal communication, 1990; Rosenthal et al. 1980; Van Praag and Nijo 1984; Winokur et al. 1990) (Table 28–3). Outcome was measured in many different ways, and no single outcome measure was common across all reports. In general, we used the best single "general measure" that reflected both psychosocial and symptomatic outcome. One exception was the report of Coryell and Tsuang, which presented such a rich array of comparisons that we were forced to compile a "box score" of the comparisons of four different outcome dimensions across five diagnostic classes. In addition to reports with numerical results, one report that used RDC (Grossman et al. 1984) found no significant differences ($P > .20$) in outcome between patients with MICPAI and schizoaffective disorder patients. Two articles (Van Praag and Nijo 1984; Winokur et al. 1990) reported separate results for patients with manic and depressive syndromes.

Hypothesis 1. Seven comparisons were available between MICP and nonpsychotic affective illness (Abrams and Taylor 1983; Brockington et al. 1982, 1983; Coryell and Tsuang 1985; Coryell et al. 1982; Van Praag and Nijo 1984; Winokur et al. 1990), and in all but one of them (Abrams and Taylor 1983) the MICP group had a worse outcome. However, in only three of these studies were the differences statistically significant (Coryell and Tsuang 1985; Coryell et al. 1982; Van Praag and Nijo 1984). Twelve studies produced 14 comparisons in outcome between MCP

Table 28–3. Studies reporting outcome of patients with mood-incongruent psychotic affective illness

Study	Polarity	Outcome measure	Proband diagnoses: NPAI	MCPAI	MICPAI	SA	SCH	Comment
Rosenthal et al. 1980[a]	B	Mean social functioning score	—	2.70[b]	3.00	—	—	Assessed at interview; higher scores mean worse outcome
Coryell et al. 1982	U	Short-term outcome % recovered	69[c]	44	33	—	7[c]	Coded from hospital charts; 2- to 3-year follow-up
Brockington et al. 1982	U	Mean general outcome regression score	1.38	1.49	1.60	—	—	Personal follow-up; higher scores mean poorer outcome
Abrams and Taylor 1983	U	Improvement (%)	81	93	—	—	35	Improvement in global severity score from admission to discharge (%)
Brockington et al. 1983	B	Mean general outcome regression score	1.31	1.25	1.39	—	—	Personal follow-up; higher scores mean worse outcome
Van Praag and Nijo 1984	U,B	Mean residual psychopathology score						Idiosyncratic criteria approximate DSM-III; 4- to 7-year follow-up
		Depression	1.8[c]	1.6	2.3	—	4.0[c]	
		Mania	—	1.4	2.3	—	1.0[c]	
Coryell and Tsuang 1985	U	Of 8 comparisons, number significantly different from MICPAI						
		Better	4	4	—	—	0	
		Worse	0	0	—	—	7	
Coryell et al. 1986	U	Recovered (%)	—	55	33	—	—	6-month follow-up

Coryell and Zimmerman 1987[d]	—	Recovered (%)	—	76[c]	39	—	6[c]	6-month personal follow-up
Coryell and Zimmerman 1988[a,d]	U	Recovered (%)	—	—	67	29[c]	—	At 1-year follow-up
Winokur et al. 1990	U,B	Marked improvement (%)						At discharge
		Depression	61	68	57	—	—	
		Mania	61	64	58	—	—	
Coryell et al. 1990a[a]	—	Recovered (%)	—	89	82	56	—	Recovery from index episode; from Collaborative Study of Depression
Coryell et al. 1990b[a]	B	Recovered (%)	—	95	67	100	—	5-year personal follow-up
M. Harrow, personal communication, 1990	U,B	Poor outcome (%)	—	21	47	—	56[c]	5-year global outcome from Chicago follow-up study

Note. NPAI = nonpsychotic affective illness. MCPAI = mood-congruent psychotic affective illness. MICPAI = mood-incongruent psychotic affective illness. SA = schizoaffective disorder. SCH = schizophrenia. B = bipolar illness only. U = unipolar illness only. U,B = both unipolar and bipolar illness.

[a]Research Diagnostic Criteria used.

[b]Mixed nonpsychotic and mood-congruent psychotic patients.

[c]$P < .05$ from MICPAI.

[d]Coryell and Zimmerman 1987 and Coryell and Zimmerman 1988 analyze the same data set. Only in the latter article are schizoaffective patients subdivided into mainly affective and mainly schizophrenic types.

and MICP groups (Brockington et al. 1982, 1983; Coryell and Tsuang 1985; Coryell and Zimmerman 1987; Coryell et al. 1982, 1986, 1990a, 1990b; M. Harrow, personal communication, 1990; Rosenthal et al. 1980; Van Praag and Nijo 1984; Winokur et al. 1990). In *all of them,* the MICP group had the worse outcome. However, the differences tended to be small, and were statistically significant in only two of the studies (Coryell and Zimmerman 1987; Coryell and Tsuang 1985). These results argue strongly against subhypothesis 1A, but are consistent with subhypothesis 1B. That is, MICP patients have a consistently worse outcome than more typical patients with affective illness, although the difference may not be very large.

Hypothesis 2. Only three comparisons of outcome were found between MICPAI and schizoaffective patients (Coryell and Zimmerman 1988; Coryell et al. 1990a, 1990b). In two of these studies, the schizoaffective patients had worse outcome: one was statistically significant (Coryell and Zimmerman 1988) and one nonsignificant (Coryell et al. 1990a). In one study (Coryell et al. 1990b) based on a very small sample of schizoaffective patients ($N = 4$), the schizoaffective group had a nonsignificantly better outcome. These results do not provide strong evidence for or against the validity of hypothesis 2.

Hypothesis 3. Six studies yielded seven comparisons of the outcome of MICPAI and schizophrenia (Abrams and Taylor 1983; Coryell and Tsuang 1985; Coryell and Zimmerman 1987; Coryell et al. 1982; M. Harrow, personal communication, 1990; Van Praag and Nijo 1984). In *all of them,* schizophrenic patients had worse outcomes. The differences tended to be substantial and reached statistical significance in all but one (Abrams and Taylor 1983). These results provide strong evidence against the validity of hypothesis 3.

Discussion and Recommendations

In this review, I sought to evaluate several competing hypotheses regarding the proper nosologic position of MICPAI. What conclusions can be reached from these efforts? First, the available evidence argues with substantial consistency against the validity of hypothesis 3; that is, MICPAI should not be considered a subtype of schizophrenia, as defined by DSM-III. This conclusion is most strongly supported by the results of the studies of family history and outcome, but also by demographic data and results from the DST.

Second, the evidence is relatively consistent in rejecting subhypothesis 1A; contrary to the conclusions of Pope and Lipinski (1978), the presence of MICP features in the setting of affective illness does appear to have clinical significance. It predicts lower rates of affective illness and higher rates of schizophrenia in relatives, lower rates of melancholic symptoms, and a poorer outcome.

Third, the available results tend to argue against hypothesis 2. When schizoaffective disorder is defined as in DSM-III-R (and in the mainly schizophrenic subtype in the RDC), there are nontrivial differences in several classes of validators between MICPAI and schizoaffective disorder. It is important to note, however, that relatively few studies have addressed this question.

Fourth, the results are broadly consistent with subhypothesis 1B. Across most validators, MICPAI tended 1) to differ modestly from cases of more typical affective illness but 2) to differ considerably more from cases of schizophrenia (and sometimes, of schizoaffective illness). This pattern is most clearly seen with family history, the DST, and outcome. Although readers may fairly reach a different conclusion, the accumulated evidence supports the decision of the framers of DSM-III and DSM-III-R in considering MICPAI to be a subtype of affective illness.

The hypotheses tested assumed that cases of MICPAI are etiologically homogeneous. This assumption may be incorrect. In particular, patients with MICPAI may represent a mixture of individuals with "true" schizophrenia and "true" affective illness. If this "admixture" model is correct, then the results of this review could be interpreted somewhat differently. They suggest that in cohorts of patients with MICPAI, patients with true affective illness considerably outnumber those with true schizophrenia. Although it is theoretically possible to discriminate this admixture model from subhypothesis 1B, this would require statistical techniques, such as admixture analysis of the distribution of quantitative validators in MICPAI patients, that were not presented in any of the articles reviewed.

References

Abrams R, Taylor MA: The importance of mood-incongruent psychotic symptoms in melancholia. J Affective Disord 5:179–181, 1983

American Psychiatric Association: Diagnostic and Statistical Manual: Mental Disorders. Washington, DC, American Psychiatric Association, 1952

American Psychiatric Association: Diagnostic and Statistical Manual of Mental Disorders, 2nd Edition. Washington, DC, American Psychiatric Association, 1968

American Psychiatric Association: Diagnostic and Statistical Manual of Mental Disorders, 3rd Edition. Washington, DC, American Psychiatric Association, 1980

American Psychiatric Association: Diagnostic and Statistical Manual of Mental Disorders, 3rd Edition, Revised. Washington, DC, American Psychiatric Association, 1987

Ayuso-Gutierrez JL, Almoguera MI, Garcia-Camba E, et al: The dexamethasone suppression test in delusional depression: further findings. J Affective Disord 8:147–151, 1985

Baron M, Gruen R, Asnis L, et al: Schizoaffective illness, schizophrenia and affective disorders: morbidity risk and genetic transmission. Acta Psychiatr Scand 65:253–262, 1982
Bleuler E: Textbook of Psychiatry, 4th Edition. New York, Macmillan, 1924
Breslau N, Meltzer HY: Validity of subtyping psychotic depression: examination of phenomenology and demographic characteristics. Am J Psychiatry 145:35–40, 1988
Brockington IF, Helzer JE, Hillier VF, et al: Definitions of depression: concordance and prediction of outcome. Am J Psychiatry 139:1022–1027, 1982
Brockington IF, Hillier VR, Francis AF, et al: Definitions of mania: concordance and prediction of outcome. Am J Psychiatry 140:435–439, 1983
Caroff S, Winokur A, Rieger W, et al: Response to dexamethasone in psychotic depression. Psychiatry Res 8:59–64, 1983
Coryell W, Tsuang MT: Major depression with mood-congruent or mood-incongruent psychotic features: outcome after 40 years. Am J Psychiatry 142:479–482, 1985
Coryell W, Zimmerman M: Progress in the classification of functional psychoses. Am J Psychiatry 144:1471–1474, 1987
Coryell W, Zimmerman M: Diagnosis and outcome in schizo-affective depression: a replication. J Affective Disord 15:21–27, 1988
Coryell W, Tsuang MT, McDaniel J: Psychotic features in major depression: is mood congruence important? J Affective Disord 4:227–236, 1982
Coryell W, Endicott J, Keller M, et al: Phenomenology and family history in DSM-III psychotic depression. J Affective Disord 9:13–18, 1985
Coryell W, Pfohl B, Zimmerman M: Heterogeneity in psychotic depression. Compr Psychiatry 27:430–438, 1986
Coryell W, Keller M, Lavori P, et al: Affective syndromes, psychotic features and prognosis, I: depression. Arch Gen Psychiatry 47:651–657, 1990a
Coryell W, Keller M, Lavori P, et al: Affective syndromes, psychotic features and prognosis, II: mania. Arch Gen Psychiatry 47:658–662, 1990b
Grossman LS, Harrow M, Fudala JL, et al: The longitudinal course of schizoaffective disorders: a prospective follow-up study. J Nerv Ment Dis 172:140–149, 1984
Katona CLE, Roth M: The dexamethasone suppression test in schizo-affective depression. J Affective Disord 8:107–112, 1985
Kraepelin E: Manic-Depressive Insanity and Paranoia. Edinburgh, Scotland, ES Livingston, 1921
Lewis A: Melancholia: a clinical survey of depressive states. Journal of Mental Science 80:277–378, 1934
Lewis A: Melancholia: prognostic study and case material. Journal of Mental Science 82:488–558, 1936
Maj M: Response to the dexamethasone suppression test in schizoaffective disorder, depressed type. J Affective Disord 11:63–67, 1986
Maj M: Lithium prophylaxis of schizoaffective disorders: a prospective study. J Affective Disord 14:129–135, 1988
Maj M, Arena F, Lovero N, et al: Factors associated with response to lithium prophylaxis in DSM III major depression and bipolar disorder. Pharmacopsychiatry 18:309–313, 1985
Minter RE, Mandel MR: The treatment of psychotic major depressive disorder with drugs and electroconvulsive therapy. J Nerv Ment Dis 167:726–733, 1979
Pope HG, Lipinski JF: Diagnosis in schizophrenia and manic-depressive illness: a reassessment of the specificity of "schizophrenic" symptoms in the light of current research. Arch Gen Psychiatry 35:811–828, 1978

Rosenthal NE, Rosenthal LN, Stallone F, et al: Toward the validation of RDC schizoaffective disorder. Arch Gen Psychiatry 37:804–810, 1980

Sauer H, Koehler KG, Sass H, et al: The dexamethasone suppression test and thyroid stimulating hormone response to TRH in RDC schizoaffective patients. Eur Arch Psychiatry Neurol Sci 234:264–267, 1984

Spitzer RL, Endicott J, Robins E: Research Diagnostic Criteria: rationale and reliability. Arch Gen Psychiatry 35:773–782, 1978

Van Praag HM, Nijo L: About the course of schizoaffective psychoses. Compr Psychiatry 25:9–22, 1984

Winokur G, Black D, Nasrallah A: The schizoaffective continuum: non-psychotic, mood-congruent, and mood incongruent, in Schizoaffective and Affective Disorders: Similarities and Differences. Edited by Marneros A, Tsuang MT. New York, Springer-Verlag, 1990, pp 23–32

Chapter 29

Trait Markers in Schizophrenia

Are They Diagnostic?

Sally Szymanski, D.O.
John Kane, M.D.
Jeffrey Lieberman, M.D.

Statement of the Issues

Should DSM-IV include biological indicators of pathophysiology as trait markers for schizophrenia?

Significance of the Issues

Due to the presumed heterogeneity of the etiology of schizophrenia, a search for trait markers that will help to define valid subtypes and the biological basis of the disorder is ongoing. Psychiatric diagnostic categories can then be developed that will more accurately reflect the pathophysiologic and clinical nature of the illness.

Abnormalities in eye movement, electrodermal activity, event-related brain potentials, attention and informational processing, and brain imaging have been described as promising trait markers for schizophrenia. In this chapter we review the current research on the relationship of these putative trait markers to clinical characteristics of schizophrenia such as symptoms. In the future, multiple biological measures may describe specific psychiatric syndromes with greater precision that the current use of clinical criteria alone.

This work was supported in part by the Mental Health Clinical Research Center at Hillside Hospital (MH41960) and a Research Scientist Development Award to Dr. Lieberman (MH100537). We thank Dr. Deborah Levy, Dr. Robert Bilder, Dr. Corrine Manetto, Dr. Bernhard Bogerts, and Dr. Gustav Degreef for their expert advice on certain areas of this chapter.

METHODS

Utilizing 15 searches, the English-language literature over the past 20 years on biological studies of schizophrenia was systematically reviewed. In this report we focus on those biological indicators of pathophysiology (e.g., eye-tracking abnormalities) that best met the definition of a possible trait marker for schizophrenia. Due to the broad nature of the literature, space considerations did not allow for discussion of studies in electroencephalography (EEG), computerized EEG, single photon emission computed tomography, cerebral blood flow, or soft signs, or for a more extensive review of possible attention and informational processing markers such as reaction time. This review was intended to be selective and directed toward a discussion of the most promising "leads" in the search for a trait marker for schizophrenia.

RESULTS

According to Buchsbaum and Haier (1983), a biological marker is a measurable indicator of a disease, which can be state dependent (state marker) or trait dependent (trait marker). Garver (1987) described the following criteria for a trait marker to detect biological risk: the trait marker 1) distributes differently in psychotic individuals than in control populations; 2) has a greater prevalence in family members of identified psychotic patients than in the general populations and is associated with psychotic spectrum disorder in family members; 3) is correlated with subsequent development of psychotic spectrum illness in high-risk children and occurs preceding the development of clinical manifestations of psychotic spectrum disease; and 4) is reliable and stable over time. A number of potential trait markers in schizophrenia show promise for meeting Garver's criteria. In this chapter we review the evidence for abnormalities in eye movement, electrodermal activity, event-related brain potentials, attention and informational processing disturbances, and brain imaging studies as putative trait markers for schizophrenia.

Eye Movement Dysfunction (EMD)

Traditionally, EMD has been a qualitative rating based on the similarity between eye position and target as the eye follows the target with deviations of eye position from the target pattern considered to be indicative of impairment. In studies of schizophrenic patients, the prevalence of EMD has ranged from 50% to more than 85%, which is significantly higher than the prevalence of EMD in nonschizophrenic psychotic patients (22%) and in nonpsychotic control subjects (8%) (Holzman 1987). There have been more than 20 replications of the association of EMD with schizophrenia, with no failures to replicate (Holzman et al. 1988). The specificity of EMD for schizophrenia (Holzman 1987) has been questioned by the findings of similar rates of EMD in patients with affective disorders (Lipton et al. 1980). However, this apparent nonspecificity seems to be a function of treatment with lithium carbonate (Levy et al. 1985). In 1987, Holzman observed that factors such as clinical status, neuroleptic medication, fluctuating levels of attention, and changes in target and measurement characteristics did not affect the replicability of eye movements, although Clementz and Sweeney (1990) disagreed.

Holzman and colleagues (1984) reported that 34% of the parents of schizophrenic patients showed EMD compared with 10% of the parents of manic depressive patients. Furthermore, the proportion of first-degree family members of schizophrenic patients who exhibit qualitatively abnormal pursuit has been reported to range from 34% to 58%, in contrast to the prevalence of 5%–13% of abnormal pursuit in first-degree relatives of persons with other psychiatric disorders (Clementz and Sweeney 1990). In two twin studies done by Holzman and colleagues in 1977 and 1980, the results showed that clinically discordant monozygotic twin pairs for schizophrenia had greater eye-tracking similarity than clinically discordant dizygotic pairs. The concordance rates in both types of twins was noted to be about 80% of the theoretically predicted values for a trait under polygenic control.

In further work, Holzman and colleagues (1988) applied the latent trait model to the distribution of EMD and schizophrenia in nuclear families of twin pairs discordant for functional psychosis to determine the mode of transmission of the schizophrenia-EMD complex. The investigators compared the offspring of twins discordant for schizophrenia with the offspring of twins discordant for manic-depressive disorder or reactive psychosis. Their analysis was consistent with a single autosomal dominant gene transmission of a latent trait, when both schizophrenia and EMD are considered as two independent manifestations of that trait. This model was shown not to account for the distribution of either mania or reactive psychosis and EMD. Since EMD can occur in nonpsychiatric control subjects, patients with bipolar disorder, patients with certain central nervous system diseases, and asymptomatic relatives of schizophrenic patients, the presence of EMD cannot be considered to be wholly specific for schizophrenia (Holzman 1987). EMD may, however, be one possible manifestation of a "latent trait," with schizophrenic symptoms being one of several possible phenotypic expressions of that trait. Overall, EMD is a robust candidate in the search for a trait marker but not a confirmatory test for schizophrenia.

Electrodermal Activity

The decreased skin conductance orienting response (a pattern of electrodermal activity) has been found to characterize 40%–50% of schizophrenic patients and

5%–10% of nonpsychiatric control subjects; it is also present in patients with affective disorder (Erlenmeyer-Kimling 1987; Holzman 1987). Studies of orienting nonresponding in children of schizophrenic patients have found conflicting results (Olbrich 1989), although an association with a family history of schizophrenia has been reported (Alm et al. 1984).

Research studies that have examined positive and negative symptoms in an effort to define a subgroup of schizophrenic patients who might be orienting nonresponding have had mixed results. Straube (1979) and Bernstein and colleagues (1981) found orienting nonresponding schizophrenic patients to be anhedonic and cognitively disorganized. Alm and colleagues (1984) reported nonresponding patients to have positive symptoms, such as delusions and auditory hallucinations. However, Green and colleagues (1989) observed that nonresponding patients showed a nonsignificant tendency to have both more positive and negative symptoms than responding patients.

Research has been contradictory as to whether electrodermal nonresponsivity is affected by neuroleptic medication (Green et al. 1989; Spohn et al. 1989; Zahn et al. 1981) and is stable over time (Mednick and McNeil 1968; Mednick and Schulsinger 1974; Mednick et al. 1978; Nuechterlein 1987). Other factors that can also affect electrodermal measures include sweat gland activity, arousal states of the autonomic and central nervous system, attention, emotion, and informational processes (Olbrich 1989). The influence of these factors on electrodermal nonresponsivity requires clarification in longitudinal studies to verify whether electrodermal activity abnormalities constitute a state or trait marker for schizophrenia.

Event-Related Brain Voltage Potentials (ERPs)

The P300 endogenous brain potential is a large late positive potential that reaches a peak between 300 and 500 milliseconds poststimulus (Pritchard 1986) and that is generated whenever infrequently occurring sensory stimuli are correctly detected or when unexpected and highly unusual stimuli are delivered to a subject (Mesulam 1985). The P3 refers to the major positive aspect of the P300 after the stimulus presentation. In schizophrenic patients, smaller P300 amplitudes and delays in latency have been reported versus control subjects (St. Clair et al. 1989). Prolonged P300 latencies have also been found in a group of hospitalized schizophrenic patients, persisting in patients after they had achieved clinical remission (Blackwood et al. 1987). Results have varied among studies associating high-risk children or siblings of schizophrenic patients with reduced P300 amplitudes (Pritchard 1986). Factors that may affect P300 amplitude are the presence of neuroleptics (Blackwood et al. 1987; St. Clair et al. 1989) and task requirements (Pfefferbaum et al. 1989).

The correlation of P300 abnormalities with symptomology or diagnosis is unclear. Reduced auditory- and visual-evoked P3 amplitudes have been correlated with negative symptoms in unmedicated schizophrenic patients (Pfefferbaum et al. 1989), and increased auditory P300s also have been associated with positive symptoms (Shenton et al. 1989). Clinical subtypes such as paranoid and nonparanoid schizophrenia have been reported to have similar frequencies of P300 abnormalities (St. Clair et al. 1989). P300 abnormalities appear nonspecific for schizophrenia; they have been found in patients with borderline and schizotypal personality disorders (Blackwood et al. 1986; Kutcher et al. 1987) as well as dementia (Goodin et al. 1978).

The N100 is an earlier occurring endogenous event potential that has been studied in schizophrenia. A visual-reducing pattern has been reported in acute schizophrenia that is not seen in chronic and paranoid patients (Landau et al. 1975; Schooler et al. 1976). Studies with schizophrenic patients have been confounded by the differences in paradigms measuring this ERP component as well as by possible medication effect (Pritchard 1986).

Contingent negative variation (CNV) is a slowly building negative voltage shift that begins after presentation of a warning stimulus. Reduction in amplitude in schizophrenic patients compared with control subjects has been reported (Pritchard 1986). A decreased CNV not associated with symptoms or remission status has been observed in chronic but not in acute schizophrenic patients (Pritchard 1986). However, CNV reduction appears nonspecific; it has been reported in both anxiety states and affective disorders (Claveric et al. 1984; McCallum and Walter 1968).

Sensory-gating defects in schizophrenic patients are thought to be due to perceptual and attentional disturbances resulting from difficulties filtering or gating sensory afferent input, causing hyperalertness and discrimination problems (Baker et al. 1987), which may lead to stimulus overload and cognitive fragmentation (Braff and Geyer 1990). Sensory-gating abnormalities have been tested in multiple ways, for example, by means of a two-stimulus conditioning ERP paradigm using auditory stimuli with a second stimulus-evoked P50 wave (Adler et al. 1982). P50 wave suppression has been seen in nonpsychiatric, nonmedical control subjects (Freedman et al. 1983), although, using a slightly different methodological approach, Kathmann and Engel (1990) failed to replicate this finding. Lack of P50 wave suppression in schizophrenic patients has been reported (Adler et al. 1982; Freedman et al. 1983; Siegel et al. 1984). The decreased auditory P50 wave suppression found in schizophrenic patients has also been seen in more than half of their first-degree relatives (Siegel et al. 1984). Even so, decreased P50 wave suppression of the auditory-evoked potentials appears nonspecific; it has been reported in other illnesses such as mania (Franks et al. 1983).

P300, N100, CNV, and sensory-gating abnormalities are present in a portion of schizophrenic patients. The variety of paradigms utilized in these studies, the conflicting results, and the nonspecificity of the findings for schizophrenia make the abnormalities interesting but inconclusive trait markers.

Attention and Information Processing

Deficits in attentional processes have been observed in numerous studies of schizophrenic patients (Cornblatt et al. 1989; Erlenmeyer-Kimling 1987; Nuechterlein and Dawson 1984). Sustained focused attention on complex tasks with high processing demands as measured by the visual continuous performance tests (CPTs) may be a promising trait marker for the attentional problems manifested by schizophrenic patients. Other potential markers include measures of reaction time, selective attention, short-term recall memory, early processing stages (as measured by forced-choice of apprehension testing or by backward masking), and concept formation (Erlenmeyer-Kimling 1987).

The CPT is a visual vigilance task, which was originally developed to detect deficits in sustained alertness in subjects with brain damage. Some 40%–50% of schizophrenic patients have been reported to show impaired performance, but not high-risk children on simple versions of the CPT (Erlenmeyer-Kimling and Cornblatt 1987). When more complex CPT versions with higher processing loads were given to high-risk individuals, significant differences were seen between these individuals as compared with control subjects (Erlenmeyer-Kimling and Cornblatt 1987). In two studies of schizophrenic offspring, the performance of such children on the CPT was found to be abnormal relative to children of parents with other psychiatric disorders (Nuechterlein et al. 1986). Nuechterlein and colleagues (1989) observed that cross-sectional studies of symptomatic and remitted schizophrenic patients and high-risk children demonstrate a consistent pattern of CPT abnormalities, but that high processing loads are needed to detect deficits in high-risk children and remitted schizophrenic patients. Overall, sustained focused attention as measured by CPT appears to be the most robust candidate in the search for a trait marker in the attentional and processing area in schizophrenia.

Brain Imaging Procedures: Computed Tomography (CT), Magnetic Resonance Imaging (MRI), and Positron-Emission Tomography (PET)

A large number of CT studies have described lateral and third ventricular enlargement and reduction in cortical volume in schizophrenic patients, although negative studies have also been reported (Raz and Raz 1990; Shelton and Weinberger 1986). Cerebral asymmetry, cerebellar volume reduction, and brain density changes have also been observed (Andreasen 1989). In a meta-analysis of CT and MRI studies in schizophrenia, ventriculomegaly was found to be a more prevalent abnormality as compared with third ventricular dilatation or cortical volume reduction (Raz and

Raz 1990). Longitudinal studies to determine when in the course of illness morphological brain abnormalities occur and whether they change over time have demonstrated conflicting results (Woods et al. 1990). Moreover, CT abnormalities appear nonspecific for schizophrenia; they have also been reported in affective disorders, alcoholism, dementia, anorexia nervosa, and autism (Andreasen 1989).

CT studies of siblings (Weinberger et al. 1981), twins (Reveley et al. 1982), and offspring of schizophrenic patients have suggested at least a partial genetic component to ventricular enlargement (Erlenmeyer-Kimling 1987), although environmental factors such as perinatal injury also appear to be associated with the development of schizophrenia. An inverse relationship between ventricular enlargement and family history of schizophrenia has been reported (Reveley et al. 1984), although some studies have failed to demonstrate this association (Miller 1989; Owen et al. 1989).

Neither ventricular enlargement nor cortical volume reduction has been conclusively associated with a particular diagnostic subtype of schizophrenia (Goetz and Van Kammen 1986). Imaging studies have suggested a possible association between ventricular enlargement and particular clinical characteristics such as negative symptoms, cognitive impairment, hypofunction of the monoamine system, and a poor neuroleptic response and outcome (Cazzullo et al. 1989; Goetz and Van Kammen 1986). In contrast, certain studies have demonstrated the absence of a correlation between negative symptoms and ventricular dilatation (Bishop et al. 1983; Keilp et al. 1988; Losonczy et al. 1986; Luchins et al. 1984; Nasrallah et al. 1983a; Pandurangi et al. 1988). In other studies, negative symptoms have been associated with cortical volume reduction (Nasrallah et al. 1983b; Pandurangi et al. 1988). In a review of the relationship between brain imaging findings and psychopathology, Marks and Luchins (1990) found that in 18 of 28 CT studies, an association existed between ventriculomegaly or cortical atrophy with less positive or increased negative symptoms.

MRI studies have confirmed the CT findings of cerebral ventriculomegaly in schizophrenia (Andreasen et al. 1989). Midsagittal, coronal, cerebral, frontal, and cerebellar structure volume reduction (Nasrallah 1989), corpus callosal area, length and thickness differences (Andreasen 1989), temporal lobe abnormalities (Rossi et al. 1990; Suddath et al. 1989), hippocampal volume reduction (Suddath et al. 1990), and signal intensity value alterations (Nasrallah 1989) have been reported. Preliminary MRI studies of twins have reported bilateral hippocampal-amygdala complex and parahippocampal gyrus area reduction in siblings of schizophrenic patients (DeLisi et al. 1987), corpus callosal anterior and middle segmental shape differences (Casanova et al. 1990), and hippocampal volume reduction as well as third and lateral ventriculomegaly (Suddath et al. 1990) in the affected twin in discordant monozygotic twin pairs.

Research attempting to correlate symptomology or diagnosis with brain abnormalities seen on MRI has produced mixed results. Initially, Andreasen and colleagues (1986) found that decreased cerebral and cranial size was correlated with negative symptoms, although frontal lobe volume reduction was not. In further work, Andreasen and colleagues (1990) reported that patients with prominent negative symptoms possessed larger ventricles than those with mixed or positive subtypes, but these authors were unable to reproduce their earlier findings of decreased frontal cerebral and cranial size. In Bogerts and colleagues' (1990) study of hippocampal-amygdala complex volumes and adjacent temporal horns measurements, no correlation with either positive or negative symptoms was found. Using a different methodology, Besson and colleagues (1987) reported increased T_1 relaxation times in the left frontal and the left medial temporal lobe, correlating with increased negative symptoms and increased positive symptoms, respectively. Attempting to correlate certain MRI abnormalities with diagnosis, Johnstone and colleagues (1989) found that temporal lobe volume reduction, not lateral ventricular or temporal horn area, separated schizophrenic patients from bipolar and control subjects.

PET is a relatively new technique that has shown metabolic activity abnormalities in schizophrenic patients versus control subjects. In reviewing PET studies in schizophrenia, Andreasen (1989) observed that reduced frontal lobe glucose utilization activity, altered utilization activities with tasks, and a reversal of subcortical-cortical relationships have been found in schizophrenic patients. Decreased glucose consumption in the basal ganglia, which normalizes after neuroleptic treatment, has also been reported in schizophrenic patients (Buchsbaum and Haier 1987). In quantitative imaging studies of neuroreceptors, elevated D_2 dopamine receptor densities in the caudate-putamen of drug-naive, first-episode schizophrenic patients were found using [^{11}C] *N*-methylspiperone (Wong et al. 1986). However, using a different ligand, ^{11}C-labeled raclopride, Farde and colleagues (1990) failed to replicate this finding. Methodological differences between the two studies include the use of [^{11}C] raclopride versus [^{11}C] *N*-methylspiperone as ligands that have different D_2 dopamine receptor affinities, patient age and psychological status, experimental design, and the method of calculating receptor density (Sedvall 1990).

Structural brain imaging abnormalities revealed by imaging techniques (CT and MRI) such as ventricular enlargement appear to be relatively robust but not invariant findings in schizophrenic patients. However, the relation of these neuropathological changes to clinical symptoms, phase of illness, and diagnostic subtype remains unclear. Twin and longitudinal studies of adults and high-risk children of schizophrenic patients, standardization of imaging technique, and studies to differentiate further the neuromorphologic basis of schizophrenia from other psychiatric syndromes are needed so that definitive trait markers in brain imaging for schizophrenia can be developed.

Other Studies of Potential Trait Markers for Schizophrenia

Multiple possible neurotransmitter-related enzymatic activity markers have been studied, which include platelet monoamine oxidase (MAO type B) and plasma dopamine beta hydroxylase (Baron 1986). Platelet MAO activity levels initially were reported to be significantly lower in chronic schizophrenic patients versus nonpsychiatric, nonmedical control subjects by approximately 30% (DeLisi et al. 1987). Subsequent findings disputed this theory, including reports that neuroleptics may reduce platelet MAO activity levels, that low platelet MAO levels occur frequently in the general population, that patients in other diagnostic groups such as bipolar patients can have low platelet MAO levels, and that studies on the relationship between platelet MAO activity and family history of schizophrenia were inconclusive (Baron 1986; Erlenmeyer-Kimling 1987; Siever and Coursey 1985). Preliminary studies of other potential markers include elevated ^{3}H-spiperone–binding sites in lymphocytes (Bondy and Ackenheil 1987); reduced levels of peptide YY (Widerlov et al. 1988); increased skeletal creatinine phosphokinase activity (Meltzer 1987); lower active uptake of serotonin by platelets (Rotman et al. 1982); decreased methionine adenosine transferase activity (Smythies 1984); mixed findings concerning cerebrospinal fluid levels of 5-hydroxyindoleacetic acid and homovanillic acid (Van Kammen et al. 1986); and various immune abnormalities (reduced number of peripheral blood lymphocytes, antibrain antibodies, and decreased interleukin-2 production) (Villemain et al. 1989).

Discussion

Promising trait markers for schizophrenia have been selectively reviewed. All studies of potential markers suffer from a lack of standardized methodology, which limits comparisons of results across studies. None of the current possible trait markers completely meet Garver's (1987) criteria. Longitudinal studies in high-risk children and adults utilizing multiple biological measures may eventually define specific psychiatric syndromes with greater precision than clinical criteria or single biological markers. Biological assessment may then become a useful method in differentiating psychiatric diagnoses.

Recommendations

In reviewing this literature, the DSM-IV Psychotic Disorders Work Group suggested that, although some markers such as smooth-pursuit EMD or increased ventricular brain ratio may in some cases be associated with a schizophrenic illness, they may lack sufficient sensitivity and specificity to be useful in the diagnostic process.

At present, there are no abnormal physical, radiologic, or laboratory findings that can be employed in establishing a diagnosis of schizophrenia.

References

Adler LE, Pachtman E, Franks RD, et al: Neurophysiological evidence for a defect in neuronal mechanisms involved in sensory gating in schizophrenia. Biol Psychiatry 17:639–654, 1982

Alm I, Lindström LH, Öst L, et al: Electrodermal nonresponding in schizophrenia: relationships to attentional, clinical, biochemical, computed tomographic, and genetic factors. Int J Psychophysiol 1:195–208, 1984

Andreasen NC: Brain Imaging: Applications in Psychiatry. Washington, DC, American Psychiatric Press, 1989

Andreasen NC, Nasrallah HA, Dunn V, et al: Structural abnormalities in the frontal system in schizophrenia. Arch Gen Psychiatry 43:136–144, 1986

Andreasen NC, Ehrhardt J, Yuh W, et al: Magnetic resonance imaging in schizophrenia: an update, in Schizophrenia: Scientific Progress. Edited by Schultz SC, Tamminga CA. New York, Oxford University Press, 1989

Andreasen NC, Ehrhardt JC, Swayze VW, et al: Magnetic resonance imaging of the brain in schizophrenia. Arch Gen Psychiatry 47:35–44, 1990

Baker N, Adler LE, Franks RD, et al: Neurophysiological assessment of sensory gating in psychiatric inpatients: comparison between schizophrenia and other diagnoses. Biol Psychiatry 22:603–617, 1987

Baron M: Genetics of schizophrenia, II: vulnerability traits and gene markers. Biol Psychiatry 21:1189–1211, 1986

Bernstein A, Taylor K, Starkey P, et al: Bilateral skin conductance, finger pulse volume, and EEG orienting response to tone of differing intensities in chronic schizophrenics and controls. J Nerv Ment Dis 169:513–528, 1981

Besson JAO, Corrigan FM, Cherryman GR, et al: Nuclear magnetic resonance brain imaging in chronic schizophrenia. Br J Psychiatry 150:161–163, 1987

Bishop RJ, Golden CJ, MacInnes WD, et al: The relationship of cerebral ventricular size in a population of acute and chronic schizophrenics. Psychiatry Res 9:225–231, 1983

Blackwood DHR, St. Clair DM, Kutcher SP: P300 event related potential abnormalities in borderline personality disorder. Biol Psychiatry 21:557–560, 1986

Blackwood DHR, Whalley LJ, Christie JE, et al: Changes in auditory P3 event related potential in schizophrenia and depression. Br J Psychiatry 150:154–160, 1987

Bogerts B, Ashtari M, Degreef G, et al: Reduced temporal limbic structure volumes on magnetic resonance images in first episode schizophrenia. Psychiatry Res: Neuroimaging 35:1–13, 1990

Bondy B, Ackenheil M: ^{3}H-Spiperone binding sites in lymphocytes as possible vulnerability marker for schizophrenia. J Psychiatr Res 21:521–529, 1987

Braff DL, Geyer MA: Sensorimotor gating and schizophrenia. Arch Gen Psychiatry 47:181–188, 1990

Buchsbaum MS, Haier RJ: Psychopathology: biological approaches. Annu Rev Physiol 34:401–430, 1983

Buchsbaum MS, Haier RJ: Functional and anatomical brain imaging: impact on schizophrenia research. Schizophr Bull 13:115–132, 1987

Casanova MF, Sanders RD, Goldberg TE, et al: Morphometry of the corpus callosum in monozygotic twins discordant for schizophrenia: a magnetic resonance imaging study. J Neurol Neurosurg Psychiatry 53:416–421, 1990

Cazzullo CL, Vita A, Sacchetti E: Cerebral ventricular enlargement in schizophrenia: prevalence and correlates, in Schizophrenia: Scientific Progress. Edited by Schultz SC, Tamminga CA. New York, Oxford University Press, 1989, pp 163–166

Claverie B, Brun A, Nizard A, et al: Multiparametric outlines with CNV: applications to depressive syndromes, in Brain and Information: Event-Related Potentials. Edited by Karrer R, Cohen J, Tueting P. New York, New York Academy of Sciences, 1984

Clementz BA, Sweeney JA: Is eye movement dysfunction a biological marker for schizophrenia? a methodological review. Psychol Bull 108:77–92, 1990

Cornblatt B, Winters L, Erlenmeyer-Kimling L: Attentional markers of schizophrenia: evidence from the New York high-risk study, in Schizophrenia: Scientific Progress. Edited by Schultz SC, Tamminga CA. New York, Oxford University Press, 1989

DeLisi LE, Golden LR, Gershon ES: Studies of biological factors associated with the inheritance of schizophrenia: a selective review. J Psychiatr Res 21:507–513, 1987

Erlenmeyer-Kimling L: Biological markers for the liability to schizophrenia, in Biological Perspectives of Schizophrenia (Dahlem Workshop Reports). Edited by Helmchen H, Henn FA. New York, Wiley, 1987

Erlenmeyer-Kimling L, Cornblatt B: High-risk research in schizophrenia: a summary of what has been learned. J Psychiatr Res 21:401–411, 1987

Farde L, Wiesel FA, Stone-Elander S, et al: D_2 dopamine receptors in neuroleptic-naive schizophrenic patients. Arch Gen Psychiatry 47:213–219, 1990

Franks RD, Adler LE, Waldo MC, et al: Neurophysiological studies of sensory gating in mania: comparison with schizophrenia. Biol Psychiatry 18:989–1005, 1983

Freedman R, Adler LE, Waldo MC, et al: Neurophysiological evidence for a defect in inhibitory pathways in schizophrenia: comparisons of medicated and drug-free patients. Biol Psychiatry 18:537–551, 1983

Garver DL: Methodological issues facing the interpretation of high-risk studies: biological heterogeneity. Schizophr Bull 13:525–529, 1987

Goetz KL, Van Kammen DP: Computerized axial tomography and subtypes of schizophrenia. J Nerv Ment Dis 174:31–41, 1986

Goodin DS, Squires KC, Starr A: Long latency event related components of the auditory evoked potential in dementia. Brain 101:635–648, 1978

Green MF, Nuechterlein KH, Satz P: The relationship of symptomatology and medication to electrodermal activity in schizophrenia. Psychophysiology 26:148–157, 1989

Holzman PS: Recent studies of psychophysiology in schizophrenia. Schizophr Bull 13:49–75, 1987

Holzman PS, Kringlen E, Levy DL, et al: Abnormal-pursuit eye movements in schizophrenia. Arch Gen Psychiatry 34:802–805, 1977

Holzman PS, Kringlen E, Levy DL, et al: Deviant eye tracking in twins discordant for psychosis: a replication. Arch Gen Psychiatry 37:627–631, 1980

Holzman PS, Solomon C, Levin S, et al: Pursuit eye movement dysfunctions in schizophrenia: family evidence for specificity. Arch Gen Psychiatry 41:136–139, 1984

Holzman PS, Kringlen E, Matthysse S, et al: A single dominant gene can account for eye tracking dysfunctions and schizophrenia in offspring of discordant twins. Arch Gen Psychiatry 45:641–647, 1988

Johnstone EC, Owens DG, Crow TJ, et al: Temporal lobe structure as determined by nuclear magnetic resonance in schizophrenia and bipolar affective disorder. J Neurol Neurosurg Psychiatry 52:736–741, 1989

Kathmann N, Engel RR: Sensory gating in normals and schizophrenics: a failure to find strong P50 suppression in normals. Biol Psychiatry 27:1216–1226, 1990

Keilp JG, Sweeney JA, Jacobsen P, et al: Cognitive impairment in schizophrenia: specific relations to ventricular size and negative symptomatology. Biol Psychiatry 24:47–55, 1988

Kutcher SP, Blackwood DHR, St. Clair D, et al: P3 abnormality in borderline personality disorder and schizophrenia. Arch Gen Psychiatry 44:645–650, 1987

Landau SG, Buchsbaum MS, Carpenter W, et al: Schizophrenia and stimulus intensity control. Arch Gen Psychiatry 32:1239–1245, 1975

Levy DL, Dorus E, Shaughnessy R, et al: Pharmacological evidence for specificity of pursuit dysfunction to schizophrenia: lithium carbonate associated with abnormal pursuit. Arch Gen Psychiatry 42:335–341, 1985

Lipton RB, Levin S, Holzman PS: Horizontal and vertical smooth pursuit eye movements, the oculocephalic reflex, and the functional psychoses. Psychiatr Res 3:193–203, 1980

Losonczy MF, Song IS, Mohs RC, et al: Correlates of lateral ventricular size in chronic schizophrenia, I: behavioral and treatment response measures. Am J Psychiatry 143:976–981, 1986

Luchins DJ, Levine RR, Meltzer HY: Lateral ventricular size psychopathology and medication response in the psychoses. Biol Psychiatry 19:29–44, 1984

Marks RC, Luchins DJ: Relationship between brain imaging findings in schizophrenia and psychopathology, in Schizophrenia: Positive and Negative Symptoms and Syndromes: Modern Problems of Pharmacopsychiatry, Vol 24. Edited by Andreasen NC. Basel, Switzerland, Karger, 1990, pp 89–123

McCallum WC, Walter W: The differential effects of distraction on the contingent negative variation in normal subjects and psychiatric patients. Electroencephalogr Clin Neurophysiol 24:593, 1968

Mednick SA, McNeil TF: Current methodology in research on the etiology of schizophrenia: serious difficulties which suggest the use of the high risk method. Psychol Bull 70:681–693, 1968

Mednick SA, Schulsinger F: Studies of children at high risk for schizophrenia, in Genetics Environment and Psychopathology. Edited by Mednick SA, Schulsinger F, Higgins J, et al. Amsterdam, North Holland, 1974, pp 103–116

Mednick SA, Schulsinger F, Teasdale TW, et al: Schizophrenia in high risk children: sex differences in predisposing factors, in Cognitive Defects in the Development of Mental Illness. Edited by Serban G. New York, Brunner/Mazel, 1978, pp 168–169

Meltzer HY: Biological studies in schizophrenia. Schizophr Bull 13:77–114, 1987

Mesulam MM: Principles of Behavioral Neurology. New York, FA Davis, 1985

Miller R: Schizophrenia as a progressive disorder: relations to EEG, CT, neuropathological and other evidence. Prog Neurobiol 33:17–44, 1989

Nasrallah HA: Magnetic resonance brain imaging: clinical and research application in schizophrenia. Paper presented at the Second Heidelberg Symposium "Search for the Causes of Schizophrenia," Heidelberg, Germany, May 24–26, 1989

Nasrallah HA, Kuperman S, Jacoby CG, et al: Clinical correlates of sulcal widening in chronic schizophrenia. Psychiatry Res 10:237–242, 1983a

Nasrallah H, Kuperman S, Hamra B, et al: Clinical differences between schizophrenic patients with and without large cerebral ventricles. J Clin Psychiatry 44:407–409, 1983b

Nuechterlein KH: Vulnerability models for schizophrenia, state of the art, in Search for the Causes of Schizophrenia. Edited by Hafner H, Gattaz NF. Heidelberg, Germany, Springer-Verlag, 1987, pp 297–316

Nuechterlein KH, Dawson ME: Information processing and attentional functioning in the developmental course of schizophrenic disorders. Schizophr Bull 10:160–202, 1984

Nuechterlein KH, Edell WS, Norris M, et al: Attention vulnerability indicators, thought disorder, and negative symptoms. Schizophr Bull 12:408–426, 1986

Nuechterlein KH, Dawson ME, Ventura J, et al: Testing vulnerability models: stability of potential vulnerability indicators across clinical state. Paper presented at the Second Heidelberg Symposium "Search for the Causes of Schizophrenia," Heidelberg, Germany, May 24–26, 1989

Olbrich R: Electrodermal activity and its relevance to vulnerability research in schizophrenics. Br J Psychiatry 155 (suppl 5):40–45, 1989

Owen MJ, Lewis SW, Murray RM: Family history and cerebral ventricular enlargement in schizophrenia: a case control study. Br J Psychiatry 154:629–634, 1989

Pandurangi AK, Bilder RM, Rieder RO, et al: Schizophrenic symptoms and deterioration: relation to computed tomographic findings. J Nerv Ment Dis 176:200–206, 1988

Pfefferbaum A, Ford JM, White PM, et al: P3 in schizophrenia is affected by stimulus modality, response requirements, medication status and negative symptoms. Arch Gen Psychiatry 46:1035–1044, 1989

Pritchard WS: Cognitive event-related potential correlates of schizophrenia. Psychol Bull 100:43–66, 1986

Raz S, Raz N: Structural brain abnormalities in the major psychoses: a quantitative review of the evidence from computerized imaging. Psychol Bull 108:93–108, 1990

Reveley AM, Reveley MA, Clifford CA, et al: Cerebral ventricular size in twins discordant for schizophrenia. Lancet 1:540–541, 1982

Reveley AM, Reveley MA, Murray RM: Cerebral ventricular enlargement in non-genetic schizophrenia: a controlled twin study. Br J Psychiatry 144:89–93, 1984

Rossi A, Stratta P, D'Albenzio L, et al: Reduced temporal lobe areas in schizophrenia: preliminary evidences from a controlled multiplanar magnetic resonance imaging study. Biol Psychiatry 27:61–68, 1990

Rotman A, Zemishlany Z, Munitz H, et al: The active uptake of serotonin by platelets of schizophrenic patients and their families: possibility of a genetic marker. Psychopharmacology 77:171–174, 1982

Schooler C, Buchsbaum MS, Carpenter WT: Evoked response and kinesthetic measures of augmenting/reducing in schizophrenics: replications and extensions. J Nerv Ment Dis 163:221–232, 1976

Sedvall G: PET imaging of dopamine receptors in human basal ganglia: relevance to mental illness. Trends in International Neuroscience 13:302–307, 1990

Shelton RC, Weinberger DR: X-ray computerized tomography studies in schizophrenia: a review and synthesis, in Handbook of Schizophrenia, Vol 1. Edited by Nasrallah HA, Weinberger DR. New York, Elsevier, 1986, pp 207–250

Shenton ME, Faux SF, McCarley RW, et al: Correlations between abnormal auditory P300 topography and positive symptoms in schizophrenia: a preliminary report. Biol Psychiatry 25:710–716, 1989

Siegel C, Waldo M, Mizner G, et al: Deficits in sensory gating in schizophrenic patients and their relatives. Arch Gen Psychiatry 41:607–612, 1984

Siever LJ, Coursey RD: Biological markers for schizophrenia and the biological high-risk approach. J Nerv Ment Dis 173:4–16, 1985

Smythies JR: The role of the one-carbon cycle in neuropsychiatric disease. Biol Psychiatry 19:755–758, 1984

Spohn HE, Coyne L, Spray L: Eye tracking and skin conductance in schizophrenia: the role of neuroleptics and tardive dyskinesia, in Schizophrenia: Scientific Progress. Edited by Schulz SC, Tamminga CA. New York, Oxford University Press, 1989, pp 110–114

St. Clair D, Blackwood D, Muir E: P300 abnormality in schizophrenic subtypes. J Psychiatr Res 23:49–55, 1989

Straube E: On the meaning of electrodermal nonresponding in schizophrenia. J Nerv Ment Dis 167:601–611, 1979

Suddath RL, Casanova MF, Goldberg TE, et al: Temporal lobe pathology in schizophrenia: a quantitative magnetic resonance imaging study. Am J Psychiatry 146:464–472, 1989

Suddath RL, Christison GW, Torrey EF, et al: Anatomical abnormalities in the brains of monozygotic twins discordant for schizophrenia. N Engl J Med 322:789–794, 1990

Van Kammen DP, Peters JP, Van Kammen WB: Cerebrospinal fluid studies of monoamine metabolism in schizophrenia. Psychiatr Clin North Am 1:81–97, 1986

Villemain F, Chatenoud L, Galinowski A, et al: Aberrant T cell-mediated immunity in untreated schizophrenic patients: deficient interleukin-2 production. Am J Psychiatry 146:609–616, 1989

Weinberger DR, DeLisi LE, Neophytides AN, et al: Familial aspects of CT scans abnormalities in chronic schizophrenia patients. Psychiatry Res 4:65–71, 1981

Widerlov E, Lindstrom LH, Wahlestedt C, et al: Neuropeptide Y and peptide YY as possible cerebrospinal fluid markers for major depression and schizophrenia, respectively. J Psychiatr Res 22:69–79, 1988

Wong DE, Wagner HN, Tune LE, et al: Position emission tomography reveals elevated D2 dopamine receptors in drug-naive schizophrenics. Science 234:1558–1563, 1986

Woods B, Yurgelun-Todd D, Benes FM, et al: Progressive ventricular enlargement in schizophrenia: comparison to bipolar affective disorder and correlation with clinical course. Biol Psychiatry 27:341–352, 1990

Zahn TP, Carpenter WT, McGlashan TH: Autonomic nervous system activity in acute schizophrenia, II: relationships to short-term prognosis and clinical state. Arch Gen Psychiatry 38:260–266, 1981

Section IV

Medication-Induced Movement Disorders

Contents

Section IV
Medication-Induced Movement Disorders

Introduction to Section IV

Medication-Induced Movement Disorders

Allen J. Frances, M.D.
Peter J. Weiden, M.D.
Ruth Ross, M.A.

Most users of DSM-IV are familiar with the standard psychiatric indications for neuroleptic treatment, which include Schizophrenia, Schizoaffective and Schizophreniform Disorders, Major Depression with psychotic features, manic disorders, Delusional Disorders, and Tourette's Disorder. DSM-III-R (American Psychiatric Association 1987) did not include any special provision for coding the presence of medication-induced movement disorders and did not provide text and criteria to guide medical judgment in this area. Unfortunately, there is considerable evidence that these side effects are often not recognized. In this section, the authors examine the question of whether increased clinical attention to this problem provided by inclusion in DSM-IV would assist clinicians in identifying medication-induced movement disorders and more accurately differentiating between them and primary psychiatric diagnoses.

Suggested Reasons for the Inclusion of Medication-Induced Movement Disorders in DSM-IV

- Medication-induced movement disorders are a common cause of iatrogenic morbidity.
- Patients receiving neuroleptics are often psychotic and are poor historians. They commonly do not report symptoms that would distress nonpsychotic individuals, or may report symptoms in a psychotic and unintelligible manner.
- There is a tremendous overlap between medication-induced movement disorders and Axis I primary mental disorders. This overlap makes careful consideration of medication-induced movement disorders a crucial step for

clinicians when considering whether a patient meets criteria for an Axis I mental disorder. For example, behavior syndromes of psychomotor retardation may occur in depression, psychotic states, and drug-induced akinesia. Similarly, bizarre movements may represent acute dystonia, chronic dyskinesia, or psychotic stereotyped movements.

- No physical finding is unique or pathognomonic for medication-induced movement disorders. All movements are also found in other neurologic, degenerative, toxic, and metabolic syndromes. Furthermore, many diseases that cause primary motoric disorders also have psychiatric manifestations (e.g., Huntington's disease, idiopathic Parkinson's disease). A neurologic disorder with psychiatric symptoms will often lead to treatment of the patient with a neuroleptic, so that the presence of a neuroleptic-induced movement disorder may be the indirect consequence of a primary neurologic illness.
- In general medical practice, many neuroleptics are used for other indications or may appear in combination prescriptions. For example, amitriptyline-perphenazine accounts for 24% of all outpatient prescriptions, yet one-half of resident internists did not know that this drug has neuroleptic properties.
- Accurate drug histories that would reveal neuroleptic exposure may not be forthcoming in certain groups. Individuals who abuse substances may inadvertently buy a street drug that is really a neuroleptic; individuals with dementia may forget what medications they are taking.

Since available research suggests that these conditions are often underrecognized and undertreated in clinical practice, it has been proposed that medication-induced movement disorders be listed with codes and a brief description under Other Conditions That May Be a Focus of Clinical Attention; the criteria sets and texts would be placed in an appendix for further study.

Proposed Description

It has been proposed that the following description appear in DSM-IV in the section on Other Conditions That May Be a Focus of Clinical Attention:

Medication-Induced Movement Disorders

The following medication-induced movement disorders are included because of their frequent importance in 1) the management of individuals treated with medication for mental disorders and 2) the differential diagnosis with Axis I disorders (e.g., Anxiety Disorder versus Neuroleptic-Induced Akathisia, Catatonia versus Neuroleptic Malignant Syndrome). Medication-induced movement disorders should be coded on Axis I. Although these disorders are labeled "medication-induced," it is often difficult to establish the causal relationship between medication exposure and the development of the movement disorder, especially since some of these movement disorders occur in the absence of medication exposure.

332.1 Neuroleptic-Induced Parkinsonism

Parkinsonian tremor, muscular rigidity or akinesia developing within a few weeks of starting or raising the dose of a neuroleptic medication, or reducing medication used to treat extrapyramidal symptoms.

333.92 Neuroleptic Malignant Syndrome

Severe muscle rigidity, elevated temperature, and other related findings (e.g., diaphoresis, dysphagia, incontinence, changes in level of consciousness ranging from confusion to coma, mutism, elevated or labile blood pressure, elevated creatine phosphokinase [CPK]) developing in association with the use of neuroleptic medication.

333.7 Neuroleptic-Induced Acute Dystonia

Abnormal positioning or spasm of the muscles of the head, neck, limbs, or trunk developing within a few days of starting or raising the dose of a neuroleptic medication, or reducing medication used to treat extrapyramidal symptoms.

333.99 Neuroleptic-Induced Acute Akathisia

Subjective complaints of restlessness accompanied by observed movements (e.g., fidgety movements of the legs, rocking from foot to foot, pacing, or inability to sit or stand still) developing within a few weeks of starting or raising the dose of a neuroleptic medication, or reducing medication used to treat extrapyramidal symptoms.

333.82 Neuroleptic-Induced Tardive Dyskinesia

Involuntary choreiform, athetoid, or rhythmic movements (lasting at least a few weeks) of the tongue, jaw, or extremities developing in association with the use of neuroleptic medication for at least a few months (may be for a shorter period of time in the elderly).

333.1 Medication-Induced Postural Tremor

Fine tremor occurring during attempts to maintain a posture and developing in association with the use of medication (e.g., lithium, antidepressants, valproate).

333.90 Medication-Induced Movement Disorder Not Otherwise Specified

This category is for medication-induced movement disorders not classified by any of the specific disorders listed above. Examples include parkinsonism, acute akathisia, acute dystonia, dyskinetic movement, or a neuroleptic malignant syndrome-like presentation associated with a medication other than a neuroleptic; tardive dystonia.

Literature reviews on the prevalence, importance, degree of underrecognition, and definitional features of each of these disorders were completed. A major goal of these reviews has been to identify criteria that would provide a balance between discouraging false positives and providing a specific enough definition to facilitate research ensuring that the diagnosis is not overlooked and undertreated in the clinical setting.

Statement of the Issues and Significance of the Issues

In each literature review in this section, the issue of whether the particular movement disorder being discussed should be included in DSM-IV is addressed. To address this issue, authors review the literature concerning prevalence, morbidity, underrecognition, and differential diagnosis, as well as specific criteria for each disorder. Because of frequent misuse of neuroleptics in certain high-risk populations and also frequent underrecognition of medication-induced movement disorders by clinicians, it was proposed that these disorders be included in DSM-IV to facilitate recognition and treatment of these problems.

Neuroleptic-Induced Parkinsonism

In Chapter 30, Weiden discusses neuroleptic-induced parkinsonism. The literature review investigated rates of neuroleptic-induced parkinsonism in the psychiatric patient population, clinical underrecognition of neuroleptic-induced parkinsonism, direct morbidity, and behavioral toxicity and indirect morbidity (using a meta-analysis of the neuroleptic treatment literature). Ninety articles fulfilled the selection criteria, and a total of 6,366 patients were included. The combined estimate of neuroleptic-induced parkinsonism prevalence was 40.4%, with rigidity being the most frequently reported individual parkinsonian symptom, followed by tremor and akinesia, with cogwheel rigidity and gait disturbance receiving far fewer mentions. The literature emphasizes that underrecognition of neuroleptic-induced parkinsonism is very common and that serious complications are not uncommon.

Morbidity from nonrecognition can be life threatening since diagnostic delays may lead to symptom progression from neuroleptic-induced parkinsonism to fulminant neuroleptic malignant syndrome. Direct complications of neuroleptic-induced parkinsonism are similar to those seen with idiopathic Parkinson's disease. Indirect complications include unrecognized behavioral syndromes, depression, suicide, dysphoria, vocational impairment, and social stigma. Unrecognized parkinsonism may lead to noncompliance, and a psychotic relapse because of neuroleptic refusal may be a lethal, but indirect, complication. Neuroleptic-induced parkinsonism is common, not often recognized, and overlaps with and mimics psychiatric symptoms.

Based on the literature review, it was recommended that neuroleptic-induced parkinsonism be included in DSM-IV to improve diagnostic rates and help clinicians accurately differentiate between schizophrenia, catatonia, depression, and neuroleptic-induced parkinsonism. The inclusion appears to be justified because neuroleptic-induced parkinsonism is prominent in the differential diagnosis of many other mental disorders, and its diagnosis requires special skills. Specific criteria are proposed based on the literature review and designed to avoid both false positives and false negatives. The proposed criteria would require that one of the following signs or symptoms developed within a few weeks of starting or raising the dose of a neuroleptic medication, or reducing medication used to treat extrapyramidal symptoms: 1) parkinsonian tremor, 2) parkinsonian muscular rigidity, or 3) akinesia. The criteria would specify that the symptoms are not better accounted for by a mental disorder and are not due to a neurologic disorder or other general medical condition.

Neuroleptic Malignant Syndrome

In Chapter 31, Addonizio and Susman discuss neuroleptic malignant syndrome. Neuroleptic malignant syndrome is a potentially lethal disorder estimated to develop in 0.07%–1.4% of patients on neuroleptics, with mortality rates ranging between 10% and 20%. In the literature review, it was found that there is consensus that much of the mortality and morbidity associated with neuroleptic malignant syndrome has been the result of lack of recognition of the syndrome. Early recognition and intervention have the potential to alter the course significantly, making it important that accurate diagnostic information be readily available. Fulminant cases are easily recognized, and there is little debate about the validity of the diagnosis in such cases; however, there is considerable controversy over whether mild or partial syndromes exist in addition to the full-blown disorder. The literature was reviewed to determine which symptoms are essential for making the diagnosis, which are associated but nonessential features, and what the threshold should be for the severity of symptoms.

Based on the literature review, the authors recommend that neuroleptic malignant syndrome be included in DSM-IV. They propose criteria that would be as specific as possible, but skewed toward the clinical goal of not overlooking any potential case. They stress the importance of differential diagnosis to distinguish the symptoms of neuroleptic malignant syndrome from those that might be caused by another disorder requiring very different treatment. The proposed criteria would require the development of severe muscle rigidity and elevated temperature associated with the use of neuroleptic medication and not attributable to other medical conditions. In addition to the above criteria, two items from the following list of symptoms identified from the literature review would have to be present: diaphoresis, dysphagia, tremor, incontinence, changes in level of consciousness ranging from confusion to coma, mutism, tachycardia, elevated or labile blood pressure, leukocytosis, or laboratory evidence of muscle injury such as elevated CPK. The criteria would specify that the symptoms are not due to a neurologic disorder or other general medical condition (such as viral encephalitis) and are not better accounted for by a mental disorder (such as Mood Disorder with catatonic features).

Neuroleptic-Induced Acute Dystonia

In Chapter 32, Casey discusses neuroleptic-induced acute dystonia. A review of the literature from 1952 through mid-1991 was done to ascertain what is known about neuroleptic-induced acute dystonia, to determine whether it should be included in DSM-IV, and to establish an acceptable definition of the syndrome. Neuroleptic-induced acute dystonia is a common problem with neuroleptic treatment, occurring in more than 50% of patients in the high-risk group and 10% or less in the low-risk group. Severity of symptoms can range from a minor inconvenience to a life-threatening situation, which is uncommon but merits full medical supervision and immediate treatment with parenteral drugs. Visibility in DSM-IV will increase recognition and accurate diagnosis of neuroleptic-induced acute dystonia and reduce misdiagnoses of hysteria, malingering, or catatonia in patients who appear to have bizarre postures early in their neuroleptic treatment course. Increased awareness will also alert clinicians to the risk for recurrence in patients with a history of neuroleptic-induced acute dystonia and the need to consider appropriate use of prophylaxis in high-risk patients.

A criteria set for neuroleptic-induced acute dystonia is proposed that it is hoped will be objective enough to avoid overdiagnosis, which could lead to incorrect treatment or overuse of prophylaxis. The proposed criteria would require objective signs of muscular contractions that produce abnormal positioning or dysfunction of the body parts. Subjective complaints alone would not be sufficient to qualify for the diagnosis because of the difficulty in distinguishing such complaints from those that are unrelated to drug therapy and may be part of the underlying mental disorder. Subjective complaints can be useful as indicators of the prodrome leading to objective signs, however. Objective signs and symptoms would include abnormal positioning of the head and neck in relation to the body (e.g., retrocollis, torticollis); spasms of the jaw muscles (trismus, gaping, grimacing); impaired swallowing (dysphagia), speaking, or breathing (laryngeal-pharyngeal spasm, dysphonia); thickened or slurred speech due to hypertonic or enlarged tongue (dysarthria, macroglossia); tongue protrusion or tongue dysfunction; eyes deviated up, down, or sideward (oculogyric crisis); or abnormal positioning of the distal or proximal limbs or the trunk. These should occur within 7 days of starting neuroleptic therapy, rapidly raising an existing neuroleptic dose, continuing a depot neuroleptic injection schedule, or suddenly stopping medicines that are treatments for acute extrapyramidal syndromes, such as anticholinergic, antihistaminic, or dopamine agonist agents. The criteria would specify that the symptoms are not better accounted for by a mental disorder and are not due to a neurologic disorder or other general medical condition.

Neuroleptic-Induced Acute Akathisia

In Chapter 33, Adler and Angrist discuss neuroleptic-induced acute akathisia. Akathisia, a frequent and disturbing side effect of neuroleptic treatment, literally means an inability to remain seated. Patients with neuroleptic-induced akathisia have subjective complaints of restlessness, usually referable to the legs, and often have characteristic objectively discernible movements. The subjective distress of akathisia is significant and can lead to refusal of neuroleptic treatment or a worsening of psychosis. The syndrome can be so dysphoric that it has been associated with violence or aggression or suicide attempts. This significant distress makes recognition of akathisia very important. Worsening of psychosis or behavioral dyscontrol are frequently perceived by clinicians as indications for increasing the dose of neuroleptics. If akathisia is the cause, this response will likely lead to an escalating cycle of akathisia, clinical worsening, dose increase, and further deterioration. A variety of psychiatric conditions and other movement disorders may appear similar to neuroleptic-induced acute akathisia; the authors recommend that suspected akathisia should be clinically treated given the significant morbidity if left untreated.

The reported prevalence of neuroleptic-induced acute akathisia varies widely, probably due to a lack of recognition, a lack of standard criteria for diagnosis, and the potency of the neuroleptics used. A fairly liberal threshold is proposed for diagnosing neuroleptic-induced acute akathisia, using sensitive but not specific criteria that include milder forms of the condition to encourage recognition and treatment since the clinical consequences of missing a diagnosis are significant and the risks of treating akathisia are minimal. Therefore, the risk-benefit ratio in treating a suspected case of akathisia is fairly high. Anticholinergic medications, and most recently beta-blockers, have often been found to be effective treatments for neuroleptic-induced acute akathisia. The proposed criteria require a diagnosis of mild akathisia on the global rating using criteria derived from the Barnes akathisia scale (Barnes 1989). These criteria would use cutoffs that include severity for both subjective complaints and objective movements.

The proposed criteria would require the development of subjective complaints of restlessness after exposure to a neuroleptic medication, as well as the observation of one of the following: 1) fidgety movements or swinging of the legs, 2) rocking from foot to foot while standing, 3) pacing to relieve restlessness, or 4) inability to sit or stand still for at least several minutes. The criteria would specify onset of symptoms within 4 weeks of initiating or increasing the dose of the neuroleptic, or reducing medication used to treat extrapyramidal symptoms. Symptoms must not be better accounted for by a mental disorder and not be due to a neurologic disorder or other general medical condition.

Neuroleptic-Induced Tardive Dyskinesia

In Chapter 34, Jeste and Yassa discuss neuroleptic-induced tardive dyskinesia. Neuroleptic-induced tardive dyskinesia is relatively common and potentially persistent and irreversible. The literature was reviewed to determine if tardive dyskinesia should be included in DSM-IV, what criteria should be used, and at what level the threshold should be set. All available prevalence studies through 1989 were reviewed, and 76 published studies including 39,187 patients were found that met the selection criteria. The questions addressed were whether tardive dyskinesia would be included in DSM-IV, and if so what criterion for severity should be used and should a subtyping system be employed.

The overall prevalence of tardive dyskinesia in patients treated long term with neuroleptics was approximately 24.2%. Since spontaneous dyskinesia unrelated to neuroleptic use occurs in more than 5%, it may be difficult to prove that neuroleptics produced tardive dyskinesia in a specific individual, necessitating the development of specific diagnostic criteria for tardive dyskinesia. The authors conclude that the risk of overdiagnosis due to lack of a severity criterion could be reduced by ruling out conditions in the differential diagnosis and by including a criterion for a minimum duration of at least 4 weeks. They conclude that, although providing subtypes would prevent viewing tardive dyskinesia as a homogeneous condition, there is not enough literature validating (or even reliably identifying) specific subtypes of tardive dyskinesia at this time. The proposed diagnostic criteria for tardive dyskinesia require use of neuroleptics or related compounds for at least 3 months (or 1 month in patients age 60 or older) with onset of dyskinetic movements while on neuroleptics or within a few weeks of withdrawal. There must be involuntary movements present that are choreiform (nonrepetitive, rapid, jerky, quasipurposive), athetoid (slow, sinuous, continuous, purposeless), or rhythmic (stereotypies) in nature and affect at least one of the following parts: tongue, jaw, or extremities. Symptoms must be present for at least 4 weeks and must not be due to other causes of dyskinesia.

Lithium Tremor

In Chapter 35, Gelenberg and Jefferson discuss lithium tremor. To determine whether lithium tremor should be included in DSM-IV, a literature review was done to examine the data on the nature, incidence, consequences, and treatment of tremor caused by lithium therapy. Tremor is a common, usually benign and well-tolerated side effect of therapeutic amounts of lithium. However, it is possible that lithium tremor may sometimes cause noncompliance. A worsening of tremor may be indicative of impending lithium intoxication.

The reported prevalence of lithium tremor varies widely (4%–65%). Nontoxic lithium tremor may improve spontaneously over time despite continued lithium treatment. If treatment intervention is necessary, there are a number of nonpharmacologic and pharmacologic approaches that may be beneficial.

Including a diagnosis of lithium tremor in DSM-IV could enhance clinicians' recognition of this side effect and lead to improved management. Criteria would need to be specific enough to limit false positives while encouraging accurate diagnosis of the syndrome. The proposed criteria for medication-induced postural tremor would require the presence of a fine tremor (i.e., a regular, rhythmic oscillation of a body part about a point) of about 8–12 cycles per second, most easily observed when the affected body part is held in a sustained posture. The criteria would specify that the tremor must be related to treatment with lithium or other medication, and not be due to a preexisting nonpharmacologically induced tremor and not be better accounted for by neuroleptic-induced parkinsonism.

Conclusion

Based on the results of the literature reviews, it was proposed that the medication-induced movement disorders reviewed in this section be placed in DSM-IV and listed with codes and brief descriptions with Other Conditions That May Be a Focus of Clinical Attention. Since the criteria sets are still preliminary, it was proposed that criteria sets and texts for these disorders be placed in an appendix for further study and research. It is hoped that the inclusion of this new category in DSM-IV will result in greater recognition of these important syndromes and better patient management and will lead to new research in this area and the development of more precise diagnostic criteria for DSM-V.

References

American Psychiatric Association: Diagnostic and Statistical Manual of Mental Disorders, 3rd Edition, Revised. Washington, DC, American Psychiatric Association, 1987

Barnes TRE: A rating scale for drug-induced akathisia. Br J Psychiatry 154:672–676, 1989

Chapter 30

Neuroleptic-Induced Parkinsonism

Peter J. Weiden, M.D.

Statement of the Issues

The issue addressed in this chapter is whether a diagnosis of neuroleptic-induced parkinsonism (NIP) should be included in DSM-IV. To address this issue, I review the literature concerning 1) the pharmaco-epidemiology of neuroleptic use in psychiatric practice, 2) rates of NIP among psychiatric patient populations, 3) morbidity from NIP, 4) clinical underrecognition of NIP, and 5) overlap between NIP and primary psychiatric diagnoses.

Significance of the Issues

The purpose here is to consider the clinical significance of the proposal to include NIP in DSM-IV. The disadvantage of this proposal is that NIP may be more appropriately conceptualized as a neurologic complication than a mental disorder, and thus be inappropriate for DSM-IV. Also, including a side effect of psychotropic medication could conceivably open a Pandora's box that could overwhelm future editions of the DSM. These concerns are important; therefore, including NIP is potentially controversial. The advantages of inclusion need to be compelling enough to warrant including this syndrome in DSM-IV. Relevant questions include the following:

1. How often are neuroleptics prescribed? Who receives neuroleptic treatment?
2. Are rates of NIP high enough and morbidity great enough to warrant consideration in DSM-IV?
3. Are neuroleptics properly prescribed? Is NIP currently underrecognized by the psychiatric community? If so, what are the underrecognition rates? Should improving current practice be a goal for the profession?

4. How do symptoms of NIP overlap with symptoms of DSM-IV mental disorder diagnoses? In other words, how frequently will the differential between NIP and established DSM-IV diagnoses occur?
5. Can NIP be reliably defined? What constitutes definitive symptoms versus associated features? What are the minimal thresholds for NIP symptoms? How can NIP be distinguished from other parkinsonian syndromes and other mental disorders that have similar clinical presentations?
6. Would inclusion of NIP improve the accuracy of DSM-IV diagnoses, or might it distract the clinician from making the proper psychiatric diagnosis? Would inclusion of NIP improve cross-linkage with ICD-10 (World Health Organization 1992)?

I address the first four sets of questions and outline the general approach that was undertaken in the literature review to evaluate these issues.

Unnecessary Neuroleptic Exposure and Underrecognition of NIP

NIP is, by definition, iatrogenic. Thus, the responsibility for proper diagnosis of NIP and minimizing exposure to neuroleptic agents rests with the practitioner and, on a larger scale, with the psychiatric profession. Justifying the use of DSM-IV as a vehicle for clinician education about NIP depends in part on whether the psychiatric community is now adequately addressing this complication. Unfortunately, there is strong evidence suggesting that current practice does not succeed in this goal. In particular, the literature indicates misuse of neuroleptics for certain high-risk populations and high rates of diagnostic errors—especially underrecognition—of NIP in common clinical situations.

Neuroleptic misuse. Most users of DSM-IV will be familiar with the standard psychiatric indications for neuroleptic treatment. The most definitive indications are the acute psychotic phases of schizophrenic, schizoaffective, and schizophreniform disorders; major depression with psychotic features; and manic disorders. There is evidence that neuroleptic dosages are often too high during the inpatient treatment of acute psychosis, increasing the likelihood of developing NIP. There is a mismatch in dosage prescribing practices for schizophrenia between the optimal doses of 300–500 mg of chlorpromazine (CPZ) equivalents (Baldessarini et al. 1988; Davis 1976) and doses used in actual clinical practice. High-potency agents are a risk factor for prescribing dosages beyond the standard accepted ranges (Baldessarini et al. 1984). Neuroleptics are not indicated but prescribed for the following disorders: primary substance abuse disorders without psychotic symptoms, anxiety disorders, insomnia, and somatization disorders.

Medical indications for neuroleptic drugs are primarily for treatment of nausea and vomiting (Davidson et al. 1975; Derogatis et al. 1979). Unfortunately, these indications may blur with vague psychosomatic complaints. Also, neuroleptics may be prescribed indefinitely—and without adequate review—in medical settings where the risk of NIP and other movement disorders is not considered. Elderly patients seem to be at high risk for receiving inappropriate neuroleptic treatment; for example, in 48 consecutive cases of NIP in the elderly studied by Stephen and Williamson (1984), "In no case did this drug [neuroleptic] seem to be indicated" (p. 1082). Efforts have been focused on overuse of neuroleptics among nursing home populations (Avorn et al. 1989).

Underrecognition of NIP. Another major problem is underrecognition of NIP in settings where the neuroleptic is indicated but the side effect is missed. Despite having a clear responsibility to recognize and treat NIP (Wettstein 1985), there is strong evidence that NIP is underrecognized by the psychiatric community at large, and that at least 50% of all clinically significant NIP diagnoses are missed (Hansen et al. 1992; Weiden et al. 1987).

Morbidity From NIP

There is strong evidence that NIP is a most serious complication, resulting in direct patient morbidity (e.g., neuroleptic malignant syndrome) and indirectly leading to other complications (e.g., medication noncompliance).

Overlap Between Symptoms of NIP and Psychiatric Disorders

There is a great deal of overlap between NIP and primary psychiatric symptoms. Symptoms of NIP include behavioral toxicities that resemble depression (Siris 1987; Van Putten and May 1978a, 1978b) and negative symptoms of schizophrenia (Carpenter et al. 1985). Furthermore, patients may manifest difficulties that seem to be psychosocial complications of their psychiatric disorder but actually result from altered appearances related to NIP. For example, a complaint of stigma about treatment may really be from a patient's akinetic appearance (e.g., "looking like a zombie").

Methods

Overview

As outlined in the section on significance earlier, I attempt to address four issues in this review: 1) rates of NIP in the psychiatric patient population, 2) clinical underrecognition of NIP recognition rates, 3) direct morbidity, and 4) behavioral toxicity and indirect morbidity.

Prevalence of NIP

How often is NIP a complication of neuroleptic treatment? Prevalence of NIP was studied with a meta-analysis of the neuroleptic-treatment literature. Many neuroleptic treatment studies systematically evaluate for parkinsonian side effects, even if side effects are not the central focus of the study. Unfortunately, quantity of studies does not guarantee that a thorough or systematic approach was used to diagnosis NIP. Methodological validity checks were used to estimate whether some of these studies met minimal quality criteria.

The problems with a literature-based review of NIP rates included 1) lack of standardized assessments or accepted cutoff criteria for what is a threshold severity; 2) the relative absence of data about functional disability or distress arising from NIP (Hogan et al. 1983); 3) the fact that studies do not always report rates of individual NIP symptoms; 4) variations in prescribed drug dosages, drug potency, and length of treatment time; and 5) differences in study patient populations. These variables affected data on individual patient vulnerability to NIP and limited the goals of this broad-based literature review.

Achievable goals for the purposes of this DSM-IV review were to 1) establish the overall range of global NIP diagnoses, 2) determine the relative frequencies of individual NIP symptoms, 3) attempt to understand better the risk factors for NIP, and 4) estimate behavioral toxicity rates. Behavioral toxicity is reported from rates and number of studies found reporting behavioral toxicity in the NIP rate review and includes effects on control subjects (e.g., Anderson et al. 1981). It is not possible to estimate morbidity or disability from a review of NIP rates; therefore, I review morbidity and indirect complications using data based on case report literature later.

NIP Prevalence Review

Many studies that report NIP rates did not appear on a Medline computer-based literature review (using key words *extrapyramidal, parkinsonism,* and *major tranquilizer*). The problem was that NIP, although often reported, usually was not the major focus of the article. To compensate for this problem, the literature review for NIP base rates was done manually. To avoid bias in the manual search, the journals and time period covered were set beforehand. The methodology for the literature review is described below.

Time period. The year 1970 was chosen because that time period reflected a resurgence of interest in the problem of NIP. Earlier studies on this topic (e.g., Ayd

1961) were not used because, in general, standardized parkinsonism scales (e.g., the Simpson-Angus Scale for Rating NIP [Simpson and Angus 1970]) were not routinely used before the 1970s.

Journal selection. All articles published between 1970 and 1991 in one of the following journals were manually screened: *Acta Psychiatrica Scandinavica, American Journal of Psychiatry, Archives of General Psychiatry, British Journal of Psychiatry, Comprehensive Psychiatry, Journal of Clinical Psychopharmacology,* and *Journal of Nervous and Mental Disease.* There were some additions from other sources. Several important references for special groups (e. g., studies of child, geriatric, and mentally retarded patient populations) came from other journal sources because of the scarcity of appropriate studies available in the primary journal source.

Screening criteria. An article was included when it studied the effects of neuroleptic treatment and systematically evaluated for NIP. The research focus of the publication was coded into one of the following: 1) a primary study on extrapyramidal symptoms, 2) an anticholinergic withdrawal study, 3) an acute inpatient drug trial, 4) a maintenance outpatient drug trial, 5) a Tourette's syndrome drug trial, 5) a study on neuroleptics for medical indications, or 6) other. Any study that used duplicated subjects from another study in this meta-analysis was excluded.

Diagnostic methods. Parkinsonism diagnoses were based on motor examination. From there, however, study methods diverge. The assessment methods included quantitative assessments (such as tremor accelerometer), anchored standardized rating scale (e.g., the Simpson-Angus), qualitative assessments, or psychometric assessments. A study could have more than one assessment modality.

Rates of NIP and individual NIP symptoms. Overall rates of NIP were estimated from the study report or calculated from the individual item data. A "zero prevalence" study (e.g., a study that found no cases of the NIP in question despite a statement in its methods section that the NIP was evaluated) would not be averaged into the prevalence estimate. Excluding such studies can lead to inflated estimates of prevalence; including them could distort the prevalence the other way. One way this problem was addressed was to report the number of studies with zero prevalence next to the prevalence estimates. It is strongly suggested that you evaluate both of these numbers before drawing your own conclusions.

Rates of subcomponents of NIP (akinesia, rigidity, tremor, cogwheeling, gait disturbance, and behavioral toxicity) were also recorded. Symptoms of drooling and postural instability were not coded because of the infrequency with which these particular symptoms were reported. Studies that did not report the specific subsyndrome rates were not used in this part of the analysis; however, the absolute number of studies that report on specific subsyndromes can give indirect evidence of their perceived importance. Therefore, the subcomponents of parkinsonism are reported as 1) the number of studies from the available pool of studies reporting the presence of a particular sign or symptom and 2) the average of the prevalence of the symptoms for those studies that reported that symptom. (Exclusion of other studies not reporting the particular symptom may artificially increase prevalence of individual symptoms but should not affect the relative frequencies of occurrence.)

Coding criteria. Parkinsonism rates were extracted from the primary journal articles into a Quattro Pro spreadsheet. When possible, the data were transformed and recorded into 1) the number of subjects at risk for the report of side effect, 2) the overall percentage of parkinsonism experienced by the study population, and 3) the rates of the main features of parkinsonian syndromes. Most of the time, the overall parkinsonism rates excluded acute dystonic reactions and akathisia; however, these side effects were not clearly separated from overall parkinsonism rates in some studies. Therefore, the overall parkinsonism rates may include, in some studies, cases of akathisia and acute dystonia (not tardive dyskinesia). Table 30–1 reports the coded variables with comments.

Clinical underrecognition of NIP. There are many case reports and clinical impressions of NIP underrecognition but few systemized studies with base-rate population. They are subdivided into medically ill (primarily geriatric patients with NIP misdiagnosed as idiopathic) and psychiatric populations (primarily acutely psychotic schizophrenic inpatients). The studies that were found were located by the author of this report. The literature review for NIP rates did not reveal any additional studies.

Morbidity from NIP. Criteria for reporting direct morbidity include 1) at least two cases reported in the psychiatric literature, and 2) the complication was clearly associated with neuroleptic exposure.

Like the prevalence analysis, because base rates were not possible to estimate, morbidity rates in psychiatric populations are not known.

Complications

Rates of behavioral toxicity were obtained from the NIP rate review. Such an estimate is, at best, an approximation. A more qualitative description of the forms of NIP behavioral toxicity rates was obtained from another, less systematic review

Table 30–1. Variables coded from each study

Domain	Variable	Definition
Patient population	Responsive schizophrenia; refractory schizophrenia; affective psychosis; Tourette's; geriatric; child	*Responsive schizophrenia* includes studies with short length of stay (< 6 months) and/or patients who are responsive to short-term neuroleptic trial (includes all outpatient studies). *Refractory schizophrenia* is defined as long-term inpatients (> 6 months) and/or unresponsive to acute neuroleptic trial. Studies of subjects who were ≤ 16 years of age were categorized as *child*, and *geriatric* for ≥ 60 years.
Purpose of study	Anticholinergic; acute; maintenance	*Anticholinergic* is defined as a study whose primary research goal was either 1) determine the effects of anticholinergic withdrawal, or 2) test efficacy of adjuvant anticholinergic therapy. An *acute study was when the neuroleptic treated acted psychosis. Maintenance* corresponds to studies of prophylactic neuroleptic therapy of schizophrenic outpatients.
Hospital status	Inpatient; outpatient	Primary setting of where the study took place.
Neuroleptic dose	mg/neuroleptic/day	Mean daily neuroleptic dose given to the study sample converted to CPZ equivalents as per methods of Baldessarini et al. (1988). Fluphenazine decanoate doses were converted to oral equivalents as 50 mg im every month = 15 mg oral fluphenazine/day. Haloperidol decanoate was converted from 100 mg im every month to 10 mg oral haloperidol/day.
Neuroleptic class	High potency; intermediate (or mixed); low; long-acting	Examples of *high* include haloperidol, fluphenazine, and pimozide. Examples of *intermediate* include trifluoperazine, thiothixine, and loxapine, or when neuroleptics of different classes were not reported separately. Examples of *low* include chlorpromazine and thioridazine. Examples of *long-acting* include fluphenazine decanoate, haloperidol decanoate, pimozide decanoate, and flupenthixol decanoate.

Note. CPZ = chlorpromazine.

of the literature on neuroleptic compliance, neuroleptic dysphoria, and akinetic depression. The clinical forms behavioral toxicity can take include 1) neuroleptic-induced dysphoria, 2) neuroleptic-induced depression, 3) suicide, 4) immediate noncompliance, and 5) delayed noncompliance. These "indirect" aspects of NIP morbidity are reviewed.

Results and Discussion

Prevalence

Ninety articles fulfilled the selection criteria. Several articles could be subdivided into more than one study; these were counted as separate studies. A total of 6,366 patients were included. Table 30–2 shows the major domains of this analysis with the number of studies and patients used during the analysis of the particular domain. (A complete list of references is available on request from the author.)

NIP rates. The combined estimate of NIP prevalence (average of the percentages) was 40.4% (63 studies, 3,556 patients). Rigidity was the most frequently reported individual parkinsonian symptom (23 studies, 640 patients, 31.02% average prevalence) followed by tremor (21 studies, 648 patients, 25.95% average prevalence), akinesia (19 studies, 553 eligible patients, 33.95% average prevalence), cogwheel rigidity (7 studies, 293 eligible patients, 19.6% average prevalence), and gait disturbance (1 study, 75 patients, 11% prevalence). Because cogwheel rigidity and gait disturbance received far fewer mentions as specific NIP symptoms, they were excluded from further analysis.

Table 30–2. Number of studies and subjects for major variables

Domain	Number of studies[a]	Number of patients
All studies	92	6,366
By patient population[b]	88	3,556
By purpose of study[b]	66	2,141
Inpatient versus outpatient	79	3,378
By neuroleptic class[b]	84	5,346
By neuroleptic dose[b]	53	3,583

[a]Number of studies available for analysis in the particular domain. Studies were omitted when the relevant data could not be obtained.
[b]See Table 30–1.

Study methodology. The most common assessment method of evaluation for NIP was using an anchored rating scale (57 studies), usually the Simpson-Angus. The second most common method was a qualitative evaluation for NIP (35 studies), either alone (28 studies) or in conjunction with anchored measure (7 studies). There were very few reports using quantitative (e.g., accelerometer) (4 studies) or psychometric (3 studies) measures.

NIP rates from qualitative studies were suspect. Qualitative studies were compared with anchored studies as a validity check. A secondary goal was to see whether these two methods had similar or different emphasis on the makeup of NIP. In particular, some anchored rating scales tend to weigh rigidity more heavily than akinesia. Table 30–3 compares overall NIP and individual NIP symptoms.

The 35 studies that used qualitative methods found lower overall average prevalence rates of NIP than the 52 studies using anchored scales (28% versus 49%). However, the odds that a qualitative study would report finding any NIP were similar to anchored studies (26/35 versus 37/52). Furthermore, qualitative studies did not always report lower symptom prevalence. In particular, qualitative studies found higher rates of akinesia (44.8% versus 28.9%) than did the studies using anchored scales. These results are inconclusive. They are compatible with two possible explanations: 1) qualitative measures do not pick up the physical signs of NIP as readily as anchored scales, or 2) qualitative assessments may be more

Table 30–3. Study patient population and reported rates of neuroleptic-induced parkinsonism

Diagnosis	N of studies[a]	Neuroleptic-induced parkinsonism %[b]	N[c]	Akinesia %[b]	N[c]	Rigidity %[b]	N[c]	Tremor %[b]	N[c]
Responsive schizophrenia	47	49.6	28	31.3	10	35.2	13	24.5	10
Refractory schizophrenia	17	26	13	40.3	3	29.8	5	35.5	4
Affective disorder	10	33.9	8	—	0	8.2	2	—	0
Tourette's	5	57.3	2	49.5	3	—	0	20	2

[a]The number of studies that were relevant to each symptom.
[b]Average of prevalence for the studies with greater-than-zero prevalence.
[c]The number of studies (out of the eligible N) that reported greater-than-zero prevalence of the symptom.

sensitive for akinesia than currently used anchored scales. In this chapter I include qualitative studies because the reported NIP rates are not vastly different.

Patient population. The most common patient population was responsive schizophrenia (47 studies), followed by refractory schizophrenia (17 studies), affective disorders (10 studies), Tourette's syndrome (5 studies), children (3 studies), geriatric (2 studies), and mentally retarded (2 studies). Table 30–3 shows the NIP prevalence rates and proportion of studies reporting NIP symptoms for the first four populations; the other patient populations had too few studies to be meaningful.

Several findings are worth mentioning. First, the chances that a study will report at least one case of NIP do not seem to be influenced by the patient population. What does vary between patient populations is the average prevalence rates for those studies reporting NIP (approximately 60% of all study groups reported at least one case of NIP). The differences in average prevalence are most striking when comparing the neuroleptic-responsive population with the refractory schizophrenic population. The NIP prevalence in neuroleptic-responsive patients was almost twice that of refractory patients (49.6% versus 26%). This effect does not seem to be an artifact of neuroleptic dose, which was slightly lower in the responsive population (814 versus 575 mg CPZ equivalents). Another interesting finding is the high rate of akinesia reported in the Tourette's syndrome studies. The number of studies reporting akinesia and the average prevalence of akinesia is higher for Tourette's syndrome than for all other patient populations.

NIP and study purpose. The primary goal of the study was evaluated, using schizophrenic patients only. The four most common study types were 1) prevalence of extrapyramidal symptoms, 2) anticholinergic withdrawal, 3) acute inpatient drug trial, and 4) maintenance outpatient drug trial. Table 30–4 shows the relationship between study purpose and NIP rates.

Several patterns can be seen from Table 30–4. First, the range of overall NIP rates does not seem to differ between studies whose primary focus is on NIP rates versus neuroleptic treatment efficacy studies where NIP is an outcome variable. However, NIP prevalence studies and anticholinergic withdrawal studies seem to report higher average prevalence rates of akinesia and behavioral toxicity, whereas neuroleptic treatment studies are more likely to report tremor and rigidity as the most common forms of NIP.

NIP and neuroleptic dose. Nineteen studies reported the mean dose of neuroleptic and overall NIP rates. This analysis did not find any correlation between neuroleptic dose and NIP rates. This is not surprising since there are so many confounding factors (e.g., neuroleptic class, anticholinergic treatment). A further analysis tried to address some of these confounds. Studies were categorized into the subjects' primary diagnosis, inpatient versus outpatient status, and class of neuroleptic used in treatment.

There were some dose effects under certain conditions. Outpatient maintenance neuroleptic studies showed a tendency toward a relationship between dose and side effects. Two studies that used maintenance neuroleptic doses 500 mg CPZ equivalents had an average overall NIP rate of 5% compared with six studies where subjects were maintained at doses 500 mg CPZ equivalents and had an average NIP rate of 74%. Anticholinergic withdrawal was the other type of study that seemed to show a positive neuroleptic dose-side effect relationship. Of five anticholinergic withdrawal studies included here, three had subjects on an average dose 700 mg CPZ equivalents. Two studies had subjects maintained on CPZ doses 1,500 mg. After anticholinergic withdrawal, the corresponding NIP rates were 13% versus 77%. The small numbers of studies involved and the nature of the post hoc analyses make this association speculative at best. However, it seems possible that dose-side effect relationships are more discernible for schizophrenic outpatients and when anticholinergics are discontinued.

In contrast, a relationship between inpatient neuroleptic dose and side effects is either nonexistent or obscured by other factors not evaluated in this analysis. Six inpatient studies of acutely psychotic, neuroleptic-responsive inpatients failed to show any dose-response relationship (mean dose range, 255–1,800 mg CPZ equivalents; parkinsonism rates range, 24%–96%). Similarly, seven studies of chronic

Table 30–4. Purpose of the study

Study type[a]	*N* of studies[b]	Neuroleptic-induced parkinsonism		Akinesia		Rigidity		Tremor	
		%[c]	*N*[d]	%[c]	*N*[d]	%[c]	*N*[d]	%[c]	*N*[d]
Prevalence	16	61.4	10	33.4	5	52	3	23	2
Anticholinergic	9	31.6	8	20	3	26	2	11.5	2
Inpatient	7	47.2	4	—	0	28.8	4	21.2	4
Outpatient	7	67.6	5	26	1	11	1	32.5	2

[a]Only neuroleptic-responsive schizophrenia studies were used for this analysis.
[b]The number of studies that were relevant to each symptom.
[c]Average of prevalence for the studies with greater-than-zero prevalence. Studies reporting zero rates were not included because of difficulty ascertaining whether the symptom was evaluated.
[d]The number of studies (out of the eligible *N*) that reported greater-than-zero prevalence of the symptom.

neuroleptic-nonresponsive inpatients showed no relationship (dose range, 230–1,000 mg CPZ equivalents; overall NIP rates of 0%–66%).

NIP and neuroleptic class. The association between class of neuroleptic and NIP seems to be stronger than dose effects. As Table 30–5 shows, NIP is less likely to be reported in studies using low-potency neuroleptics (versus all other classes) and, when reported, occurs less frequently. The differences do not seem to be an artifact of absolute dose effect difference. The so-called medium-potency neuroleptics are equivalent to low-potency vis-à-vis average dose used, yet the medium-potency agents seem to behave more like higher-potency drugs in terms of propensity to cause NIP.

Behavioral toxicity. Of the 92 studies, 21 reported NIP presenting with behavioral symptoms. The average of the neuroleptic dose used was 404 mg CPZ equivalents, and the patient number totaled 1,137. The associated physical findings of NIP were not very different from those in the majority of studies that did not report behavior toxicities. The overall rate of behavioral toxicity was 45.9%. The average of the more typical NIP symptoms was 44% (8 studies), akinesia 36% (3 studies), rigidity 15% (1 study), and tremor 15.5% (1 study). Notably, most behavior-toxicity studies were done on neuroleptic-responsive schizophrenic patients. Outpatient settings ($N = 6$) reported higher average rates of behavioral toxicity than did inpatient studies ($N = 7$, 55.8% versus 35.6%) despite outpatient studies using lower neuroleptic doses (478 versus 610 mg CPZ equivalents).

Table 30–5. Neuroleptic class and parkinsonism

Neuroleptic class[a]	*N* of studies[b]	Mean dose (CPZ)	Neuroleptic-induced parkinsonism %[c]	Neuroleptic-induced parkinsonism N[d]
High	37	635	42.9	25
Medium	20	459	34.8	15
Low	12	470	18.2	9
Intramuscular	15	1,475[e]	64.7	11

Note. CPZ = chlorpromazine.
[a]See Table 30–1 for definitions of neuroleptic class studies.
[b]The number of studies that were relevant to each symptom.
[c]Average of prevalence for the studies with greater-than-zero prevalence.
[d]The number of studies (out of the eligible *N*) that reported greater-than-zero prevalence of the symptom.
[e]See Table 30–1 for how intramuscular doses were estimated to comparable oral doses.

Underrecognition

Underrecognition of NIP is very common. This problem has been anecdotally reported for many years. At least five systematic studies have documented this problem (Table 30–6). This literature emphasizes that the underrecognition is not trivial. The cases described in these studies frequently had serious consequences. Morbidity from nonrecognition can be life threatening. For example, diagnostic delays may lead to symptom progression from NIP to fulminant neuroleptic malignant syndrome.

Morbidity

Objective morbidity from NIP resembles that of parkinsonian syndrome. However, there are noticeable differences between the neurologic and psychiatric literature. The major difference is that morbidity is much better documented in the neurologic literature, and complications of idiopathic Parkinson's disease are often more life threatening than NIP (e.g., dysphagia, falling). It is not clear whether the difference in symptom distribution is secondary to age effects (idiopathic Parkinson's disease occurs in the geriatric population) or because idiopathic Parkinson's disease is progressive. Several standard textbooks report that tremor is more common in idiopathic Parkinson's disease than NIP and that akinesia is more frequent in NIP. Immobility from akinesia can cause hip fractures (Boyce and Vessey 1988) or pulmonary emboli. It is also thought that NIP is relatively more responsive to anticholinergics, whereas L-dopa is more effective for idiopathic

Table 30–6. Medical and psychiatric reports of underrecognition of neuroleptic-induced parkinsonism

Study	*N*	Error rate (%)	Comments
Neurologic			
Indo and Ando 1982	282	11	Parkinson clinic; mostly metoclopramide; akinesia predominant symptom
Stephen and Williamson 1984	98	49	Parkinson clinic; thioridazine and prochlorperazine predominant; 15% mortality
Grimes 1982	39	36	Elderly patients
Psychiatric			
Weiden and Harrigan 1986	29	41	Prospectively rated parkinsonism compared with chart diagnoses in a private hospital setting
Hansen et al. 1992	26	56	Similar methodology in a Veterans Administration setting

Parkinson's disease. In contrast to idiopathic Parkinson's disease, NIP occurs more often in younger individuals, is not progressive, and is reversible on discontinuation of the offending drug. The following reports of morbidity are for patients with known NIP.

Hospital admissions. Complications from neuroleptic treatment are by far the most common iatrogenic cause of psychiatric admission (Wolf et al. 1989). Neuroleptics are the most common cause of serious morbidity in inpatients (Grohmann et al. 1984). These reactions lead to admission in 1% of all cases and account for 40% of all serious adverse drug reactions.

Medical sequelae. Medical complications are usually secondary to the decreased motor activity found with akinetic states, which include pulmonary emboli, contractures, and bedsores. Stephen and Williamson (1984) found a 15% mortality rate for NIP in elderly patients. Kennedy and colleagues (1971) showed that up to 75% of cases of NIP had morbidity including difficulty with speaking, dressing, feeding, or writing. Falling and hip fractures are complications of parkinsonism (Grisso et al. 1991), especially for elderly patients. Neuroleptic exposure has been associated with increased rates of hip fractures in the elderly. Decreased gag reflex and dysphagia from parkinsonism can be life threatening (Weiden and Harrigan 1986) and may present as aspiration pneumonia or unexplained weight loss. Urinary incontinence was found in 50% of an NIP elderly sample. When milder forms of NIP are unrecognized and the neuroleptic dose is raised, they may progress to more dangerous forms (e.g., catatonia or neuroleptic malignant syndrome).

Vocational disability. The motoric impairment can cause vocational disability, especially when manual dexterity is necessary. Rigidity, tremor, and decreased coordination can all be factors. What is most striking is the almost complete void in the literature on vocational and functional impairment from NIP.

Complications

The indirect consequences of NIP can be severe. Symptoms of behavioral toxicity can include worsening of depression, negative symptoms of schizophrenia, and suicidal despair. What many of these symptoms have in common is the great degree of overlap with primary psychiatric symptoms. The onset may be insidious, may be unrecognized, and may erode the therapeutic relationship. Behavioral toxicity can be difficult to diagnose, especially in the psychotic, neurologic, or mentally retarded patient populations given neuroleptics (Chadsey-Rusch and Sprague 1989).

Depression. Akinesia can cause depression. Depression in schizophrenia is common and has several etiologies. Depression can represent a prodromal sign of relapse, can be a part of the acute psychosis, can be an independent syndrome (postpsychotic depression), or can be a behavioral component of akinesia. Epidemiologic studies of depression in schizophrenia suggest that akinetic depression is not the most common cause of postpsychotic depression (Drake and Cotton 1986). Nonetheless, since neuroleptic-induced akinesia is readily treatable, akinetic depression remains an important differential diagnosis (Rifkin et al. 1975; Van Putten and May 1978a, 1978b).

Psychosocial complications. The psychosocial complications include stigma from a patient's akinetic appearance (e.g., "looking like a zombie"). Sometimes it is the drug effect, not the illness itself, that makes it readily apparent to others that the person suffers from a major mental disorder. Subtle behavioral disturbance can erode the relationship between the patient and the family. For example, Kreisman and colleagues (1988) found that families had greater satisfaction levels with the relatives on low-dose treatment despite higher relapse rates. Weiden and colleagues (1991) found that distress from akinesia at the time of discharge from the hospital predicted erosion of family support for the continued neuroleptic treatment of schizophrenic outpatients.

Suicide. Suicide is the most extreme form of behavioral toxicity. Neuroleptic-induced suicidal behavior can be directly mediated through neuroleptic-induced depression (Van Putten and May 1978a, 1978b), akathisia (Drake and Ehrlich 1985), or other behavioral toxicities (e.g., dysphoria) (Bruun 1988). The notion that suicide can be neuroleptic induced began after a study reported higher rates of suicide in schizophrenia when, because of policy changes, patients were converted from oral to intramuscular fluphenazine (Alarcon and Carney 1969). Another study of schizophrenic patients on depot fluphenazine found a greater preoccupation with death or suicide in patients with severe side effects (66% versus 4% of control patients) (Blum 1980). Therefore, although akinesia cannot explain the high suicide rates in recently discharged schizophrenic outpatients, anecdotal reports and clinical experience suggest that akinesia may promote suicidal behavior for a few vulnerable individuals.

Immediate noncompliance. Patients who are distressed by the behavioral symptoms of neuroleptics may become noncompliant. In turn, noncompliance in schizophrenia will increase the risk of relapse. Therefore, the study of morbidity from NIP needs to include noncompliance. In a series of studies, Van Putten and colleagues (Van Putten 1974; Van Putten and May 1978a, 1978b) found that early-onset akinesia (also akathisia) predicted future medication refusal. Hogan and colleagues (1983) found that the self-report of "feeling like a zombie" (presumably subjective akinesia) was a predictor of outpatient neuroleptic noncompliance. Marder and colleagues (1984) reported a greater dropout rate of high-dosage patients in a controlled outpatient fluphenazine trial; they postulated that the differential dropout rate was from akinesia. It seems to be the subjective distress from parkinsonism rather than objective physical signs of parkinsonism that "drives" the noncompliance. Many studies do not report the subjective distress from neuroleptics, but single-dose studies in control subjects show significant negative subjective responses to neuroleptics (Henninger et al. 1965).

Long-term noncompliance. Long-term neuroleptic refusal can result from acute parkinsonism, even if short-lived. This phenomenon can be viewed as an example of conditioned avoidance. The acute noxious stimuli produces long-term aversive behavior, similar to when a person avoids a restaurant for years after a single episode of food poisoning. Evidence for this effect is supported by several studies. Schooler (1988) reported that noncooperative outpatients for a maintenance treatment study had higher parkinsonism scores around the time of study entry. Van Putten and colleagues (1990) found higher dropout rates during a fixed-dose acute treatment study when patients were given daily doses of 20 mg of haloperidol compared with those receiving 10 mg and 5 mg a day. In support of the notion that adverse parkinsonian effects are remembered, Seltzer and colleagues (1980) identified fearful anticipation of extrapyramidal symptoms as the most commonly given reason for neuroleptic noncompliance in outpatients, and Finn and colleagues (1990) showed that neuroleptics commonly interfere with perceived goals and needs.

Summary of complications. NIP is a most common cause of patient morbidity. Direct complications of NIP are similar to those seen with idiopathic Parkinson's disease. Indirect complications include unrecognized behavioral syndromes, depression, suicide, dysphoria, vocational impairment, and social stigma. Furthermore, unrecognized parkinsonism may alienate the patient and family from treatment, and a psychotic relapse because of neuroleptic refusal may be a lethal, but indirect, complication. For such cases, even "mild" parkinsonian symptoms can be a tragedy. In summary, NIP is common, is not often recognized, and overlaps with and mimics psychiatric symptoms.

Definition

Parkinsonian syndrome is characterized by rigidity, tremor, akinesia (also called bradykinesia), cogwheeling, masked facies, drooling, and postural instability. The hallmark of NIP are the same signs and symptoms that characterize parkinsonian syndrome. Therefore, it makes sense to look at the neurologic literature for diagnostic approaches used by neurologists for parkinsonian syndrome. The neurologic literature uses a syndromal, not quantitative, approach. For example, a leading neurologic text (Adams and Victor 1989) introduces the parkinsonian syndrome with "The picture of the Parkinson Syndrome, with its slowness of movement, poverty of facial expression, flexed posture, immobility and static tremor should be fixed in the mind; it is the particular combination of these features that stamps the patient unmistakably as parkinsonian" (p. 67). The *Textbook of Neuropsychiatry* defines parkinsonian syndrome patients who "exhibit with tremor, rigidity, bradykinesia, as well as disturbance of posture, gait and autonomic functions" (Hales and Yudofsky 1987, p. 258). A more quantitative description of parkinsonian syndrome was found in *Diseases of the Nervous System: Clinical Neurobiology* (Asbury et al. 1986); parkinsonian syndrome was described as "Four cardinal motor features, 1) resting tremor, 2) rigidity, 3) bradykinesia, and 4) loss of postural reflexes. . . . For practical purposes *at least two* of these should be present before a firm diagnosis of parkinsons is made" (p. 1217). Since the definition of NIP is a parkinsonian syndrome that is caused by exposure to neuroleptic drugs, a syndromal approach to NIP could parallel the syndromal approach for parkinsonian syndrome. This does not mean that NIP is identical to parkinsonian syndrome due to other causes. The exact weighing of syndromal criteria could differ between parkinsonian syndrome and NIP. Although the signs and symptoms of parkinsonian syndrome are the same as NIP, individual symptoms may have different frequencies of occurrence or modes of presentation. Possible symptom differences between parkinsonian syndrome and NIP are outlined in detail below.

Differential Diagnosis

The differential diagnosis between NIP, other neurologic disorders, and primary psychiatric symptoms is covered here.

Akinesia. Akinesia is a state of decreased spontaneous motor activity. Patients are globally slowed and show slowness in initiating and executing a movement. Normal behaviors of everyday life (e.g., grooming) are reduced. Rigidity often coexists with akinesia but is not necessary for the clinician to diagnose a neuroleptic-induced akinesia. Akinesia can be a purely subjective experience without any evidence of motoric slowing. Patients may complain of feeling listless, lacking spontaneity and drive, oversleeping, and depression. There may be few physical signs to confirm these complaints. Patients can often distinguish between the sedative effects and the akinetic effects. "Thorazine makes me sleepy . . . Haldol makes me a zombie." With akinesia, the patient is slowed from baseline. Establishing the "baseline" motor state may not be easy if the examiner has never seen the patient unmedicated. The patient's age, cultural background, and motivation affect baseline spontaneity.

False-positive akinesia. Akinesia and depression have many overlapping symptoms. Patients with primary or postpsychotic depression are more likely to have associated vegetative signs (e.g., early morning awakening). Hopelessness and despair are found in depression; apathy is more typical of either akinesia or negative symptoms of schizophrenia. This important differential diagnosis usually cannot be based on the interview alone. Patients suffering from neuroleptic malignant syndromes are akinetic, but have additional physical and laboratory findings (e.g., fever, increased creatine phosphokinase). Primary catatonic states arising from schizophrenic or manic-depressive disorders can be indistinguishable from severe akinesia. However, a patient with primary catatonia may have additional signs of psychosis not normally associated with akinesia (gegenhalten, echolalia). Waxing and waning of symptoms is not helpful in distinguishing primary catatonia from neuroleptic-induced catatonia. A person with severe withdrawal from psychosis may show "breakthrough" signs of psychosis, such as the frequent eye-darting seen with paranoia. Pharmacologic history can be helpful. A severely withdrawn psychosis should improve with neuroleptics, whereas akinesia would worsen. Focal neurologic signs are not a part of akinesia. Strokes and other focal lesions of the central nervous system cause immobility from flaccid or spastic paralysis, whereas muscle strength is normal on formal testing in patients with akinesia.

Rigidity. Rigidity is defined as a motoric state where the patient's muscles are firm and tense. The muscle rigidity can affect all skeletal muscle or involve only discreet muscle groups, sparing some of the limbs and affecting others. Rigidity may be unilateral or bilateral. Parkinsonian rigidity has two classic forms: lead pipe and cogwheel. Both of these forms have a kind of rigidity that is continuous from the beginning to the end of the muscle movement. This continuity of rigidity, regardless of joint position, distinguishes parkinsonian rigidity from spastic rigidity and the rigidity that appears to be associated with anxiety or psychosis. Resistance to passive motion is constant whether the extremity is moved slowly or rapidly. The lead-pipe form is so called because, after being moved, the limb or joint may retain its position with the same resistance to movement noted in the original position. Cogwheel rigidity is seen when the muscle is passively stretched. There is a rhythmically interrupted, ratchet-like resistance that is felt on the tendons of the muscles being pulled. The wrists and elbows are the most common site for cogwheel rigidity. Deep tendon reflexes are normal. Lead-pipe rigidity is persistent; cogwheel rigidity often waxes and wanes. The wrist can be a more sensitive location for rigidity than the elbow. Rapid alternating movements and repeating fine finger movements are excellent ways of detecting subtle parkinsonian rigidity, which may come out only after repetitive motor tasks. This easy fatigability and clumsiness secondary to rigidity will appear only after repeated fast-action movements. Patients with milder forms of rigidity may have problems with repetitive, fast tasks even when obvious rigidity is not there (Hoffman 1981). Patients will describe parkinsonian rigidity as generalized stiffness, body aching, lack of coordination during sports, muscle or joint pain, or muscle tenderness.

False-positive rigidity. The patient must be relaxed to test for parkinsonian rigidity. Anxiety about the physical examination can be mistaken as parkinsonian rigidity; the examiner should take this into account and try to put the patient at ease. Diseases that interfere with the patient's ability to attend or concentrate (e.g., acute psychosis or dementia) can lead to false-positive rigidity. Rigidity from parkinsonism needs to be differentiated from the "clasp knife" phenomenon found in pyramidal lesions and oppositional behavior (gegenhalten). Conversion disorders may present with parkinsonism-like findings of mutism and catatonia. However, conversion symptoms are a diagnosis of exclusion and are associated with severe dissociative states. Paradoxically, physical findings in conversion disorders are less likely to fluctuate during the physical examination than will true parkinsonian symptoms. Also, in conversion syndromes, the rigidity will disappear when the patient thinks he or she is alone (this should not be confused with worsening of rigidity with anxiety, which is typical of true parkinsonism).

Parkinsonian tremor. Parkinsonian tremor is a steady, rhythmic oscillatory movement. The parkinsonian type of tremor is typically slow (2–6 cycles/second). The tremor is suppressible, especially when the patient attempts to perform a task with the tremulous limb. Tremor will be described by patients as shaking, especially during times of stress or fatigue. It may be intermittent, unilateral, or dependent on location of the affected limb (e.g., positional). Parkinsonian tremor can wax and wane and may be unilateral or positional. A lip tremor, also known as "rabbit syndrome," is simply a parkinsonian tremor of the oral area. Head and tongue tremor may occur and have motor characteristics and pharmacologic response similar to the better recognized hand tremor. There is disagreement over the relative frequency of tremor in NIP versus other parkinsonian syndrome etiologies. Some authors believe it is more common in NIP, others less common.

False-positive parkinsonian tremor. The differential diagnosis of tremor includes NIP, a coexisting lithium or tricyclic tremor, familial tremor, and drug withdrawal. Lithium and tricycles cause tremor. Typically, nonparkinsonian tremors are finer (e.g., smaller amplitude), faster (10 cycles/second), and worsen on intention (e.g., when the patient reaches out to hold a cup). A drug or alcohol withdrawal tremor will usually have associated hyperreflexia and increased autonomic signs. Cerebellar tremor will be intentional and may have associated nystagmus, ataxia, or scanning speech. The choreiform movements associated with tardive dyskinesia can, at first glance, resemble tremor. However, the dyskinetic movements associated with tardive dyskinesia will be less regular and rhythmic (e.g., intermittent). The steady, rhythmicity of a parkinsonian tremor is a good way to distinguish it from dyskinesia.

Gait abnormalities. Observing the patient while walking is a most sensitive test for early signs of rigidity and tremor. Abnormalities associated with parkinsonism can be seen with gait, length of stride, arm swing, and overall spontaneity of walking, especially during turns. The gait can be considered in the context of that expected for the patient's age and physical shape. An early sign of parkinsonism is a decrease in arm swing. The elbows can remain partly flexed and frozen even if the arm swing is intact. More obvious signs of parkinsonism include a bent-over neck, stooped shoulders, and small shuffling steps.

Oropharyngeal involvement. Drooling may be a symptom of parkinsonism and is thought to arise from a general decrease in pharyngeal motor activity. Drooling may be less common for neuroleptic-induced cases than for other causes of parkinsonism because of the anticholinergic properties of neuroleptic drugs. Swallowing dysfunction may be from parkinsonism and may cause dysphagia. The gag reflex may be impaired, and the patient may be at risk for aspiration.

Other features. Other signs and symptoms of parkinsonism include small handwriting (micrographia), dysphagia, postural instability, inhibited blinking in response to glabellae tapping, and seborrhea. These features will not be discussed in any more detail because they do not represent the most common features of parkinsonian syndrome as it presents in the psychiatric population.

Neuroleptic versus other etiologies. Many of the physical signs of other primary neurologic diseases and psychiatric syndromes have already been covered. There are other indications that the symptoms are from other neurologic diseases. Recent exposure to a dopamine-blocking or dopamine-depleting drug is essential for diagnosing a parkinsonian syndrome as NIP. In terms of whether or not unique symptoms of NIP exist that distinguish NIP from other causes of parkinsonian syndrome, I agree with Kaufman (1981), who stated that "the similarity between parkinsonian syndrome and NIP is so great that the distinction [on clinical examination] is almost impossible" (p. 315). Neuroleptic exposure is necessary but not sufficient, and for NIP the symptoms cannot be due to another organic or neurologic cause. Although it is beyond the scope of this review to cover in detail the neurologic differential diagnosis, some indications that the parkinsonian syndrome is not from neuroleptic exposure include

- The presence of a family history of an inherited neurologic disorder.
- Rapidly progressive parkinsonism that cannot be explained by recent psychopharmacologic changes that would occur in NIP.
- The presence of other nonextrapyramidal neurologic signs (e.g., frontal release signs, cranial nerve abnormalities, or a positive Babinski sign).

Recommendations

Should NIP be included in DSM-IV? The advantages of adding NIP to DSM-IV include

1. Increase of general awareness that the signs of NIP often resemble the criteria for other diagnoses, such as the negative symptoms of schizophrenia. Current underrecognition of NIP can lead to an overdiagnosis of these disorders.
2. Decrease of morbidity from NIP by encouraging its diagnosis, especially in those settings that rely heavily on DSM-IV as the primary guide to differential diagnosis.
3. Reassurance of consumer and family advocacy groups that the American Psychiatric Association is concerned about the public health problems posed by iatrogenic complications of treatment.
4. Encouragement of future research in the epidemiology and differential diagnosis of NIP.
5. Greater compatibility with ICD-10, which includes NIP as a diagnostic entity.

The disadvantages of including NIP in DSM-IV include

1. Inclusion of a neurologic side effect may be considered beyond the scope of DSM-IV.
2. Inclusion of any side effect, even if justifiable in its own right, will open the "floodgates" to other side effects and psychopharmacologic treatment issues.
3. Inclusion of NIP in DSM-IV, while solving some false-positive diagnostic problems, will cause new ones. In particular, there may be inappropriate overdiagnosis of NIP at the expense of the Axis I disorders in the differential. Another concern is the possibility that clinicians would assume that neurologic

symptoms are from medication, and not consider other neurologic etiologies of parkinsonian syndrome.

4. It is not clear that inclusion of NIP in DSM-IV would definitely improve recognition of this side effect or encourage a more accurate differential diagnosis of other Axis I disorders.

Balancing the Advantages and Disadvantages

In my opinion, NIP should be included in DSM-IV. There is ample evidence that physicians are not well trained in neuroleptic effects (Weiner and Schumacher 1976) and that increased attention to NIP improves diagnostic rates (Dixon et al. 1989). The clinician's ability to make an informed and accurate differential between schizophrenia, catatonia, depression, and NIP is vital to the patient's welfare. Therefore, I think that the advantages to the profession are real, and the claims are not overstated. The disadvantages, for the most part, seem remediable. The inclusion of a side effect is justifiable because of its prominence in the differential diagnosis of so many other mental disorders. Unlike other medical "rule-outs" (e.g., hyperthyroidism presenting as a panic disorder), the diagnosis of NIP requires special diagnostic skills that cannot be delegated to general medical or neurologic colleagues. Because of this, it is my view that NIP (and other extrapyramidal symptoms) represents a special case where the inclusion of a medication side effect in DSM-IV can readily be justified. I am not aware of any other iatrogenic condition in psychiatry that presents with symptoms that are so close to primary psychiatric symptoms; thus, the special circumstances of NIP would not open up a so-called floodgate of requests for including other side effects.

False-Positive and False-Negative Problems

The most serious problem, it seems, is the danger that including NIP will cause a new set of diagnostic errors. This potential problem requires careful consideration in formulating the criteria set and is discussed in detail.

False-positive problem: psychiatric symptom versus NIP. There is a potential danger in setting criteria too wide because of the behavioral overlap with depression and negative symptoms. One could argue that the criteria need to be based strictly on physical findings.

False-positive problem: neurologic etiology versus NIP. In my judgment, this problem is outside the scope of DSM-IV.

False-negative problem. The false negatives seem to arise, based on this review, from excessive reliance on physical findings of tremor and rigidity and an underemphasis on akinesia as a hallmark symptom of NIP.

Choice of NIP symptoms. It seems clear that rigidity, akinesia, and tremor should form the essential physical findings that constitute NIP. The diagnosis of NIP should not be made unless one of these characteristic symptoms is present. The neurologic literature emphasizes parkinsonism as a syndrome and emphasizes the dichotomous nature of the individual symptoms. I recommend that DSM-IV take that approach and just use presence or absence of the sign as the cutoff point. A more difficult issue is whether to allow the use of historical information, subjective complaints, and behavioral symptoms as substitutes for clear-cut physical findings of NIP. The pros and cons of this problem have already been mentioned. Because behavioral or subjective symptoms of parkinsonism are very difficult to distinguish from primary psychiatric syndromes, behavioral symptoms should be downplayed to safeguard against making excessive NIP diagnoses and underdiagnosing other conditions (e.g., postpsychotic depression or psychotic withdrawal). The advantage of including rigidity and tremor as criteria is that both have clear physical signs. Akinesia is more challenging because it can be either a physical finding or subjective complaint. In my opinion, it may be better to use only objective criteria that can be validated by abnormal physical findings for the akinesia criteria (e.g., complaints of depression would not be used as a proxy for akinesia).

Can DSM-IV Help Address Underrecognition of NIP?

If DSM-IV includes NIP, the criteria and text will have to be written in a way that implicitly addresses the problem of underrecognition and misdiagnosis of NIP. The reasons behind the high rates of misdiagnoses need to be understood. There are many obstacles to the evaluation for NIP:

- There are not many systematic training programs on movement disorders available for clinicians working with the seriously ill.
- Clinicians, by force of habit, may minimize distress from NIP.
- NIP symptoms wax and wane. Physical findings may be absent during any given examination.
- Patients receiving neuroleptics are often very poor historians, limiting the amount of historical information that can be obtained.
- Behavioral symptoms from NIP and primary psychiatric symptoms overlap. For example, psychomotor retardation can be a symptom of depression or psychosis, as well as akinesia.

- Parkinsonian symptoms arise from many neurologic diseases; no physical finding is unique to neuroleptic-induced states.

The criteria set for NIP will need to address these issues, while maintaining a high enough threshold for the NIP diagnosis to avoid overdiagnosing NIP.

Threshold Issues

The major threshold problems that need to be addressed in establishing DSM-IV criteria for NIP include the following:

1. Do the physical findings for NIP need to be above some cutoff on a continuum (e.g., above a certain threshold on a parkinsonian rating scale) or dichotomous (e.g., the NIP symptom is judged to be either present or absent)?
2. Should the criteria rely only on definitive physical findings or should they allow subjective complaints and behavioral symptoms to be included? If so, should subjective or behavioral symptoms be weighted equally with physical findings?
3. Should the use of historical information be permitted if the patient does not have any current physical findings?

The threshold problems should be considered in light of the false-positive and false-negative issues in NIP diagnosis. In my opinion, criteria should be conservatively set to include only signs and symptoms that are considered essential for the neurologic diagnosis of parkinsonian syndrome and are less likely to cause false-positive NIP diagnoses.

Example of a Possible Criteria Set for NIP

One of the following signs or symptoms of neuroleptic-induced parkinsonism is necessary to make the diagnosis if a physical finding is present.

1. Parkinsonian Tremor. A coarse, rhythmic (2–6 HZ) resting tremor. The tremor may be unilateral or bilateral and can wax and wane. It may affect the limbs, head, mouth, or tongue.
2. Parkinsonian Rigidity. Parkinsonian rigidity has two major forms:

   - Cogwheel rigidity, a ratchet-like motion when joints are passively fled or ended. Cogwheeling may be unilateral and preferentially affect certain joints, usually wrists, elbows, shoulder, and knees.
   - Continuous muscular rigidity, lead-pipe rigidity. This kind of rigidity can be diagnosed by palpating the resting, relaxed muscle or by observing stiff movements during motoric activity (e.g., no arm swing when walking).

3. Akinesia represents a decrease in spontaneous facial expressions, gestures, or body movements from the patient's baseline state. Akinesia can be seen in one of three ways:

   - Motoric slowing, especially on initiating new tasks.
   - Decrease, from baseline, in spontaneity of speech and facial expressions.
   - Decrease, from baseline, in motivation, desire, and capacity for emotions and spontaneity.

Definition of Neuroleptic Exposure

To make an NIP diagnosis, there needs to be a recent history of exposure to an offending dopamine-blocking drug. The propensity of neuroleptics to cause parkinsonian syndrome may persist for some time after discontinuation of the drug. The persistence of these drugs means that NIP can last for months after discontinuation. The trade-off here is false-positive attribution of parkinsonian symptoms to neuroleptics. The longer time elapsed since last neuroleptic exposure, the more likely the symptoms are to be from other causes. Thus, the choice of time criteria cutoffs for neuroleptic exposure will have false-positive and false-negative diagnosis trade-offs. Too short an exclusionary time period between neuroleptic discontinuation and the NIP diagnosis can lead to unnecessary neurologic workups. Too long a waiting period might lead to primary neurologic disease being overlooked. The time period of 3 months after last dose is a compromise. It acknowledges the existence of persistent NIP, but keeps the waiting time reasonably short.

Extra time (12 months) is given for long-acting injectable forms of neuroleptics, which remain active for much longer time periods than oral forms. For example, the text would contain a statement such as:

> To distinguish NIP from other causes of parkinsonian syndrome, the neuroleptic exposure should have occurred within 3 months for oral agents and within 12 months of administration of a long-acting parenteral neuroleptic agent. If the parkinsonian symptoms were present before neuroleptic treatment, or the drug history is equivocal, then a diagnosis of neuroleptic-induced parkinsonism cannot be made.

Whatever the decision, there should be a clear statement in DSM-IV addressing this problem.

Summary of Recommendations

NIP is common, leads to substantial morbidity, and is not recognized by psychiatric clinicians. This lack of recognition arises, in part, from the overlap between NIP and primary psychiatric symptoms. Omission of NIP in DSM-III-R (American Psychiatric Association 1987) has not helped matters, and including NIP in DSM-IV may be a very effective way of addressing this public health problem. Including NIP in DSM-IV should increase the sophistication of the DSM-IV differential diagnosis decision tree for primary psychiatric disorders that have symptoms overlapping with NIP. Symptoms of NIP should become explicit exclusionary criteria for other primary psychiatric diagnoses found in DSM-IV. In particular, clinicians who need DSM-IV to diagnose schizophrenia will also need DSM-IV to diagnose or rule out neuroleptic-induced parkinsonism. The major problem in making this addition will be to construct criteria for NIP that do not cause the opposite problem: overdiagnosis of NIP relative to Axis I disorders. A proposed conservative solution is to limit the criteria to the three most common signs: rigidity, akinesia, and tremor. Behavioral toxicity would be omitted. In conclusion, the availability of specific and objective criteria for NIP within the body of the DSM-IV text will improve clinical recognition of this complication and improve DSM-IV's usefulness to our profession.

References

Adams RD, Victor M: Principles of Neurology. New York, McGraw-Hill, 1989

Alarcon R, Carney MWP: Severe depressive mood changes following slow-release intramuscular fluphenazine injection. BMJ 3:569–677, 1969

American Psychiatric Association: Diagnostic and Statistical Manual of Mental Disorders, 3rd Edition, Revised. Washington, DC, American Psychiatric Association, 1987

Anderson BC, Reber D, Volavka J, et al: Prolonged adverse effects from haloperidol in normals. N Engl J Med 205:643–644, 1981

Asbury A, McKhann G, McDonald I: Diseases of the Nervous System: Clinical Neurobiology. Philadelphia, PA, WB Saunders, 1986

Avorn J, Dreyer P, Connelly K, et al: Use of psychoactive medication and the quality of care in rest homes. N Engl J Med 320:227–232, 1989

Ayd FJ Jr: A survey of drug-induced extrapyramidal reactions. JAMA 175:1054–1060, 1961

Baldessarini RJ, Katz B, Cotton P: Dissimilar dosing with high-potency and low-potency neuroleptics. Am J Psychiatry 141:748–752, 1984

Baldessarini RJ, Cohen BM, Teicher MH: Significance of neuroleptic dose and plasma level in the pharmacological treatment of psychoses. Arch Gen Psychiatry 45:79–91, 1988

Blum A: Patients at risk of developing severe side effects from depot fluphenazine treatment. Am J Psychiatry 137:254–255, 1980

Boyce NJ, Vessey MP: Habitual physical inertia and other factors in relation to the risk of fracture of the proximal femur. Age Ageing 17:319–327, 1988

Bruun R: Subtle and underrecognized side effects of neuroleptic treatment in children with Tourette's Disorder. Am J Psychiatry 145:621–624, 1988

Carpenter WT, Heinrichs DW, Alphs LD: Treatment of negative symptoms. Schizophr Bull 11:440–452, 1985

Chadsey-Rusch J, Sprague RI: Maladaptive behaviors associated with neuroleptic drug maintenance. Am J Ment Retard 93:607–617, 1989

Davidson JRT, Raft D, Lewis BF, et al: Psychotropic drugs on general medical and surgical wards of a teaching hospital. Arch Gen Psychiatry 32:507–511, 1975

Davis JM: Comparative doses and costs of antipsychotic medication. Arch Gen Psychiatry 33:858–861, 1976

Derogatis LR, Feldstein M, Morrow G, et al: A survey of psychotropic drug prescriptions in an oncology population. Cancer 44:1919–1929, 1979

Dixon L, Weiden PJ, Frances A, et al: Management of neuroleptic-induced movement disorders: effects of physician training. Am J Psychiatry 146:104–105, 1989

Drake R, Cotton PC: Depression, hopelessness and suicide in chronic schizophrenia. Br J Psychiatry 148:554–559, 1986

Drake R, Ehrlich J: Suicide attempts associated with akathisia. Am J Psychiatry 142:499–501, 1985

Finn SE, Bailey JM, Schultz RT, et al: Subjective utility ratings of neuroleptics in treating schizophrenia. Psychol Med 20:843–848, 1990

Grimes JD: Drug-induced parkinsonism and tardive dyskinesia in nonpsychiatric patients. Can Med Assoc J 126:468, 1982

Grisso JA, Kelsey JL, Strom BL, et al: Risk factors for falls as a cause of hip fracture in women. N Engl J Med 324:1326–1331, 1991

Grohmann R, Hippius H, Muller B, et al: Assessment of adverse drug reactions in psychiatric hospitals. Eur J Clin Pharmacol 26:727–734, 1984

Hales RE, Yudofsky SC (eds): Textbook of Neuropsychiatry. Washington, DC, American Psychiatric Press, 1987

Hansen TE, Brown WL, Weigel RM, et al: Underrecognition of tardive dyskinesia and neuroleptic-induced parkinsonism. Gen Hosp Psychiatry 14:340–344, 1992

Henninger G, DiMascio A, Klerman GL: Personality factors in variability of response to phenothiazines. Am J Psychiatry 121:1091–1094, 1965

Hoffman BF: The diagnosis and treatment of neuroleptic-induced parkinsonism. Hosp Community Psychiatry 32:110–114, 1981

Hogan TD, Awad AC, Eastwood R: A self-report scale predictive of drug compliance in schizophrenics: reliability and discriminative validity. Psychol Med 13:177–183, 1983

Indo T, Ando K: Metoclopramide-induced parkinsonism, clinical characteristics of ten cases. Arch Neurol 39:494–496, 1982

Kaufman DM: Clinical Neurology for Psychiatrists. New York, Grune & Stratton, 1981

Kennedy PF, Hershon HI, McCuire RJ: Extrapyramidal disorders after prolonged phenothiazine therapy. Br J Psychiatry 118:509–518, 1971

Kreisman D, Blumenthal R, Borenstein M, et al: Family attitudes and patient social adjustment in a longitudinal study of outpatient schizophrenics receiving low-dose neuroleptics: the family's view. Psychiatry 51:3–13, 1988

Marder SR, Van Putten T, Mintz J, et al: Costs and benefits of two doses of fluphenazine. Arch Gen Psychiatry 41:1025–1029, 1984

Rifkin A, Quitkin F, Klein DF: Akinesia: a poorly recognized drug-induced extrapyramidal behavioral disorder. Arch Gen Psychiatry 32:672–674, 1975

Schooler N: Predictors of stabilization in schizophrenia. Paper presented at the American Psychiatric Association annual meeting, Montreal, Canada, May 1988

Seltzer A, Roncari I, Garfinkel P: Effect of patient education on medication compliance. Am J Psychiatry 25:638–645, 1980

Simpson G, Angus J: Drug-induced extrapyramidal disorders. Acta Psychiatr Scand 45 (suppl 212):11–19, 1970

Siris SC: Akinesia and post-psychotic depression: a difficult differential diagnosis. J Clin Psychiatry 48:240–243, 1987

Stephen PJ, Williamson J: Drug-induced parkinsonism in the elderly. Lancet 1:1082–1083, 1984

Van Putten T: Why do schizophrenic patients refuse to take their drugs? Arch Gen Psychiatry 31:67–72, 1974

Van Putten T, May PRA: "Akinetic depression" in schizophrenia. Arch Gen Psychiatry 35:1101–1107, 1978a

Van Putten T, May PRA: Subjective response as a predictor of outcome in pharmacotherapy. Arch Gen Psychiatry 35:477–480, 1978b

Van Putten T, Marder SR, Mintz JA: A controlled dose comparison of haloperidol in newly admitted schizophrenic patients. Arch Gen Psychiatry 47:754–758, 1990

Weiden PJ, Harrigan M: A clinical guide for diagnosing and managing patients with drug-induced dysphagia. Hosp Community Psychiatry 37:396–398, 1986

Weiden PJ, Mann JJ, Haas G, et al: Clinical nonrecognition of neuroleptic-induced movement disorders: a cautionary study. Am J Psychiatry 144:1148–1153, 1987

Weiden PJ, Dixon L, Frances A, et al: Neuroleptic noncompliance in schizophrenia, in Advances in Neuropsychiatry and Psychopharmacology, Vol 1, Schizophrenia Research. Edited by Tamminga C, Schulz C. New York, Raven, 1991

Weiner J, Schumacher GE: Psychotropic drug therapy knowledge of health care practitioners. Am J Hosp Pharm 33:237–241, 1976

Wettstein R: Legal aspects of neuroleptic-induced movement disorders, in Legal Medicine. Edited by Wecht C. New York, Praeger Scientific, 1985

Wolf B, Grohmann R, Schmidt LG, et al: Psychiatric admissions due to adverse drug reactions. Compr Psychiatry 30:534–545, 1989

World Health Organization: The ICD-10 Classification of Mental and Behavioural Disorders: Clinical Descriptions and Diagnostic Guidelines. Geneva, World Health Organization, 1992

Chapter 31

Neuroleptic Malignant Syndrome

Gerard Addonizio, M.D.
Virginia L. Susman, M.D.

Statement of the Issues

The purpose of this review is to address the issue of whether DSM-IV should include a diagnosis of neuroleptic malignant syndrome (NMS) and, if so, to develop criteria that will be broad enough to identify mild or partial syndromes while not including other disorders that require different treatments. We attempt to define criteria that are narrow and specific enough to facilitate research but also broad and sensitive enough to ensure that the diagnosis is not overlooked in the clinical setting.

Significance of the Issues

NMS has been estimated to develop in 0.07%–1.4% of patients on neuroleptics. The significant difference in frequency rates is probably due to a lack of consistency across studies in diagnostic criteria in neuroleptic prescribing practices, in study design, and in the demographics of the study populations. Mortality rates have also been variable, most often ranging between 10% and 20%. This variability can be attributed to the same factors that have produced the different rates of frequency of the syndrome. Additionally, there is consensus in the literature that much of the mortality and morbidity associated with NMS has been the result of a lack of recognition of the syndrome. Indirect evidence for this premise can be derived from the observed trend toward lower mortality rates, which occurred during the years in which awareness of NMS increased dramatically. (In a 1986 review of 320 cases in the literature and 10 of his own, Pearlman found two separate mortality rates: 22% for cases reported through 1980 and only 4% for the last 50 cases he reviewed.)

Clearly, NMS is a clinically significant phenomenon that carries a risk of substantial morbidity. The complications that have been associated with NMS include pneumonia, renal failure, cardiac arrest, seizures, sepsis, and pulmonary embolism. It is important to distinguish NMS from severe extrapyramidal symptoms (EPS) because the conventional treatments for severe EPS have been largely ineffective in NMS. Early recognition and intervention have the potential to alter the course significantly.

Methods

The following journals were reviewed since 1984: *American Journal of Psychiatry, Archives of General Psychiatry, Hospital and Community Psychiatry, Biological Psychiatry, Journal of Nervous and Mental Disease, Journal of Clinical Psychiatry, British Journal of Psychiatry, Journal of Clinical Psychopharmacology, Comprehensive Psychiatry, New England Journal of Medicine, Acta Psychiatrica Scandinavica, Psychiatric Annals, Canadian Journal of Psychiatry, Psychosomatics, Neurology,* and *Annals of Neurology.*

Index Medicus was reviewed back to 1974. A MEDLARS search was done back to 1976. Cases were reviewed based on "neuroleptic malignant syndrome" in the title of the article; cases of catatonia and cases of severe EPS were reviewed. Most of the literature on NMS involves case reports and analysis of collections of case reports. There are a few retrospective and prospective studies.

Results

Incidence

The incidence of NMS in inpatients on neuroleptics has been estimated to be between 0.07% and 1.4% (Delay et al. 1962; Friedman et al. 1988; Gelenberg et al. 1988; Keck et al. 1987, 1989a, 1989b; Pope et al. 1986). An incidence of 2.4% was found in a retrospective study (Addonizio et al. 1986) designed to maximize the discovery of NMS cases by restricting the population to acutely psychotic young men. Pope and colleagues (1986) found an incidence of 1.4% in a retrospective review of 500 inpatients treated with neuroleptics at McLean Hospital, a private psychiatric hospital in Belmont, Massachusetts. The same investigators then did a prospective study (Keck et al. 1987) and found a lower incidence of 0.9% among 679 patients. Two subsequent prospective studies found lower incidences of 0.2% among 495 patients (Friedman et al. 1988) and 0.07% among 1,470 patients (Gelenberg et al. 1988). A retrospective study at a state hospital found a 0.9% incidence among a population of 551 patients (Keck et al. 1989a). Discrepant results may be explained by different patient populations, lengths of stay, and medication practices.

Another major source of variance in incidence may be method of diagnosis. In performing their studies, the McLean group developed operational criteria for NMS (Pope et al. 1986):

> All three items are required for a definite diagnosis. 1) Hyperthermia: oral temperature of at least 37.5°C in the absence of another known etiology. 2) Severe extrapyramidal effects characterized by two or more of the following: lead-pipe muscle rigidity, pronounced cogwheeling, sialorrhea, oculogyric crisis, retrocollis, opisthotonus, trismus, dysphagia, choreiform movements, dyskinetic movements, festinating gait, and flexor-extensor posturing. 3) Autonomic dysfunction characterized by two or more of the following: hypertension (at least 20 mm rise in diastolic pressure above baseline), tachycardia (at least 30 beats/minute above baseline), tachypnea (at least 25 respirations/minute), prominent diaphoresis, and incontinence. In retrospective diagnosis, if one of these three items has not been specifically documented, a probable diagnosis is still permitted if the remaining two criteria are clearly met and the patient displays one of the following characteristic signs: clouded consciousness as evidenced by delirium, mutism, stupor, or coma; leukocytosis (more than 15,000 WBC [white blood cell count]/mm^3); and serum creatine kinase level greater than 300 U/ml. (p. 1233)

In 1989 these criteria were revised (Keck et al. 1989a) to require a temperature of at least 38.0°C and a serum creatine kinase level greater than 1,000 U/ml.

Age and Sex

Caroff's 1980 review of 60 NMS cases in the literature indicated that NMS was predominantly a disorder of young men since 80% of the cases he reviewed were age 40 years or younger, and male patients outnumbered females 2:1. Of the 320 cases reported by Pearlman (1986) in his literature review, the male-to-female ratio was approximately 1.4:1, and the median age was 36 (1–78 years). Men constituted 63% of the 115 case reports reviewed by Addonizio and colleagues (1987a) and 68% of the 47 cases for whom sex was identified in Levenson's (1985) review. Subsequent case reports have described NMS in patients in their 80s and 90s (Osser and Stewart 1988; Rosebush and Stewart 1989). Of the 115 NMS patients reviewed by Addonizio and colleagues (1987a), 16% were 60 years or older. Reasons for NMS occurring more often in young patients are unclear but may be related to the use of larger neuroleptic doses with more frequent dosage increments in young patients. Additionally, male patients may be seen as more threatening than females and thus may be given more medication.

Signs and Symptoms

The classic case of NMS includes hyperthermia, EPS, autonomic instability, and altered consciousness. There is little debate that essential features are EPS and elevated temperature. There is debate about how many features must be present to diagnose the syndrome and the degree of severity of each sign necessary to consider it present (Guze and Baxter 1985; Levenson 1985; Roth et al. 1986; Shalev and Munitz 1986). There is also debate about the possibility that mild or partial forms of NMS exist (Addonizio et al. 1986, 1987b; Adityanjee 1987; Adityanjee and Singh 1988). Some investigators feel that NMS is underdiagnosed because partial syndromes are disregarded (Keck et al. 1987; Pope et al. 1986); others claim that NMS is too readily diagnosed and that other causes of the patients' symptoms are overlooked (Levinson and Simpson 1986). The possible existence of mild or partial forms has complicated the study of NMS because this idea has led to an increasing number of case reports that diagnose NMS using various criteria that lack consensus by investigators.

Levenson (1985) proposed the following criteria for NMS. Major manifestations include fever, rigidity, and elevated creatine phosphokinase (CPK) level. Minor manifestations include tachycardia, abnormal blood pressure, tachypnea, altered consciousness, diaphoresis, and leukocytosis. The presence of all three major, or two major and four minor, manifestations indicates a high probability of the presence of NMS, if supported by clinical history. Designating elevated levels of CPK as a major manifestation and allowing NMS to be diagnosed in the absence of elevated temperature or rigidity has been disputed (Roth et al. 1986). Keck and colleagues (1989a) proposed operational criteria for NMS (see earlier section on incidence) that are more rigorous than Levenson's criteria.

Elevated Temperature

Addonizio and colleagues (1987a) reviewed 115 case reports of NMS and found 106 examples of increased temperature (≥ 38°C, 100.4°F); 15 patients had temperatures ≥ 41°C (105.8°F), and 46 patients had temperatures ≥ 40°C (104°F). In a separate review (Caroff and Mann 1988), 190 of 194 patients (98%) with reported temperatures had temperature elevations. Of the patients with elevated temperature, 39% had elevations greater than 40°C.

Extrapyramidal Symptoms

Rigidity was identified in 89% of 53 patients in Levenson's (1985) literature review, in 91% of the patients in the review by Addonizio and colleagues (1987a), in 92% of the 52 patients reviewed by Kurlan and colleagues (1984), and in 97% of the 187 patients for whom these data were presented in the review by Caroff and Mann

(1988). A prospective analysis of 24 episodes of NMS in 20 patients over a 6-year period identified rigidity in 96% of their patients (Rosebush and Stewart 1989). Other types of EPS have been reported, although as with any of these tallies of symptom occurrence, variable amounts of clinical detail in published cases limit the meaningfulness of these frequency rates. Tremor was seen in 45% of the case reports reviewed by Levenson (1985), 48% of the cases reviewed by Addonizio and colleagues (1987a), and 56% of the cases reviewed by Kurlan and colleagues (1984). In their prospective study, Rosebush and Stewart (1989) found tremor in 92% of their patients.

Dystonia was less frequently mentioned. Addonizio and colleagues (1987a) found a 29% occurrence of dystonia in their review of published cases; Kurlan and colleagues (1984) found 33%. Rosebush and Stewart (1989) found dystonic posturing or choreiform movements in 59% of their patients.

Autonomic Instability

In NMS, elevated or labile blood pressure, tachycardia, profuse diaphoresis, incontinence, and pallor are the most frequently reported autonomic signs. In published case reports, they are very poorly and infrequently documented, making frequency rates based on reviews of published case reports questionably accurate. In one review, Addonizio and colleagues (1987a) pointed out that only 63 of 115 patients (55%) had actual blood pressure values reported. They found that, of these 63 patients, 35 (55%) had systolic values greater than 140; 31 (49%) had diastolic values over 90; 27 (43%) had both systolic and diastolic elevations; and 24 (38%) were normotensive. In their literature review, Caroff and Mann (1988) found actual vital sign values available for only 153 of 256 cases. Of the 153 patients, 146 (95%) had evidence of autonomic problems. Kurlan and colleagues (1984) reported lability of blood pressure in 59% of patients. Levenson (1985) reported abnormal blood pressure in 79%. In the 24 episodes of NMS prospectively analyzed by Rosebush and Stewart (1989), 44% had high blood pressure and 33% had labile blood pressure.

Tachycardia is frequently reported in cases of NMS. Rosebush and Stewart (1989) reported tachycardia in all of their 24 patients. Kurlan and colleagues (1984) reported 79% had this sign. Addonizio and colleagues (1987a) had pulse rate data for 85 of the 115 case reports they reviewed, but in these patients found 97% had elevated pulse.

Diaphoresis was reported in all patients studied by Rosebush and Stewart (1989), in 60% of the case reports reviewed by Kurlan and colleagues (1984), in 67% of the case reports reviewed by Levenson (1985), and in 57% of the case reports reviewed by Addonizio and colleagues (1987a).

Incontinence was noted in 55% of the cases of Rosebush and Stewart (1989), in 15% of the cases reviewed by Kurlan and colleagues (1984), and in 21% of the cases reviewed by Levenson (1985).

Altered Consciousness

Caroff and Mann (1988) found information on mental status changes for 167 of the 256 case reports they reviewed. Of the 167, 164 (98%) had changes ranging from stupor with mutism to coma. Levenson (1985) found altered levels of consciousness in 84% of the cases he reviewed. Kurlan and colleagues (1984) found that 27% of the patients had coma, 27% experienced stupor, and 12% experienced "lethargy." In addition, 38% had mutism. In their prospective study, Rosebush and Stewart (1989) found that all 24 episodes of NMS exhibited delirium.

Laboratory Findings

Muscle CPK is frequently reported to be elevated in NMS. In some cases the rise is slight, but sometimes it is significantly elevated. In one review of 115 case reports (Addonizio et al. 1987a), CPK values were available for 67 patients, and CPK values were elevated in 65 patients (97%). In their prospective analysis of 24 episodes of NMS, Rosebush and Stewart (1989) found that CPK was elevated in all 21 cases for which serial values were available. CPK was greater than 10,000 IU/L in 7 cases and greater than 1,000 IU/L in 18 cases. Caroff and Mann (1988) reviewed 256 NMS cases in the literature from 1980 to 1987. Serum CPK was measured in 140 cases and was elevated in 133 cases (95%). Harsch (1987) reported on findings in nine cases of NMS. CPK values were elevated in all cases, with levels ranging from 432 IU/L to 189,000 IU/L. CPK levels were not related to the degree or duration of rigidity or to the degree of temperature elevation. In his review of 53 cases of NMS, Levenson (1985) found CPK data on 32 patients and found elevations in 31 (97%); most patients had levels in the range of 2,000–15,000 IU/L, but 6 had levels below 600 IU/L, and 2 had values that exceeded 100,000 IU/L.

Elevated WBC

Leukocytosis is a frequently mentioned finding in cases of NMS. In a review of 115 cases in the literature, Addonizio and colleagues (1987a) found WBC data for 59 patients, and 46 (78%) were elevated. The reported range was 10,000–40,000/mm^3, with 33 of the 46 (72%) having mild elevations between 10,000 and 20,000. Levenson (1985) found WBC elevations in 19 (79%) of 24 cases in which the data were reported. Levels ranged from minor elevations to 29,000/mm^3. In their prospective analysis of 24 episodes of NMS, Rosebush and Stewart (1989) found WBC elevations in 18 cases (75%). Caroff and Mann (1988) found leukocytosis in 105 (98%) of 107 case reports. In nine cases of NMS, Harsch (1987) reported leukocytosis in eight patients, with a range of 12,400 to 38,000 cu/mm.

Myoglobinuria

Testing for myoglobin is so infrequently mentioned in case reports that the data are relatively scanty. Nevertheless, as myoglobinuria is a harbinger of renal failure, it is a very important piece of clinical information to ascertain. Caroff and Mann (1988) found myoglobin levels reported in 30 out of 256 case reports and found myoglobinuria in 20 of the 30 (67%). Rosebush and Stewart (1989) prospectively found myoglobinuria in 16 (67%) of 24 cases. Levenson (1985) found myoglobinuria in only one of eight patients for whom such information was given. Shalev and colleagues (1989) reviewed 202 published case reports and found 19 patients in whom myoglobinemia was reported. Of the patients, nine (47%) died.

Neuroleptics

Reviews of series of case reports have led people to believe that high-potency neuroleptics are more likely to cause NMS. These conclusions may not be warranted and may only reflect prescribing practices. Keck and colleagues (1988) reviewed haloperidol use at their institution over 30 months. They found that of approximately 1,162 patients on neuroleptics, 21% received haloperidol, yet this medication was implicated in the development of NMS in 35% of the episodes. However, this increased rate may be the result of dosing practices. In reviewing 115 case reports, Addonizio and colleagues (1987a) found that the large majority of NMS cases occurred on high-potency neuroleptics. A prospective study by Deng and colleagues (1990) of 9,792 inpatients found 12 cases of NMS. They did not find that use of oral high-potency neuroleptics was a risk factor for NMS. On the other hand, depot fluphenazine decanoate, especially if used without an antiparkinsonian agent, was a risk factor. Keck and colleagues (1989b) did a case control study comparing 18 patients with NMS and 36 matched neuroleptic-treated control patients with no known history of NMS. They found that patients with NMS were on significantly higher doses of neuroleptics at greater rates of dosage increase, and they received a greater number of intramuscular injections. Gelenberg and colleagues (1988) found an annual NMS frequency of 0.07%, a statistic lower than other reports. They also found that their psychiatrists generally prescribed modest doses of neuroleptics. This led them to conclude that higher drug doses potentially predispose the patient to NMS. In a review of 120 published case reports, Shalev and Munitz (1986) found that doses were increased in 91% of cases to an equivalent of 40–6,000 mg/day of chlorpromazine. They concluded that a positive loading rate was a major contributing factor to the development of NMS.

Kurlan and colleagues (1984) reviewed 52 cases of NMS and found that 5 developed NMS within 24 hours of their first lifetime exposure to neuroleptics. Also, the onset of NMS occurred within 2 weeks of the initiation of neuroleptic treatment or an increase in the dosage in 47 patients (90%). In reviewing 115 case reports, Addonizio and colleagues (1987a) reported that 66% of 86 patients, for whom information existed, experienced NMS within the first 2 weeks of neuroleptic treatment. Shalev and Munitz (1986) found that in reviewing 65 case reports, 59 cases (91%) had NMS begin within 10 days of starting treatment with a new neuroleptic, and the mean time between starting neuroleptic and developing NMS was 4.8 days. Caroff and Mann (1988) reviewed 256 cases and found sufficient data on 136 patients. Of these patients, 16% developed NMS within 24 hours of starting neuroleptics, 30% within 48 hours, 66% within 1 week, and 96% within 30 days. Rosebush and Stewart (1989) found adequate dosing data on 22 of 24 prospectively followed patients and determined that 11 either restarted treatment with neuroleptics or received them for the first time the week before the onset of NMS.

In their review, Caroff and Mann (1988) reported a mean duration from termination of neuroleptic treatment to resolution of NMS of 9.6 ± 9.1 days, with 23% recovered within 48 hours, 63% within 1 week, 82% within 2 weeks, and 97% within 1 month. Shalev and Munitz (1986) found a range of 4–40 days (mean 14.73 ± 9.8 days for oral neuroleptics and 17.5 ± 10 days for long-acting preparations). Addonizio and colleagues (1987a) found a mean duration of 13 days for oral and 26 days for depot neuroleptics.

Mortality

Literature reviews of case reports of NMS between 1977 and 1989 document declining fatality rates. Shalev and colleagues (1989) found an overall fatality rate of 18.8% from 1959 through 1987, with 27.7% before 1980, 22.6% between 1980 and 1983, and 11.6% after 1984. Pearlman's (1986) extensive literature review found a mortality rate of 22% for cases reported through 1980 and 4% among the last 50 cases. Addonizio and colleagues (1987a) found a fatality rate of 10% in their review. In their review of 256 NMS case reports, Caroff and Mann (1988) found that 25 cases (10%) resulted in death. The above fatality rates are based on reviews of published case reports and therefore may grossly distort the true incidence of mortality in NMS. In six studies of NMS (Friedman et al. 1988; Gelenberg et al. 1988, 1989; Keck et al. 1987, 1989a; Pope et al. 1986), four of which were prospective, 24 cases of NMS were found, with 2 cases resulting in death. This represents a mortality rate of 8.3%.

Medical Complications

In their review of 115 case reports, Addonizio and colleagues (1987a) found that 15 patients developed pneumonia, 9 developed renal failure (usually due to rhabdomyolysis and myoglobinuria), 7 developed cardiac arrest, 4 developed seizures, 3 developed sepsis, 3 developed pulmonary embolism, and 2 developed pulmonary edema. Rosebush and Stewart (1989) reported finding prerenal azotemia in 16 of 24 cases (67%) prospectively studied and renal failure in 7 (29%). Shalev and Munitz (1986) found 12% of their 120 cases demonstrated pulmonary insufficiency. Various other complications may be seen, such as disseminated intravascular coagulation, myocardial infarction, and myoneuropathies in small numbers of cases.

Discussion

NMS is a potentially fatal reaction to neuroleptic medication. As neuroleptics have widespread use in psychiatry, knowledge of NMS is critical to the clinician. Underrecognition of NMS in the past led to significant morbidity and mortality. It appears from reported cases that mortality has decreased as the psychiatric community has become more aware of this disorder. In an effort to disseminate widely an understanding of this potentially fatal reaction, we feel it would be important to include NMS in DSM-IV.

There is little controversy over the core signs and symptoms, which include elevated temperature, rigidity, autonomic instability, and altered consciousness. On the other hand, there has been debate about whether each of the features must be present, about the sequence in which the features develop, and about the degree of symptom severity necessary to make the diagnosis (Guze and Baxter 1985; Levenson 1985; Roth et al. 1986; Shalev and Munitz 1986). Disagreement also continues about the likelihood of NMS being a spectrum disorder with milder or self-limited variants (Addonizio et al. 1986, 1987b; Adityanjee 1987; Adityanjee and Singh 1988). In attempting to describe and study NMS further, several investigators have proposed their own sets of criteria for establishing the diagnosis. However, there has not been any rigorous test of the proposed criteria nor has there been any study comparing or contrasting the various proposals.

In 1985, Levenson outlined a schema for diagnosing NMS that involved so-called major and minor manifestations and a formula that required varying numbers of symptoms from each category. He proposed fever, rigidity, and elevated CPK as major manifestations and several autonomic signs and altered consciousness as minor manifestations. According to Roth and colleagues (1986), two weaknesses of Levenson's schema were designating elevated CPK as a major manifestation and the formula that permitted diagnosing NMS in the absence of either elevated temperature or rigidity.

Keck and colleagues (1989a) refined and made more stringent their earlier proposed criteria. The revised criteria included: 1) temperature elevation—38°C, 2) at least two of a number of severe extrapyramidal side effects, and 3) at least two clinically significant disturbances of autonomic function. They added the corollary that NMS could be retrospectively diagnosed if certain additional signs and symptoms were present in those cases that documented only two of the three core criteria.

Since there has been no study of the validity of any diagnostic criteria, it is important to consider the conflicting needs of research and clinical practice in the establishment of such criteria. Research would be advanced by clear, rigorous criteria that minimize the chance of including cases that are not truly NMS. Good clinical care dictates that criteria be more broad and general so that no case is missed even at the expense of applying the diagnosis erroneously. In other words, research criteria should be highly specific, whereas clinical criteria should be highly sensitive. Ideal criteria would, of course, be as specific and sensitive as possible. The criteria proposed herein draw from the proposals of others and attempt to be as specific and sensitive as possible, but are skewed toward the clinical goal of not overlooking any potential case of NMS. The evidence for NMS being a spectrum disorder adds to the need for making the criteria particularly sensitive because milder or indolent cases of NMS can progress to severe NMS and, to date, there is no way to predict the course or outcome of any given case of NMS. On the other hand, it is also imperative that other medical conditions not be misdiagnosed as NMS because these disorders can also be life threatening, and they require significantly different treatment strategies.

In summary, the criteria proposed include elevated temperature and rigidity, unlike the less stringent criteria of Levenson (1985), which require only one of those. However, the autonomic signs and other EPS outlined by Keck and colleagues (1989a) are not required. Careful ruling out of other potential medical disorders is another central feature of these criteria. It is intended that these criteria will direct clinicians toward recognizing NMS as early and as frequently as it occurs without overlooking other serious disorders.

Recommendations

Although there is relative unanimity in the literature that NMS is a valid clinical entity, disagreement exists about essential features and about symptom severity. As NMS is potentially fatal, we feel that the threshold for diagnosis should be relatively low to avoid false negatives. On the other hand, having too low a threshold could lead to morbidity by prematurely terminating neuroleptic use. Based on our review of the literature, we feel the proposed criteria (Table 31–1) will capture cases of NMS while limiting false negatives.

Our approach to the diagnosis of NMS is much more consistent with NMS as

Table 31–1. Proposed DSM-IV diagnostic criteria for Neuroleptic Malignant Syndrome

A. The development of severe muscle rigidity and elevated temperature are associated with the use of neuroleptic medication.

B. Two of the following:
   (1) diaphoresis
   (2) dysphagia
   (3) tremor
   (4) incontinence
   (5) changes in level of consciousness ranging from confusion to coma
   (6) mutism
   (7) tachycardia
   (8) elevated or labile blood pressure
   (9) leukocytosis
   (10) laboratory evidence of muscle injury (e.g., elevated CPK)

C. The symptoms in A and B are not due to neurologic or other general medical conditions (e.g., viral encephalitis).

D. The symptoms in A and B are not better accounted for by a mental disorder (e.g., mood disorder with catatonic features or phencyclidine psychotic disorder).

Note. CPK = creatine phosphokinase.

a spectrum disorder rather than an acute fulminant reaction. Although some cases occur in an explosive way, many do not. Even though this view of NMS may allow for occasional false positives, we feel that it is clinically the safer route to follow. It would be important for future research to examine prospectively the validity of proposed criteria.

References

Addonizio G, Susman VL, Roth SD: Symptoms of neuroleptic malignant syndrome in 82 consecutive inpatients. Am J Psychiatry 143:1587–1590, 1986

Addonizio G, Susman VL, Roth SD: Neuroleptic malignant syndrome: review and analysis of 115 cases. Biol Psychiatry 22:1004–1020, 1987a

Addonizio G, Susman VL, Roth SD: Reply to diagnosing and defining neuroleptic malignant syndrome. Am J Psychiatry 144:1370–1371, 1987b

Adityanjee: Diagnosing and defining neuroleptic malignant syndrome. Am J Psychiatry 144:1370–1371, 1987

Adityanjee, Singh S: Spectrum concept of neuroleptic malignant syndrome. Br J Psychiatry 153:107–111, 1988

Caroff SN: The neuroleptic malignant syndrome. J Clin Psychiatry 41:79–83, 1980

Caroff SN, Mann SC: Neuroleptic malignant syndrome. Psychopharmacol Bull 24:25–29, 1988

Delay J, Pichot P, Lemperiere T, et al: L'emploi des butyrophenones en psychiatrie etude statistique et psychometrique. Symposium Internazionale Sull'Haloperidole E Triperidol, Milano, November 18, 1962, pp 305–319

Deng MZ, Chen GQ, Phillips MR: Neuroleptic malignant syndrome in 12 of 9,792 Chinese inpatients exposed to neuroleptics: a prospective study. Am J Psychiatry 147:1149–1155, 1990

Friedman JH, Davis R, Wagner RL: Neuroleptic malignant syndrome: the results of a 6-month prospective study of incidence in a state psychiatric hospital. Clin Neuropharmacol 11:373–377, 1988

Gelenberg AJ, Bellinghausen B, Wojcik JD, et al: A prospective survey of neuroleptic malignant syndrome in a short-term psychiatric hospital. Am J Psychiatry 145:517–518, 1988

Gelenberg AJ, Bellinghausen B, Wojcik JD, et al: Patients with neuroleptic malignant syndrome histories: what happens when they are rehospitalized? J Clin Psychiatry 50:178–180, 1989

Guze BH, Baxter LR Jr: Neuroleptic malignant syndrome. N Engl J Med 313:1292–1293, 1985

Harsch HH: Neuroleptic malignant syndrome: physiological and laboratory findings in a series of nine cases. J Clin Psychiatry 48:328–333, 1987

Keck PE Jr, Pope HG Jr, McElroy SL: Frequency and presentation of neuroleptic malignant syndrome: a prospective study. Am J Psychiatry 144:1344–1346, 1987

Keck PE Jr, Pope HG Jr, McElroy SL: Haloperidol and neuroleptic malignant syndrome. Am J Psychiatry 145:654, 1988

Keck PE Jr, Sebastianelli J, Pope HG Jr, et al: Frequency and presentation of neuroleptic malignant syndrome in a state psychiatric hospital. J Clin Psychiatry 50:352–355, 1989a

Keck PE Jr, Pope HG Jr, Cohen BM, et al: Risk factors for neuroleptic malignant syndrome: a case-control study. Arch Gen Psychiatry 46:914–918, 1989b

Kurlan R, Hamill R, Shoulson I: Neuroleptic malignant syndrome. Clin Neuropharmacol 7:109–120, 1984

Levenson JL: Neuroleptic malignant syndrome. Am J Psychiatry 142:1137–1145, 1985

Levinson DF, Simpson GM: Neuroleptic-induced extrapyramidal symptoms with fever. Arch Gen Psychiatry 43:839–848, 1986

Osser DN, Stewart TD: Agitation associated with dementia: neuroleptic malignant syndrome and fatal outcome in an 84-year old man. J Clin Psychopharmacol 8:443–444, 1988

Pearlman CA: Neuroleptic malignant syndrome: a review of the literature. J Clin Psychopharmacol 6:257–273, 1986

Pope HG Jr, Keck PE Jr, McElroy SL: Frequency and presentation of neuroleptic malignant syndrome in a large psychiatric hospital. Am J Psychiatry 143:1227–1232, 1986

Rosebush P, Stewart T: A prospective analysis of 24 episodes of neuroleptic malignant syndrome. Am J Psychiatry 146:717–725, 1989

Roth SD, Addonizio G, Susman VL: Diagnosing and treating neuroleptic malignant syndrome. Am J Psychiatry 143:673, 1986

Shalev A, Munitz H: The neuroleptic malignant syndrome: agent and host interaction. Acta Psychiatr Scand 73:337–347, 1986

Shalev A, Hermesh H, Munitz H: Mortality from neuroleptic malignant syndrome. J Clin Psychiatry 50:18–25, 1989

Chapter 32

Neuroleptic-Induced Acute Dystonia

Daniel E. Casey, M.D.

Statement of the Issues

Adding treatment-induced syndromes, such as neuroleptic-induced acute dystonia, to DSM-IV has been suggested. In any discussion of the issues for and against this proposal, it is necessary to review thoroughly what is known about neuroleptic-induced acute dystonia to weigh adequately the merits of inclusion or exclusion. If neuroleptic-induced acute dystonia is included, it will first be essential to establish an accepted definition of the syndrome. Additionally, it will be necessary to create criteria that are broad enough to encompass the wide array of symptoms associated with neuroleptic-induced dystonia, yet are narrow enough to include only bona fide acute dystonic reactions and exclude the ambiguous or irrelevant symptoms.

Significance of the Issues

Neuroleptic-induced acute dystonic reactions most commonly occur during the early phases of drug treatment (Ayd 1961; Donlon et al. 1980; Keepers et al. 1983; Singh et al. 1990). Their presentations can be sufficiently complex to lead occasionally to misdiagnoses of hysteria, malingering, catatonia, or seizures (Casey 1992). The most common complications of acute dystonic reactions are fear instilled in the patients about what is happening to them and the consequent issues of treatment noncompliance. Rarely, acute dystonic reactions can be dangerous and life threatening (Flaherty and Lahmeyer 1978; H. Freed 1958; Koek and Pi 1989; Mann

This work was supported in part by funds from the Veterans Administration Research Program and by NIMH Grant 36657.

et al. 1979; Waugh and Metts 1960). Additionally, it is highly valuable to identify those patients who have experienced neuroleptic-induced acute dystonic reactions so that they will be recognized as patients who are at high risk for another dystonic reaction with subsequent neuroleptic treatment. For those at high risk, alternate treatment strategies are available to reduce the likelihood that they will develop another dystonic reaction with future neuroleptic treatment (Arana et al. 1988; Casey 1992; Keepers and Casey 1991; Keepers et al. 1983; Koek and Pi 1989; Sramek et al. 1986; Winslow et al. 1986).

Methods

The material generated for this literature review was primarily obtained through a MEDLARS search from 1952 to mid-1991. A computer-based search was conducted for the years 1966–1991. Key terms for the computer-based search were *dystonia, chemically induced, neuroleptics, psychotropic drugs, drug-induced dyskinesias,* and *movement disorders.* Prior to the computer-based search, a manual review of *Index Medicus* was done using the key terms of *antipsychotic drugs, dyskinesia, dystonia, motor skills, movement, movement disorders, neuroleptics, parasympatholytics, psychotropic, schizophrenia therapy,* and *side effects.* A secondary source of information was a search of the references in the literature reviewed to identify articles that may have been missed through the MEDLARS and *Index Medicus* searches.

Very few studies have solely investigated neuroleptic drug-induced dystonia. Even fewer have studied this syndrome in well-controlled, blind protocols. Thus the data must often be extracted from reports that evaluated the extrapyramidal syndromes as a group or investigated neuroleptic drugs in treating psychoses. Not all references are included because of the large repetition of similar findings, particularly in case reports. However, reviews, well-controlled studies, and early reports of new findings are included.

Results

Clinical Presentation

Neuroleptic-induced acute dystonia can present in a wide variety of ways. The breadth of the syndrome encompasses both subjective complaints and objective signs, which range from the straightforward classic presentations to symptoms that may appear to be bizarre (Casey 1992; Owens 1990). The involuntary muscular contractions of acute dystonia produce briefly sustained or fixed abnormal posture(s) in one or more body areas that are associated with functional impairment.

Signs include retrocollis, torticollis, trismus, grimacing or jaw gaping, oculogyric crises, laryngeal-pharyngeal constriction, dysphagia, dysphonia, tongue protrusion or tongue swelling, dysarthria, and opisthotonos or bizarre positions of the limbs and trunk. When the throat and pharynx are involved, it is difficult to observe the abnormal muscular contractions, so the diagnosis must rely on both the patient's complaints, such as difficulty swallowing, tightening in the throat, or a feeling of being strangled, and clearly observed difficulty swallowing or breathing. Protrusion, incoordination, or swelling of the tongue may lead to dysarthria or an increase in the appearance of tongue thickness. If the limbs and trunk are affected by dystonia, the patient may walk with a bizarre gait or sit and lie in peculiar postures. When these symptoms appear without prior warning, it can have a negative effect on the mental status because patients often believe that something external is controlling their body. In addition to sometimes producing pain or cramps in the affected muscles, dystonia may make some patients quite fearful or anxious and lead to additional feelings of paranoia and to delusional ideas.

One of the hallmarks of acute dystonia is that symptoms in the early phases of the reaction may come and go. If this is not accurately recognized, it may lead to a delay in the appropriate diagnosis and treatment. Another feature of the syndrome is that patients can often temporarily overcome the symptoms and assume a normal posture and gait. Yet within a few seconds to a few minutes, the symptoms may return again when patients can no longer voluntarily interrupt the muscular contractions. The combination of a waxing and waning course coupled with the apparent volitional control may lead some to conclude that the patient is manipulating to obtain some secondary gain. However, this is rarely the case. Patients should be given the benefit of the doubt, and caregivers should have a high index of suspicion for drug-induced acute dystonia during the first 7 days of neuroleptic treatment (Ayd 1961; Keepers et al. 1983; Singh et al. 1990), following a large neuroleptic dose increase, after receiving a depot neuroleptic injection (Johnson 1973), or after anticholinergic or antihistaminic drugs have been abruptly discontinued (Arana et al. 1988).

The range of symptom severity also varies widely. Mild symptoms may be present only as an extended thumb and first finger coupled with flexed second, third, and fourth fingers, which can best be seen when the patient walks. Other mild symptoms could include a slight slurring or thickening of speech or be limited to subjective complaints of throat tightening or difficulty swallowing. In contrast, severe symptoms may completely impair a patient so that the patient is not able to get out of bed, walk, swallow, or speak. Although these latter, most severe syndromes are rare, they do occur frequently enough and are of such potential danger that it is important for them to be recognized early and treated immediately with appropriate drug interventions.

Differential Diagnosis

The variety of clinical presentations of neuroleptic-induced acute dystonia requires a knowledge of differential diagnosis. First, for the diagnosis of acute neuroleptic drug-induced dystonia to be valid, a patient must have been exposed to neuroleptic drugs within the past several days. Sometimes patients are not aware of receiving neuroleptic drugs, cannot accurately report which drugs they have received, or intentionally mislead the evaluator. Another clinical situation to consider includes the patient who may have received a depot neuroleptic injection within the past week but does not know the name of the medicine or is too psychotic to give a useful history. Or a patient may have ingested someone else's medicine, either at home, in an institution, or on the street, and cannot report what drug he or she took. Children may also unwittingly take some medicine they find in the home and subsequently develop acute dystonic reactions. Occasionally children present for emergency care with acute dystonic reactions when they have received antiemetic syrup, pills, or suppositories because of other illnesses, which subsequently greatly complicates the differential diagnosis (Anderson 1959; Gupta and Lovejoy 1967).

Other psychiatric syndromes must be differentiated from neuroleptic-induced acute dystonia, such as hysteria or malingering (Angus and Simpson 1970). Catatonia needs to be distinguished from the immobilized posture of drug-induced acute dystonia, which can be a difficult discrimination in the first few treatment days of a severely ill psychotic patient who has shown some symptoms of catatonia prior to drug therapy.

Sustained dystonic postures can be one of several extrapyramidal symptoms associated with fever in the neuroleptic malignant syndrome. However, acute drug-induced dystonia does not have fever or the generalized increased muscular tone seen with the neuroleptic malignant syndrome. Tardive dystonia is a syndrome complex of persisting dystonic symptoms that occur in association with tardive dyskinesia. It is differentiated from acute dystonia by its onset late in the course of neuroleptic treatment and persistence for weeks, months, or years (Burke and Kang 1988; Burke et al. 1982).

Other drugs besides those typically used to treat schizophrenia can cause acute dystonia. Any compound with dopamine receptor-blocking properties has the potential to produce acute dystonia, especially in the high-risk patient. Antiemetic compounds, which are most commonly dopamine receptor antagonists, such as prochlorperazine (Compazine), promethazine (Phenergan), trimethobenzamide (Tigan), and thiethylperazine (Torecan), are well recognized for their dystonia-producing capacity (Anderson 1959; Christian and Paulson 1958; DeGrandi and Simon 1987; Khanderia 1985; Preswick and McClatchie 1965; Swaiman 1960; Waugh and Metts 1960). This is particularly common in children, adolescents, and young adults. Metoclopramide (Reglan), another dopamine antagonist that is used for diabetic gastroparesis, esophageal reflux, and as an antiemetic, can cause acute dystonia (Kris et al. 1983; Pollera et al. 1984) as well as other extrapyramidal syndromes of akathisia, drug-induced parkinsonism, and tardive dyskinesia, when used on a chronic basis (Casey 1983). Amoxapine (Asendin) is also a dopamine receptor antagonist that is marketed as an antidepressant, but it causes acute dystonia, other extrapyramidal syndromes, and tardive dyskinesias like all other typical neuroleptics (Hunt-Fugate et al. 1984; Lapierre and Anderson 1983; Steele 1982). Droperidol (Inapsine), also a dopamine receptor antagonist, is used as a pre-anesthetic antianxiety agent and precipitates acute dystonic reactions (Taylor 1969). Alcohol ingestion may trigger dystonia in patients who are receiving neuroleptics but who have not previously experienced dystonic episodes (E. Freed 1981).

Anticonvulsant drugs at normal or toxic doses, such as phenytoin (Dilantin) and carbamazepine (Tegretol) can produce dystonic postures that are often a part of a much broader clinical picture of neurological dysfunction (Chadwick et al. 1976; Jacome 1979; Lazaro 1982). Rarely, diazepam has been associated with inducing acute dystonia (Hooker and Danzl 1988), but this has been questioned. Chronic antihistaminic drug use has also been rarely associated with a persisting dystonic syndrome that resembles tardive dyskinesia (Powers 1982; Thatch et al. 1975).

Other less common idiopathic neurological syndromes have dystonia as a component symptom. These include focal or regional dystonias such as torticollis, oromandibular dystonia, blepharospasm, laryngeal or pharyngeal dystonias, and severe writer's cramp (Calne and Lang 1988; Fahn et al. 1987). These are usually distinguishable by the absence of neuroleptic treatment as well as the slow onset of symptoms spanning weeks to months. Endocrinological disorders, such as hyperthyroidism, hypoparathyroidism, and hypocalcemia, have been infrequently associated with dystonic symptoms (Baldessarini 1985; Davis 1985; Weiner 1979). Additionally, other central nervous system disorders, such as temporal lobe seizures, may produce bizarre behavior as well as peculiar postures. Infections, both viral and bacterial, as well as trauma or space-occupying lesions, are also capable of producing dystonic symptoms (Calne and Lang 1988; Owens 1990). Tetanus, although rare, must also be distinguished from a drug-induced "pseudo-tetanus" syndrome (Melvin 1962).

Rating Scales

Unlike many of the other neuroleptic drug-induced extrapyramidal syndromes, there is no uniformly accepted or widely used rating scale for assessing drug-induced dystonia. It does appear as an isolated item on several rating scales that are primarily dedicated to assessing neuroleptic drug-induced parkinsonism. Such scales include the Neurological Rating Scale (Simpson and Angus 1970), the Extrapyramidal Syndrome Rating Scale (Chouinard et al. 1980), and the Saint Hans Dyskinesia Rating Scale (Gerlach 1979) as well as a few others. However, none are widely recognized for their application to neuroleptic-induced acute dystonia.

Epidemiology

The incidence (number of new cases within a specific time) and prevalence (number of existing cases at a given time) are nearly identical because acute dystonia occurs at only a few time points during neuroleptic therapy (see later). The changing patterns of neuroleptic use over the past three and a half decades since neuroleptics were introduced have profoundly affected the frequency of acute dystonia as well as other acute extrapyramidal syndromes. In the early 1960s, a survey of all extrapyramidal syndromes noted a 2.3% rate of acute dystonia (Ayd 1961). As a historical note, it is worthwhile to observe that what is now referred to as acute dystonia was often referred to as dyskinesia or acute dyskinesia in the 1950s and early 1960s since tardive dyskinesia was not labeled as such until 1964 (Faurbye et al. 1964). In the 1960s and 1970s, acute dystonia usually occurred in 10% or fewer of patients receiving neuroleptics (National Institute of Mental Health 1964; Swett 1975). However, the steady increase in the use of low-milligram, high-potency neuroleptics, such as haloperidol, and the use of higher and higher neuroleptic drug dosages led to much higher rates of acute dystonia. Surveys in 1980 observed prevalence rates of acute dystonia ranging from 39% (Keepers et al. 1983) to 70% in patients receiving high neuroleptic doses (Donlon et al. 1980). A later study of high-potency neuroleptics in high-risk patients observed an acute dystonia rate of 90% (Boyer et al. 1987).

Risk Factors

Three separate categories of risk factors determine the vulnerability to acute dystonia: patient characteristics, drug factors, and temporal aspects.

Patient characteristics. Age is the most important risk factor in neuroleptic-induced dystonia. Children and young adults are highly vulnerable to acute dystonia, whereas there is a near absence of this syndrome in the elderly (Addonizio and Alexopoulos 1988; Ayd 1961; Keepers et al. 1983; Singh et al. 1990; Swett 1975). Although this may be explained by the observation that the elderly get lower neuroleptic doses than young adults, it is surely not the sole explanation, since the elderly tend to get another extrapyramidal syndrome, neuroleptic drug-induced parkinsonism, very frequently at the low neuroleptic doses they customarily receive (Keepers et al. 1983; Richardson and Craig 1982). Gender also plays an important role; males are nearly twice as susceptible to acute dystonia (Ayd 1961; Keepers et al. 1983; Swett 1975). This contrasts with the apparent increased risk in females for tardive dyskinesia (Casey 1987). A past history of dystonic reactions with neuroleptics is a potent predictor of future vulnerability. In a study evaluating the ability to predict dystonia with future treatments when the vulnerability to dystonia from prior neuroleptic treatment was known, it was possible to predict with approximately 75% accuracy which patients would or would not develop neuroleptic-induced acute dystonia on subsequent treatment with the same drug dose and type (Keepers and Casey 1986, 1991). Race has also been suggested as a risk factor, especially for Asians (Binder and Levy 1981), but this has not been consistently observed (Keepers and Casey 1989) or systematically studied. Stimulant abuse, such as of cocaine or amphetamines, may also increase the vulnerability to neuroleptic drug-induced dystonia (Kumor et al. 1986). Finally, there are conflicting data about whether patients with affective disorders are more likely than schizophrenic patients to develop neuroleptic drug-induced dystonia (Nasrallah et al. 1988; Remington et al. 1990).

Drug factors. Neuroleptic drug characteristics strongly influence acute dystonia rates. The association with dosage is complicated. There is an inverted U-shaped curve function between the prevalence of dystonia and neuroleptic dose (Keepers et al. 1983). Most dystonia occurs with moderate to high doses of neuroleptics. Subsequently, there is a decrease in the incidence of dystonia when megadoses (approximately over 2,000 mg/day of chlorpromazine equivalence) are used. Thus, the very low doses and the very high doses of neuroleptics produce the least dystonia (Keepers and Casey 1986; Keepers et al. 1983; Tesar et al. 1985).

Drug potency is predictably correlated with acute dystonia. The low-milligram, high-potency compounds (e.g., haloperidol, fluphenazine) produce higher rates of dystonia, whereas the high-milligram, low-potency compounds (e.g., thioridazine, chlorpromazine) produce much lower rates (Keepers et al. 1983; Snyder et al. 1974). The relative balance of dopamine receptor blocking and anticholinergic properties intrinsic to each neuroleptic drug also correlates with both milligram potency and capacity to produce acute dystonia.

Clozapine, a compound with low acute extrapyramidal syndrome rates and no documented cases of clozapine-induced acute dystonia (Casey 1989a), has been explained on the basis of several proposals. The low dopamine-to-acetylcholine antagonism ratio is commonly offered as an explanation for the exceptionally low rate of acute extrapyramidal syndromes and dystonia. Alternatively, the ratio between dopamine and serotonin receptor blockade has been proposed as an explanation for the low extrapyramidal syndrome liability (Casey 1989b; Meltzer et al. 1989). Yet other explanations include specific ratios between blocking receptors of dopamine subtypes, such as the D_1 and D_2 receptor (Casey 1989a, 1989b, 1991), and specific antagonism of the D_4 receptor (VanTol et al. 1991).

Temporal aspects. Time since the last neuroleptic exposure is an essential aspect in understanding drug-induced acute dystonia. The vast majority (approximating 95%) of all dystonia cases occur within the first 7 days of starting or rapidly increasing neuroleptic dose (Ayd 1961; Donlon et al. 1980; Garver et al. 1976; Keepers et al. 1983; Prien et al. 1969; Singh et al. 1990). Acute dystonic reactions may also develop in the third to seventh day after receiving each depot neuroleptic injection. Only rarely is neuroleptic-induced acute dystonia encountered as a recurring problem with stable neuroleptic treatment (Gardos 1981). If such dystonic symptoms do develop, this should lead one to a high index of suspicion and search for alternate explanations. Perhaps the patient has taken a larger neuroleptic dose than prescribed, has combined his or her neuroleptic with other neuroleptics or alcohol, or has suddenly discontinued anticholinergic or antihistaminic medicines. Perhaps the patient is showing the first signs of tardive dystonia or has a separate underlying etiology of dystonia (see Differential Diagnosis earlier).

Treatment

Treatment approaches to acute dystonia are twofold. Either one waits for symptoms to develop and then initiates appropriate treatment, or prophylaxis with anticholinergic or antihistaminic medicines may be used to prevent the onset of symptoms. Both strategies have advantages and disadvantages.

Treating neuroleptic-induced acute dystonia is straightforward and highly successful once an accurate diagnosis has been made. Parenteral or oral administration of anticholinergics (e.g., benztropine mesylate [Cogentin], biperiden [Akineton], procyclidine [Kemadrin], trihexyphenidyl hydrochloride [Artane]) or antihistaminics (e.g., diphenhydramine [Benadryl]) is nearly uniformly effective in reversing acute dystonia (H. Freed 1958; Freyhan 1958; Waugh and Metts 1960). A failure of symptoms to improve substantially or to resolve after one to three doses over a 30- to 90-minute period should stimulate the search for other less common causes of dystonia associated with unrecognized illnesses. Only in rare situations may it be necessary to try a parenteral benzodiazepine (Korczyn and Goldberg 1972) or barbiturate sedative like amobarbital (Christian and Paulson 1958) after the anticholinergics have failed. Other treatments that have no advantage over standard approaches include caffeine (Kulenkampff and Tarnow 1956) and methylphenidate (Fann 1966).

Prophylaxis against acute dystonia is controversial. Proponents of prophylaxis argue that dystonic episodes can be dangerous, such as the laryngeal-pharyngeal dystonia; may often be a harbinger of other extrapyramidal syndromes that will develop later; and may lead to patient noncompliance. Opponents of prophylaxis argue that the prophylactic medicines have their own drawbacks, such as memory impairment, blurred vision, dry mouth, and constipation. As expected, both sides of the controversy contend that their approach is the best method for achieving the maximum benefit with the minimum side effects. Therefore, each group claims that their strategy best fosters a therapeutic alliance with the patient that encourages treatment compliance.

Prophylaxis is highly appropriate when there is 1) a high risk of acute dystonia; 2) a predisposition to acute dystonia; and 3) detrimental sequelae, such as paranoid patients believing that external forces are controlling them (Casey 1992; Casey and Keepers 1988). A review of the studies examining the effectiveness of prophylaxis at the initiation of neuroleptic treatment indicates that it is clearly efficacious (Casey and Keepers 1988; Lake et al. 1986; McEvoy 1983). Both prospective and retrospective studies have consistently found a statistically significant benefit of prophylaxis (Boyer et al. 1987; Hanlon et al. 1966; Keepers et al. 1983; Manos et al. 1981, 1986; Sramek et al. 1986; Stern and Anderson 1979; Winslow et al. 1986). However, it is obvious that not all patients require prophylaxis against acute dystonia. If there is a low likelihood of dystonia risk, treatment with only a neuroleptic drug and no prophylactic agent is the preferred approach because the risk of undesirable side effects from the prophylactic drug outweighs the limited potential benefit of this agent. A reasoned strategy about whether to use prophylaxis is best made by considering the relative contributions of patient characteristics (age, gender, prior dystonic reactions), drug properties (milligram potency, dosage, intrinsic anticholinergic activity), and temporal aspects when neuroleptic drugs are initiated (Casey and Keepers 1988; Keepers et al. 1983). If initial prophylaxis is used for acute dystonia, these agents should be gradually tapered after the first 7–14 days of treatment because acute dystonia rarely occurs beyond the fifth to seventh day of neuroleptic therapy. It is critically important to taper the anti-extrapyramidal syndrome drugs slowly because sudden discontinuation may cause a rebound acute dystonic reaction (Arana et al. 1988).

Discussion and Recommendations

Should Neuroleptic-Induced Acute Dystonia Be Included in DSM-IV?

The preponderance of the data indicate that neuroleptic drug-induced dystonia should be included in DSM-IV. Neuroleptic drug-induced dystonia is a common problem with neuroleptic treatment. It occurs frequently, often in more than 50% of the patients who are in the high-risk group (Donlon et al. 1980; Keepers et al. 1983; Singh et al. 1990; Sramek et al. 1986). In contrast, the frequency of neuroleptic-induced acute dystonia may be 10% or less in low-risk patients (Keepers et al. 1983; Singh et al. 1990; Swett 1975). Severity of symptoms can range from a minor inconvenience to a life-threatening situation requiring emergency intervention. Although this life-threatening severity is uncommon, it occurs frequently enough to merit full medical supervision and immediate treatment with parenteral drugs. Since underrecognition is a real possibility with neuroleptic-induced acute dystonia as well as with other drug-induced movement disorders, visibility in DSM-IV will increase the likelihood of recognition and accurate diagnoses. This should also reduce the misdiagnoses of hysteria, malingering, or catatonia in patients who appear to have bizarre postures early in their neuroleptic treatment course. Increased awareness and visibility of dystonia will alert future caregivers to have a high vigilance level for the reoccurrence of this syndrome in patients who have had prior neuroleptic-induced acute dystonic reactions. Finally, it is critically important to consider that these dystonic reactions are potentially preventable with a reasoned consideration of the risk factors of patient characteristics, drug factors, temporal aspects, and the appropriate utilization of prophylaxis against these reactions.

There are also disadvantages to including neuroleptic drug-induced dystonia in DSM-IV. If criteria for inclusion are too subjective, then dystonia may be overdiagnosed. This would lead to patients being exposed to additional drug treatment with antidotes that are unnecessary. Similarly, prophylaxis may be overutilized, which would lead to unnecessary drug exposure.

Definition of Neuroleptic-Induced Acute Dystonia

It is proposed that neuroleptic-induced acute dystonia be defined as the briefly sustained or fixed abnormal posture(s) that occurs in relation to starting or substantially raising neuroleptic drug levels or abruptly discontinuing anticholinergic or antihistaminic agents or dopamine agonists that are used as anti-extrapyramidal medicines.

The advantage of employing this broad-based definition is that it would encompass the wide breadth of symptoms that can occur with the flexion or extension of focal or segmental muscle groups. The disadvantage of a narrow syndrome definition is that it would exclude bona fide dystonic reactions that produce apparently bizarre positioning of parts of the body, which might then be incorrectly attributed to nonorganic causes.

Establishing Criteria for a Diagnosis of Neuroleptic-Induced Acute Dystonia

The proposed criteria for diagnosing this syndrome would require objective signs of muscular contractions that produce abnormal positioning or dysfunction of the body parts. Although it is tempting to accept only subjective complaints to qualify for a dystonic reaction, this would set too low a threshold level for a diagnosis. The central problem with utilizing only subjective complaints is the difficulty associated with distinguishing complaints that are related to neuroleptic drug administration from complaints that are unrelated to drug therapy and may be part of the underlying psychiatric illness. However, subjective complaints can be useful indicators of the prodrome that leads to objective signs. These subjective reports can include tightness in the throat, awareness that the eyes want to roll to the side or upward, a feeling of increased muscle tone, or an awareness of an inability to make the muscles do exactly what the patient wants them to do.

The objective criteria proposed for a diagnosis of neuroleptic drug-induced dystonia would meet one or more of the indicators for each of the three categories of signs and symptoms, drug treatment, and time.

Signs and symptoms would include abnormal positioning of the head and neck in relation to the body (e.g., retrocollis, torticollis); spasms of the jaw muscles (trismus, gaping, grimacing); impaired swallowing (dysphagia), speaking, or breathing (laryngeal-pharyngeal spasm, dysphonia); thickened or slurred speech secondary to hypertonic or enlarged tongue (dysarthria, macroglossia); tongue protrusion or tongue dysfunction; eyes deviated up, down, or sideward (oculogyric crises); or abnormal positioning of the distal or proximal limbs or the trunk.

These should occur in relation to starting neuroleptic drug therapy, raising rapidly an existing neuroleptic dose, continuing a depot neuroleptic injection schedule, or stopping suddenly medicines that are treatments for acute extrapyramidal syndromes, such as anticholinergic, antihistaminic, or dopamine agonist agents. These should occur within 7 days of starting or altering neuroleptic treatment.

Future Research

The increased attention to neuroleptic-induced dystonia from inclusion in DSM-IV may stimulate additional research in this area. Several topics are worth pursuing. Research diagnostic criteria should be developed so that reliable and valid dystonia scales can be developed to aid diagnostic consistency. Patient characteristics need to be developed for prospectively identifying those at risk. Perhaps biological markers will be found that indicate individual vulnerability. Drug factors such as critical blood levels, rates of drug dose adjustment, and mechanisms of producing dystonia are a few important areas to pursue. Finally, issues of timing of dystonic reactions and the eventual development of tolerance to this syndrome should be investigated.

References

Addonizio G, Alexopoulos GS: Drug-induced dystonia in young and elderly patients. Am J Psychiatry 145:869–871, 1988

Anderson WO: Antinauseant drugs in treatment of epidemic or virus gastritis? Pediatrics 23:1015–1016, 1959

Angus JWS, Simpson GM: Hysteria and drug-induced dystonia. Acta Psychiatr Scand Suppl 212:52–58, 1970

Arana G, Goff DC, Baldessarini RJ, et al: Efficacy of anticholinergic prophylaxis for neuroleptic-induced dystonia. Am J Psychiatry 145:993–996, 1988

Ayd FJ: A survey of drug-induced extrapyramidal reactions. JAMA 175:1054–1060, 1961

Baldessarini RJ: Antipsychotic agents, in Chemotherapy in Psychiatry: Principles and Practice. Cambridge, MA, Harvard University Press, 1985, pp 14–92

Binder RL, Levy R: Extrapyramidal reactions in Asians. Am J Psychiatry 138:1243–1244, 1981

Boyer WF, Bakalar NH, Lake CR: Anticholinergic prophylaxis of acute haloperidol-induced acute dystonic reactions. J Clin Psychopharmacol 7:164–166, 1987

Burke RE, Kang UJ: Tardive dystonia: clinical aspects and treatment, in Advances in Neurology, Vol 49: Facial Dyskinesias. Edited by Jankovic J, Tolosa E. New York, Raven, 1988, pp 199–210

Burke RE, Fahn S, Jankovic J, et al: Tardive dystonia: late-onset and persistent dystonia caused by antipsychotic drugs. Neurology 32:1335–1346, 1982

Calne DB, Lang AE: Secondary dystonia, in Advances in Neurology, Vol 50: Dystonia 2. Edited by Fahn S, Marsden CD, Calne DB. New York, Raven, 1988, pp 9–33

Casey DE: Metoclopramide side effects. Ann Intern Med 98:673–674, 1983

Casey DE: Tardive dyskinesia, in Psychopharmacology: The Third Generation of Progress. Edited by Meltzer H. New York, Raven, 1987, pp 1411–1419

Casey DE: Clozapine: neuroleptic-induced EPS and tardive dyskinesia. Psychopharmacology 99:S47–S53, 1989a

Casey DE: Serotonergic aspects of acute extrapyramidal syndromes in nonhuman primates. Psychopharmacol Bull 25:457–459, 1989b

Casey DE: Neuroleptic drug-induced extrapyramidal syndromes and tardive dyskinesia. Schizophrenia Research 4:109–120, 1991

Casey DE: Neuroleptic-induced acute dystonia, in Drug-Induced Movement Disorders. Edited by Lang AE, Weiner WJ. New York, Futura Press, 1992

Casey DE, Keepers GA: Neuroleptic side effects: acute extrapyramidal syndromes and tardive dyskinesia, in Psychopharmacology: Current Trends. Edited by Casey DE, Christensen AV. Berlin, Springer-Verlag, 1988, pp 74–93

Chadwick D, Reynolds EH, Marsden CD: Anticonvulsant-induced dyskinesias: a comparison with dyskinesias induced by neuroleptics. J Neurol Neurosurg Psychiatry 1976; 39:1210–1218

Chouinard G, Ross-Chouinard A, Annable L: Extrapyramidal symptom rating scale. Can J Neurol Sci 7:233, 1980

Christian CD, Paulson G: Severe motility disturbance after small doses of prochlorperazine. N Engl J Med 259:828–830, 1958

Davis JM: Antipsychotic drugs, in Comprehensive Textbook of Psychiatry. Edited by Kaplan HI, Sadock BJ. Baltimore, MD, Williams & Wilkins, 1985, pp 1507–1508

DeGrandi T, Simon JE: Promethazine-induced dystonic reaction. Pediatr Emerg Care 3:91–92, 1987

Donlon PT, Hopkin JT, Tupin JP, et al: Haloperidol for acute schizophrenic patients: an evaluation of three oral regimens. Arch Gen Psychiatry 37:691–695, 1980

Fahn S, Marsden CD, Calne DB: Classification and investigation of dystonia, in Movement Disorders, Vol 2. Edited by Marsden CD, Fahn S. London, Butterworths, 1987

Fann WE: Use of methylphenidate to counteract acute dystonic effects of phenothiazines. Am J Psychiatry 122:1293–1294, 1966

Faurbye A, Rasch PJ, Bender Peterson P, et al: Neurological symptoms in the pharmacotherapy of psychoses. Acta Psychiatr Scand 40:10–26, 1964

Flaherty JA, Lahmeyer HW: Laryngeal-pharyngeal dystonia as a possible cause of asphyxia with haloperidol treatment. Am J Psychiatry 135:1414–1415, 1978

Freed E: Alcohol-triggered neuroleptic-induced tremor, rigidity and dystonia. Med J Aust 2:44–45, 1981

Freed H: On special uses of diphenhydramine hydrochloride in the somatic therapy ward of a psychiatric hospital. Am J Psychiatry 115:359–360, 1958

Freyhan FA: Occurrence and management of extrapyramidal syndromes in psychiatric treatment with trifluoperazine, in Extrapyramidal Symptoms and Other Side Effects. Philadelphia, PA, Lea & Febiger, 1958

Gardos G: Dystonic reaction during maintenance antipsychotic therapy. Am J Psychiatry 138:114–115, 1981

Garver DL, Davis JM, Dekirmenjian H, et al: Dystonic reactions following neuroleptics: time course and proposed mechanisms. Psychopharmacology 47:199–201, 1976

Gerlach J: Tardive dyskinesia. Dan Med Bull 26:209–245, 1979

Gupta JM, Lovejoy FH: Acute phenothiazine toxicity in childhood: a five year study. Pediatrics 39:771–774, 1967

Hanlon TE, Schoenrich C, Freinek W, et al: Perphenazine-benztropine mesylate treatment of newly admitted psychiatric patients. Psychopharmacologia 9:328–339, 1966

Hooker EA, Danzl DF: Acute dystonic reaction due to diazepam. J Emerg Med 6:491–493, 1988

Hunt-Fugate AK, Zander J, Lesar TS: Adverse reactions due to dopamine blockade by amoxapine. Pharmacotherapy 4:35–39, 1984

Jacome D: Carbamazepine-induced dystonia. JAMA 241:2263, 1979

Johnson DAW: The side-effects of fluphenazine decanoate. Br J Psychiatry 123:519–522, 1973

Keepers GA, Casey DE: Clinical management of acute neuroleptic-induced extrapyramidal syndromes, in Current Psychiatric Therapies. Edited by Masserman JH. New York, Grune & Stratton, 1986, pp 139–157

Keepers GA, Casey DE: Prediction of dystonia. J Clin Psychopharmacol 9:307–308, 1989

Keepers GA, Casey DE: Use of neuroleptic-induced extrapyramidal symptoms to predict future vulnerability to side effects. Am J Psychiatry 148:85–89, 1991

Keepers GA, Clappison VJ, Casey DE: Initial anticholinergic prophylaxis for neuroleptic-induced extrapyramidal syndromes. Arch Gen Psychiatry 40:1113–1117, 1983

Khanderia U: Recurrent dystonic reactions induced by thiethylperazine. Drug Intelligence and Clinical Pharmacy 19:550–551, 1985

Koek RJ, Pi EH: Acute laryngeal dystonic reactions to neuroleptics. Psychosomatics 30:359–364, 1989

Korczyn AD, Goldberg GJ: Intravenous diazepam in drug-induced dystonic reactions. Br J Psychiatry 121:75–77, 1972

Kris MG, Tyson LB, Gralla RJ, et al: Extrapyramidal reactions with high-dose metoclopramide. N Engl J Med 309:433–434, 1983

Kulenkampff C, Tarnow G: Ein eigentümliches syndrom im oralen bereich bei megaphenapplikation. Nervenarzt 27:178–180, 1956

Kumor K, Sherer M, Jaffe J: Haloperidol-induced dystonia in cocaine addicts. Lancet 2:1341–1342, 1986

Lake CR, Casey DE, McEvoy JP, et al: Anticholinergic prophylaxis in young adults treated with neuroleptic drugs. Psychopharmacol Bull 22:981–984, 1986

Lapierre YD, Anderson K: Dyskinesia associated with amoxapine antidepressant therapy. Am J Psychiatry 140:493–494, 1983

Lazaro RP: Involuntary movements induced by anticonvulsant drugs. Mt Sinai J Med 49:274–281, 1982

Mann SC, Cohen MP, Boger WP: The danger of laryngeal dystonia. Am J Psychiatry 136:1344–1345, 1979

Manos N, Gkiouzepas J, Tzotzoras T, et al: Gradual withdrawal of antiparkinson medication in chronic schizophrenics: any better than the abrupt? J Nerv Ment Dis 169:659–661, 1981

Manos N, Lavrentiadis G, Gkiouzepas J: Evaluation of the need for prophylactic antiparkinsonian medication in psychotic patients treated with neuroleptics. J Clin Psychiatry 47:114–116, 1986

McEvoy JP: The clinical use of anticholinergic drugs as treatment for extrapyramidal side effects of neuroleptic disorders. J Clin Psychopharmacol 3:288–302, 1983

Meltzer HY, Matsubara S, Lee JC: Classification of typical and atypical antipsychotic drugs on the basis of dopamine D-1, D-2 and serotonin pKi values. J Pharmacol Exp Ther 251:238–246, 1989

Melvin KEW: Tetanus-like reactions to the phenothiazine drugs: "the grimacing syndrome." N Z Med J 61:90, 1962

Nasrallah HA, Churchill CM, Hamdan-Allan GA: Higher frequency of neuroleptic-induced dystonia in mania than in schizophrenia. Am J Psychiatry 145:1455–1456, 1988

National Institute of Mental Health, Psychopharmacology Service Center Collaborative Study Group: Phenothiazine treatment in acute schizophrenia. Arch Gen Psychiatry 10:246–261, 1964

Owens DGC: Dystonia—a potential psychiatric pitfall. Br J Psychiatry 156:620–634, 1990

Pollera CF, Cognetti F, Nardi M, et al: Sudden death after acute dystonic reaction to high-dose metoclopramide. Lancet 2:460–461, 1984

Powers JM: Decongestant-induced blepharospasm and orofacial dystonia. JAMA 247:3244–3245, 1982

Preswick G, McClatchie G: Acute dystonic reaction following thiethylperazine ("Thorecan") therapy. Med J Aust 1:623–624, 1965

Prien RF, Cole JO, Belkin NF: Relapse in chronic schizophrenia following abrupt withdrawal of tranquillizing drugs. Br J Psychiatry 115:679–686, 1969

Remington GJ, Voineskos G, Pollock B, et al: Prevalence of neuroleptic-induced dystonia in mania and schizophrenia. Am J Psychiatry 147:1231–1233, 1990

Richardson MA, Craig TJ: The coexistence of parkinsonism-like symptoms and tardive dyskinesia. Am J Psychiatry 139:341–343, 1982

Simpson GM, Angus JWS: A rating scale for extrapyramidal side-effects. Acta Psychiatr Scand Suppl 212:11–19, 1970

Singh H, Levinson DF, Simpson GM, et al: Acute dystonia during fixed-dose neuroleptic treatment. J Clin Psychopharmacol 10:389–396, 1990

Snyder S, Greenberg D, Yamamura H: Antischizophrenic drugs and brain cholinergic receptors. Arch Gen Psychiatry 31:58–61, 1974

Sramek JJ, Simpson GM, Morrison RL, et al: Anticholinergic agents for prophylaxis of neuroleptic-induced dystonic reactions: a prospective study. J Clin Psychiatry 47:305–309, 1986

Steele TE: Adverse reactions suggesting amoxapine-induced dopamine blockade. Am J Psychiatry 139:1500–1501, 1982

Stern TA, Anderson WH: Benztropine prophylaxis of dystonic reactions. Psychopharmacology 61:261–262, 1979

Swaiman KF: Acute neurologic reaction to promethazine. N Engl J Med 263:747, 1960

Swett C: Drug-induced dystonia. Am J Psychiatry 132:532–533, 1975

Taylor JFN: Tranquillising drugs and dystonia. Lancet 2:159–160, 1969

Tesar GE, Murray GB, Cassem NH: Use of high-dose intravenous haloperidol in the treatment of agitated cardiac patients. J Clin Psychopharmacol 5:344–347, 1985

Thatch BT, Chase TN, Bosma JF: Oral facial dyskinesia associated with prolonged use of antihistaminic decongestants. N Engl J Med 293:486–487, 1975

VanTol HHM, Bunzow JR, Guan H-C, et al: Cloning of the gene for a human dopamine D_4 receptor with high affinity for the antipsychotic clozapine. Nature 350:610–614, 1991

Waugh WH, Metts JC Jr: Severe extrapyramidal motor activity induced by prochlorperazine: its relief by the intravenous injection of diphenhydramine. N Engl J Med 262:353–354, 1960

Weiner MF: Haloperidol, hyperthyroidism, and sudden death. Am J Psychiatry 136:717–718, 1979

Winslow RS, Stillner V, Coons DJ, et al: Prevention of acute dystonic reactions in patients beginning with high-potency neuroleptics. Am J Psychiatry 143:706–710, 1986

Chapter 33

Neuroleptic-Induced Acute Akathisia

Lenard A. Adler, M.D.
Burt Angrist, M.D.

Statement of the Issues

The purpose of this chapter is to discuss whether the neuroleptic side effect of akathisia should be included in DSM-IV. To address this issue, data concerning diagnostic features, epidemiology, clinical significance, and treatment of the syndrome are reviewed.

Significance of the Issues

Akathisia has important clinical consequences. The distress it causes may limit the doses of antipsychotic drugs administered to a suboptimal range, may result in neuroleptic noncompliance, may exacerbate psychotic symptoms, and, in some patients, may lead to violence or suicide attempts. At the same time, the condition is usually, although not always, briskly responsive to rather benign treatments. It is therefore important that clinicians be aware of akathisia and its treatment.

Inclusion of akathisia in DSM-IV would emphasize the clinical importance of the syndrome and encourage its diagnosis and treatment. Conversely, this benefit also carries the risk of possible overdiagnosis and patients receiving pharmacologic treatment that is not needed.

Methods

More than 150 articles were reviewed. Although computer searches using *akathisia* as the index word were completed, these were not the main source of familiarity with the literature. Rather, this was the result of approximately 7 years of work in this area in the course of which more than 12 papers on akathisia and its treatment have been written, including an earlier review article (Adler et al. 1989) and a book chapter (Adler et al. 1992).

Results

Diagnosis

Essential Features

The akathisia syndrome is composed of both subjective complaints of restlessness and objective movements. It may be difficult to diagnosis akathisia in patients with the mild form of the syndrome, who exhibit only subjective complaints, without showing objective movements (Barnes and Braude 1986; Van Putten and Marder 1987). However, objective movements almost always accompany subjective restlessness in moderate and severe akathisia.

Subjective complaints (Gibb and Lees 1986; *Lancet* 1986; Van Putten 1975) include 1) a sense of inner restlessness, most often referable to the legs; 2) a compulsion to move one's legs; 3) distress if one is asked not to move one's legs; and 4) dysphoria and anxiety.

Objective movements (Barnes 1989; Braude et al. 1983; Gibb and Lees 1986; Van Putten and Marder 1987) include 1) rocking from foot to foot or "walking on the spot" while standing; 2) repetitive movements of the legs while seated, including swinging of the legs; 3) pacing; and 4) in its most severe form, tasikinesia, an inability to maintain any position.

Differential Diagnosis

Agitation seen with other psychiatric disorders. Major depression, mania, or psychosis may all result in agitation. Thus, it may be difficult to distinguish agitation from akathisia in patients who are receiving neuroleptics. However, a pattern in which agitation worsens with increasing doses of neuroleptics may particularly alert the clinician to suspect akathisia. In such cases, treatment of the suspected akathisia is warranted.

Patients with generalized anxiety disorder may be restless and pace. Some patients can differentiate akathisia from generalized anxiety, since they experience akathisia as being "driven," "unnatural," or different from previously experienced feelings (Kendler 1976; Van Putten 1975). However, not all patients can make this distinction. Again, treatment response may help differentiate these conditions.

Drug withdrawal states. Restlessness, painful sensations in the legs, and leg movements are common symptoms of opiate withdrawal. However, in practice, most patients in opiate withdrawal know what is wrong and in fact "make the diagnosis" themselves. Interestingly, however, the same agents have been found to be effective in treating both conditions. The alpha$_2$ agonist clonidine has been found to improve both opiate withdrawal (Gold et al. 1978) and akathisia (Adler et al. 1987; Zubenko et al. 1984c). Additionally, low doses of the beta-blocker propranolol have been reported to improve the restlessness of opiate withdrawal (Roehrich and Gold 1987) as well as akathisia (Adler et al. 1985, 1986, 1991c; Kramer et al. 1988; Lipinski et al. 1983, 1984).

Chronic akathisia. Chronic akathisias occur late in the course of treatment, unlike acute akathisia, which is an early effect. In both forms of the syndrome, patients have subjective complaints of restlessness along with objective movements. Barnes and Braude (1985) defined chronic akathisia as occurring more than 6 months after initiation of, or increase in the dose of, neuroleptic. Chronic akathisia may be more difficult to treat than acute akathisia (Simpson 1977).

Pseudoakathisia. Patients with pseudoakathisia have objective movements of akathisia, without subjective complaints of restlessness. It has been hypothesized that acute akathisia, chronic akathisia, pseudoakathisia, and tardive dyskinesia may be points in a continuum (Chouinard et al. 1979; Munetz 1986; Munetz and Cornes 1982; Stahl 1985). This supposition is based on several studies finding present pseudoakathisia and a history of acute akathisia on the one hand, and a relationship between pseudoakathisia and dyskinetic movements on the other. Munetz and Cornes (1982) studied 45 patients with tardive dyskinesia; they found that 21 patients had an acute akathisia at some prior time and that 11 of these 21 had a pseudoakathisia at the time of the examination. Barnes and Braude (1985) studied 39 patients who had akathisia. They divided the patients according to whether they had acute akathisia, chronic akathisia, or pseudoakathisia. None of the patients with acute akathisia had tardive dyskinesia, whereas more than half of the patients with chronic akathisia or pseudoakathisia also had dyskinesias.

Tardive akathisia. Tardive akathisia is a chronic form of akathisia that behaves like tardive dyskinesia, in that it is improved by increasing the dose of neuroleptic and worsened by dose reduction (Braude and Barnes 1983; Jeste and Wyatt 1982; Kruse 1960; Weiner and Luby 1983). However, tardive akathisia, like the acute form of the syndrome, has been reported to respond to treatment with beta-blockers (Yassa et al. 1988).

Tardive dyskinesia. Tardive dyskinesia often also has a component of generalized restlessness that may coexist with akathisia in a patient receiving neuroleptics. In such cases, it may be impossible to say what restlessness is due to tardive dyskinesia and what is due to akathisia. Response patterns of akathisia variants to pharmacologic treatment are not well established at this time; therefore, if the patient is experiencing distress, a trial of treatment seems warranted.

Epidemiology

Timing of Onset and Relation to Dose

Akathisia can develop very rapidly after initiating or increasing neuroleptics or other dopamine antagonists. Barnes and colleagues (1982) reported akathisia developing within an hour of receiving preoperative medication with droperidol and metoclopramide. The development of akathisia also appears to be dose dependent.

Ayd (1961) surveyed 3,775 patients receiving neuroleptics and found that patients started on higher doses of neuroleptics were more likely to develop akathisia than patients started on lower doses. Braude and colleagues (1983) prospectively studied the development of akathisia in 109 inpatients followed over 23 days and also found a dose-dependent relationship. Acute akathisia tends to persist, although fluctuating in intensity over time for as long as neuroleptics are continued (*Lancet* 1986).

Prevalence of Acute Akathisia

The reported prevalence of akathisia in patients receiving neuroleptics varies widely. Lower estimates of prevalence (3%–13%) were found in earlier studies (Freyhan 1958; Goldman 1961; National Institute of Mental Health 1964). More recent investigations have found higher prevalences. Van Putten (1975) and Gibb and Lees (1986) found figures in the 40%–45% range. Van Putten and colleagues (1984) studied 32 patients diagnosed with schizophrenia who were taken off neuroleptics and then treated with haloperidol 10 mg/day for 7 days and found a 75% incidence of akathisia. The most common estimate of prevalence is 20% (Ayd 1961; Braude et al. 1983; Marsden and Jenner 1980). Several factors may account for this wide variability in prevalence (Adler et al. 1989): 1) lack of recognition of akathisia (Weiden et al. 1987); 2) the fact that some investigators exclude patients who present with only subjective complaints of restlessness, without classic objective movements (as may exist in mild forms of the syndrome); and 3) the degree to which high- versus low-potency neuroleptics are used. Although all neuroleptics can cause akathisia, the syndrome appears to occur more frequently with higher-potency agents (Ayd 1960, 1961).

Clinical Significance

The subjective distress resulting from akathisia is significant and can lead to refusal of neuroleptics or a worsening of psychosis. In a study of 85 patients, Van Putten (1974) found that akathisia was significantly more prevalent in patients who refused medication than in those who were compliant with neuroleptics. Van Putten and colleagues (1974) coined the term *phenothiazine-induced decompensation* to refer to an increase in psychosis associated with akathisia. They found that such decompensations were similar to the original psychosis and that "thought processes became disorganized, secondary symptoms recurred, quality of contact deteriorated, and many complained of an abject fear or terror that was difficult to articulate" (p. 70). Additionally, the syndrome can be so dysphoric that it has been associated with violence or aggression (Keckich 1978; Kumar 1979; Schulte 1985) or suicide attempts (Drake and Ehrlich 1985; Schulte 1985; Shaw et al. 1986; Shear et al. 1983; Weiden 1985).

It is important that akathisia be recognized because of this distress. Clinicians often perceive worsening of psychosis or behavioral dyscontrol as indications for increasing the dose of neuroleptics. If akathisia is the cause for this exacerbation, this response is likely to lead to further deterioration of the patient's status and still further increases in dose. Such escalating cycles of akathisia, clinical worsening, dose increase, and further deterioration are not uncommon in our experience.

Treatment of Akathisia

Treatment of akathisia is covered extensively in a review (Adler et al. 1989) and a chapter (Adler et al. 1992) on akathisia. The reader is referred to these for further details.

Adjusting the Dose of Neuroleptic Medication

The simplest treatment of acute akathisia is to lower the dose of neuroleptics (Braude et al. 1983). Obviously, however, dose reduction is not always a viable strategy in floridly psychotic patients. Switching the patient to a lower-potency neuroleptic is another potential strategy (Ayd 1961).

Pharmacologic Treatment of Akathisia

The agents that have been used to treat neuroleptic-induced akathisia include 1) antiparkinsonian agents, including anticholinergics and amantadine; 2) benzodiazepines; and 3) agents that affect noradrenergic function, such as beta-blockers and clonidine (Adler et al. 1989).

Antiparkinsonian agents. Antiparkinsonian medications are commonly used to treat akathisia. However, there are few formal prospective studies of these agents in akathisia. Many clinicians feel that antiparkinsonian agents are only partially effective; in addition, their use is limited by anticholinergic side effects (Ayd 1960, 1961) or tolerance to the therapeutic effect of amantadine (Zubenko et al. 1984b).

Benzodiazepines. Several benzodiazepines such as diazepam (Donlon 1973; Gagrat et al. 1978), lorazepam (Adler et al. 1985; Bartels et al. 1987), and clonazepam (Kutcher et al. 1987, 1989) have been found to be helpful in treating akathisia. Longer-term studies have not been performed to determine whether tolerance develops to improvement in akathisia, as occurs with the use of benzodiazepines as hypnotics.

Beta-blockers. Beta-blockers are currently considered to be the most promising treatments for akathisia. The beta-blocker that has been most extensively studied in akathisia is propranolol, which nonselectively blocks both $beta_1$ and $beta_2$ receptors. The use of propranolol in states of pathologic restlessness was first reported by Strang (1967), who described the beneficial effects of propranolol (5–30 mg/day) in parkinsonian patients who had restless leg syndrome. Lipinski and colleagues (1983) noted this report and were the first to assess propranolol as a treatment for akathisia due to neuroleptics. Another case of neuroleptic-induced akathisia successfully treated with propranolol was reported by Kulik and Wilbur (1983) in the same year. Subsequently, there have been two noncontrolled investigations (Adler et al. 1988; Lipinski et al. 1984) and five controlled studies of propranolol in akathisia (Adler et al. 1985, 1986, 1991c; Kramer et al. 1988; J. F. Lipinski, G. Mallya, B. Cohen, et al., A double-blind, placebo-controlled study of propranolol in neuroleptic-induced akathisia, unpublished manuscript). Propranolol (30–80 mg/day) has been generally effective in treating akathisia and has been well tolerated by patients in all of these studies, although rarely patients have had decreased blood pressure at these doses. Propranolol should not be used to treat akathisia in patients who have contraindications to receiving beta-blockers, such as cardiac conduction delays, hypotension, insulin-dependent diabetes mellitus, or, above all, asthma.

$Beta_1$ selective agents, such as betaxolol (Adler et al. 1991a; Dupuis et al. 1987) and metoprolol (Adler et al. 1990; Kim et al. 1989) and an investigational $beta_2$-blocker (Adler et al. 1991b) have also been found to be effective in treating neuroleptic-induced akathisia. However, these studies have generally been less well controlled and conducted with smaller patient samples than the studies with propranolol. Additionally, Zubenko and colleagues (1984a) found that metoprolol was effective only when given in doses (i.e., greater than 200 mg/day) where both

$beta_1$ and $beta_2$ receptors are blocked. Therefore, if one is going to use a beta-blocker to treat neuroleptic-induced akathisia, we believe that propranolol presently remains the agent of choice.

Discussion

Akathisia is a complication of neuroleptic treatment that can profoundly compromise treatment. At the same time, the syndrome is often briskly responsive to anticholinergics or low doses of beta-blockers, treatments that in themselves are rather benign if medical contraindications are respected. Thus, it is extraordinarily important for clinicians to be keenly alert to the development of akathisia and ways to treat it.

The proper mechanism to accomplish this goal is the question raised in this chapter. As noted earlier, inclusion of akathisia in DSM-IV would emphasize the syndrome to clinicians and encourage its diagnosis and treatment. Although this is desirable, overdiagnosis and resulting unnecessary treatment is also a potential concern. Finally, akathisia is clearly not a psychiatric disorder per se, but rather, a common side effect of a widely used and in fact indispensable class of therapeutic agents. Thus, it might well be more appropriate to include discussion of akathisia under "other clinically significant problems that may be a focus of treatment." The risk in doing so is loss of emphasis to busy clinicians who may not read this section closely.

Recommendations

As noted earlier, we feel that the clinical significance of akathisia is such that it should be continuously assessed in patients receiving neuroleptics, and, if suspected, a trial of treatment should be undertaken. Because the treatments are safe (if medical contraindications are respected), we feel that the potential benefits probably outweigh the risks. Inherent in this position is the assumption that clinicians will assess the effects of their interventions and not continue them if no benefit is noted.

Thus our recommendation is that the potential benefits of inclusion outweigh the risks.

Threshold Criteria

We believe that the threshold for diagnosing neuroleptic-induced akathisia should be fairly liberal or, using epidemiologic terms, utilize sensitive but not specific criteria. In this regard, the number of false positives (patients diagnosed as having the syndrome who actually do not) would be fairly high, whereas the number of false negatives (patients who do have the syndrome, but are not diagnosed) would be fairly low. The rationale for setting sensitive but not specific criteria is that the consequences of missing a diagnosis of akathisia are significant, and we believe the emphasis should be on treating the syndrome when it is suspected. As noted in the literature review, akathisia can have important clinical consequences. Anticholinergic medications, and most recently beta-blockers, have often been found to be effective treatments for neuroleptic-induced akathisia. Therefore, the benefit-risk ratio in treating a suspected case of akathisia is fairly high.

Accordingly, the criteria we propose require a diagnosis of mild akathisia on the global rating from the Barnes akathisia scale (Barnes 1989). These criteria would use both a severity cutoff in subjective complaints ("Awareness of restlessness in the legs and/or inner restlessness worse when required to stand still. . . . Condition causes little or no distress") and objective movements ("Fidgety movements present, but characteristic movements of restlessness not necessarily observed"). By encouraging the diagnosis of mild akathisia, we hope that clinicians will err on the side of treating the syndrome. It should also be noted that this proposed threshold would not include a diagnosis of pseudoakathisia—as the definition of mild akathisia is specifically based on subjective complaints of restlessness in the legs, which are absent in pseudoakathisia. We feel that this exclusion is appropriate since it is not clear whether the morbidity, pathophysiology, or response to medications of pseudoakathisia is similar to that of more classic akathisias.

Thus, we are proposing a liberal threshold for diagnosis, based on criteria that are sensitive, rather than specific, and that will specifically include milder forms of the syndrome.

Future Educational and Research Directions

A workshop project has begun at the National Institute of Mental Health in which a videotape library is being prepared showing patients with akathisia of varying degrees of severity before and after treatment. A preliminary review of these tapes (Kane et al. 1993) by a group of rather sophisticated psychopharmacologically oriented clinicians and subsequent discussions reinforce our impression that akathisia is readily diagnosed in its more severe forms, but more difficult to diagnose when milder. Thus moderate and mild presentations will be particularly emphasized as tapes are collected in the future.

The response patterns of akathisia variants (i.e., chronic akathisia, tardive akathisia, pseudoakathisia, restlessness in the context of tardive dyskinesia) to specific pharmacologic treatments are not well defined at present. Thus guidelines for treatment and risk-benefit ratios are not known. Finally, large prospective studies comparing the most commonly used treatments of acute akathisia, anticholinergics and beta-blockers, are yet to be reported.

References

Adler LA, Angrist B, Peselow E, et al: Efficacy of propranolol in neuroleptic-induced akathisia. J Clin Psychopharmacol 5:164–166, 1985

Adler LA, Angrist B, Peselow E, et al: A controlled assessment of propranolol in the treatment of neuroleptic-induced akathisia. Br J Psychiatry 149:42–45, 1986

Adler LA, Angrist B, Peselow E, et al: Clonidine in neuroleptic-induced akathisia. Am J Psychiatry 144:235–236, 1987

Adler L, Reiter S, Corwin J, et al: Propranolol and benztropine in neuroleptic-induced akathisia. Biol Psychiatry 23:211–213, 1988

Adler LA, Angrist B, Reiter S, et al: Neuroleptic-induced akathisia: a review. Psychopharmacology 97:1–11, 1989

Adler LA, Angrist B, Rotrosen J: Metoprolol versus propranolol. Biol Psychiatry 27:673–675, 1990

Adler LA, Angrist B, Rotrosen J: Betaxolol in neuroleptic-induced akathisia. Psychiatry Res 39:193–198, 1991a

Adler L, Duncan E, Angrist B, et al: Effects of a specific -2 receptor blocker in neuroleptic-induced akathisia. Psychiatry Res 27:1–4, 1991b

Adler LA, Angrist B, Fritz P, et al: Lack of efficacy of *d*-propranolol in neuroleptic-induced akathisia. Neuropsychopharmacology 4:109–115, 1991c

Adler LA, Angrist B, Rotrosen J: Acute neuroleptic-induced akathisia, in Drug-Induced Movement Disorders. Edited by Lang AE, Weiner WJ. New York, Futura Press, 1992

Ayd FJ: Drug-induced extrapyramidal reactions: their clinical manifestations and treatment with akineton. Psychosomatics 1:143–150, 1960

Ayd FJ: A survey of drug-induced extrapyramidal reactions. JAMA 175:1054–1060, 1961

Barnes TRE: A rating scale for drug-induced akathisia. Br J Psychiatry 154:672–676, 1989

Barnes TRE, Braude WM: Akathisia variants and tardive dyskinesia. Arch Gen Psychiatry 42:874–878, 1985

Barnes TRE, Braude WM: Toward a more reliable diagnosis of akathisia (in reply). Arch Gen Psychiatry 43:1016, 1986

Barnes TRE, Braude WM, Hill DJ: Acute akathisia after oral droperidol and metoclopramide preoperative medication. Lancet 2:48–49, 1982

Bartels M, Heide K, Mann K, et al: Treatment of akathisia with lorazepam: an open trial. Pharmacopsychiatry 20:51–53, 1987

Braude WM, Barnes TRE: Late onset akathisia—an indicant of covert dyskinesia: two case reports. Am J Psychiatry 140:611–612, 1983

Braude WM, Barnes TRE, Gore SM: Clinical characteristics of akathisia. Br J Psychiatry 143:134–150, 1983

Chouinard G, Annable L, Ross-Chouinard A, et al: Factors related to tardive dyskinesia. Am J Psychiatry 136:79–83, 1979

Donlon P: The therapeutic use of diazepam for akathisia. Psychosomatics 14:222–225, 1973

Drake RE, Ehrlich J: Suicide attempts associated with akathisia. Am J Psychiatry 142:499–501, 1985

Dupuis B, Catteau J, Dumon J-P, et al: Comparison of propranolol, sotalol and betaxolol in the treatment of neuroleptic-induced akathisia. Am J Psychiatry 144:802–805, 1987

Freyhan FA: Extrapyramidal Symptoms and Other Side Effects of Trifluoperazine: Clinical and Pharmacologic Aspects. Philadelphia, PA, Lea & Febiger, 1958

Gagrat D, Hamilton J, Belmatier R: Intravenous diazepam in the treatment of neuroleptic-induced dystonia or akathisia. Am J Psychiatry 135:1232–1233, 1978

Gibb WR, Lees AJ: The clinical phenomenon of akathisia. J Neurol Neurosurg Psychiatry 49:861–866, 1986

Gold MS, Redmond DE, Kleiber HD: Clonidine blocks the acute opiate withdrawal syndrome. Lancet 2:403–405, 1978

Goldman D: Parkinsonism and related phenomena from administration of drugs: their production and control under clinical conditions and possible relation to therapeutic effect. Rev Can Exp Biol 20:549–560, 1961

Jeste DV, Wyatt RJ: Understanding and Treating Tardive Dyskinesia. New York, Guilford, 1982

Kane JM, Dauphinais D, Barnes TRE, et al: Assessing negative symptoms and extrapyramidal side-effects in schizophrenia: workshop report. Psychopharmacol Bull 29:45–49, 1993

Keckich WA: Violence as a manifestation of akathisia. JAMA 240:2185, 1978

Kendler K: A medical student's experience with akathisia. Am J Psychiatry 133:454–455, 1976

Kim A, Adler L, Angrist B, et al: Efficacy of low-dose metoprolol in neuroleptic-induced akathisia. J Clin Psychopharmacol 9:294–296, 1989

Kramer SM, Gorkin RA, DiJohnson C, et al: Propranolol in the treatment of neuroleptic-induced akathisia (NIA) in schizophrenics: a double-blind, placebo-controlled study. Biol Psychiatry 24:823–827, 1988

Kruse W: Persistent muscular restlessness after phenothiazine treatment: report of three cases. Am J Psychiatry 11:152–153, 1960

Kulik AV, Wilbur R: Case report of propranolol (Inderal) pharmacotherapy for neuroleptic-induced akathisia and tremor. Prog Neuro-psychopharmacol Biol Psychiatry 7:223–225, 1983

Kumar BB: An unusual case of akathisia. Am J Psychiatry 136:1088, 1979

Kutcher SP, Mackenzie S, Galarraga W, et al: Clonazepam treatment of adolescents with neuroleptic-induced akathisia. Am J Psychiatry 144:823–824, 1987

Kutcher S, Williamson P, MacKenzie S, et al: Successful clonazepam treatment of neuroleptic-induced akathisia in older adolescents and young adults: a double-blind study. J Clin Psychopharmacol 9:403–406, 1989

Lancet: Akathisia and antipsychotic drugs (editorial). Lancet 2:1131–1132, 1986

Lipinski JF, Zubenko GS, Barriera P, et al: Propranolol in the treatment of neuroleptic-induced akathisia. Lancet 2:685–686, 1983

Lipinski JF, Zubenko GS, Cohen BM, et al: Propranolol in the treatment of neuroleptic-induced akathisia. Am J Psychiatry 141:412–415, 1984

Marsden CD, Jenner P: The pathophysiology of extrapyramidal side-effects of neuroleptic drugs. Psychol Med 10:55–72, 1980

Munetz MR: Akathisia variants and tardive dyskinesia. Arch Gen Psychiatry 43:1015, 1986

Munetz MR, Cornes CL: Distinguishing akathisia and tardive dyskinesia: a review of the literature. J Clin Psychopharmacol 3:343–350, 1982

National Institute of Mental Health: Psychopharmacology survey center collaborative study group: phenothiazine treatment in acute schizophrenia. Arch Gen Psychiatry 10:246–261, 1964

Roehrich H, Gold MS: Propranolol as adjunct to clonidine in opiate detoxification. Am J Psychiatry 144:1099–1100, 1987

Schulte JR: Homicide and suicide associated with akathisia and haloperidol. American Journal of Forensic Psychiatry 6:3–7, 1985

Shaw ED, Mann JJ, Widen P, et al: A case of suicidal and homicidal ideation and akathisia in a double-blind neuroleptic crossover study. J Clin Psychopharmacol 6:196–197, 1986

Shear K, Frances A, Weiden P: Suicide associated with akathisia and depot fluphenazine treatment. J Clin Psychopharmacol 3:235–236, 1983

Simpson GM: Neurotoxicity of major tranquilizers, in Neurotoxicology. Edited by Roizin L, Shiroki H, Grcevic N. New York, Raven, 1977, p 3

Stahl SM: Akathisia and tardive dyskinesia: changing concepts. Arch Gen Psychiatry 42:915–917, 1985

Strang RR: The symptom of restless legs. Med J Aust 24:1211–1213, 1967

Van Putten T: Why do schizophrenic patients refuse to take their drugs? Arch Gen Psychiatry 31:67–72, 1974

Van Putten T: The many faces of akathisia. Compr Psychiatry 16:43–47, 1975

Van Putten T, Marder SR: Behavioral toxicity of antipsychotic drugs. J Clin Psychiatry 48 (suppl):13–19, 1987

Van Putten T, Mutalipassi LR, Malkin MD: Phenothiazine induced decompensation. Arch Gen Psychiatry 30:102–105, 1974

Van Putten T, May PRA, Marder SR: Akathisia with haloperidol and thiothixene. Arch Gen Psychiatry 41:1036–1039, 1984

Weiden P: Akathisia from prochlorperazine. JAMA 253:635, 1985

Weiden P, Mann JJ, Haas G, et al: Clinical nonrecognition of neuroleptic-induced movement disorders: a cautionary study. Am J Psychiatry 144:1148–1153, 1987

Weiner WJ, Luby ED: Persistent akathisia following neuroleptic withdrawal. Ann Neurol 13:466–467, 1983

Yassa R, Iskandar H, Nastase C: Propranolol in the treatment of tardive akathisia: a report of two cases. J Clin Psychopharmacol 8:283–285, 1988

Zubenko GS, Lipinski JF, Cohen BM, et al: Comparison of metoprolol and propranolol in the treatment of akathisia. Psychiatry Res 11:143–148, 1984a

Zubenko GS, Barreira P, Lipinski JF: Development of tolerance to the therapeutic effect of amantadine on akathisia. J Clin Psychopharmacol 4:218–219, 1984b

Zubenko GS, Cohen BM, Lipinski JF, et al: Use of clonidine in the treatment of akathisia. Psychiatry Res 13:253–259, 1984c

Chapter 34

Neuroleptic-Induced Tardive Dyskinesia

Dilip V. Jeste, M.D.
Ramzy Yassa, M.D.

Statement of the Issues

Neuroleptic-induced tardive dyskinesia (TD) is one of the most important iatrogenic disorders in psychiatry. It is relatively common, is potentially persistent and even irreversible, and has resulted in a number of malpractice suits. Yet it was not included in DSM-III-R (American Psychiatric Association 1987). There is an important need for developing a standardized set of diagnostic criteria for TD.

There are three main questions: 1) does TD belong in DSM-IV; 2) what are the criteria for a clinical diagnosis (as opposed to a strict research diagnosis) of TD; and 3) should the threshold for the diagnosis be low or high?

Significance of the Issues

The reported prevalence of TD increased progressively from 1960 through 1980 (Jeste and Wyatt 1982). During the past 15 years, the American Psychiatric Association has appointed two Task Forces (Baldessarini 1980; Kane et al. 1992) to study and make recommendations regarding prevention and treatment of TD. The ongoing debate and controversy about the need to obtain an informed consent for neuroleptic use can be traced primarily to the problem of TD. TD has become an important medicolegal issue. Not only has there been an increase in the number of lawsuits resulting from the development of TD (Tancredi 1988), but the awards in some of these cases have also been large. Furthermore, plaintiffs are successful in approximately 50% of all TD-related malpractice cases, compared with only about 10%–20% of all medical malpractice suits, according to Heaton (1990). There are reports of increased morbidity and possibly even mortality associated with TD.

One frequently encountered problem in this area is underdiagnosis, reflected by a lack of documentation of TD in the patients' charts. Absence of TD in the DSM nomenclature has contributed to that problem in a major way. Similarly, a lack of DSM-approved diagnostic criteria for TD has hampered cross-study comparison of many epidemiologic and clinical investigations on TD.

Methods

We selected a number of well-cited review articles and books on TD (e.g., Baldessarini 1980; Jeste and Wyatt 1982; Kane et al. 1988). In addition, we reviewed all the available prevalence studies on TD published through 1989. These studies were retrieved through a Medline search as well as through references quoted in books and major review articles on TD. We reviewed only articles published in English and French (or in other languages, if there was a detailed summary of the study given in English or French). To be included in our survey, a study needed to have 50 patients or more, to include both genders in its sample, and to specify the number of men and women affected by TD.

We ended up with a total of 76 prevalence studies comprising 39,187 patients (Yassa and Jeste 1992).

Results

Prevalence and Incidence

The overall prevalence of TD in patients treated long-term with neuroleptics was approximately 24.2%.

Kane and Smith (1982) found that the average unweighted prevalence of TD in 56 studies was 20%. Jeste and Wyatt (1982), reviewing selected studies, found that the weighted mean prevalence of TD was 25.7% in the 1976–1980 articles. This closely resembles our calculated value from 76 published studies in which mean prevalence of TD was 24.2%.

Although these prevalence figures apply to the general population receiving neuroleptic drugs, elderly patients seem to develop TD more often, and these figures are around 50% (Barnes 1987; Yassa et al. 1988). However, the prevalence of TD varied greatly from one study to another (2%–62%), depending on the type of patients studied, the inclusion criteria used, and the type of setting in which TD was studied (e.g., inpatient, outpatient, psychiatric institution, general hospital).

Proper prospective studies have only recently begun (Weiner and Lang 1989). Kane and colleagues (1982, 1984, 1986, 1988) have been conducting incidence studies for several years now and have found that the overall incidence of TD is 40% ± 7% after 8 years of cumulative exposure to neuroleptics (the annual incidence being 4%–5%). This figure has been confirmed by Chouinard and colleagues (1986), who also found an incidence of 40% after 8 years of neuroleptic exposure. This figure is much higher in psychogeriatric patients and amounts to almost 50% after an average of 10-month cumulative exposure to neuroleptics (Saltz et al. 1989).

In an ongoing study, Harris and colleagues (1992) have evaluated 75 older psychiatric outpatients, with the largest group having a diagnosis of dementia (mean age, 76 years), followed by psychotic disorders (mean age, 62 years) and mood disorders (mean age, 68 years). Of the patients followed for a mean of 6 months, 13.6% developed TD. An additional 7.8% patients developed borderline TD over that period.

Etiological Association With Neuroleptics

A large number of epidemiologic studies have established the etiological relationship between neuroleptic use and TD. Nonetheless, any dyskinesia seen in a neuroleptic-treated patient is not necessarily neuroleptic-induced TD. As spontaneous dyskinesia occurs in more than 5% of persons (and is also more common in the elderly), it may be difficult to *prove* that neuroleptics produced TD in a given patient.

Onset

The onset of TD is almost always insidious. First signs of dyskinesia may appear either while a patient is on stable doses of neuroleptics or within a few weeks of neuroleptic-withdrawal or tapering (i.e., within 4 weeks of withdrawal from oral medication, and 8 weeks of withdrawal from parenteral depot medication). "Neuroleptics" include typical and atypical antipsychotic agents, as well as prochlorperazine and metoclopramide, which are commonly used for nausea and gastroparesis, respectively. The withdrawal-emergent type of dyskinesia may remit with continued withdrawal from neuroleptics, or may persist and warrant a diagnosis of TD.

Symptoms

Of the TD patients, 81% have abnormal orofacial movements, 51% have limb involvement, and 23% trunk-axial dyskinesia. All three regions are affected in 11% of the patients (Jeste and Wyatt 1982). Involvement of other muscle groups (e.g., pharyngeal, abdominal) in the absence of dyskinesia of orofacial region, limbs, or trunk is quite rare.

Severity

In general, severe TD is rare (3% in a study by Yassa et al. 1990). Yet, when present, severe TD causes great discomfort and physical complications and may be the source of serious litigation. Interestingly, there is no unified manner by which to define severe TD. Some authors (Yesavage et al. 1982) use the total score on a scale as their criterion of severity. Others (Gardos et al. 1987) consider the level of subjective and objective distress and degree of functional impairment as a measure of severity. Still others (Smith et al. 1978; Yassa et al. 1990) base the severity criterion on any one body area. There are problems with each system of evaluation. Severity of TD frequently changes from day to day (Jeste and Wyatt 1982; Singh and Simpson 1988). Also, not all patients with severe TD complain of their movements (Rosen et al. 1982; Yassa et al. 1990). Thus, there is no reliable measure that will consistently evaluate severe TD. Of course, the more severe the TD the less prevalent the condition in a given study. In addition, in those studies where older women were not included, severe TD was noted to be absent (Gardos et al. 1980; Mukherjee et al. 1982).

What is considered to be a minimum severity for the diagnosis of a case of TD? There is no consensus on this issue. According to Schooler and Kane (1982), a minimum score of 2 in two different areas of the body or one score of 3 in one body area on the Abnormal Involuntary Movement Scale (AIMS) is necessary for the diagnosis of TD. Although this is a criterion for the research diagnosis of TD, Jeste and Wyatt (1982) suggested no need for a criterion of minimum severity of TD from the viewpoint of a clinical diagnosis.

Yassa and colleagues (1990) conducted an 8-year follow-up study of 20 patients who were previously diagnosed as suffering from mild TD (i.e., a score of 2 on the AIMS) in one body area and found that 55% showed no change in their TD, whereas 20% had a disappearance of TD, and 25% had a worsening of their TD. The authors suggested that patients with one AIMS rating of 2 in one body area should also be included in the category of TD.

Risk Factors for TD

Of the suggested risk factors, only old age has been consistently found to be associated with an increased frequency of TD, especially severe TD. Female gender, mood disorders (particularly unipolar depression), "brain damage," greater cumulative amount of neuroleptics, early development of extrapyramidal side effects, and frequent and lengthy drug-free intervals have also been proposed by some (but not all) investigators as risk factors for TD.

Course

Typically, the signs of TD at onset are minimal to mild in severity and escape notice except by a keen observer. They remain mild in a majority of cases; in a minority they increase in severity and may spread to other parts of the body. If a patient is kept off neuroleptics, the dyskinesia remits within 3 months in a little more than

33% of the patients, although this percentage tends to be lower in the elderly. The longer the period of neuroleptic withdrawal, the greater the chance of remission of TD. Even if neuroleptics are continued in patients with TD, the dyskinesia tends to remain stable or may even improve. In a proportion of patients (more so among the elderly), TD becomes more severe or more generalized with continued neuroleptic use.

A number of studies have been published in which either neuroleptics were discontinued or the TD examined periodically for periods up to 7 years. Neuroleptic withdrawal has been reported to lead to improvement in up to 55% of the patients whose neuroleptics were discontinued (Jeste et al. 1988). Improvement may be apparent even after 5 years of neuroleptic withdrawal (Klawans et al. 1984). On the other hand, discontinuation of neuroleptics is associated with a risk of psychotic relapse, and thus neuroleptic withdrawal may not be feasible in many cases where exacerbation of psychosis warrants the restarting of neuroleptics (Glazer et al. 1984; Seeman 1981).

In patients who were assessed periodically while receiving neuroleptics, TD was found to be stable over time in about 50%, about 25% of patients seemed to get worse, and the rest seemed to improve (Fornazzari et al. 1989; Yassa et al. 1984b). In general, younger patients tended to improve more readily than older ones.

Thus, TD improves when neuroleptics are discontinued in a higher percentage than when they are continued.

Subtypes

TD that resolves within 3 months of diagnosis, whether or not neuroleptics are continued, may be called reversible TD, whereas TD that persists for longer than 3 months may be called persistent TD. Persistent TD is, however, not synonymous with irreversible TD because TD may remit months or even years after its onset, especially in neuroleptic-withdrawn patients.

Clinical usefulness of subtyping TD according to its localization (orofacial versus limb-truncal) is unclear.

It is possible that there are neurochemical subtypes of TD (e.g., those with noradrenergic hyperactivity, gamma-aminobutyric acid or GABA-ergic hypoactivity). At present, however, it is difficult to identify these clinically.

Differential Diagnosis

TD needs to be distinguished from other causes of orofacial and body dyskinesias. These conditions include Huntington's disease; Wilson's disease; Sydenham's (rheumatic) chorea; thyrotoxicosis; heavy metal poisoning; dyskinesias due to other drugs such as L-dopa, bromocriptine, or amantadine; ill-fitting dentures; and spontaneous dyskinesias that are not secondary to any known brain pathology. The differentiation is based not so much on the descriptive characteristics of the abnormal movements, as on the history, physical examination, and appropriate laboratory tests (Baldessarini et al. 1980; Kane et al. 1992).

Morbidity and Mortality

In a majority of cases, TD is mild and is not associated with any significant morbidity, except from a cosmetic or psychosocial viewpoint (Kaufman 1989).

In severe cases, however, TD may be associated with medical complications such as ulcers in cheeks and tongue; ill-fitting dentures; loss of teeth; macroglossia; difficulty in walking, swallowing, or breathing; weight loss; depression; and suicidal ideation (Jeste and Wyatt 1982; Yassa and Nair 1987; Youssef and Waddington 1989). Two studies have found patients with TD to show a greater susceptibility to infections (McClelland et al. 1986; Youssef and Waddington 1987).

Excessive mortality has also been studied in relation to TD. Three studies have found that patients with TD have a higher mortality rate than patients without TD (McClelland et al. 1986; Mehta et al. 1978; Youssef and Waddington 1987); two other studies failed to confirm this finding (Kucharski et al. 1979; Yassa et al. 1984a).

Discussion

At this stage, there are two main options. One is to continue to exclude TD from DSM. The advantage of this option is the maintenance of the status quo. The disadvantage is the loss (or at least delay) of the opportunity to advance the field.

The second option is to include TD and a set of standardized diagnostic criteria for TD in DSM-IV. The advantages of this approach for clinical, research, and medicolegal purposes have been discussed earlier. The disadvantage is that no set of criteria is perfect, and there would be some criticism of the criteria proposed.

As far as the proposed criteria are concerned, the two main concerns could be a criterion for severity of TD and subtyping of TD.

Criterion for Severity of TD

The main argument in favor of including a criterion for severity of TD is that it would reduce the chances of overdiagnosis. Without a minimum level of severity, questionable cases might be included, and there could be a number of false positives. The research diagnosis of TD, according to the criteria of Schooler and

Kane (1982), does include specified minimum scores on the AIMS.

The argument on the opposite side is that although a severity criterion is useful for research purposes, it is not necessary for a clinical diagnosis of TD. In clinical practice the focus should be on diagnosis of early or mild TD. The main problem in clinical practice is underdiagnosis (and not overdiagnosis) of TD. In some cases, TD starts out at minimal or mild level of severity and then progresses to become more severe (Yassa et al. 1990). Discontinuation of neuroleptics or some other therapeutic measure at an early stage of TD development could conceivably prevent progression (and persistence) of TD in a proportion of such cases. Hence, an important goal in clinical practice should be early detection of TD. (On the other hand, a research study would generally require definitive cases of TD and would want to incorporate a criterion of minimum severity.)

The risk of overdiagnosis of TD due to a lack of a severity criterion can be reduced by ruling out conditions in the differential diagnosis and by including a criterion for a minimum duration of TD (at least 4 weeks). It is also worth noting that the DSM diagnosis of conditions such as schizophrenia and depression does not depend on minimum scores on rating scales (e.g., the Brief Psychiatry Rating Scale [Overall and Gorham 1962] or the Hamilton Rating Scale for Depression [Hamilton 1960]). For research purposes, however, investigators may use an additional criterion of a certain minimum score. Likewise, the clinical diagnosis of TD should not require a rating scale score cutoff, although researchers may use it. (Furthermore, there is no standardized rating scale that is diagnostic for TD.)

Subtyping of TD

In terms of subtyping of TD, we have already mentioned different ways of subtyping TD. The advantage of subtyping is that it would prevent viewing TD as a homogeneous condition with uniform course, prognosis, and treatment. For both clinical and research purposes, subtyping TD would be helpful.

The disadvantage of subtyping TD at this stage is that there is not enough literature on validating (or even reliably identifying) specific subtypes of TD. Defining TD subtypes in DSM-IV would suggest the availability of a far greater data base on the subtypes than there is in reality. Going from DSM-III-R, which did not include TD at all, the first step should be to define TD. In subsequent classifications (e.g., DSM-V), TD subtypes may be included if the data permit.

Recommendations

Proposed Diagnostic Criteria for TD

Table 34–1 provides proposed diagnostic criteria for TD.

Table 34–1. Proposed DSM-IV diagnostic criteria for Tardive Dyskinesia

A. Use of neuroleptics or related compounds for at least 3 months (or 1 month in patients age 60 or older) with onset of dyskinetic movements while on neuroleptics, or within a few weeks of withdrawal (i.e., within 4 weeks of withdrawal from oral medication, and 8 weeks of withdrawal from parenteral depot medication).

B. Presence of involuntary movements that are choreiform (nonrepetitive, rapid, jerky, quasipurposive), athetoid (slow, sinuous, continuous, purposeless), or rhythmic in nature. These affect at least one of the following parts: tongue, jaw, or extremities. Tremor, acute dystonia, mannerism, compulsion, and myoclonus are not a part of the tardive dyskinesia syndrome.

C. Symptoms present over a period of at least 4 weeks.

D. Not due to other causes of dyskinesia (e.g., Huntington's disease, Wilson's disease, Sydenham's chorea, hyperthyroidism, heavy metal toxicity, ill-fitting dentures, medications such as L-dopa and bromocriptine, or spontaneous dyskinesia).

Associated Features:

Worsened by stress, voluntary movements in unaffected parts of the body, stimulants, neuroleptic withdrawal, anticholinergic medications (except in cases of tardive dystonia).

Reduced by relaxation, voluntary movements in affected parts of the body.

Absent during sleep.

Masked by increasing doses of neuroleptic medications, sedatives.

Risk Factors:

The only established risk factor is old age. Other suggested risk factors include mood disorder, increased cumulative amount of neuroleptics, female gender, early development of extrapyramidal side effects, and frequent and lengthy drug-free periods.

Course:

Discontinuation of neuroleptics results in remission of tardive dyskinesia within 3 months in about one-third of patients. The longer the patients can be maintained off neuroleptics, the greater the chances of remission of tardive dyskinesia. Continuation of neuroleptics has variable effects and may cause aggravation of tardive dyskinesia in a minority of patients.

References

American Psychiatric Association: Diagnostic and Statistical Manual of Mental Disorders, 3rd Edition, Revised. Washington, DC, American Psychiatric Association, 1987

Baldessarini RJ: Tardive Dyskinesia (Task Force Report No 18). Washington, DC, American Psychiatric Association, 1980

Barnes TRE: The present status of tardive dyskinesia and akathisia in the treatment of schizophrenia. Psychiatr Dev 4:301–309, 1987

Chouinard G, Annable L, Mercier P, et al: A five-year follow-up study of tardive dyskinesia. Psychopharmacol Bull 22:259–263, 1986

Fornazzari S, Grossman H, Thornton J, et al: Tardive dyskinesia: a five-year follow-up. Can J Psychiatry 34:700–703, 1989
Gardos G, Samu I, Kallos M: Absence of severe TD in Hungarian schizophrenic outpatients. Psychopharmacology 71:29–34, 1980
Gardos G, Cole JO, Salomon M: Clinical forms of severe tardive dyskinesia. Am J Psychiatry 144:895–902, 1987
Glazer WM, Moore DC, Schooler NR: Tardive dyskinesia: a discontinuation study. Arch Gen Psychiatry 41:623–627, 1984
Hamilton M: A rating scale for depression. J Neurol Neurosurg Psychiatry 23:56–62, 1960
Harris MJ, Panton D, Krull AJ, et al: A high incidence of tardive dyskinesia in older psychiatric outpatients on low does of neuroleptics. Psychopharmacol Bull 28:87–92, 1992
Heaton H: Plaintiffs win half of suits involving tardive dyskinesia. Clinical Psychiatry News 18:12–17, 1990
Jeste DV, Wyatt RJ: Understanding and Treating Tardive Dyskinesia. New York, Guilford, 1982
Jeste DV, Lohr JB, Clark K, et al: Pharmacological treatment of tardive dyskinesia in the 1980s. J Clin Psychopharmacol 8:38S–48S, 1988
Kane JM, Smith JM: Tardive dyskinesia: prevalence and risk factors, 1959–1979. Arch Gen Psychiatry 39:473–481, 1982
Kane JM, Woerner M, Weinhold P, et al: A progressive study of tardive dyskinesia development: preliminary results. J Clin Psychopharmacol 2:345–349, 1982
Kane JM, Woerner M, Weinhold P, et al: Incidence of tardive dyskinesia: five-year data from a prospective study. Psychopharmacol Bull 20:387–389, 1984
Kane JM, Woerner M, Borenstein M, et al: Integrating incidence and prevalence of tardive dyskinesia. Psychopharmacol Bull 22:254–258, 1986
Kane JM, Woerner M, Lieberman J: Tardive dyskinesia: prevalence, incidence and risk factors. J Clin Psychopharmacol 8 (suppl):52S–56S, 1988
Kane JM, Jeste DV, Barnes TRE, et al: Report of the American Psychiatric Association Task Force on Tardive Dyskinesia. Washington, DC, American Psychiatric Press, 1992
Kaufman DM: Facial dyskinesias. Psychosomatics 30:263–269, 1989
Klawans HL, Tanner CM, Barr A: The reversibility of "permanent" tardive dyskinesia. Clin Neuropharmacol 7:153–159, 1984
Kucharski LT, Smith JM, Dunn DD: Mortality and tardive dyskinesia. Am J Psychiatry 136:1228, 1979
McClelland HA, Dulta D, Metcalfe A, et al: Mortality and facial dyskinesia. Br J Psychiatry 148:310–316, 1986
Mehta D, Mallya A, Volavka J: Mortality of patients with tardive dyskinesia. Am J Psychiatry 135:371–372, 1978
Mukherjee S, Rosen AM, Cardenas C: Tardive dyskinesia in outpatients: a study of prevalence and association with demographic, clinical and drug history variables. Arch Gen Psychiatry 39:466–469, 1982
Overall JE, Gorham DR: The Brief Psychiatric Rating Scale. Psychol Rep 10:799–812, 1962
Rosen AM, Mukherjee S, Olarte S: Perception of tardive dyskinesia in outpatients receiving maintenance neuroleptics. Am J Psychiatry 139:372–374, 1982
Saltz BL, Kane JM, Woerner MG: Prospective study of tardive dyskinesia in the elderly. Psychopharmacol Bull 25:52–56, 1989
Schooler NR, Kane JM: Research diagnosis for tardive dyskinesia. Arch Gen Psychiatry 39:486–487, 1982

Seeman MV: Tardive dyskinesia: two-year recovery. Compr Psychiatry 22:189–192, 1981

Singh H, Simpson GM: Tardive dyskinesia: clinical features, in Tardive Dyskinesia: Biological Mechanisms and Clinical Aspects. Edited by Wolf ME, Mosnaim AD. Washington, DC, American Psychiatric Press, 1988, pp 67–86

Smith JM, Oswald WT, Kucharski T: Tardive dyskinesia: age and sex differences in hospitalized schizophrenics. Psychopharmacology 58:207–211, 1978

Tancredi LR: Malpractice and tardive dyskinesia: a conceptual dilemma. J Clin Psychopharmacol 8:71S–76S, 1988

Weiner WJ, Lang AE: Movement Disorders: A Comprehensive Survey. New York, Futura, 1989

Yassa R, Jeste DV: Gender differences in tardive dyskinesia: a critical review of the literature. Schizophr Bull 18:701–715, 1992

Yassa R, Nair NPV: The effect of tardive dyskinesia on body weight. Acta Psychiatr Scand 75:209–211, 1987

Yassa R, Mobelsky H, Dimitry R, et al: Mortality rate in tardive dyskinesia. Am J Psychiatry 141:1018–1019, 1984a

Yassa R, Nair V, Schwartz G: Tardive dyskinesia: a two-year follow-up study. Psychosomatics 25:852–855, 1984b

Yassa R, Nastase C, Camille Y, et al: Tardive dyskinesia in a psychogeriatric population, in Tardive Dyskinesia: Biological Mechanisms and Clinical Aspects. Edited by Wolf ME, Mosnaim AD. Washington, DC, American Psychiatric Press, 1988, pp 123–133

Yassa R, Nair NPV, Iskandar H, et al: Factors in the development of severe forms of tardive dyskinesia. Am J Psychiatry 147:1156–1163, 1990

Yesavage JA, Becker J, Werner PD, et al: Serum level monitoring of thiothixene in schizophrenia: acute single-dose levels at fixed doses. Am J Psychiatry 139:174–178, 1982

Youssef HA, Waddington JL: Morbidity and mortality in tardive dyskinesia: associations in chronic schizophrenia. Acta Psychiatr Scand 75:74–77, 1987

Youssef HA, Waddington YL: Characterization of abnormal respiratory movements in schizophrenic, bipolar and mentally handicapped patients with typical tardive dyskinesia. J Clin Psychopharmacol 4:55–59, 1989

Chapter 35

Lithium Tremor

Alan J. Gelenberg, M.D.
James W. Jefferson, M.D.

Statement of the Issues

In this chapter, we address the issue of whether a diagnosis of lithium tremor should be included in DSM-IV by reviewing data on the nature, incidence, consequences, and treatment of tremor caused by lithium therapy.

Significance of the Issues

Tremor is a common side effect of lithium therapy. It can be embarrassing and may interfere with daily activities. It may cause noncompliance. Many knowledgeable clinicians believe that when it is recognized, however, it can be effectively managed, thus allowing lithium treatment to continue.

Inclusion of this diagnosis in DSM-IV could lead to enhanced recognition of the syndrome and, therefore, improve treatment of patients requiring lithium. An alternative classification would be to include this side effect, along with other movement disorders caused by psychotropic medications, in a separate section – "other clinically significant problems that may be a focus of diagnosis and treatment."

Methods

The computerized data base of the Lithium Information Center (Department of Psychiatry, University Hospital, 600 Highland Avenue, Madison, Wisconsin 53792) contains more than 21,000 references to lithium and its role in medicine. The data base was searched using the subject and title term *lithium tremor.* A printout containing 300 references was generated. Pertinent articles from this listing were obtained from the information center to address issues related to definition, recognition, risk factors, impact, and treatment of lithium-induced tremor.

Results

In 1959, Schou wrote

> A fine tremor of the hands is extremely frequent and may be observed even in patients who receive very small lithium doses. When present in slight degree it must be considered entirely innocuous. If, on the other hand, the tremor becomes so pronounced that it interferes with the patients' eating or needlework, or if the lower jaw also starts to tremble, one may usually take these symptoms as a warning that the lithium concentration in blood and tissues is about to reach toxic levels. (pp. 72–73)

Tremor caused by therapeutic amounts of lithium is common, often socially embarrassing and occupationally compromising, and sometimes the reason for noncompliance with treatment. This tremor may worsen or generalize as serum lithium levels approach toxic levels. Tremor of another type is characteristic of the permanent neurological impairment that may follow lithium poisoning.

Defining Lithium Tremor

"Tremor is involuntary movement characterized by rhythmic oscillations of a part of the body. The differential diagnosis is lengthy and complex" (Hallett 1986, p. 583). Hallett classified lithium tremor as a "postural tremor" and subcategorized it as an "exaggerated physiologic tremor" with a frequency of 8–12 Hz in the hands. Other factors that increase physiologic tremor are emotion, exercise fatigue, hypoglycemia, thyrotoxicosis, pheochromocytoma, hypothermia, alcohol withdrawal, and a wide variety of drugs (Hallett 1986) and should be considered part of the differential diagnosis of lithium tremor (and as potential contributors to the severity of an existing lithium tremor).

A closely related postural tremor is essential tremor, the frequency of which ranges from 4 to 9 Hz. According to Hallett (1986), differentiating exaggerated postural tremor from essential tremor is often difficult, and some authors consider the former a subtype of the latter. The tremor caused by lithium is usually classified in one or both of these categories and distinguished from tremors at rest such as those seen with parkinsonism (usually a 4–5 Hz frequency tremor), other postural tremors such as those of cerebellar origin, and intention tremors commonly seen with cerebellar disease. Van Putten (1978) described six patients with either preexisting essential tremor or a family history of essential tremor who developed disabling tremors at relatively low serum lithium levels (0.5–0.8 mEq/L). One patient had "tremor so severe he could no longer write or drink from a cup and his voice became quavery" (p. 27).

Tyrer and colleagues (1981) reported that chronic lithium therapy shifts tremor frequency from the range of exaggerated physiologic tremor *toward* the parkinsonism range. When compared to age- and sex-matched control subjects, 23 patients on lithium for 1/2 to 9 years (mean, 43 months) had a mean tremor frequency that was about 1/2 Hz slower ($P < .05$). This observation is consistent with other reports of extrapyramidal side effects associated with lithium use (Jefferson et al. 1987).

Prevalence of Lithium Tremor

Several factors affect the reported prevalence of lithium tremor. First, studies usually assume tremor not to be present prior to taking lithium, yet Vestergaard and colleagues (1988) found that 5% (24/471) of patients complained of hand tremor at baseline. Therefore, studies may overestimate the true prevalence of lithium tremor.

Next, studies tend to base estimates of tremor on patient complaints (subjective) rather than observation (objective). Which approach is more accurate is not known. It is generally assumed that the absence of tremor during evaluation does not exclude a tremor from being present (and possibly troublesome) at other times. On the other hand, physical examination for tremor may be positive in the absence of subjective complaints. Also, the frequency of tremor may be mood-state dependent. Bone and colleagues (1980) found tremor to be more common in noneuthymic patients as compared with euthymic patients who were taking lithium as the only medication (50% versus 24.6%).

Next, studies may not mention the presence of other tremor-producing medications that might either cause or contribute to a tremor in a patient taking lithium. Bone and colleagues (1980) found that tremor prevalence in the presence of lithium plus other psychotropic medication exceeded that associated with lithium alone in both euthymic (61.9% versus 24.6%) and noneuthymic (62.2% versus 50%) patients.

Finally, in a study of 265 lithium clinic patients, Simhandl and colleagues (1988) found that although 23.7% of patients taking lithium listed tremor as a subjective complaint, when they were interviewed independently by two doctors to determine whether the complaint was truly lithium related, the percentages dropped to 13.9% (doctor 1) and 8.6% (doctor 2).

Goodwin and Jamison (1990) reported a wide range of tremor complaints—from 4% to 65%—across 13 studies with a pooled sample size of more than 1,000 patients. Although the studies listed were not all-inclusive (examples of omitted reports include Jarrett et al. 1975; Simhandl et al. 1988; Spaulding et al. 1975; Vestergaard et al. 1988), they provided a reasonable representation of the prevalence of tremor.

Also of importance is whether a tremor is truly troublesome or merely an observation made in passing. Again, there is a paucity of data. Vestergaard and colleagues (1980) reported that 45% of 237 patients on lithium for at least 6 months described a tremor that was socially embarrassing or professionally troublesome. Many clinicians, however, find this figure to be exceptionally high. Indeed, the pooled percentage for any complaint of tremor in 1,094 patients was only 26.6%. Jamison and Goodwin (1990) reported that 32% of patients felt that incoordination or tremor was "very important" and likely to lead to noncompliance. This figure represents patient speculation rather than the actual occurrence of noncompliance because of tremor. Although it is generally accepted that tremor has caused noncompliance in a substantial number of lithium patients, quantitative data to support and better define this opinion are not available.

A variety of factors have been identified as increasing the risk of lithium tremor. These include increasing age, high serum lithium levels, antidepressant drugs, neuroleptic drugs, excessive caffeine intake, personal or family history of tremor, presence of alcoholism, and associated anxiety. Several authors (Bech et al. 1979; Simhandl et al. 1988) did not find increasing age to be a factor. The frequency of tremor complaints appears to decrease with duration of lithium treatment (Vestergaard et al. 1988).

Treatment of Lithium Tremor

Nontoxic lithium tremor is usually well tolerated and often improves with time on lithium. Additional treatment measures include reduction in serum lithium level (at the risk of losing the therapeutic effect), single daily dosing, or a change in lithium preparation. It should be noted, however, that Vestergaard and colleagues (1988) did not find a correlation between tremor frequency and lithium preparation or number of daily doses. Favorably modifying factors that aggravate physiologic or essential tremor should also be of help. These include reducing or eliminating other drugs that could be worsening the tremor (e.g., caffeine, neuroleptics, antidepressants, beta agonists) and treating anxiety. Although a reduction in caffeine intake would be expected to improve a tremor, under extreme conditions the opposite may occur. Caffeine, like other methylated xanthines, increases renal lithium clearance. It is possible that eliminating large amounts of caffeine would decrease renal lithium clearance, increase serum lithium level, and worsen a tremor (Jefferson 1988).

Beta receptor-blocking drugs have been the agents of choice for treatment of lithium tremor. Various beta-blockers have been used successfully, but most reports have involved single cases or a small number of patients administered drug openly. For example, Perez-Cruet and Ananth (1975) treated nine patients in open fashion with 30–80 mg/day of propranolol and found good control of tremor in all immediately after the first dose. Kellett et al. (1975) gave 15 patients propranolol

(40 mg), practolol (120 mg) (a beta-blocker that does not readily cross the blood-brain barrier), or placebo in random order on 3 consecutive days with nonblind objective measurements. Both drugs produced *more* tremor than placebo.

Another study (Brosteanu et al. 1977) involved 15 patients in a double-blind, crossover comparison of oxprenolol (80 mg twice daily) and placebo and found that the former was more effective. Kirk and colleagues (1973) compared propranolol (30–80 mg/day) to placebo in a single-blind, crossover trial and found benefit from propranolol. Lapierre (1976) treated five patients openly with 30–40 mg/day of propranolol, and all responded positively. Studies with metoprolol (a cardioselective drug that enters the central nervous system) have been both positive (Gaby et al. 1983 [$N = 2$], Zubenko et al. 1984 [$N = 4$]) and negative (North and Roerig 1982 [$N = 1$]). Beta-blockers with poor central nervous system penetration have also been reported to be beneficial in open studies—for example, nadolol (Kruse et al. 1984 [$N = 6$]) and atenolol (Salzman 1982 [$N = 1$])—suggesting a peripheral mechanism of action.

All in all, there have not been well-designed, double-blind, placebo-controlled studies of adequate sample size to confirm the value of beta-blockers for treating lithium tremor. Nonetheless, the usefulness of these drugs for treating similar neurological tremors (essential tremor) has been more firmly established (Hubble et al. 1989), and clinical experience with beta-blockers for lithium tremor support their continued recommendation.

Schou and Vestergaard (1987) suggested that beta-blockers be used on an "as needed" basis rather than a scheduled basis because of observations that propranolol lowers glomerular filtration rate and may be associated with a 19% reduction in renal lithium clearance.

Another drug that may be of value in treating lithium tremor is primidone. It has been shown to be as effective as propranolol in treating essential tremor (Hubble et al. 1989), but it has not been formally studied for lithium tremor. In a case report, a woman with tricyclic-lithium tremor responded dramatically to treatment with 62.5 mg/day of primidone (Goumentouk et al. 1989).

Lieb and Horrobin (1981) claimed that "there can be no doubt that the treatment with essential fatty acids is successful in controlling tremors caused by lithium, alcohol withdrawal and familial essential tremor" (p. 536). Seven patients with lithium tremor responded to treatment with safflower oil or evening primrose oil. The study, however, was uncontrolled, and only two of the lithium patients were described. Schou (1980), on the other hand, had negative results using safflower oil in five patients with lithium tremor and did not feel a double-blind study was worth pursuing.

Finally, Cummings and colleagues (1988) described a patient whose tremor and ankle edema improved when treated with 16 mEq/day of oral potassium, recurred when potassium was stopped, and improved again when it was restarted. Whether oral potassium supplementation is beneficial to lithium tremor requires further study.

Tremor and Lithium Toxicity

Severe tremor associated with lithium toxicity was recognized as early as 1898 by Kolipinski. In a toxic octogenarian "the upper extremities, particularly the hands, presented a constant fine tremor of acute onset and so severe he could no longer write his name" (p. 4). The patient recovered completely 3–4 days after discontinuation of lithium. As lithium intoxication develops, the exaggerated physiologic tremor commonly seen in the hands at therapeutic levels may become more exaggerated and coarser and may generalize to other parts of the body.

If permanent neurological complications follow lithium intoxication, a cerebellar tremor is commonly seen. In fact, "the type of permanent impairment most characteristic of lithium intoxication is cerebellar in nature with findings of ataxia, dysarthria, nystagmus, and intention tremor" (Jefferson 1991, p. 21).

Summary

Although tremor is usually considered a benign, well-tolerated side effect of therapeutic amounts of lithium, it is sometimes problematic socially and occupationally. It is assumed that tremor of this type is sometimes the cause of noncompliance with lithium therapy, although just how often this occurs is not known. Evaluating patients for lithium tremor on a regular basis is highly recommended, not only because the tremor may cause personal discomfort and interfere with functioning, but also because a worsening of tremor may be indicative of impending lithium intoxication.

Nontoxic lithium tremor may improve spontaneously over time, despite continued lithium treatment. If treatment intervention is necessary, there are a number of nonpharmacologic and pharmacologic approaches that may be of benefit. Beta-blocking drugs have been widely recommended for treating lithium tremor, and although their benefit has not been firmly substantiated in well-designed clinical studies, clinical experience supports their continued recommendation. Having reviewed the literature on lithium tremor, we found that there is less known about its role in noncompliance and about the effectiveness of drugs to treat it than previously believed.

Discussion

One advantage of including lithium tremor in DSM-IV is the likelihood of enhancing clinicians' recognition of this side effect and thereby improving its management. The appearance of lithium tremor can herald the onset of lithium toxicity. The generally accepted clinical wisdom is that lithium tremor is common and should respond to lowering the lithium blood level or introducing a contra-active agent, such as a beta-blocker. On the other hand, as our literature review indicates, the estimated frequency of this adverse reaction varies widely, and its effects on patients are unclear. Furthermore, there are many unknowns about the factors that influence lithium tremor, and knowledge about its treatment is much less solidly grounded than most clinicians believe. It is possible that inclusion of this category in the psychiatric nomenclature should await further systematic research. An additional argument against the inclusion of this and other side effects in the mainstream psychiatric nomenclature is the potentially endless stream of adverse drug reactions that would crowd and thereby dilute psychiatric diagnostic categories.

Recommendations

We believe that drug-induced side effects should not be part of the main body of DSM-IV but, if included at all, they should be in a section separate from the primary diagnostic categories. Furthermore, although simple criteria for lithium tremor can be proposed, the data base at this time is insufficient for anything but a very tentative entry. Possible criteria for diagnosing lithium tremor are presented in Table 35–1.

For future research, we believe that a collaborative multicenter study of many patients taking lithium could standardize the diagnostic criteria for lithium tremor

Table 35–1. Proposed DSM-IV diagnostic criteria for Lithium Tremor

1. The patient has a fine tremor (i.e., a regular, rhythmic oscillation of a body part about a point) of about 8–12 cycles per second, most easily observed when the affected body part is held in a sustained posture (e.g., hands outstretched, mouth held open).
2. The tremor bears an obvious relation to lithium therapy (e.g., it was not present before lithium treatment was instituted, it correlates positively with the serum lithium concentration, and/or it disappears after discontinuation of lithium).
3. If the patient has a preexisting, nonpharmacologically induced tremor (i.e., a "benign," "essential," "familial," or "senile" tremor) that worsens during lithium treatment, it may be considered a lithium-aggravated tremor but not, strictly speaking, a lithium tremor.
4. If the patient describes a tremor consistent with the criteria above, but the examiner does not directly observe the tremor, the examiner should ask the patient to try to recreate the situation in which the tremor occurred (e.g., drinking from a cup and saucer). If the examiner still does not see the tremor, the designation may be made "*possible* lithium tremor."

(probably working with neurological consultants), identify correlates (e.g., serum lithium levels), and address putative treatments (especially propranolol) in a rigorous, double-blind, and random-assignment fashion.

References

Bech P, Thomsen J, Prytz S, et al: The profile and severity of lithium-induced side effects in mentally healthy subjects. Neuropsychobiology 5:160–166, 1979

Bone S, Roose SP, Dunner DL, et al: Incidence of side effects in patients on long-term lithium therapy. Am J Psychiatry 137:103–104, 1980

Brosteanu ER, Floru L, Kaiser H: Double-blind trial with oxprenolol versus placebo in the treatment of lithium-induced tremor, in Beta-Blockers and the Central Nervous System. Edited by Kielholz P. Stuttgart, Wien, Hans Huber, 1977

Cummings MA, Cummings KL, Haviland MG: Use of potassium to treat lithium's side effects. Am J Psychiatry 145:895, 1988

Gaby NS, Lefkowitz DS, Israel JR: Treatment of lithium tremor with metoprolol. Am J Psychiatry 140:593–595, 1983

Goodwin FK, Jamison KR: Manic Depressive Illness. New York, Oxford University Press, 1990

Goumentouk AD, Hurwitz TA, Zis AP: Primidone in drug-induced tremor. J Clin Psychopharmacol 9:451, 1989

Hallett M: Differential diagnosis of tremor, in Handbook of Clinical Neurology, Vol 49. Edited by Vinken PJ, Bruyn GW, Klawans HL. New York, Elsevier, 1986

Hubble JP, Busenbark KL, Koller WC: Essential tremor: a review. Clin Neuropharmacol 12:453–482, 1989

Jamison KR, Goodwin FK: Medication compliance, in Manic-Depressive Illness. Edited by Jamison KR, Goodwin FK. New York, Oxford University Press, 1990

Jarrett DB, Serry J, Burrows GD: Lithium-induced tremor. Med J Aust 1:21, 1975

Jefferson JW: Lithium tremor and caffeine intake: two cases of drinking less and shaking more. J Clin Psychiatry 49:72–73, 1988

Jefferson JW: Lithium poisoning. Emergency Care Quarterly 7:18–28, 1991

Jefferson JW, Greist JH, Ackerman DL, et al: Lithium Encyclopedia for Clinical Practice, 2nd Edition. Washington, DC, American Psychiatric Press, 1987

Kellett JM, Metcalfe M, Bailey J, et al: Beta blockade in lithium tremor. J Neurol Neurosurg Psychiatry 38:719–721, 1975

Kirk L, Baastrup PC, Schou M: Propranolol treatment of lithium-induced tremor. Lancet 2:1086–1087, 1973

Kolipinski L: Note on some toxic effects from the use of citrate of lithium tablets. Md Med J 40:4–5, 1898

Kruse JM, Ereshefsky L, Scavone M: Treatment of lithium-induced tremor with nadolol. Clinical Pharmacology 3:299–301, 1984

Lapierre YD: Control of lithium tremor with propranolol. Can Med Assoc J 114:619–624, 1976

Lieb J, Horrobin DF: Treatment of lithium-induced tremor and familial essential tremor with essential fatty acids. Prog Lipid Res 20:535–537, 1981

North DS, Roerig JL: Ineffectiveness of metoprolol in controlling lithium-induced tremor. Clinical Pharmacology 1:264–266, 1982

Perez-Cruet J, Ananth J: Control of lithium tremors not due to lithium intoxication with propranolol. Clin Res 23:223A, 1975

Salzman C: A primer on geriatric psychopharmacology. Am J Psychiatry 139:67–74, 1982

Schou M: Lithium in psychiatric therapy: stock-taking after ten years. Psychopharmacology 1:65–78, 1959

Schou M: Linoleic acid in the treatment of lithium-induced tremor: a pilot trial with negative outcome. Prostaglandins Medicine 5:343–344, 1980

Schou M, Vestergaard P: Use of propranolol during lithium treatment: an inquiry and a suggestion. Pharmacopsychiatry 20:131, 1987

Simhandl CH, Thau K, Spiel CH, et al: Side effects (self rating and objective rating) in 265 patients under lithium long-term therapy, in Lithium: Inorganic Pharmacology and Psychiatric Use. Edited by Birch NJ. Oxford, England, IRL Press, 1988

Spaulding SW, Ramey JN, Burrow GN, et al: Antithyroid synergism of iodides in patients on chronic lithium therapy. Clin Res 23:243A, 1975

Tyrer P, Lee I, Trotter C: Physiological characteristics of tremor after chronic lithium therapy. Br J Psychiatry 139:59–61, 1981

Van Putten T: Lithium-induced disabling tremor. Psychosomatics 19:27, 31, 1978

Vestergaard P, Amdisen A, Schou M: Clinically significant side effects of lithium treatment: a survey of 237 patients in long-term treatment. Acta Psychiatr Scand 62:193–200, 1980

Vestergaard P, Poulstrup I, Schou M: Prospective studies on a lithium cohort. Acta Psychiatr Scand 78:434–441, 1988

Zubenko GS, Cohen BM, Lipinski JF: Comparison of metoprolol and propranolol in the treatment of lithium tremor. Psychiatry Res 11:163–164, 1984

Section V

Sleep Disorders

Contents

Section V
Sleep Disorders

Introduction to Section V

Sleep Disorders

David J. Kupfer, M.D.
Daniel J. Buysse, M.D.
Eric A. Nofzinger, M.D.
Charles F. Reynolds III, M.D.

The purpose of this introduction is to provide an executive summary of the proceedings and initial proposals of the DSM-IV Work Group on Sleep Disorders. To present a brief overview of the options and proposals presented in the *DSM-IV Options Book* (American Psychiatric Association 1991), along with their rationale and support, we have chosen to present the results of our work within the historical context of specific sleep-disorder nosologies published over the past 13 years. We also indicate which issues were identified for each disorder and the rationale for why each was chosen. Findings from the ongoing DSM-IV field trial on the diagnosis of insomnia will be published elsewhere.

The field of sleep disorders medicine is in its relative infancy, having existed only for about 25 years. Throughout this period, the field has fortunately remained truly interdisciplinary, including specialists from psychiatry, psychology, neurology, pulmonary medicine, and otolaryngology. These two factors have led to special challenges in the development of nosologies for the classification of sleep disorders. Nevertheless, a good deal of progress has been made, due in part to important lessons learned from previous versions of the DSM.

Issues in the Classification of Sleep Disorders

As we have pointed out elsewhere (Buysse et al. 1993), many of the problems confronting sleep disorders classifications are similar to those faced by more traditional classifications of mental disorders. First, "sleep disorders" include a wide variety of conditions, ranging from those with well-defined clinical and pathophysiological features (such as narcolepsy and obstructive sleep apnea syndrome) to those with less certain validity (such as the various types of insomnia).

Similar to classifications for mental disorders, sleep disorders nosologies must confront heterogeneous clinical constructs, evaluating the differential weight of supporting evidence for various disorders. In addition, no structural pathology has been identified for most sleep disorders, meaning that classification usually rests on clinical features and abnormal physiology.

A second problem facing sleep disorders nosologies is that of "caseness": when do clinical features constitute a disorder? For instance, this problem is especially relevant to the sleep symptoms of mental disorders. When does the symptom become a disorder in its own right? Similarly, the boundary between a "long sleeper" and a patient with "idiopathic" or "primary" hypersomnia may be very difficult to discern on clinical grounds. Likewise, periodic limb movements can occur during sleep in persons without sleep disorders as well as patients complaining of insomnia or excessive sleepiness, but there is no precise threshold for how many limb movements constitute abnormality, which may differ at different points in the life cycle. Indeed, most subjective and objective measures of sleep show wide variability even in the normal population.

A third problem for sleep disorders classifications is the lack of data supporting the interrater or test-retest reliability for specific diagnoses. In this sense, sleep disorders classification lags behind the classification of other mental disorders. However, in terms of establishing empirical validity of specific disorders, the field is in some ways ahead. For example, evidence of genetic linkage in narcolepsy is much stronger than for most medical or mental disorders. In addition, laboratory-based sleep studies (polysomnography) allows for objective quantification of variables, such as sleepiness, sleep disruption, and sleep-disordered breathing, which is not possible for most other mental symptoms or disorders.

Previous and Current Classifications (Table 1)

Comparative features of major sleep disorders classifications are presented in Table 1. The first widely used classification of sleep disorders was published in 1979 by the Association of Sleep Disorders Centers (ASDC). This system included four major sections of disorders, organized on the basis of primary presenting symptom. The individual categories were derived from a consensus of expert opinion. In summary, the major problems of the ASDC nosology were 1) overlap and redundancy, 2) the lack of operationalized diagnostic criteria using clinical symptoms or laboratory findings, and 3) the lack of data on the reliability and validity of most ASDC diagnoses.

The ASDC classification has been superseded by the International Classification of Sleep Disorders (ICSD) (American Sleep Disorders Association 1990). Like

Table 1. Classification systems for sleep disorders

Attribute	ASDC	ICSD	ICD-10	DSM-III-R	DSM-IV
Derivation of categories	Expert opinion and consensus	Expert opinion and consensus	Expert opinion and consensus	Expert and psychiatric opinion	Expert opinion and consensus; literature reviews
Organizing principles	Major presenting symptom	Pathophysiology and presumed etiology	Presumed etiology	Pathophysiology and presenting symptoms	Pathophysiology and presumed etiology
Major categories	Disorders of initiating and maintaining sleep; disorders of excessive somnolence; disorders of the sleep-wake schedule; parasomnias	Dyssomnias: intrinsic, extrinsic, circadian rhythm sleep disorders; parasomnias; medical/psychiatric sleep disorders; proposed sleep disorders	Psychogenic sleep disorders; organic sleep disorders	Dyssomnias: insomnias, hypersomnias, sleep-wake schedule disorders; parasomnias	Primary sleep disorders: dyssomnias, parasomnias; sleep disorders related to another mental disorder; secondary sleep disorders; substance-induced sleep disorders
Breath of categories	Detailed	Detailed	General	General	Intermediate
Operational clinical criteria	No	Yes	Yes, for sleep disorders due to emotional causes	Yes	Yes
Operational polysomnographic criteria	No	Yes (for most disorders)	No	No	No, except for breathing-related sleep disorder
Multiaxial diagnosis	No	Yes, with different axes than DSM	No	Yes	Yes
Reliability data available	No, but prevalence data available	No	No	Yes (unpublished)	From DSM-IV field trial
Number of distinct categories (including subtypes)	68	88	18	14	23

Note. ASDC = Association of Sleep Disorders Centers. ICSD = International Classification of Sleep Disorders.

its predecessor, the ICSD is based on a consensus of expert opinion. Unlike its predecessor, the ICSD constitutes its major categories on the basis of pathophysiology and presumed etiology. The dyssomnias are disorders that produce either difficulty initiating or maintaining sleep, or excessive sleepiness; they are further divided into disorders originating from "intrinsic" physiological disturbances, "extrinsic" factors, and circadian rhythms disturbances. The parasomnias are abnormal behaviors or physiological events that occur during sleep, but do not produce a primary complaint of insomnia or excessive sleepiness. The other two major categories in ICSD are sleep disorders arising from medical or psychiatric disorders and proposed sleep disorders. In the ICSD, no disorder is represented more than once (unlike the ASDC classification). Furthermore, the ICSD establishes operational criteria based on clinical and polysomnographic data, and it includes codes for severity and duration of the disorders.

The International Classification of Diseases, 9th Edition (ICD-9-CM) (World Health Organization 1980) and 10th Edition (ICD-10-M) (World Health Organization 1992), set forth fairly general classification schemes for sleep disorders. These are broadly divided into sleep disorders due to emotional causes and organic sleep disorders. The ICD includes very general categories relative to ICSD.

DSM-III-R (American Psychiatric Association 1987) was the first edition of the DSM to include a specific section for sleep disorders within the text. (DSM-III [American Psychiatric Association 1980] contained a summary version of the ASDC classification as an appendix.) DSM-III-R organizes sleep disorders into dyssomnias (disturbances in the amount, timing, or quality of sleep) and parasomnias (abnormal events occurring during sleep, or at the threshold of sleep and wakefulness, in which the predominant complaint is the disturbance itself). Dyssomnias are further divided into insomnias, hypersomnias, and sleep-wake schedule disturbances. DSM-III-R preceded ICSD and resembles it in several respects, including the organization into dyssomnias and parasomnias, the use of specified clinical criteria, and pathophysiological organization. It differs in the scope of disorders represented and the absence of specific criteria based on polysomnography. Although DSM-III-R appears to be applicable and "user-friendly" in most psychiatric settings, it has been criticized by sleep medicine specialists for not specifically including some well-recognized sleep disorders, such as narcolepsy and sleep apnea, and for "lumping" disorders into overly broad categories.

For the sleep disorders section of DSM-IV, an overriding question has been whether a more detailed classification (such as ICSD) or a more general one (such as DSM-III-R) should be adopted. The literature reviews for DSM-IV support the clinical utility and validity of some more specific disorders, such as narcolepsy and sleep apnea syndrome, while maintaining a more conservative stance on other disorders, such as subtypes of insomnia. This overall general versus specific tension is especially obvious in considering insomnia diagnoses (Reynolds et al. 1991). On the one hand there is a danger of reifying the general DSM-III-R category of "primary insomnia" into a single disorder, and providing insufficient attention to legitimate subtypes of insomnia. On the other hand, although it is likely that many factors can contribute to insomnia disorders, it is less obvious whether each of these factors could be conceptualized as a separate disorder, as in ICSD.

Analysis of data supports the notion that the general classification of DSM-III-R is associated with greater interrater reliability than a more specific system such as ASDC (D. J. Buysse, C. F. Reynolds, D. J. Kupfer, unpublished observations, 1991). Other data demonstrate that the use of a structured sleep disorders interview for DSM-III-R produces excellent rates of test-retest and interrater reliability (Schramm et al. 1993). These issues are addressed in the DSM-IV insomnia field trial.

Organizing Principles

The proposed DSM-IV classification of sleep disorders includes a larger number of disorders than DSM-III-R, but far fewer than ICSD (Table 2). Like ICSD, DSM-IV is organized by pathophysiology and presumed etiology, although the general categories differ. Basically, DSM-IV would include four general categories: primary sleep disorders, sleep disorders related to another mental disorder, secondary sleep

Table 2. Proposed DSM-IV categories for sleep disorders

- Primary sleep disorders
  - Dyssomnias
    - Primary insomnia
    - Primary hypersomnia
    - Narcolepsy
    - Breathing-related sleep disorder
    - Circadian rhythms sleep disorder[a]
    - Dyssomnia NOS
  - Parasomnias
    - Nightmare disorder
    - Sleep terror disorder
    - Sleepwalking disorder
    - Parasomnia NOS
- Sleep disorders related to another mental disorder
  - Insomnia related to Axis I or Axis II disorder
  - Hypersomnia related to Axis I or Axis II disorder
- Secondary sleep disorder due to an Axis III condition
  - Insomnia type
  - Hypersomnia type
  - Parasomnia type
  - Mixed type
- Substance-induced sleep disorder
  - Insomnia type
  - Hypersomnia type
  - Parasomnia type

Note. NOS = not otherwise specified.
[a]Two options for specific types are under consideration.

disorders (due to an Axis III disorder), and substance-induced sleep disorders. This organization makes the sleep disorders section compatible with other sections of DSM-IV. Within the four major categories, DSM-IV would include subsections for dyssomnias and parasomnias. Specific disorders with well-established clinical validity, such as narcolepsy and breathing-related sleep disorder (sleep apnea), would be included. Like DSM-III-R, DSM-IV would rely on clinical criteria and would not require specific polysomnographic criteria except for breathing-related sleep disorder. Polysomnographic characteristics for other disorders would also be discussed in the text.

The proposals concerning sleep terror disorder and sleepwalking disorder are not covered by a literature review, because no substantive changes were proposed for them in DSM-IV, given the absence of new research that would have supported such changes.

Issues for Each Sleep Disorder

In the following, the specific issues identified for each disorder and the rationale for the choice of each are summarized.

Primary Sleep Disorders: Dyssomnias

F51.0 Primary Insomnia

DSM-III-R uses the term *primary insomnia* to indicate insomnia that lasts longer than 1 month and is not related to other diagnosable medical or mental disorders. This has caused controversy among psychiatric sleep researchers and clinicians, some of whom have objected that the term is difficult to interpret and groups together patients with widely differing complaints of insomnia.

The controversy revolves around three major issues: 1) the extent to which sleep disorders, particularly those involving insomnia, can be classified into subtypes; 2) the feasibility and utility of more differentiated versus general classifications in the practice of psychiatry; and 3) the value and place of the sleep laboratory in the differential diagnosis of insomnia complaints.

Although the Work Group acknowledges the clinical utility of the ICSD subtypes of primary insomnia (childhood-onset, psychophysiological, and subjective insomnia without objective findings), as well as their probable heuristic value, it appears that the available empirical evidence on the reliability and validity of these subtypes may not yet provide a compelling basis for abandoning the DSM-III-R concept of primary insomnia (Reynolds et al. 1991).

The proposed revisions to the criteria set for primary insomnia presented in the *Options Book* are minor and are intended mostly for clarification and to reduce redundancy or "pseudo-precision." A field trial is being conducted to compare methods of defining insomnia as these are rendered in ICD-10, the ICSD, and proposed for DSM-IV.

F51.1 Primary Hypersomnia

G47.4 Narcolepsy

G47.3 Breathing-Related Sleep Disorder

The major issues addressed by the Work Group were 1) whether to include narcolepsy in DSM-IV and 2) whether to subsume Breathing-Related Sleep Disorder under dyssomnia related to a known organic factor.

Narcolepsy was not included in DSM-III-R but is proposed for inclusion in DSM-IV because of its importance in the differential diagnosis of excessive sleepiness. It is distinguished from primary hypersomnia by the presence in narcolepsy of sleep attacks, cataplexy, and other specific clinical features. Accordingly, the proposed changes in the diagnostic criteria for primary hypersomnia were made to accommodate the addition of narcolepsy.

In DSM-III-R, breathing-related sleep disorder was subsumed under the two disorders "Insomnia Related to a Known Organic Factor" and "Hypersomnia Related to a Known Organic Factor." The Work Group has now proposed that breathing-related sleep disorder be added as a separate disorder to the Sleep Disorders section of DSM-IV because of its clinical significance (both prognostically and for its treatment implications). Since breathing-related sleep disorder is a common cause of symptoms of insomnia and excessive sleepiness, symptoms frequently encountered in clinical psychiatric practice, the clinical psychiatrist should be aware of their features. Also, the clinical picture and treatment are very distinct from other organic causes. Finally, it should be noted that this proposed diagnosis may require laboratory confirmation of the presence of a breathing disorder (a discussion of this point would be included in the text).

F51.2 Circadian Rhythm Sleep Disorder

In DSM-III-R this disorder was known as "Sleep-Wake Schedule Disorder." The Work Group proposes to change the name to "Circadian Rhythm Sleep Disorder" because this term is more familiar and more indicative of the physiological problem. The most common situations involving a circadian rhythm disturbance are jet lag and shift work. In recognition of this fact, the Work Group now proposes two different options: 1) to split the DSM-III-R "Frequently Changing Type" (of sleep-wake schedule disorder) into "Jet Lag Type" and "Shift Work Type"; or 2) to substitute "Desynchronized Type" for the DSM-III-R "Frequently Changing Type." Finally, a criterion is proposed that requires impairment or distress. The Work Group concluded that as a clinical phenomenon, sleep altered by shift work is common and varied, probably expresses nonphysiological sleep-wake scheduling, and is rarely treated (Regestein and Monk 1991). Further study of its health effects and consideration of whether it is a "disorder" or a "problem" seem warranted.

Parasomnias

F51.5 Nightmare Disorder (Dream Anxiety Disorder)

F51.4 Sleep Terror Disorder

F51.3 Sleepwalking Disorder

The Work Group proposes a name change from the DSM-III-R "Dream Anxiety Disorder" to "Nightmare Disorder" to maintain consistency with the ICSD and the ICD-10. No other substantive changes are proposed in the diagnostic criteria for any of these parasomnias.

Sleep Disorders Related to Another Mental Disorder

F51.0 Insomnia Related to [Axis I or Axis II Disorder]

F51.1 Hypersomnia Related to [Axis I or Axis II Disorder]

This category was introduced in the Sleep Disorders section in DSM-III-R to provide a comprehensive differential diagnosis for Sleep Disorders. The fact that the DSM-III-R criteria set provides no guidelines concerning the circumstances for assigning this diagnosis creates serious problems because sleep problems are so frequently encountered as a symptom of other mental disorders. It is therefore being suggested that criterion D in insomnia and criterion C in hypersomnia be modified to indicate that the sleep disorder must be the *primary* complaint. The reliability of this judgment is being studied in the field trial.

The Work Group recommends that future research efforts should focus on 1) further clarification of the specificity of sleep findings for individual disorders; 2) further definition of sleep disorders related to mental disorders versus associated sleep symptoms of mental disorders; 3) the clinical relevance of individual sleep findings with respect to clinical course and treatment response; 4) the role of disrupted sleep as an etiologic factor, associated feature, or lasting scar of mental disorder; and 5) the impact of disrupted sleep on the functional capacity of the individual (Nofzinger et al. 1993).

G47. Secondary Sleep Disorder Due to a General Medical Condition

F—.8 Substance-Induced Sleep Disorder

DSM-III-R included categories for Insomnia and Hypersomnia "Related to a Known Organic Factor." The Work Group recommends that these categories be split according to etiology but joined with respect to phenomenology. Thus we propose that DSM-IV include categories for secondary sleep disorder due to a general medical condition and for substance-induced sleep disorder to facilitate differential diagnosis. Subtypes are added to indicate the specific sleep disturbance associated with each category. The specific medical condition would be specified on Axis III.

(Note that "Secondary Sleep Disorder" is used in the *DSM-IV Options Book.* However, it was subsequently decided to refer to these disorders simply as "Sleep Disorders Due to a General Medical Condition." Since these chapters were written in support of the *Options Book,* "Secondary Sleep Disorder" is used here.)

The Work Group is also proposing a new method for coding substance-induced disorders in DSM-IV. Under this scheme, the diagnosis is constructed by indicating the type of substance used, the context in which the substance-induced disorder has developed (i.e., during intoxication or withdrawal), and the specific phenomenologic description. For example, insomnia that occurs during cocaine intoxication would be diagnosed as follows: F14.8 cocaine intoxication sleep disorder, insomnia type.

What arises most clearly from the literature review is that there is not sufficient basis for singling out the sleep disorder(s) associated with any one medical or neurological condition by establishment of separate criteria. For the most part, the sleep disorders observed are not specific to the medical or neurological condition in question, and diagnostic criteria would, of necessity, be more strongly oriented toward characteristics of the medical or neurological condition—a practice that would be inappropriate for DSM-IV.

Summary

The changes proposed for DSM-IV sleep disorders represent evolutionary rather than revolutionary changes relative to DSM-III-R. The Work Group hopes that the DSM-IV classification will entice clinicians to consider sleep disorders from an etiological and pathophysiological perspective and to make the most specific appropriate diagnoses. In this sense, also, we hope that the DSM-IV classification of sleep disorders will serve an educational function, as well as a communicative one.

References

American Psychiatric Association: Diagnostic and Statistical Manual of Mental Disorders, 3rd Edition. Washington, DC, American Psychiatric Association, 1980

American Psychiatric Association: Diagnostic and Statistical Manual of Mental Disorders, 3rd Edition, Revised. Washington, DC, American Psychiatric Association, 1987

American Psychiatric Association: DSM-IV Options Book: Work in Progress 9/9/91. Washington, DC, American Psychiatric Association, 1991

American Sleep Disorders Association, Diagnostic Classification Steering Committee: International Classification of Sleep Disorders: Diagnostic and Coding Manual. Rochester, MN, American Sleep Disorders Association, 1990

Association of Sleep Disorders Centers: Diagnostic classification of sleep and arousal disorders. Sleep 2:1–137, 1979

Buysse DJ, Reynolds CF, Kupfer DJ: Classification of sleep disorders: a preview of the DSM-IV, in Current Psychiatric Therapy. Edited by Dunner DL. Philadelphia, PA, WB Saunders, 1993, pp 360–361

Nofzinger EA, Buysse DJ, Reynolds CF, et al: Sleep disorders related to another mental disorder: a literature review for the DSM-IV Workgroup on sleep disorders. J Clin Psychiatry 54:244–255, 1993

Regestein QR, Monk TH: Is the poor sleep of shift workers a disorder? Am J Psychiatry 148:1487–1493, 1991

Reynolds CF, Kupfer DJ, Buysse DJ, et al: Subtyping DSM-III-R "primary insomnia": usefulness, reliability, and validity. Am J Psychiatry 148:432–439, 1991

Schramm E, Hohagen F, Grasshoff U, et al: Test-retest reliability of the Structured Interview for Sleep Disorders according to DSM-III-R. Am J Psychiatry 150:867–872, 1993

World Health Organization: Manual of the International Classification of Diseases, 9th Revision, Clinical Modification. Washington, DC, U.S. Government Printing Office, 1980

World Health Organization: The ICD-10 Classification of Mental and Behavioural Disorders: Clinical Descriptions and Diagnostic Guidelines. Geneva, World Health Organization, 1992

Chapter 36

Subtyping DSM-III-R Primary Insomnia

Charles F. Reynolds III, M.D.
David J. Kupfer, M.D.
Daniel J. Buysse, M.D.
Patricia A. Coble, R.N.
Amy Fasiczka, B.A.

Statement of the Issues

DSM-III-R (American Psychiatric Association 1987) uses the term "Primary Insomnia" to indicate insomnia that lasts longer than 1 month and is not related to other diagnosable medical or psychiatric disorders. This has caused controversy among psychiatric sleep researchers and clinicians, some of whom have objected that the term is difficult to interpret, and groups together patients with widely differing complaints of insomnia.

The controversy revolves around three major issues: 1) the extent to which sleep disorders, particularly those involving insomnia, can be classified into subtypes; 2) the feasibility and utility of more differentiated versus general classifications in the practice of psychiatry; and 3) the value and place of sleep laboratory data in the differential diagnosis of insomnia complaints.

Significance of the Issues

The critical issue is whether subtyping primary insomnia enhances communication, clinical utility, or validity of the diagnostic process. A related, and equally

The authors thank Thomas Roth, Ph.D., Howard Roffwarg, M.D., Peter Hauri, Ph.D., and Ralph Pascualy, M.D., for reviewing and commenting on this manuscript. Supported in part by NIMH Grants 00295, 37869, and 30915.

important, issue is whether the subgroups of primary insomnia elaborated in the International Classification of Sleep Disorders (ICSD) (American Sleep Disorders Association 1990) are clinically relevant to the practice of psychiatry and can be used reliably by psychiatrists. For example, do the ICSD subgroups of primary insomnia denote clinical conditions that have developed in response to distinct etiologic factors? Do they predict a differential response to specific therapeutic interventions? Is a different family history of sleep disorders associated with each? In asking whether there is empirical support for the ICSD subtypes of primary insomnia, as well as for the ICSD subtypes of extrinsic insomnia, it is important to remember that clinical constructs, such as those proposed by the ICSD, may have considerable heuristic value and, as such, may drive clinical investigation in psychiatric sleep research and sleep disorders medicine (Buysse and Reynolds 1990).

As noted by Hauri (1983), the 1979 Association of Sleep Disorders Centers' (ASDC) Diagnostic Classification of Sleep and Arousal Disorders and its successor ICSD are both based on extensive clinical experience and appear to represent the consensus of most active sleep research clinicians in psychiatry. When one contrasts the classification of insomnia in DSM-III-R with the classification in the ASDC and ICSD, the critical issue is to determine the number of groups, or "clusters," of patients with insomnia not related to diagnosable medical or psychiatric disorders ("primary insomnia"). Hauri stated the issue and the dilemma well: "With too few clusters, interpretation is difficult because many widely differing patients are lumped together. With too many clusters, interpretation is also difficult, because some of the differences between clusters become minute and esoteric" (p. 328).

Methods

We reviewed all of the primary source references in the bibliography for each insomnia disorder in the ICSD. We then pursued all the additional primary sources cited in each of these referenced papers. Our third step was to conduct an automated literature search using Medline. We found a total of 48 primary sources published over the last two decades in the English-language literature. Each of these 48 reports was then coded according to the following eight criteria: 1) type of publication (i.e., peer-reviewed, research abstract, or review); 2) number of subjects; 3) use of specific diagnostic criteria (e.g., ASDC, DSM-III-R, Research Diagnostic Criteria [Spitzer et al. 1978]); 4) use of diagnostic reliability procedures; 5) inclusion of control or contrast groups; 6) inclusion of follow-up data; 7) inclusion of polysomnographic data, as well as anamnestic data; and 8) inclusion of treatment outcome data.

None of the reports reviewed met all of these criteria. Accordingly, we gave the greatest weight to 27 studies that were reported in peer-reviewed journals, had the most subjects, and met most of the criteria (such as diagnostic reliability procedures and inclusion of comparison groups).

Results

The three ICSD disorders most closely related to the DSM-III-R concept of primary insomnia will be reviewed first: idiopathic insomnia (also known as "childhood-onset insomnia"), sleep state misperception (also known as "subjective insomnia without objective findings"), and psychophysiological insomnia. After the review of these three intrinsic insomnia disorders, we review the literature related to three ICSD extrinsic disorders: inadequate sleep hygiene, insufficient sleep syndrome, and adjustment sleep disorder. Altitude insomnia and environmental insomnia will be briefly touched on, followed by two of the pediatric insomnias, sleep-onset association disorder and limit-setting sleep disorder.

Intrinsic Insomnia Disorders

Idiopathic insomnia. The ICSD notes that idiopathic insomnia (ASDC "childhood-onset insomnia") is rarely seen in its pure form. The ICSD distinguishes it from psychophysiological insomnia, which is diagnosed if the inherent predisposition toward poor sleep is mild and requires the stress of maladaptive conditioning to manifest itself. Idiopathic insomnia is, rather, conceptualized as a more chronic and stable form of insomnia appearing first in early childhood and persisting unrelentingly. The ICSD indicates that patients with idiopathic insomnia are psychologically healthy.

The ICSD concludes that idiopathic insomnia is a lifelong, serious disorder that cannot be explained by psychological trauma in early childhood or by medical disorders. However, the ICSD notes that idiopathic insomnia is likely to be complicated by poor sleep hygiene, learned maladaptive associations, or psychiatric disturbances. This statement raises the possibility of an age-related or developmental continuum in the ICSD types of insomnia, as well as the probability of overlap between these proposed types of insomnia.

The best data source for idiopathic insomnia was the study by Hauri and Olmstead (1980), which contrasted 20 patients with childhood-onset insomnia and 39 patients with adult-onset (psychophysiological) insomnia. External validation of the distinction between idiopathic and adult psychophysiological insomnia was provided by polysomnographic evidence of less sleep continuity and less rapid eye movement (REM) density in the childhood-onset group. The authors also reported a higher prevalence of soft neurological signs in the patients with childhood-onset insomnia. A subsequent cluster analysis reported by Hauri (1983) supported the distinction between childhood-onset insomnia and persistent psychophysiological insomnia. It is not clear to what extent there may have been overlap of the subjects in the two studies. We could find no replication studies of polysomnographic differences between idiopathic and psychophysiological insomnia, nor could we find studies of controlled treatment trials showing differential treatment response, long-term follow-up studies, data on diagnostic reliability, or family history studies of these two disorders.

Psychophysiological insomnia. The ICSD considers psychophysiological insomnia to be an objectively verifiable insomnia due to learned sleep-preventing associations. The patient's focus on the inability to sleep is the hallmark of psychophysiological insomnia. Apparently, compared with patients with idiopathic insomnia or sleep state misperception, patients with psychophysiological insomnia are more likely to have abnormal psychological profiles, involving malaise, guardedness, sensation avoidance, and denial (Hauri and Fisher 1986; Kales et al. 1976; Mendelson et al. 1984).

The ICSD notes that psychophysiological insomnia lies on a continuum with a number of other diagnostic categories: 1) inadequate sleep hygiene (patients with psychophysiological insomnia still sleep poorly even when they maintain adequate sleep hygiene), 2) dysthymia, 3) generalized anxiety disorder, and 4) idiopathic insomnia. The ICSD notes that patients with psychophysiological insomnia have marginal sleep during childhood and adolescence but that they get by. In contrast, patients with idiopathic insomnia sleep consistently poorly during childhood and beyond. At least two studies of patients with psychophysiological insomnia have shown that their electroencephalographic sleep profile differs from that of depressed patients (Gillin et al. 1979; Reynolds et al. 1984).

Hauri's (1983) study had the largest number of subjects, and he reported the results of a cluster analysis of insomnia involving 90 patients. Cluster 1 included both subjects with good sleep and patients diagnosed as having ASDC subjective insomnia without objective findings (ICSD "sleep state misperception"). Cluster 3 included many older patients with psychophysiological insomnia; younger patients diagnosed as having psychophysiological insomnia tended to be grouped in other clusters. Clusters 7 and 8 denoted, respectively, moderate and severe childhood-onset insomnia. Clusters 3, 7, and 8 suggested the probability of an age-related continuum in insomnia, rather than necessarily distinct disorders. The existence of idiopathic insomnia (childhood-onset insomnia) has yet to be confirmed prospectively in child patients. All of Hauri's patients, for instance, were diagnosed retrospectively on the basis of their histories of childhood onset. This is not the same thing as identifying the disorder prospectively during the first decade of life.

The importance of Hauri's (1983) study lies in the fact that it provides mathematical evidence for the validity of psychophysiological insomnia and childhood-onset insomnia as separate disorders. The question then becomes: Are these distinctions important clinically? If so, how and why? At this time this is perhaps unanswered.

Sleep state misperception. The ICSD uses the term *sleep state misperception* to mean a marked discrepancy between the subjective complaint of insomnia and the objective polysomnographic findings. The course and prevalence of sleep state misperception are unknown, but, according to the ICSD, it appears to apply to fewer than 5% of all patients with primary complaints of insomnia. In the studies to date, no typical psychological or cognitive disorder has been delineated.

There are probably fewer than 30 well-documented cases of sleep state misperception in the research literature. In a study of eight patients with sleep state misperception who were contrasted with eight patients diagnosed as having psychophysiological insomnia, Sugerman and colleagues (1985) reported no nocturnal polysomnographic abnormalities in sleep state misperception, but, surprisingly, there was evidence of impaired waking performance on an auditory vigilance task and a tendency for greater daytime sleepiness. The authors noted an absence of detectable psychopathology according to the Minnesota Multiphasic Personality Inventory (MMPI) (Hathaway and McKinley 1970). The study did not appear to control for the potentially confounding issue of motivation in the auditory vigilance task, nor did it use structured psychiatric interviewing to rule out the presence of psychopathology in the patients with sleep state misperception. We could find no other reports of treatment data for sleep state misperception, no longitudinal follow-up data, and no data on etiology. Most treatment studies of chronic insomnia probably include some of these patients, as well as patients with psychophysiological insomnia.

We believe that the salient question is: Could sleep state misperception be an extreme example of the tendency of patients with chronic insomnia to underestimate sleep time and overestimate the amount of time it takes them to get to sleep, in comparison with objective laboratory measures? In a study of this issue by Carskadon and colleagues (1976), it was observed that for fewer than one patient in five with a complaint of very short sleep or very long sleep, latency was the complaint confirmed in a laboratory sleep setting. The authors speculated that what determines the complaint of insomnia may be how the sleep loss occurs, noting that patients with insomnia have strikingly more arousals (i.e., chronic interruptions of sleep) than control subjects. Carskadon and colleagues also noted abnormal MMPI profiles in 58% of their subjects.

Further evidence of the ubiquity of sleep state misperception in chronic insomnia was provided by Frankel and colleagues (1976), who studied 18 patients with chronic primary insomnia and 18 age- and sex-matched comparison subjects. As a group, the patients with insomnia significantly overestimated sleep latency and underestimated time spent asleep and sleep efficiency. It is interesting that the comparison subjects' estimates of these variables tended to be in the opposite direction. As in the study by Carskadon and colleagues (1976), the patients with insomnia in the study by Frankel and colleagues consistently overestimated sleeplessness. To be sure, polysomnographic findings were significantly correlated with subjective estimates, but the polysomnographic findings did not necessarily explain the severity of the patient's complaint. The authors felt that night-to-night variability is critical and that the unpredictability of sleep is more important than sleeplessness-related anxiety in the pathogenesis of insomnia.

In Hauri's (1983) cluster analysis, patients with good sleep and patients with subjective complaints of insomnia without objective findings were assigned to the same cluster. When both clinical and laboratory predictor variables were used, the two groups of subjects were not separated.

Extrinsic Insomnia Disorders

Inadequate sleep hygiene. In the ICSD, disorder of sleep hygiene is constituted by various habits and activities of daily living that may promote a sleep difficulty—for example, ingestion of caffeine or taking naps at different times of the day. The ICSD recommends that sleep hygiene be evaluated in the context of every insomnia to determine how much of a contribution it is making in sustaining the sleep disturbance. The ICSD also notes that sleep hygiene "violations" may not reach sufficient severity to produce insomnia. Rather, in most cases, a confluence of factors, including inadequate sleep hygiene, produces clinically significant insomnia. The ICSD states that the usual polysomnographic features associated with sleep continuity disturbance also characterize patients with inadequate sleep hygiene. In other words, there is nothing distinctive about the polysomnographic findings in patients for whom inadequate sleep hygiene is apparently the major etiologic factor.

The ICSD cites a study by Spielman and colleagues (1986) of sleep restriction therapy as supporting the existence of a disorder of inadequate sleep hygiene. In fact, however, this study appears to be predicated on the belief that excessive time in bed is one of the important factors that perpetuates insomnia rather than being a primary cause. Moreover, the 12 subjects with persistent psychophysiological insomnia showed the same pattern of change as the entire group, including 21 patients with clinical insomnia. The authors concluded that similarities in outcome were more prominent than any differences between the diagnostic groups. Hence, no differential response to treatment was noted as a function of presumed diagnostic subtype. In a study of 44 patients with sleep-onset insomnia, 49 patients with sleep-maintenance insomnia, and 50 subjects with good sleep, Lacks and Rotert (1986) found that although the patients with insomnia had better knowledge of sleep hygiene than the comparison subjects, both insomnia groups had more deficient sleep hygiene practices regarding nicotine, sleep medication, alcohol, and exercise. The results suggested that poor sleep hygiene is not a primary cause of insomnia but may play a role in exacerbation.

Insufficient sleep syndrome. In the ICSD, the concept of insufficient sleep syndrome appears to be grounded primarily in experimental work investigating the effects of sleep deprivation and sleep restriction on physiological sleepiness the next day and on measures of mood and performance. Probably the best investigations in this area have been done by Carskadon and Dement (1981) and Friedmann and colleagues (1977). It should be noted that the initial complaint associated with insufficient sleep is more often daytime sleepiness than insomnia.

The major question is whether it is clinically useful and valid to conceptualize insufficient sleep—like poor sleep hygiene—as a separate disorder, or whether it makes more sense to consider insufficient sleep to be an important contributor to complaints of insomnia and excessive daytime sleepiness (Roehrs et al. 1983). If it were shown that some individuals have 1) short sleep duration despite adequate opportunity to sleep, 2) otherwise normal sleep study results, and 3) an objectively verified complaint of excessive daytime sleepiness, then a disorder of insufficient sleep would be more strongly supported. However, the literature review does not show this.

Adjustment sleep disorder. The ICSD uses the term *adjustment sleep disorder* to denote transient or short-term insomnia that is a reaction to stress (Beary et al. 1984). Hence, the symptoms should remit if the stressor is removed or the level of adaptation is increased. The central distinction between psychophysiological insomnia and adjustment sleep disorder is the presence of an identifiable stressor in the adjustment disorder.

The best controlled study relating to adjustment sleep disorder is probably that of Cartwright (1983), even though this study is not cited in the ICSD bibliography. Cartwright's study focused on dream reports and REM sleep changes during and after a mood-disturbing event (i.e., divorce). This study suggested that sleep physiology alterations attending a mood-disturbing event might be long-standing, particularly in patients who react with depression. Cartwright's finding of protracted sleep disturbance after divorce was similar to self-report data in longitudinal studies of bereavement, such as that of Clayton and colleagues (1972), who reported sleep disturbance to be a persistent (> 1 year) and disabling symptom in 48% of subjects whose spouses had died. Finally, in a questionnaire study involving 243 respondents, Hartmann and Brewer (1976) found that one major factor associated with an increased need for sleep was "mental or emotional stress," which correlated strongly with changes of occupation, increased mental activity, and depressed mood.

Does it make sense to distinguish the ICSD diagnosis of adjustment sleep disorder from the DSM-III-R categories of adjustment disorder with or without depressed mood and bereavement with or without complications? Would such a distinction be useful to clinical psychiatrists? If so, how? It may be possible to have a stress (e.g., medical procedure, life event) that does not lead to mood or behavioral sequelae but has insomnia as the core symptom. It is the nature of the stressor (and its meaning to the patient) that will have implications for the duration, severity, and management of the sleep complaint.

Altitude insomnia and environmental insomnia. Altitude insomnia in small groups of volunteers has been well described clinically and polysomnographically (Nicholson et al. 1988; Reite et al. 1975). It usually develops at elevations greater than 4,000 meters and may be related to normal physiological control of respiration in the presence of low inspired oxygen. The interpretation of the data appears to be partly confounded by environmental factors, such as cold, altered light and dark cycles, and possibly jet lag. In the ICSD, the concept of environmental sleep disorders is based on a handful of studies investigating the impact of ambient noise (e.g., Roth et al. 1972) and extreme temperature change (e.g., Haskell et al. 1981) on sleep.

Although these studies are of considerable experimental and scientific interest, their relevance to clinical practice appears to be limited.

Sleep-onset association disorder and limit-setting sleep disorder. The ICSD conceptualizes both of these sleep disorders as pertaining mainly to childhood (Richman 1981; Richman et al. 1975). Both represent useful clinical constructs, popularized by Ferber (1985), who wrote a self-help book for parents related to these disorders but who has not, to our knowledge, published any empirical studies. Both disorders may be conceptually similar to psychophysiological insomnia insofar as both may be related to conditioning factors adverse to sleep. In this sense, the distinction from adult psychophysiological insomnia is not supported by published empirical data.

Discussion and Recommendations

The ICSD subtypes of chronic intrinsic ("primary") insomnia are clinically appealing and represent the accumulated wisdom, the consensus, and the working diagnoses of clinical investigators and sleep disorders specialists. In our view, the ICSD subtypes embody the clinical belief that complaints of insomnia are multifactorial and that consequently treatment approaches need to be individually tailored to the specific constellation of factors found in a particular patient (Coleman et al. 1982; NIH Consensus Panel Report 1984; Zorick et al. 1981). The concepts of etiologic heterogeneity and need for treatment specificity are further supported by the work of Jacobs and colleagues (1988), who reported that polysomnographic findings resulted in the modification of the clinical diagnosis of chronic insomnia in approximately 50% of 123 consecutive patients with chronic insomnia. The concepts of heterogeneity in etiology and treatment specificity were also articulated by the National Institute of Mental Health consensus conference on drugs and insomnia (NIH Consensus Panel Report 1984).

Despite the clinical utility of the ICSD distinctions and despite the probable heuristic value, the available empirical data on the reliability and validity of these subtypes are limited and therefore do not yet provide a compelling basis for abandoning the DSM-III-R concept of primary insomnia. The clusters reported in Hauri's (1983) study need to be replicated, and their clinical validity needs to be demonstrated in studies of etiology, family history, response to treatment, and long-term course. It would serve a useful educational purpose to discuss the subtypes (idiopathic insomnia, sleep state misperception, and psychophysiological insomnia) in the DSM-IV text relating to primary insomnia and to discuss the putative roles of sleep hygiene, insufficient sleep, and environmental factors in case formulation. Similarly, the clinical importance of duration of complaint should be underscored in the text because of the greater probability of finding stressors in the lives of patients with recent-onset insomnia. The nature of the stressor, such as bereavement, will have important implications for the severity, duration, and complications of the sleep complaint and for its management. In a similar spirit of clinical relevance, pediatric sleep disturbances related to parental behaviors could be usefully discussed in the DSM-IV text. The information concerning the apparent effects of altitude change on sleep and breathing might be mentioned in the text here or discussed in relation to insomnia and medical disorders, where it seems more relevant.

In conclusion, we recommend retaining the DSM-III-R concept of primary insomnia and not adopting the ICSD subtyping of insomnia at this time. The ICSD subtyping usefully addresses factors that may be important in insomnia. As such, these factors should be considered in the text. However, on the basis of the existing empirical studies, if we were to elevate factors that disturb sleep to disorders, we might be reaching premature conclusions. At the same time, although the use of a single diagnostic category precludes the premature adoption of more differentiated diagnostic categories, it may lull clinicians into a false sense of security that might lead them to overlook clinically important heterogeneity. Accordingly, one might use the term *primary insomnias* rather than *primary insomnia* and start with two primary insomnia categories: idiopathic insomnia and psychophysiological insomnia. Although our literature review does indicate there may be valid distinctions between them, we have also suggested that further empirical validation is necessary. Such studies are crucial, we believe, to achieving the long-term goal of identifying the various clinical entities that constitute this category. The DSM-IV text should provide description of some of these entities and commentary on their potential strengths and weaknesses.

One further recommendation is in order. We do not know of any published data on the performance characteristics or the clinical and research utility of the DSM-III-R classification of insomnia. In a pilot field trial at the University of Pittsburgh, Pennsylvania, involving a review of 19 cases of chronic insomnia by six raters, interrater reliability appeared to be higher in the application of the DSM-III-R criteria than for the ASDC criteria (D. J. Buysse, C. F. Reynolds, D. J. Kupfer, unpublished data, 1991). This is perhaps not unexpected, since DSM-III-R "lumps" and ASDC "splits." On the other hand, it is also our impression that the treatment recommendations based on ASDC diagnoses were perhaps somewhat more targeted, or focused, than the treatment recommendations based on DSM-III-R diagnoses. Hence, we are conducting a field trial to evaluate the relative performance characteristics and the utility of the DSM-III-R "lumping" approach versus the ICSD "splitting" approach. Furthermore, assessment of the level of clinician expertise (sleep disorders specialist versus general psychiatrist) on interrater agreement in the application of the DSM-III-R and ICSD systems is recommended. Finally, the effect of knowledge of polysomnographic data on rates of agreement in the application of the DSM-III-R and ICSD systems needs to be assessed. It is conceivable that these data would lead to the incorporation of some ICSD subtypes (e.g., psychophysiological versus idiopathic) into DSM-IV and, at the least, would inform the discussion of these subtypes in the text.

The proposed revision to the criteria set for primary insomnia presented in the *DSM-IV Options Book* (American Psychiatric Association 1991) are minor and are intended mostly for classification and to reduce redundancy or pseudo-precision. Thus criterion A retains the focus on difficulty initiating or maintaining sleep for at least a month but deletes 1) redundant language relating to nonrestful sleep and 2) the pseudo-precise criterion of sleep disturbance three times weekly. Similarly, criterion B retains the focus on the clinically significant consequences of insomnia (daytime fatigue and impaired daytime function) and eliminates excessive language about clinical sequelae that adds nothing to the substance of the criterion. Conceptually, the criteria for primary insomnia in the *Options Book* are identical to those of DSM-III-R, a fact that reflects the conclusion of this literature review.

References

American Psychiatric Association: Diagnostic and Statistical Manual of Mental Disorders, 3rd Edition, Revised. Washington, DC, American Psychiatric Association, 1987

American Psychiatric Association: DSM-IV Options Book: Work in Progress 9/9/91. Washington, DC, American Psychiatric Association, 1991

American Sleep Disorders Association, Diagnostic Classification Steering Committee: International Classification of Sleep Disorders: Diagnostic and Coding Manual. Rochester, MN, American Sleep Disorders Association, 1990

Association of Sleep Disorders Centers: Diagnostic classification of sleep and arousal disorders. Sleep 2:1–137, 1979

Beary MD, Lacey JH, Crutchfield MB, et al: Psycho-social stress, insomnia and temazepam: a sleep laboratory evaluation in a "general practice" sample. Psychopharmacology (Berlin) 83:17–19, 1984

Buysse DJ, Reynolds CF III: Insomnia, in Handbook of Sleep Disorders. Edited by Thorpy MJ. New York, Marcel Dekker, 1990

Carskadon M, Dement W: Cumulative effects of sleep restriction on daytime sleepiness. Psychophysiology 18:107–122, 1981

Carskadon MA, Dement WC, Mitler MM, et al: Self-reports versus sleep laboratory findings in 122 drug-free subjects with complaints of chronic insomnia. Am J Psychiatry 133:1382–1388, 1976

Cartwright R: Rapid eye movement sleep characteristics during and after mood-disturbing events. Arch Gen Psychiatry 40:197–201, 1983

Clayton PJ, Halikas JA, Mauria WL: The depression of widowhood. Br J Psychiatry 120:71–78, 1972

Coleman R, Roffwarg H, Kennedy S, et al: Sleep-wake disorders based on polysomnographic diagnosis: a national cooperative study. JAMA 247:997–1003, 1982

Ferber R: Solving Your Child's Sleep Problems. New York, Simon & Schuster, 1985

Frankel B, Coursey R, Buchbinder R, et al: Recorded and reported sleep in chronic primary insomniacs. Arch Gen Psychiatry 33:615–623, 1976

Friedmann J, Globus G, Huntley A, et al: Performance and mood during and after gradual sleep reduction. Psychophysiology 14:245–250, 1977

Gillin C, Duncan W, Pettigrew K, et al: Successful separation of depressed, normal, and insomniac subjects by EEG sleep data. Arch Gen Psychiatry 36:85–90, 1979

Hartmann E, Brewer V: When is more or less sleep required? a study of variable sleepers. Compr Psychiatry 17:275–284, 1976

Haskell EH, Palca JW, Walker JM, et al: The effects of high and low ambient temperatures on human sleep stages. Electroencephalogr Clin Neurophysiol 51:494–501, 1981

Hathaway SR, McKinley JC: Minnesota Multiphasic Personality Inventory, Revised. Minneapolis, MN, University of Minnesota, 1970

Hauri P: A cluster analysis of insomnia. Sleep 6:326–338, 1983

Hauri P, Fisher J: Persistent psychophysiologic (learned) insomnia. Sleep 9:38–53, 1986

Hauri P, Olmstead E: Childhood-onset insomnia. Sleep 3:59–65, 1980

Jacobs EA, Reynolds CF III, Kupfer DJ, et al: The role of polysomnography in the differential diagnosis of chronic insomnia. Am J Psychiatry 145:346–349, 1988

Kales A, Caldwell A, Preston TA, et al: Personality patterns in insomnia: theoretical implications. Arch Gen Psychiatry 33:1128–1134, 1976

Lacks P, Rotert M: Knowledge and practice of sleep hygiene techniques in insomniacs and good sleepers. Behav Res Ther 24:365–368, 1986

Mendelson WB, Garnett D, Gillin JC, et al: The experience of insomnia and daytime and nighttime function. Psychiatry Res 12:235–250, 1984

Nicholson A, Smith P, Stone B, et al: Altitude insomnia: studies during an expedition to the Himalayas. Sleep 11:354–361, 1988

NIH Consensus Panel Report: Drugs and insomnia: the use of medications to promote sleep. JAMA 251:2410–2414, 1984

Reite M, Jackson D, Cahoon R, et al: Sleep physiology at high altitude. Electroencephalogr Clin Neurophysiol 28:463–471, 1975

Reynolds CF III, Taska LS, Sewitch DE, et al: Persistent psychophysiologic insomnia: preliminary Research Diagnostic Criteria and EEG sleep data. Am J Psychiatry 141:804–805, 1984

Richman N: A community survey of characteristics of one- to two-year-olds with sleep disruption. American Academy of Child Psychiatry 20:181–191, 1981

Richman N, Stevenson JE, Graham PJ: Prevalence of behavior problems in 3-year-old children: an epidemiological study in a London borough. J Child Psychol Psychiatry 16:277–287, 1975

Roehrs T, Zorick F, Sicklesteel J, et al: Excessive daytime sleepiness associated with insufficient sleep. Sleep 6:319–325, 1983

Roth T, Kramer M, Trinder J: The effect of noise during sleep on the sleep patterns of different age groups. Canadian Psychiatric Association Journal 17:196–201, 1972

Spielman A, Saskin P, Thorpy M: Treatment of chronic insomnia by restriction of time in bed. Sleep 10:45–46, 1986

Spitzer RL, Endicott J, Robins E: Research Diagnostic Criteria: rationale and reliability. Arch Gen Psychiatry 35:773–783, 1978

Sugerman JL, Stern JA, Walsh JK: Daytime alertness in subjective and objective insomnia: some preliminary findings. Biol Psychiatry 20:741–750, 1985

Zorick FJ, Roth T, Hartze KM, et al: Evaluation and diagnosis of persistent insomnia. Am J Psychiatry 138:769–773, 1981

Chapter 37

Primary Hypersomnia

Quentin R. Regestein, M.D.

Statement of the Issues

Concerning primary hypersomnia, there is a question of "whether this unusual condition deserves classification as a discrete symptom complex" (Mendelson et al. 1977, p. 104). The condition is presently defined largely by the absence of signs specific to other causes of sleepiness, but has had more specific criteria in the recent past.

Primary hypersomnia had been previously known as idiopathic hypersomnia (Roth 1980) or idiopathic central nervous system hypersomnia in the original Association of Sleep Disorders Centers (1979) classification and appears presently as idiopathic hypersomnia in the International Classification of Sleep Disorders (ICSD) (American Sleep Disorders Association 1990). DSM-III-R (American Psychiatric Association 1987) changed the name of the condition to primary hypersomnia, but it also lumped idiopathic hypersomnia under the same heading with any other persistent unexplained sleepiness or sleep attacks, thus changing it from a specific term to a generic term. Therefore the question arises whether idiopathic hypersomnia should denote a specific condition of unknown cause or include other excessive sleepiness problems of unknown etiology, regardless of clinical presentation.

Kleine-Levin syndrome is a well-established entity of unknown etiology that differs from idiopathic or primary hypersomnia. It was mentioned in the text, but omitted as a specific diagnosis from DSM-III-R; it was included in ICSD with its name changed to Recurrent Hypersomnia.

Significance of the Issues

Idiopathic hypersomnia has been described as "recurrent" daytime sleepiness, but classic narcoleptic sleep attacks do not occur. Naps are frequently lengthy, not refreshing, and preceded by a long period of drowsiness. Many patients report difficulties in waking up, and some complain of "sleep drunkenness" (Guilleminault and Faull 1982). Idiopathic hypersomnia involves prolonged sleepiness; attacks of diurnal sleep, usually lasting from 1 to several hours; very deep and prolonged nocturnal sleep; and, in about 60% of cases, difficult and prolonged waking in the morning, with signs of sleep drunkenness (Roth 1981). There are no laboratory findings specific to this condition alone. Guilleminault and Faull (1982) noted that "in clinical practice it is difficult to affirm the diagnosis of EDS [excessive daytime sleepiness] in borderline cases" (p. 5177). Mendelson and colleagues (1977) reserved judgment on whether the condition deserved classification as a discrete symptom complex. Thus there has been some question on whether idiopathic hypersomnia is a discrete condition. Montplaisir and colleagues (1982) defined it only in negative terms. Idiopathic hypersomnia is said to occur among EDS patients without sleep apnea; endocrine, neurological, or psychiatric disorders; or narcolepsy.

Kleine-Levin syndrome is an entity that also causes excessive sleepiness, but has a different clinical presentation. It is rarer and more incapacitating than idiopathic hypersomnia and is well-established in the medical literature. Subsuming this condition under primary hypersomnia would make a simpler classification, but it is a condition with distinct subtypes and a more heterogeneous clinical population.

Methods

The literature search for idiopathic hypersomnia and for Kleine-Levin syndrome began with a computer search (Paperchase) that used the Medline data base of items dated from 1966 to October 1990. Primary data articles relevant to diagnostic criteria were sought as cited in the Paperchase articles, limited to the major Western European languages. *Sleep Research* abstracts for 1989 and 1988 were additionally consulted. From the resulting articles, book chapters, and abstracts, diagnostic criteria were extracted. In general, the references show the basis of the literature review.

Results

Idiopathic hypersomnia is frequently compared with narcolepsy. Its clinical picture is distinguished from narcolepsy by the nature of its sleep attacks. They can be resisted for hours, often last an hour or more, and do not refresh the patient (Roth 1980). Instead, "sleep drunkenness" is often present on awakening, described as a "dissociation between awareness and motor function" (Roth et al. 1972). This is a prolonged period of grogginess and dysfunction. Nocturnal sleep is prolonged and described by the patients as very deep (Roth et al. 1972). These features contrast sharply with the irresistible but briefer and refreshing naps of narcolepsy, as well as the normal length of narcolepsy patients' night sleep and their feeling of greatest wakefulness shortly after arising from night sleep. Additionally, idiopathic hypersomnia patients lack other narcolepsy tetrad symptoms. Thus it would seem that idiopathic hypersomnia can be distinguished from narcolepsy by its clinical features.

Guilleminault (1985) subtyped idiopathic hypersomnia by clinical history into three groups. The first has no medical history but "frequently" a family history of EDS. Autonomic symptoms such as headache, orthostatic hypotension, syncope, and Raynaud's phenomenon may be present. The second group is postviral. The third have neither a family nor a viral history. Possible distinctions between postencephalitic EDS and postviral idiopathic hypersomnia are not given, but idiopathic hypersomnia is a lifelong condition unlike the sleepiness of some viral encephalopathies that gradually remits.

Polysomnographically, idiopathic hypersomnia patients have been principally compared with narcolepsy patients. On multiple sleep latency tests, they are somewhat longer to fall asleep than narcolepsy patients and do not manifest short rapid eye movement (REM) sleep latencies. During night sleep they lack myoclonus and have longer total sleep times under ad lib conditions and greater sleep efficiency (Baker et al. 1986; Canellas et al. 1989; Guilleminault and Faull 1982; Nahmias and Karetsky 1989; Van den Hoed et al. 1981). Thus they generally show sleep that is abundant, but lacking in specific diagnostic features.

Laboratory observations confirm the clinical descriptions of diffuse, mild autonomic abnormalities among idiopathic hypersomnia patients. Roth and colleagues (1972) noted higher heart and respiratory rates during the night among 48 idiopathic hypersomnia patients with sleep drunkenness, but warned that this was an unexpected result that required confirmation. One patient was reported who lacked blood pressure elevations on arousal from sleep (Schneider-Helmert et al. 1980). Baker and colleagues (1986) reported lower mean blood pressure among 74 idiopathic hypersomnia patients (127/80) compared with 257 narcolepsy patients (132/85).

Cerebral spinal fluid amine analyses have shown neurotransmitter metabolite levels to be similar in idiopathic hypersomnia and narcolepsy patients, although different from control subjects (Guilleminault and Faull 1982; Montplaisir et al. 1982). Some distinction in the pattern of amine levels was reported by Faull and colleagues (1986), who found 3-methoxy-4-hydroxyphenylglycol (MHPG) uncorrelated with other amines in six idiopathic hypersomnia patients, unlike in narcolepsy patients, where homovanillic acid (HVA) and 3,4-dihydrophenylacetic acid (DOPAC) levels departed from expected correlations. They concluded that idiopathic hypersomnia may involve abnormalities in norepinephrine as distinguished from narcolepsy, which may involve dopamine abnormalities.

Kleine (1925) originally drew five of his own cases together with four cases from the literature and called the syndrome "periodic sleeping sickness." Patients had episodes of apparently normal but prolonged sleep once or twice to several times a year. The episodes would last 2–20 days. During these episodes, when the patients were not sleeping, they were "half awake."

The patients variably had headache, weakness, and giddiness when awake. Three of his cases manifested "sexual hyperexcitability" evidenced by obscene talk, masturbation in public, and propositioning other inpatients. Levin (1936) took the two of Kleine's (1925) cases with increased appetite, added five other cases from the literature, and called the syndrome "periodic somnolence and morbid hunger." Reviewing seven patients, Gallinek (1954) called the syndrome "episodes of hypersomnia, bulimia and abnormal mental status." Each ended the bout with a depressive psychosis, however, rendering his subjects suspect for mood disorder. Rosenkoetter and Wende (1955) followed an 18-year-old man for 2.5 years. When awake during the episodes, the patient remembered that "everything seemed unreal to me"; "I didn't know whether people were really speaking to me or if I was dreaming." There were not real amnestic features in the mental status, but rather profound slowing. The patient yawned frequently, was uninterested in anything, and sat doing nothing. Repeated electroencephalograms (EEGs) in this state showed flattening of alpha waves and theta activity, with occasional sleep spindles accentuated frontally. There was a tendency to sleep during recording sessions. K-complexes were also present. As the episode developed, there was progressive slowing of the background rhythm.

Reviewing 11 personal cases and 15 from the literature, Critchley (1962) found the average episode to last a week and to appear about every 6 months. Somnolence was the most salient symptom, but truculence, confusion, dreamy states, and various affective changes, sometimes euphoria, were present. Eating became a type of compulsion that continued until no more food was available. Despite previous reports, Critchley felt only adolescent males truly fit the syndrome. Green and Crucco (1970) reported a patient with hypersomnolence attacks in which overeating was almost always present, with the other clinical features variable during attacks. The EEG showed high voltage slow waves, intermixed with theta activity, blocked temporarily by auditory stimuli during attacks, but normal EEG otherwise. Gran and Begemann (1973) reported a 32-year-old woman with 20 years of periodic sleepiness. During attacks, she evidenced headaches, spontaneous nystagmus, and left-sided intention tremor, but no more specific findings on neurological investigation. Billiard and colleagues (1975) reported a 13-year-old girl with 3- to 8-day somnolent episodes commencing at menarche and associated with menses. Uncharacteristic apathy, negativism, refusal of food and drink, and visual hallucinations were associated with these episodes; confusion was not. Exogenous estrogen but not methylphenidate relieved the symptoms, and the authors diagnosed a "variant" of Kleine-Levin syndrome.

Parkes and colleagues (1974) found extremely low levels of cerebrospinal fluid HVA and 5-hydroxyindoleacetic acid (5-HIAA) in a 13-year-old boy with Kleine-Levin syndrome after he had slept for 3 days. Yassa and Nair (1978) reported a 44-year-old man with an "abnormally slow" EEG during attacks but not otherwise. Lavie and colleagues (1979) had two patients, one with REM onset periods during symptomatic episodes. Hagel and colleagues (1980) reported on four patients and reviewed previous literature. The increased appetite as mentioned by others was evident in particular cravings for sweets—for example, heaping up sugar on cereal (Chiles and Wilkins 1976). Stealing food or eating food rejected by others (e.g., all the desserts thought unfit by mess hall diners) was also reported.

Physical findings were generally transient minor neurological signs, such as one-sided hyperreflexia; minor pyramidal tract signs; minor ophthalmoplegia (ptosis, anisocoria); spontaneous, purposeless motor movements of extremities; or perioral musculature. The EEG shows typical sleep patterns but striking findings during wakefulness, with background slowing, including intermittent delta bursts and occipital dysrhythmias.

Barontini and Zappoli (1968) described a 28-year-old man with classic symptoms: 4- to 22-day attacks twice a year, during which he slept 17–20 hours/day and ate voraciously, gaining 5 kg in one 16-day period. EEGs showed "an excess of slow waves"; a 3.5-hour polysomnography during the afternoon showed much fluctuation between light and medium sleep and brief episodes of deep sleep with only one awakening. Nocturnal polysomnography showed a normal pattern, with excessive brevity of REM periods. Reynolds and colleagues (1984) reported a patient with four sleep-onset REM periods during a symptomatic episode, but one such episode when asymptomatic.

Three cases that appeared to be secondary Kleine-Levin syndrome have been reported, one following viral encephalitis (Merriam 1986) and two following head trauma (Will et al. 1988).

Many other clinical laboratory tests were done by investigators, but no dependable findings were reported (Argentino and Sideri 1980). Hyperglycemia, a flattened glucose tolerance curve, and minimal cerebral ventricular dilations are examples.

Discussion and Recommendations

Idiopathic hypersomnia has a different clinical presentation from narcolepsy. In the laboratory it lacks the stigmata of narcolepsy and may be distinguished in its pattern of prolonged uninterrupted nocturnal sleep and its cerebrospinal fluid amine alterations. It would thus seem to be a separate entity even from "independent" or "monosymptomatic" narcolepsy (i.e., narcolepsy manifesting by sleep attacks alone). For purposes of classification, therefore, both "idiopathic" narcolepsy and idiopathic hypersomnia should be separated into different categories. This would continue a distinction commonly found in the literature. Kleine-Levin syndrome would be distinguished from primary hypersomnia by its episodic rather than continuous sleepiness, confusion during waking periods, and associations with appetite and sexual and behavioral disturbance. If it becomes subsumed under primary hypersomnia, Kleine-Levin syndrome could be described as a distinct subtype.

The past controversies about Kleine-Levin syndrome have been largely resolved. It can afflict females and may be present without gluttony. ICSD changed the name to *recurrent hypersomnia,* but this term would seem less specific than that condition described in the literature for most of the 20th century and could be confused with other conditions, such as menses-related hypersomnia, periodic hypersomnia related to infections, or other recurrent disorders that may involve a sleepiness component.

In the Work Group, written opinion generally favored retaining Kleine-Levin syndrome, although one consultant felt it could be lumped with primary hypersomnia. The proposed DSM-IV criteria for Primary (Idiopathic) Hypersomnia are provided in Table 37–1. The proposed DSM-IV criteria for Kleine-Levin Syndrome (Recurrent Hypersomnia) are provided in Table 37–2.

Table 37–1. Proposed DSM-IV diagnostic criteria for Primary (Idiopathic) Hypersomnia

A. A primary complaint of excessive sleepiness plus two of the following three symptoms:
B. Unrefreshing naps of at least 15 minutes' duration occurring almost daily.
C. Prolonged, undisturbed night sleep.
D. Sleep drunkenness.

Options:

1. Have one category for idiopathic sleepiness containing both primary (idiopathic) hypersomnia and monosymptomatic narcolepsy.
2. Have one category for idiopathic sleepiness that contains both primary (idiopathic) hypersomnia and Kleine-Levin syndrome.
3. Have one category that contains all three of these conditions.

Differences from DSM-III-R: Idiopathic hypersomnia is subsumed under "Primary Hypersomnia" but only criteria A and D above are given. Thus only sleep drunkenness is used to differentiate idiopathic hypersomnia and narcolepsy.

Table 37–2. Proposed DSM-IV diagnostic criteria for Kleine-Levin Syndrome (Recurrent Hypersomnia)

A. Bouts of almost continuous sleep, lasting a day or longer.

B. Confusion during wakeful periods.

C. Normal premorbid functioning between bouts.

D. One or more of the following:
  Onset during adolescence
  Gluttony during attacks
  Hypersexual behavior during attacks
  Uncharacteristically recalcitrant behavior during attacks
  Slowing of EEG background rhythm during attacks

Option:

Change name to "Recurrent Hypersomnia."

Differences from DSM-III-R: Kleine-Levin syndrome was mentioned only in the text.

Note. EEG = electroencephalogram.

References

American Psychiatric Association: Diagnostic and Statistical Manual of Mental Disorders, 3rd Edition, Revised. Washington, DC, American Psychiatric Association, 1987

American Sleep Disorders Association, Diagnostic Classification Steering Committee: International Classification of Sleep Disorders: Diagnostic and Coding Manual. Rochester, MN, American Sleep Disorders Association, 1990

Association of Sleep Disorders Centers: Diagnostic classification of sleep and arousal disorders. Sleep 2:1–137, 1979

Argentino C, Sideri G: Kleine-Levin syndrome. Riv Neurol 50:26–31, 1980

Baker TL, Guilleminault C, Nino-Maurcia G, et al: Comparative polysomnographic study of narcolepsy and idiopathic central nervous system hypersomnia. Sleep 9 (1 pt 2):232–242, 1986

Barontini F, Zappoli A: A case of Kleine-Levin syndrome, clinical and polygraphic study, in The Abnormalities of Sleep in Man. Edited by Gastaut H, Lugaresi E, Berti-Ceroni G, et al. Bologna, Aulo Gaggi Editore, 1968, pp 239–245

Billiard M, Guilleminault C, Dement WC: A menstruation-linked periodic hypersomnia: Kleine-Levin syndrome or a new clinical entity? Neurology 25:436–443, 1975

Canellas F, Nonquier J, Tufti M, et al: Nighttime and daytime sleep in idiopathic central nervous system hypersomnolent subjects in comparison with narcoleptic subjects. Sleep Res 18:211, 1989

Chiles JA, Wilkins RJ: Behavioral manifestations of the Kleine-Levin syndrome. Diseases of the Nervous System 37:646–648, 1976

Critchley M: Periodic hypersomnia and megaphagia in adolescent males. Brain 85:627–656, 1962

Faull KF, Thiemann S, King RJ, et al: Monoamine interactions in narcolepsy and hypersomnia: a preliminary report. Sleep 9:246–249, 1986

Gallinek A: Syndrome of episodes of hypersomnia, bulemia and abnormal mental state. JAMA 154:1081–1083, 1954

Gran D, Begemann H: New observations in a case of Kleine-Levin Syndrome. Muenschner Medijinlische Wochenschrift 115:1098–1102, 1973

Green LN, Crucco RQ: Kleine-Levin Syndrome. Arch Neurol 27:166–175, 1970

Guilleminault C: Disorders of Excessive Sleepiness. Annals of Clinical Research 17:209–219, 1985

Guilleminault C, Faull KF: Sleepiness in nonnarcoleptic EDS patients: the idiopathic CNS hypersomnolence. Sleep 5:S175–S177, 1982

Hagel K, Freytag H, Kindt H: The Kleine-Levin-Critchley syndrome: a contribution to its diagnostic classification Fortschritte der Neurologie. Psychiatrie and Ihren Grenzgebiete 48:267–278, 1980

Kleine W: Periodic sleeping sickness. Muenschner Psychiatrie und Neurologie 57:285–320, 1925

Lavie P, Gadoth N, Gordon CR, et al: Sleep patterns in Kleine-Levin syndrome. Electroencephalogr Clin Neurophysiol 47:369–371, 1979

Levin M: Periodic somnolence and morbid hunger: a new syndrome. Brain 59:494–504, 1936

Mendelson WB, Guillin JC, Wyatt RJ: Human Sleep and Its Disorders. New York, Plenum, 1977

Merriam AE: Kleine-Levin syndrome following acute viral encephalitis. Biol Psychiatry 21:1301–1304, 1986

Montplaisir J, de Champlain J, Young SN, et al: Narcolepsy and idiopathic hypersomnia: biogenic amines and related compounds in CSF. Neurology 32:1299–1302, 1982

Nahmias J, Karetsky M: Narcolepsy vs idiopathic CNS hypersomnolence: a comparison of patient and polysomnographic characteristics. Sleep Research 18:275, 1989

Parkes JD, Fenton G, Struthers G, et al: Narcolepsy and cataplexy: clinical features treatment and cerebral spinal fluid findings. Q J Med 43:5256, 1974

Reynolds CF, Kupfer DJ, Christiansen CL, et al: Multiple sleep latency test findings in Kleine-Levin Syndrome. J Nerv Ment Dis 172:41–44, 1984

Rosenkoetter L, Wende S: EEG findings in Kleine-Levin Syndrome. Muenschner Psychiatrie und Neurologie 130:107–122, 1955

Roth B: Narcolepsy and Hypersomnia. Basel, Karger, 1980

Roth B: Classifications of states of excessive sleep: a critical evaluation of the present situation, in Psychophysiological Aspects of Sleep. Edited by Karacan I. Park Ridge, IL, Noyes, 1981, pp 88–95

Roth B, Nevsimalova S, Rechtschaffen A: Hypersomnia with sleep drunkenness. Arch Gen Psychiatry 26:456–462, 1972

Schneider-Helmert D, Schenker J, Gnirss F: Deficient blood pressure regulation in a case of hypersomnia with sleep drunkenness. Electroencephalogr Clin Neurophysiol 48:230–232, 1980

Van den Hoed J, Kramer H, Guilleminault C, et al: Disorders of excessive daytime somnolence: polygraphic and clinical data for 100 patients. Sleep 4:23–37, 1981

Will RG, Young JP, Thomas DJ: Kleine-Levin syndrome: report of two cases with onset of symptoms precipitated by head trauma. Br J Psychiatry 152:410–412, 1988

Yassa R, Nair NPV: The Kleine-Levin syndrome—a variant? J Clin Psychiatry 39:254–259, 1978

Chapter 38

Narcolepsy

Quentin R. Regestein, M.D.

Statement of the Issues

As a syndrome, narcolepsy varies widely among patients. A standard definition of narcolepsy, therefore, should include the largest and exclude the smallest number of patients diagnosed by most experienced clinicians as narcoleptic. This clinical variability raises the issue of whether narcolepsy is a single entity or a syndrome provoked by multiple causes.

Although sleepiness is the signal characteristic of narcolepsy, there is a question of whether narcoleptic sleepiness is qualitatively the same or different from the sleepiness of other causes. One might ask whether any qualitative differences observed would help define diagnostic criteria.

Narcolepsy may alter laboratory test results. What might be the role of such alterations in narcolepsy diagnosis? How should patients manifesting clinical but not laboratory stigmata of narcolepsy be categorized?

These and other issues may be resolved by continually advancing descriptions of patients. At some point, however, making a standard definition facilitates communication. After diagnostic ideas have repeatedly emerged from the clinical observations made through more than a century, some standardization of diagnostic criteria would seem justified.

Significance of the Issues

Narcolepsy is a syndrome originally described as being "characterized by a pressing need to sleep, sudden and of short duration, which recurs at more or less frequent intervals" (Gelineau 1880, p. 626). A later definition was "excessive daytime sleepiness and often disturbed nocturnal sleep, and pathological manifestations of REM [rapid eye movement] sleep; which included cataplexy, sleep paralysis, hypnagogic hallucinations and sleep-onset REM periods" (Guilleminault 1976). A standardized definition of narcolepsy awaits consensus on which narcolepsy symptoms are obligatory and which facultative. "All gradations are met with, from narcolepsy without cataplexy to cataplexy without narcolepsy" (Wilson 1928). Firm clinical criteria risk excluding some patients who might benefit from narcolepsy treatment—for example, those with an average sleep latency of 5 minutes or more on multiple sleep latency testing (Richardson et al. 1978) and whose treatment might have been delayed until criteria changed, for example, to 7 minutes (Guilleminault et al. 1988), to 8 minutes (Rhodes et al. 1989), and then to 10 minutes (American Sleep Disorders Association 1990). Defining narcolepsy, therefore, involves tension between specificity and completeness.

Clinical Ambiguities and Controversy

Viewpoints have differed on whether narcolepsy should be considered a syndrome or an illness in itself. Wilson (1928) opined that narcolepsy was a syndrome destined to be expanded, whereas Henneberg (1916) argued that narcolepsy should be narrowly defined and should exclude secondary narcolepsy. Adie (1926) sought to resolve this "confusion" and distinguish narcolepsy from other causes of excessive sleepiness.

Narcolepsy was assembled feature by feature by clinical savants who noted attacks of natural sleep, named it, and emphasized its connection to cataplexy and sleep "paralysis" (Wilson 1928). The critical, classical "tetrad" was fashioned by Yoss and Daly (1960). Thus narcolepsy is basically a collection of elements from clinical histories.

Contemporary literature is relatively sparse on these clinical features. The duration of spontaneous narcolepsy naps and the magnitude of their refreshing qualities, for example, are estimated entirely by history. The clinical phenomenology of narcolepsy is based on patient descriptions and laboratory observations of induced naps. Thus some of the literature reviewed here rely on clinical impression rather than systematic observation.

Methods

The literature search for narcolepsy began with a computer search (Paperchase) that included the Medline data base since 1966 through 1990. Primary data articles relevant to diagnostic criteria were sought as cited in the Paperchase articles, limited to the Western European languages. *Sleep Research* abstracts for 1989 and 1988 were additionally consulted. Diagnostic criteria were extracted from the resulting articles, book chapters, and abstracts. The current review was editorially limited to 49 references.

Results

Sleep Attacks

"The main symptom of the narcoleptic syndrome is the narcoleptic sleep attack," according to Roth (1980, p. 64), as distinguished from "sleepiness" or "sustained drowsiness," which Yoss and Daly (1960) called "the quintessence of the disorder" (p. 955). The International Classification of Sleep Disorders (ICSD) (American Sleep Disorders Association 1990) does distinguish between "a complaint of excessive sleepiness," which is one of its minimum criteria for narcolepsy diagnosis, and "recurrent daytime naps or lapses into sleep that occur almost daily," which is not. Roth (1980) described a "sudden development of a state of sleep," as did Zarcone (1973). Cathala and colleagues (1981) described "brutal supervention" of sleep, although Dement (1976) explained reported sudden sleep onset by retrograde amnesia for sleepiness. He found that sleep could be prevented in the laboratory by a "watcher" who continually encouraged wakefulness. Thus sleep attacks were due in part to the erosion of "motivation and judgment" in patients who "give in" to the sleepiness. Even if a research assistant tries to keep them awake, and even if they try to resist an attack "by walking, getting into fresh air, washing himself in cold water, smoking, biting his cheek" (Roth 1980, p. 64), "in the end [the patient] succumbs and goes to sleep." As salient as Gelineau's "irresistible" (1880) might be Guilleminault's (1989) adjunctive "unwanted."

A sleep attack lasts 10–15 minutes on average according to Devic and colleagues (1967). By questionnaire data, Dement (1976) suggested a duration of "around 10 to 20 minutes." Although 143 of Roth's (1980) 347 patients claimed durations of 1–5 minutes, longer durations are explained by "bodily position" (Dement 1976) or "reclining" (Guilleminault 1989). Dement's 31 untreated patients averaged 2–3 attacks, and Roth's 347 patients averaged 2–5 attacks daily.

Surprisingly, narcolepsy and idiopathic hypersomnia are rarely compared in the literature. The "pathological sleep drunkenness" (Gudden 1905) or feeling "lethargic" (Mendelson 1987, p. 239) "appears at almost every awakening" (Roth 1972) in the idiopathic hypersomnia patient. This contrasts with the narcolepsy patient who "characteristically wakes up refreshed" (Guilleminault 1989) or "feels fresh on waking, and is wide awake at once" (Adie 1926).

Narcolepsy attacks occur with greater frequency 3–5 times or more (Loewenfeld 1902; Parkes et al. 1975; Rhodes et al. 1989) daily compared with once or twice in most idiopathic hypersomnia patients (Roth 1980). The diurnal sleep attacks of sleep apnea are highly variable and less predictable.

In summary, the cardinal symptom of narcolepsy is little quantified. Although authors agree that sleep attacks afflict most narcolepsy patients, some authorities find sleep attacks a sine qua non for narcolepsy (Yoss and Daly 1960), whereas others do not (American Sleep Disorders Association 1990). There is wide agreement that narcoleptic sleep attacks are relatively brief and refreshing.

For some, sleep attacks alone sufficiently diagnose narcolepsy, presumably because narcoleptic sleep attacks have specific characteristics. This has been described in 110 of 390 patients (Yoss and Daly 1960), in 113 of 360 (Roth 1980), in 54 of 75 (Sours 1963), in 8 of 51 (Ruether et al. 1972), and in 13 of 50 (Janzen and Behnsen 1940). Dement and Rechtschaffen (1968) felt that this "independent narcolepsy" was "somewhat questionable," but it represented one-quarter of their patients. They observed that such patients commonly developed cataplexy "much later" (e.g., 10–15 years). Meier-Ewert and colleagues (1975) clearly distinguished monosymptomatic or "isolated" narcolepsy from idiopathic hypersomnia by the "greater imperativeness and shorter duration of its sleep attacks" and from other narcolepsy syndromes by its more normal night sleep. Carskadon (1976) briefly quoted additional instances of this and described a case of her own. Thus "independent" or "monosymptomatic" narcolepsy may be either a prodromal state or a type of narcolepsy, depending on one's definition. So far, however, except for the DSM-IV Work Group on Sleep Disorders (American Psychiatric Association 1991), most authors have treated it as bona fide narcolepsy.

Cataplexy

The symptom of cataplexy has often been used by investigators to refine their narcolepsy populations. For example, Kales and colleagues (1987) and Broughton and colleagues (1988) used the term *narcolepsy-cataplexy* in the titles of their reports, implying that patients with cataplexy differ essentially from other narcolepsy patients. In fact, after a factor analysis of narcolepsy features, Burton and colleagues (1988) found that cataplexy correlated with daytime sleepiness, but to a small degree, about as much as did depression. Amira and colleagues (1985) found a shorter sleep latency in 31 patients with cataplexy compared with 23 without it, with a wide overlapping between the groups. Rhodes and colleagues (1989) used the term *atypical narcolepsy* for those patients who lacked cataplexy. The ICSD does not consider cataplexy a necessary feature to diagnose narcolepsy.

Cataplexy may occur independently of sleep attacks (Lhermitte and Tournay 1927; Roth 1980), possibly because of partial pathological involvement of the REM-sleep generating system (Freeman and Tant 1983), and is distinguished from gelastic-atonic seizures (Jacome and Risko 1984). Whether or not this independent cataplexy constitutes narcolepsy may be a moot question because Yoss and Daly (1960), who described the classical tetrad, defined sleep attacks as a necessary symptom and also because independent cataplexy is too rare to permit generalizations. Secondary cataplexy, principally from midbrain tegmentum lesions, has many causes, such as tumor (Stahl et al. 1980), postsurgical trauma (Schwarz et al.

1984), or lipidoses (Philippart et al. 1983).

To summarize, cataplexy helps with narcolepsy diagnosis because it is easily identified and usually associated with narcolepsy. As described by the literature, however, it is neither a necessary nor a sufficient criterion of a narcolepsy diagnosis.

Subjective Sleepiness

One possible diagnostic criterion for narcolepsy is "a complaint of excessive sleepiness." In the absence of cataplexy, sleepiness is considered necessary for a narcolepsy diagnosis in the ICSD as distinguished from "recurrent daytime naps or lapses into sleep that occur almost daily," which is not necessary. Dement (1976) distinguished the sleepiness of "inappropriate sleep episodes" from the sleepiness of "altered states of consciousness" as indicated by "automatic behavior, lapses of memory and 'blackouts.'" Automatic behavior reportedly stems from sleepiness of any cause and therefore does not distinguish narcolepsy. But some quality of the wakeful state may differentiate narcoleptic from other somnolent patients, as evidenced in evoked potential patterns that differ not only prior to REM or non–rapid eye movement (NREM) naps, but also between narcolepsy subjects and control subjects (Aguirre and Broughton 1987).

The subjective sleepiness of narcolepsy seems uncorrelated with scores on performance tests. Meier-Ewert and colleagues (1975) pointed out that evoked potential patterns differ between wakefulness after REM and after NREM sleep and raised the question whether the REM-NREM dichotomy might have some analogue during wakefulness. Since narcolepsy has many REM abnormalities, wakefulness in narcolepsy might therefore be affected. In fact, compared with control subjects, awake narcoleptic patients spend more time in active wake and less time in the quiet wake that correlates with higher vigilance.

Narcolepsy patients' measurements from visual analogue scales of wakefulness, performance tests, and Multiple Sleep Latency Test (MSLT) sleepiness vary independently. Thus subjective wakefulness, performance, and sleepiness have surprisingly little relationship. Although impaired wakefulness may be a presenting complaint, it has only been noted rather than studied as a means of diagnostic differentiation. Thus patients may be "permanently sleepy" (Roth 1980), "plodding through a haze of sleepiness" (Yoss and Daly 1960), and "spending the day at an unpleasant level of low alertness" (Guilleminault 1989). Dement (1976) stated that "there is no essential qualitative difference between normal sleepiness and pathological sleepiness."

Sleep Paralysis and Hypnagogic Hallucinations

The roles of sleep paralysis and hypnagogic hallucinations in narcolepsy diagnosis have been clear. These two symptoms have also endured as part of Yoss and Daly's

(1960) classical symptom tetrad, occur in a large minority of cases, and tend to confirm narcolepsy. Sleep paralysis has occurred in 18%–62% of reported series, and hypnagogic hallucinations in 12%–55% (Parkes et al. 1975). Independent sleep paralysis is not rare (Roth 1980); Sours (1963) found it in 5% of his narcoleptic patients. Most other authors, however, have considered sleep attacks or cataplexy as a starting point for the diagnosis of narcolepsy. Therefore it would defy convention to consider isolated sleep paralysis as even a variant of narcolepsy.

Cases have been reported in association with encephalitic, postencephalitic, diencephalic, traumatic, postsurgical neoplastic, vertebral-basilar insufficiency or atlantoaxial dislocation problems. Secondary narcolepsy accounts for 15%–25% of cases (Roth 1980).

Common idiopathic narcolepsy may be secondary to impairments marked by the presence of DR2 tissue antigens (see later). These are not specific to narcolepsy. For instance, multiple sclerosis patients also have increased DR2 antigens, which may be functionally related to the reported increase in narcolepsy symptoms among patients with multiple sclerosis. Cellular mechanisms for narcolepsy may be described in the near future (Guilleminault 1989), making narcolepsy less "idiopathic." But even if narcolepsy becomes etiologically accounted for, it may perhaps be distinguished from the present secondary narcolepsy by some term such as *sui generis* (Adie 1926; Roth 1980) to differentiate it from syndromes that appear after anatomical damage.

Narcolepsy Haplotypes

The narcolepsy-like haplotypes found in almost all narcolepsy patients suggest that genetically predisposed individuals suffer some exogenous stressor that provokes narcolepsy (Honda et al. 1986; Matsuki et al. 1987). Billiard and colleagues (1986) hypothesized that a train of etiological events may begin with a stressor falling on a DR2-positive individual, whose immune reactions include responses to some central nervous system autoantigens. They postulated a narcolepsy susceptibility gene, suggesting a genetic mechanism analogous to that of multiple sclerosis (Seboun et al. 1989). Nearly all narcolepsy patients have DR2 leukocyte antigens. Thus an absence of DR2 might be of some value in ruling out narcolepsy (Honda et al. 1986).

Polygraphic Findings

The objective verification of narcolepsy rests mostly on polygraphic methods. Although patents with narcolepsy fall asleep during the recording, they lack specific features. Using a single 45-minute afternoon nap, Roth and colleagues (1986) reported that an empirically derived score, based on sleep-stage latencies and amounts, separates patients with narcolepsy, patients with idiopathic hypersomnia, and control subjects with great clarity.

Narcolepsy patients show an individually characteristic periodicity in the timing of REM sleep episodes throughout the 24-hour day. Their REM sleep appears abnormally soon after sleep onset in longer-than-normal cycles. More fragmented and ambiguous polygraphic patterns have also been observed, such as intrusions of REM characteristics (e.g., muscle atonia or even REMs) into NREM. The most consistent impression of nocturnal REM sleep has been its wide heterogeneity (Meier-Ewert et al. 1975; Montplaisir et al. 1978; Mosko et al. 1984).

More diagnostic interest has centered on daytime laboratory naps in which short sleep latencies and frequent REM onsets are found in narcolepsy patients. Multiple nap recordings confirm or rule out narcolepsy in a large majority of cases, depending on criteria (Amira et al. 1985; Kales et al. 1987). However, most reported multiple naps were observed in narcolepsy patients who have cataplexy, that is, who are likely sleepier and who likely have more MSLT REM periods than others. Thus nap recordings may confirm the diagnosis in those narcolepsy patients whose diagnosis is clinically obvious. Mitler and colleagues (1979) suggested that two or more REM episodes on MSLT be considered a criterion for abnormality "indicative of narcolepsy." However, little literature systematically examines alternative causes for such REM abnormalities that nonspecifically occur in sleep apnea, drug withdrawal, and fragmented sleep schedules (Broughton et al. 1988). Thus some REM sleep abnormalities may be due to artifacts or other conditions, not present in many narcolepsy patients. Of 100 full-tetrad narcolepsy patients studied by MSLT, Rhodes and colleagues (1989) found that 23 of them lacked a sleep latency of less than 8 minutes and two sleep-onset REM periods. Thus false-negative and false-positive MSLT results may both occur in narcolepsy.

Opinion on the use of polygraphic recordings for narcolepsy diagnosis varies. Guilleminault and Dement (1977) found that "when the history of cataplexy is clear, no sleep recording is necessary to confirm the diagnosis." Others feel that such recordings are warranted to detect malingers, to confirm organic problems for the patient's family, or to justify stimulant drug treatment to legal authorities (Mitler et al. 1979; Thorpy et al. 1983).

Pupillography

Another laboratory method, pupillography, yields clear findings in narcolepsy (Yoss et al. 1969). Recovery of pupillary dark-adapted diameter after light exposure shows differences between narcolepsy and other sleepy patients (Schmidt and Fortin 1982), although applying such methods may be technically difficult.

Discussion

Of diagnostic interest, Rhodes and colleagues (1989) called narcolepsy patients without cataplexy "atypical" narcolepsy cases. Although approximately 15%–45% of narcolepsy patients do not have cataplexy (Amira et al. 1985; Meier-Ewert et al. 1975; Sours 1963; Yoss and Daly 1960), this designation of patients without cataplexy as atypical involves diagnostic issues that reach back to the earliest discussions of narcolepsy. Since so many investigators require cataplexy in their patient populations, those patients without cataplexy may become decreasingly investigated and eventually become either subtypes by default or the wrongful target of generalizations derived from patients with cataplexy. Should the definition of narcolepsy subsequently require cataplexy, those patients without it would be admitted to the group with primary hypersomnia, a heterogenous term that includes idiopathic hypersomnia and Kleine-Levin syndrome. However, narcolepsy would become simpler to diagnose since cataplexy is virtually pathognomonic for narcolepsy. It is far more specific than other diagnostic criteria and would render them redundant if not superfluous.

There are other operational definitions of narcolepsy (besides sleepiness with cataplexy). Multiple, irresistible brief refreshing naps have been enough for a diagnosis to some (Adie 1926; Meier-Ewert et al. 1975; Roth 1980; Wilson 1928). Others define narcolepsy as sleep attacks plus one other tetrad component (Amira et al. 1985) or even one sleep-onset REM period (SOREMP). Still others define narcolepsy according to subtypes, usually idiopathic REM or NREM types and secondary types.

For the moment, the decisions on how to classify and subtype narcolepsy will vary according to the intentions of the classifier. Those who wish maximum homogeneity for experimental purposes may require full-tetrad patients with maximally homogenous laboratory findings. Those who wish working diagnosis to indicate various treatments might accept classical descriptions of the disease. Thus early variances in how narcolepsy is viewed are likely to persist.

A hierarchy of minimal criteria may be envisioned, any level of which may be chosen for diagnostic purposes. The following would be an example.

Multiple brief, unwanted, refreshing diurnal naps in a person who, in the absence of other disorders, awakens refreshed from night sleep.

1. Plus cataplexy.
2. Without cataplexy but with another tetrad component.
3. Without another tetrad component but with positive laboratory findings reasonably specific for narcolepsy (e.g., SOREMPs, pupillary recovery pattern).

4. Without usual laboratory confirmation but with positive findings for some potentially related neurological problem.
5. Without findings for another problem.

This last level of hierarchy might be considered “monosymptomatic” (Roth 1980), “atypical” (Rhodes et al. 1989), or “independent” (Dement and Rechtschaffen 1968; Roth 1980) narcolepsy.

A conventional definition cannot conform to everyone’s definition. For instance, the above definitional scheme transgresses Wilson’s (1928) concept of isolated cataplexy defined as narcolepsy. Unlike the ICSD, which excludes “any medical or psychiatric disorder that could account for the symptoms” (American Sleep Disorders Association 1990, p. 42) that is, secondary narcolepsy—it includes narcolepsy of known medical causes. On the basis of the phenomenology of sleep attacks, it does admit those patients with the usual narcoleptic type of sleep attacks unaccompanied by other narcolepsy stigmata.

Options

There are several options.

1. Omit criteria from DSM-IV and consider narcolepsy a neurological problem. This would provide psychiatrists no information about a common cause of chronic sleepiness.
2. Require sleepiness and at least one more tetrad syndrome as, for example, Amira and colleagues (1985) have done.
3. Distinguish between probable and unequivocal narcolepsy, using the most commonly cited specific criterion, two SOREMPs on MSLT, to make this distinction. Another possibility might be to include such findings in a list of possible narcolepsy features.
4. List various narcolepsy features and designate narcolepsy as *probable* with narcoleptic-type sleep attacks, *presumed* with another tetrad symptom, and *definite* with a third tetrad feature or an additional clinical feature such as automatic behavior, family history, or disturbed nocturnal sleep or with common laboratory features such as REM-onset periods or a pathological sleep latency.

Recommendations

Narcolepsy is proposed for inclusion because it is important in the differential diagnosis of excessive sleepiness. It is distinguished from Primary Hypersomnia by specific clinical features. Table 38–1 provides proposed criteria for narcolepsy.

Table 38–1. Proposed DSM-IV diagnostic criteria for Narcolepsy

A. Irresistible attacks of refreshing sleep occurring daily over at least 3 months.
B. Cataplexy (i.e., brief episodes of sudden bilateral loss of muscle tone, most often in association with intense emotion).
C. Recurrent intrusions of elements of REM sleep into the transition between sleep and wakefulness, as manifested by either hypnopompic/hypnagogic hallucinations or sleep paralysis at the beginning or end of sleep episodes.
D. Not due to a Substance-Induced (i.e., drugs, medication) or Secondary Sleep Disorder.

Note. REM = rapid eye movement.

References

Adie WJ: Idiopathic narcolepsy: a disease sui generis. Brain 49:257–306, 1926

Aguirre M, Broughton RJ: Complex event-related potentials (P 300 and CNV) and MSLT in the assessment of excessive daytime sleepiness in narcolepsy-cataplexy. Electroencephalogr Clin Neurophysiol 67:298–316, 1987

American Psychiatric Association: DSM-IV Options Book: Work in Progress 9/9/91. Washington, DC, American Psychiatric Association, 1991

American Sleep Disorders Association, Diagnostic Classification Steering Committee: International Classification of Sleep Disorders: Diagnostic and Coding Manual. Rochester, MN, American Sleep Disorders Association, 1990

Amira SA, Johnson T, Logoniti NB: Diagnosis of narcolepsy using the multiple sleep latency test: analysis of current laboratory criteria. Sleep 8:325–331, 1985

Billiard M, Seignalet J, Besset A, et al: HLA-DR2 and narcolepsy. Sleep 9:149–152, 1986

Broughton R, Dushesne P, Dunham W, et al: A single nap is as accurate as the MSLT in diagnosing EDS in narcolepsy-cataplexy. Sleep Research 75:223–230, 1988

Burton SA, Eastman CI, Kravitz HM: Factors relating to excessive daytime sleepiness in the narcolepsy syndrome. Sleep Research 17:154, 1988

Carskadon MA: The role of sleep-onset REM periods in narcolepsy, in Narcolepsy. Edited by Guilleminault C, Dement WC, Passonant P. New York, Spectrum, 1976, p 516

Cathala HD, Laffont F, Ming M, et al: Sleep attacks and daytime somnolence. Nouvelle Presse Medicale 10:1621–1626, 1981

Dement W: Daytime sleepiness and sleep "attacks," in Narcolepsy. Edited by Guilleminault C, Dement WC, Passonant P. New York, Spectrum, 1976, pp 17–42

Dement WC, Rechtschaffen A: Narcolepsy: polygraphic aspects, experimental and theoretical considerations, in The Abnormalities of Sleep in Man. Edited by Gasteau H, Lugaresi E, Berti-Ceroni G, et al. Bologna, Aulo Gaggi Editore, 1968, pp 177–189

Devic M, Aimond P, Michael F, et al: Clinical study of the essential narcolepsy-cataplexies. Rev Neurol (Paris) 116:471–490, 1967

Freeman FR, Tant MR: Cataplexy brought on by playing checkers. South Med J 76:1193–1194, 1983

Gelineau J: On narcolepsy. Lancette Francais, Gazette des Hopitals 53:626–628, 1880

Gudden H: Physiological and pathological sleep drunkenness. Archiv fur Psychiatrie und Nervenkrankenheiten 40:989–1015, 1905

Guilleminault C: Narcolepsy syndrome, in Principles and Practice of Sleep Medicine. Edited by Cryger MH, Roth T, Dement WC. Philadelphia, PA, WB Saunders, 1989, pp 338–350

Guilleminault C, Dement WC: 235 cases of excessive daytime sleepiness. Journal of Neural Science 31:13–27, 1977

Guilleminault C, Dement WE, Passonant P: Narcolepsy (preface). New York, Spectrum, 1976

Guilleminault C, Holloman J, Grumet C, et al: HLA-DR2 and the narcolepsy syndrome: the Stamford experience in HLA, in Narcolepsy. Edited by Honda Y, Inji T. Berlin, Springer, 1988, p 109

Henneberg R: On genuine narcolepsy. Zentralblatt fur Neurologie 35:282–290, 1916

Honda Y, Juji T, Matsaki K, et al: HLA-DR2 in narcolepsy and in other disorders of excessive somnolence without cataplexy. Sleep 9:133–142, 1986

Jacome DE, Risko M: Pseudocataplexy: gelastic-atonic seizures. Neurology 34:1381–1389, 1984

Janzen R, Behnsen G: Contribution to the pathophysiology of attacks particularly of cataplectic attacks in the narcolepsy syndrome. Archiv fur Psychiatrie und Nervenkrankenheiten 111:178–189, 1940

Kales A, Bixler EO, Soldatos CP, et al: Narcolepsy/cataplexy, IV: diagnostic value of daytime nap recordings. Acta Neurol Scand 75:223–230, 1987

Lhermitte J, Tournay A: Normal and pathological. Sleep Revue Nerologique 32:751–822, 885–887, 1927

Loewenfeld L: On narcolepsy. Muenchener Medijinliche Wochenschrift 49:1041–1045, 1902

Matsuki K, Honda Y, Judi T: Diagnostic criteria for narcolepsy and HLA-DR2 frequencies. Tissue Antigens 30:155–160, 1987

Meier-Ewert K, Schoepter B, Ruether E: Three narcoleptic syndromes. Nervenarzt 46:624–635, 1975

Mendelson WB: Human Sleep. New York, Plenum, 1987

Mitler MM, Van den Hoed J, Carskadon MA, et al: REM sleep episodes during the multiple sleep latency test in narcoleptic patients. Electroencephalogr Clin Neurophysiol 46:479–481, 1979

Montplaisir J, Billiard M, Takahashi S, et al: Twenty-four hour recording in REM-narcoleptics with special reference to nocturnal sleep disruption. Biol Psychiatry 13:73–89, 1978

Mosko SS, Shampain DS, Sassin JP: Nocturnal REM latency and sleep disturbance in narcolepsy. Sleep 7:115–125, 1984

Parkes JD, Baraitser M, Marsden GD, et al: Natural history symptoms and treatment of the narcoleptic syndrome. Acta Neurol Scand 52:337–353, 1975

Philippart M, Engel J, Zimmerman EG: Gelastic cataplexy in Niemann Pick disease group C and related variants without generalized sphingomyelinase deficiency. Ann Neurol 14:492–493, 1983

Rhodes NP, Hayes B, Guilleminault C, et al: The narcoleptic tetrad and objective polysomnographic tests. Sleep Research 18:294, 1989

Richardson GS, Carskadon MA, Flagg W: Excessive daytime sleepiness in man: multiple sleep latency measurement in narcoleptic and control subjects. Electroencephalogr Clin Neurophysiol 45:621–627, 1978

Roth B: Hypersomnia with "sleep drunkenness." Arch Gen Psychiatry 26:456–462, 1972

Roth B: Narcolepsy and Hypersomnia. Karger, Basel, 1980

Roth B, Nevsimalova S, Sonka K, et al: An alternative to the multiple sleep latency test for determining narcolepsy and hypersomnia: polygraphic score of sleepiness. Sleep 9:243–245, 1986

Ruether E, Meier-Ewert K, Gallitz A: On the symptomatology of the narcoleptic syndrome. Nervenarzt 43:640–643, 1972

Schmidt HS, Fortin LD: Electronic pupillography in disorders of arousal, in Sleeping and Waking Disorders: Indications and Techniques. Edited by Guilleminault C. Menlo Park, CA, Addison-Wesley, 1982, pp 127–143

Schwarz WJ, Stakes JW, Hobson JA: Transient cataplexy after removal of a craniopharyngioma. Neurology 34:1372–1375, 1984

Seboun E, Robinson MA, Doolittle TA, et al: A susceptibility locus for multiple sclerosis is linked to the T-cell receptor chain complex. Cell 57:1095–1100, 1989

Sours JA: Narcolepsy and other disturbances in the sleep-waking rhythm: a study of 115 cases with review of the literature. J Nerv Ment Dis 137:525–542, 1963

Stahl SM, Layzer RB, Amiroff MJ, et al: Continuous cataplexy in a patient with a midbrain tumor. Neurology 30:1115–1118, 1980

Thorpy MJ, Wagner DR, Spielman AJ, et al: Objective assessment of narcolepsy. Arch Neurol 40:126–127, 1983

Wilson SAK: The Narcolepsies. Brain 51:63–109, 1928

Yoss RE, Daly DD: Narcolepsy. Med Clin North Am 44:953–968, 1960

Yoss RE, Moyer NJ, Ogle KN: The pupillogram and narcolepsy: a method to measure decreased levels of wakefulness. Neurology 19:921–928, 1969

Zarcone V: Narcolepsy. N Engl J Med 288:1156–1166, 1973

Chapter 39

Breathing-Related Sleep Disorder

Michael J. Thorpy, M.D.

Statement of the Issues

There are three forms of breathing-related sleep disorder that can produce sleep disruption and lead to complaints of insomnia or excessive sleepiness: obstructive sleep apnea syndrome, central sleep apnea syndrome, and central alveolar hypoventilation syndrome. As these disorders produce symptoms that are commonly encountered in clinical psychiatric practice, the question has been raised as to whether they should be presented in DSM-IV. They are listed as specific disorders in the newly developed International Classification of Sleep Disorders (ICSD) (American Sleep Disorders Association 1990), but were not listed in the sleep disorders section of DSM-III-R (American Psychiatric Association 1987). In DSM-III-R these breathing disorders were subsumed under the headings of "Insomnia Related to a Known Organic Factor" (p. 301) and "Hypersomnia Related to a Known Organic Factor" (p. 304). As their pathophysiology primarily affects the respiratory system, they are not regarded as being "mental disorders."

Significance of the Issues

As these disorders are common causes of symptoms of insomnia and excessive sleepiness, symptoms frequently encountered in clinical psychiatric practice, the clinical psychiatrist should be aware of their features.

Methods

The references given in the ICSD, which were the result of an evaluation of the literature concerning clinical features of the specific disorders, were used as the basis for this review (American Sleep Disorders Association 1990). Other relevant articles pertinent to the field of psychiatry were also reviewed.

Results

These three disorders—obstructive sleep apnea syndrome, central sleep apnea syndrome, and central alveolar hypoventilation syndrome—have clearly defined pathophysiological mechanisms that involve the control of respiration during sleep and are regarded as organic disorders (Guilleminault 1985; Guilleminault et al. 1976; Hudgel 1986). Their pathology can involve the upper airway, lung tissue, and lung volume or the central nervous system control of respiration and its pathways (Cherniack 1981; Guilleminault 1989; Plum and Leigh 1981). The evidence does not support the suggestion that these are mental disorders and suggests instead that they are neurological or respiratory disorders that result in symptoms of disturbed sleep. Obstructive sleep apnea syndrome is a cause of excessive sleepiness (American Sleep Disorders Association 1990; Guilleminault 1989; Guilleminault et al. 1976; Hudgel 1986; Sullivan and Issa 1985; Sullivan et al. 1984), but there are controversial opinions as to its prevalence in patients presenting with a complaint of insomnia (Guilleminault 1989; Guilleminault et al. 1973; Kales et al. 1982). Central sleep apnea syndrome and central alveolar hypoventilation syndrome are known to cause both insomnia and excessive sleepiness, but both occur less frequently than obstructive sleep apnea in patients presenting with either complaint (Bradley et al. 1986; Guilleminault et al. 1987; Issa and Sullivan 1986; Mellins et al. 1970; White 1985).

Discussion

Psychiatrists should be made aware of breathing-related sleep disorder, and it should be considered in the differential diagnosis of insomnia and excessive sleepiness.

The disorder could be written under the specific group heading "Breathing-Related Sleep Disorder," with the text emphasizing the differential diagnostic aspects with other psychiatric disorders. Alternatively, these breathing disorders could be subsumed, along with many other "organic factors," with little or no discussion, under the general headings as previously presented in DSM-III-R: "Insomnia Related to a Known Organic Factor" and "Hypersomnia Related to a Known Organic Factor." If DSM-IV contains a general text on insomnia and hypersomnia, as was contained in DSM-III-R, then these disorders should be discussed in those sections.

In addition to any of the above, or alternatively, it could be included in all discussions of the mental disorders that commonly present with symptoms of insomnia or excessive sleepiness.

Recommendations

If general descriptions of insomnia and hypersomnia are included in DSM-IV, then they should contain mention of breathing-related sleep disorder.

All disorders that produce insomnia or excessive sleepiness should contain mention of this disorder in the differential diagnosis section.

If the sleep disorders section of DSM-IV is to contain an expanded list over that contained in DSM-III-R of all disorders that can produce symptoms of insomnia or excessive sleepiness, then breathing-related sleep disorder should be listed under the heading of "Breathing-Related Sleep Disorder." Alternative consideration of terminology includes the more widely used "Sleep-Related Breathing Disorder"; however, for the purposes of DSM-IV and the listing of this disorder in the sleep disorders section, "Breathing-Related Sleep Disorder" appears more appropriate.

The majority of patients suspected of having this disorder require laboratory confirmation, which would need to be discussed in the text (Guilleminault 1989).

References

American Psychiatric Association: Diagnostic and Statistical Manual of Mental Disorders, 3rd Edition, Revised. Washington, DC, American Psychiatric Association, 1987

American Sleep Disorders Association, Diagnostic Classification Steering Committee: International Classification of Sleep Disorders: Diagnostic and Coding Manual. Rochester, MN, American Sleep Disorders Association, 1990

Bradley TD, McNicholas WT, Rutherford R, et al: Clinical and physiologic heterogeneity of the central sleep apnea syndrome. Review of Respiratory Disease 134:217–221, 1986

Cherniack NS: Respiratory dysrhythmias during sleep. N Engl J Med 305:325–330, 1981

Guilleminault C: Obstructive sleep apnea: the clinical syndrome and historical perspective. Med Clin North Am 69:1121–1359, 1985

Guilleminault C: Clinical features and evaluation of obstructive sleep apnea, in Principal and Practice of Sleep Medicine. Edited by Kryger MH, Roth T, Dement WC. Philadelphia, PA, WB Saunders, 1989, pp 552–558

Guilleminault C, Eldridge FL, Dement WC: Insomnia with sleep apnea: a new syndrome. Science 181:856–858, 1973

Guilleminault C, Tilkian A, Dement WC: The sleep apnea syndromes. Annu Rev Med 31:465–484, 1976

Guilleminault C, Quera-Salva MA, Nino-Murcia G, et al: Central sleep apnea and partial obstruction of the airway. Ann Neurol 21:465–469, 1987

Hudgel DW: Clinical manifestations of the sleep apnea syndrome, in Abnormalities of Respiration During Sleep. Edited by Fletcher EC. New York, Grune & Stratton, 1986, pp 21–37

Issa F, Sullivan C: Reversal of central sleep apnea using nasal CPAP. Chest 90:165–171, 1986

Kales A, Bixler EO, Soldatos CR, et al: Biopsychobehavioral correlates of insomnia, part 1: role of sleep apnea and nocturnal myoclonus. Psychosomatics 23:589–600, 1982

Mellins RB, Balfour HH, Turino GM, et al: Failure of automatic control of ventilation (Ondine's curse). Medicine 49:487–504, 1970

Plum F, Leigh RJ: Abnormalities of central mechanisms in regulation of breathing, part 2, in Lung Biology in Health Disease. Edited by Hornbein TF. New York, Marcel Dekker, 1981, pp 989–1067

Sullivan CE, Issa FG: Obstructive sleep apnea. Clin Chest Med 6:633–650, 1985

Sullivan CE, Issa FG, Berthon-Jones M, et al: Pathophysiology of sleep apnea, in Sleep and Breathing: Lung Biology in Health and Disease. Edited by Saunders NA, Sullivan CE. New York, Marcel Dekker, 1984, pp 299–364

White DP: Central sleep apnea. Med Clin North Am 69:1205–1219, 1985

Chapter 40

Circadian Rhythm Sleep Disorder (Sleep-Wake Schedule Disorder)

Quentin R. Regestein, M.D.

STATEMENT OF THE ISSUES

Sleep-wake disorders derive from a mismatch between the external social schedule and internal timing for the sleep-wake cycle. The question arises whether these disorders should be categorized separately or considered as variants of the same diagnosis.

One might ask whether night-shift sleep disorder is an abnormality or a normal response to schedules incompatible with optimal physiological functioning? Is it a "disorder" or a "problem"? Some workers prefer the night shift, making generalizations about the poor sleep of shift work difficult. There is but a tiny literature on the sleep of shift work relative to the vast numbers of shift workers. Thus whatever sleep changes occur may be largely accepted as an expected consequence of shift work.

Similarly, does Jet-Lag Sleep Disorder represent an actual disease process appropriately classified as a mental disorder? Given the wide variety of reactions to rapid time zone change, which ones would be judged pathological?

Irregular sleep-wake pattern is proposed by the International Classification of Sleep Disorders (ICSD) (American Sleep Disorders Association 1990) as "temporarily disorganized, variable and irregular sleep and waking behavior" (p. 125). This seems analogous to DSM-III-R (American Psychiatric Association 1987) "Sleep-Wake Schedule Disorder, Disorganized Type" (p. 307). This is described as a random and capricious sleep-wake pattern without a daily major sleep period. There is almost no literature about this proposed condition, and the available literature seems inadequate to suggest a separate dyssomnia.

Significance of the Issues

Delayed sleep phase syndrome (DSPS) is a common and well-established clinical entity. Considering that Weitzman and colleagues (1979) found 7%–10% of their insomnia patients had this disorder, relatively little clinical discussion of it has been published. Two other related disorders are vastly rarer in the literature (i.e., non-24-hour sleep phase syndrome and advanced sleep phase syndrome). Non-24-hour sleep phase syndrome, in the opinion of Weitzman and colleagues, is an extension of DSPS and probably results from either a paucity of time cues or lessened sensitivity to time cues compared with DSPS.

Thus DSPS is common, established, related to, and possibly continuous with the much rarer non-24-hour syndrome. DSPS and advanced sleep phase syndrome (ASPS) may both be considered expressions of a basic mismatch of extrinsic and intrinsic circadian rhythms. However, DSPS is more important clinically, since only one case of ASPS has been reported in the refereed literature.

Night work forces the worker to perform at the circadian nadirs for work efficiency or to change work schedules continually and thus to change sleep periods. Not surprisingly, difficulties in work performance and sleep quality arise in the majority of workers on night or rotating shifts. Webb (1989) questioned whether a sleep disorder is the same as a sleep problem, and this bears on whether these expected and statistically normal difficulties should be called a "disorder." There are other disorders based on behavior such as eating, substance abuse, and gambling disorders. As distinguished from these, shift work is imposed on the individual by organizations normally intrinsic to social maintenance. Thus to call the diminished sleep of shift work a disorder risks making a judgment from values outside the industrial culture. Values underlie judgments on whether the consequences of behavior constitute disorders (e.g., being 20% overweight, lasting less than 15 minutes on a standard treadmill test, or having low back pain), but DSM-IV seeks a base in phenomenology rather than values. To call normal, expected sleep problems of the majority of workers on certain shifts a disorder, rather than a response, expressed a value rather than a phenomenon.

The poor sleep of shift work is not analogous to the hazards of other work such as coal mining or virus research. Such hazards are really increased risks (e.g., of injury and infection) that employers seek to prevent. The sleep hazards of shift work are accepted, perhaps because they represent an acknowledged minor and temporary difficulty. It seems like a silent judgment that sleep problems are rarely discussed in the literature of industrial medicine and that no systematic research on the presumed sleep problems of sleep laboratory personnel has been published by sleep researchers who are well-positioned to observe them. It may be that shift work sleep disorder could be likened to all-night-studying disorder or having-anewborn-child disorder (i.e., a creature of definition).

Responses to shift work vary from preference to abhorrence. One might select those who base their intolerance for shift work on poor sleep and define them as night-shift disorder patients. But individual limitations exclude most people from many occupations, without their being considered disordered.

It would seem warranted for the committee to canvas experts from fields outside of psychiatry such as personnel, insurance, and industrial medicine for input into this discussion. This would prevent the committee's defining a disorder on the basis of ethnocentric judgments and might relieve the sleep disorder experts of any biases based on possible self-interest in judging an extremely common pattern of sleep-wake behavior to be a sleep disorder. No other sleep pattern has as much potential to be considered outside of medicine, and therefore the definitions made of sleep patterns related to shift work may be of particular consequence.

Transmeridian flight normally induces circadian desynchrony and commonly involves sleep impairment. Flights that are eastward, begin at night, and are relatively long produce more jet lag, as, presumably, does frequent flying. When does sleep impaired by jet lag become a disorder?

One might resolve this by a time criterion. The data indicate that there are late ripple effects on sleep quality after the worst case of a prolonged eastward flight. Subjective impairment disappears more rapidly, and Multiple Sleep Latency Test (MSLT) data show not so much increased sleepiness as a change in the shape of the sleep latency curve over the day. A time criterion cutoff (e.g., persisting after several days) might distinguish between an expected readjustment and the precipitation of a sleep disorder.

There are no clear-cut cases of irregular sleep-wake pattern in the refereed literature. There is one convincing case in the drug company pamphlet by Hauri (1982) that involved an artificial situation contrived by lawyers (see later). An ablation of circadian rhythms is presumably possible after injury to the neurological substrata of physiological timing systems, but even with severe brain impairment, sleep-wake rhythms likely entail devastations of arousal that preclude consciousness, verbal complaints of dyssomnia, and normal electroencephalogram (EEG) sleep stages. Much of the apparent irregularity of schedule meant to be covered under this diagnosis is probably referred to in night-shift or jet-lag sleep disorders.

The inclusion of this category in both DSM-III-R and in ICSD suggests that sleep disorders experts feel the need for it despite the lack of supporting literature. Although it is an axiom of sleep hygiene that regular arising times foster good sleep quality, irregularity of in-bed times is different from the described absence of a circadian sleep-wake pattern mentioned in these diagnostic schemes.

Methods

The literature search for all of the sleep-wake scheduling disorders began with a computer search (Paperchase) that includes the Medline data base since 1966 to October of 1990. Primary data articles relevant to diagnostic criteria were sought as cited in the Paperchase articles, limited to major Western European languages. *Sleep Research* abstracts of 1989 and 1988 were additionally consulted. From the resulting articles, book chapters, and abstracts, diagnostic criteria were extracted.

In general, the list of references shows the basis of the literature review. Information came from references in the text plus others, since the bibliography was editorially limited.

Results

DSPS, Hypernychthemeral Syndrome, and ASPS

Weitzman and colleagues (1979) described the DSPS as involving initial insomnia, difficulty waking mornings, and sleep undisturbed and late on vacations. Patients tended to be "evening types," and neither psychopathology nor sleep pathology was found. Inspection of sleep logs revealed "3 to 6 day sequences of a progressive delay of sleep onset of 15 to 90 minutes followed by a 1 to 2 day sleep onset advance" (p. 221). DSPS led to major work and social problems. They found 7%–10% of their insomnia patients so afflicted (Weitzman et al. 1981). Diagnosis was made primarily by sleep log. A long history of unsuccessful treatment attempts was a major feature. Childhood onset and occasional episodic reversion to longer sleep periods was also found. Five of the patients described in more detail had average bedtimes of 0415 (4:15 A.M.) and wake times of 1300 (1:00 P.M.). Surveying a population of 127 advertising respondents with DSPS diagnostic features, Joseph-Vanderpool and colleagues (1988) found a mean bedtime of 0123 on weekdays and 0223 on weekends, with wake times of 0917 on weekdays and 1053 on weekends.

The longer endogenous circadian period of youth is apparently reflected in the sleep habits of individuals exposed to normal time cues. Thus age correlates negatively with customary bedtimes (Sherman et al. 1985). Younger people might, therefore, be expected to manifest more difficulties with delayed sleep. A questionnaire survey of 109 students ages 12–19 years revealed that 16% had chronic difficulties with falling asleep and morning awakening, whereas 7.3% gave answers consistent with all the diagnostic criteria of DSPS (Pelayo et al. 1988). The distributions of DSPS scores suggested that they comprised the tail of a normal distribution. Thus DSPS may represent a normal tendency toward late bedtimes rendered inconvenient by social scheduling conventions. This suggests that DSPS is not a rare condition. Its frequency among insomnia patients (Thorpy et al. 1988; Weitzman et al. 1979) and advertisement respondents (Joseph-Vanderpool et al. 1988) confirms its common occurrence.

Among adolescents presenting with DSPS, Ferber and Boyle (1983) reported two distinct groups. The first group is motivated, cooperative, without depression, and readily relieved. The second has DSPS limited to the academic year, varying with the presence of desired morning activities, worsening if the school indulges the patient's late morning arrivals, and often associated with depression. This second type of patient proves covertly or overtly unwilling to follow a treatment program. Thus Ferber and Boyle posed a diagnostic distinction between motivated and unmotivated DSPS in that age group manifesting DSPS most commonly. It may be that the unmotivated type of DSPS would involve an additional diagnosis of Passive Aggressive Personality Disorder or Adolescent Antisocial Disorder. Alternatively, it may be that some sleep-wake scheduling disorders, like some dyssomnias, express more basic problems (e.g., psychiatric problems, drug side effects) and that DSPS might have analogous causes.

Consistent with possible mood sequelae of the syndrome is the work of Thorpy and colleagues (1988), who found psychometric features of depression in 14 of 22 adolescents presenting with DSPS symptoms, including 5 who expressed suicidal ideation. The many psychometrically normal DSPS patients (Weitzman et al. 1981) suggests that DSPS does not necessarily cause depression.

Of diagnostic criteria, the principal ones emphasized by Weitzman and colleagues (1981) were chronic inability to fall asleep at a desired clock time, normal sleep pattern when free of a strict schedule, and multiple unsuccessful attempts to relieve the problem. Joseph-Vanderpool and colleagues (1988) required disrupted work or social functioning due to sleep patterns, repeated unsuccessful attempts to sleep and wake at earlier times, and poor morning alertness at 0700–0900. The ICSD described the minimal criteria for DSPS as a complaint of chronic inability to fall asleep or to awaken spontaneously at early enough times or excessive sleepiness. Freed of an imposed schedule, patients will sleep normally and maintain a 24-hour sleep-wake cycle. Additional criteria are that data from a 2-week sleep log, 24-hour polysomnography, or ambulatory temperature monitoring should be consistent with this history. The patient should have no other difficulty initiating or maintaining sleep (DIMS) disorder.

The "non-24-hour sleep-wake syndrome" or "hypernychthemeral syndrome" (nychthemeron = a 24-hour day) involves assuming a sleep-wake pattern with a circadian period of longer than 24 hours. The first designation might allow for those with a shorter-than-24-hour pattern, but no such patients have been reported. Of those living a longer-than-24-hour day, I found seven published examples. The first of these is only briefly described (Luce 1970). A man delayed his sleep phase 65–85 minutes each day. This reportedly induced a sense of well-being that more than compensated for the inconvenience of planning long in advance for the timing of social events.

A second early case is briefly described as "a subject" who shifted his sleep progressively later "until the synchrony between his habits and those of his associates compelled him to revert abruptly to normal timing" (Eliott et al. 1971). In temporal isolation, he maintained a 26-hour activity cycle both without and with the presence of a clock.

Miles and colleagues (1977) suggested that non-24-hour sleep-wake syndrome may be frequent in the blind. They described a 28-year-old man without light perception from birth. He was an active graduate student who suffered 2- to 3-week bouts of insomnia and excessive daytime sleepiness. His sleep log suggested a free-running rhythm, and, during a hospital admission, an ad-lib schedule disclosed a 24.9-hour period. Imposing a strict schedule of bedtime, meals, and activity failed to entrain a normal sleep-wake rhythm. Subsequently the investigators found that, among 50 subjects with varying degrees of blindness, 14 of whom had no light perception, 38 complained of a significant sleep-wake disorder.

The 4-year sleep log of a student in his 20s revealed a sleep cycle of periods that varied during different epochs. These depended on his contact with others, having no scheduled classes, doing physical work with other students at a farm, and living with a woman whose sleep-wake cycles were ordinarily 24 hours, which induced varying cycle lengths from 22.9 to 40 hours (Weber et al. 1980).

A 34-year-old research analyst was a night person with significant arousal just prior to bedtime (Kokkoris et al. 1978). He maintained a 24.3-hour cycle, resetting himself to a more diurnal wake schedule when his bedtimes reached 0500–0600, by remaining awake an extra 2.5 hours until he reached a desired bedtime. The patient had a constricted affect, was socially withdrawn, lived alone, and enjoyed intellectual pursuits.

A 26-year-old man had kept his own free-running schedule of about 25 hours since age 18 (Eastman et al. 1988). He had a Minnesota Multiphasic Personality Scale (Hathaway and McKinley 1970) score consistent with a schizoid personality. Exposure to bright light for 2–3 hours on awakening slowed his delaying tendency to 5 minutes daily.

A 26-year-old student complained that he could not attend classes that were on a fixed schedule, especially those in the early morning. Psychological evaluation revealed neurotic, narcissistic, and borderline features. Analysis of his 4-year sleep diary revealed a unimodal distribution of bedtimes peaking around 0300 and total hours slept, with a broad peak between 6 and 12 hours. This case was reported as an example of "hypernychthemeral sleep-wake cycle" (Wollman and Lavie 1986), although it would seem more like a case of irregular bedtimes and sleep lengths.

The basic difficulty of non-24-hour sleep-wake syndrome may be an insensitivity to circadian time cues. The schizoid patients may have been less sensitive to societal time cues, as has been observed with others who manifest more severe psychopathology (Morgan et al. 1980). Lessened influence of time cues were present also in the blind patient, the patient whose cycles changed according to the presence of others, and the patient whose sleep-wake cycle was shortened by timed exposure to bright light. Unfortunately there is no information about use of caffeine in any of these reports, rendering the possible effect of this common long-acting stimulant that probably worsens sleep delay unaccounted for.

Weitzman and colleagues (1979) wrote that "the hypernychthemeral syndrome may be a more severe example of the same basic disorder [i.e., DSPS]." The appearance of DSPS in the early stages of what subsequently turned into non-24-hour sleep-wake syndrome (Kamgar-Parsi et al. 1983) and the easy progression of DSPS patients into an induced hypernychthemeral sleep-wake cycle would support this viewpoint. Therefore it may be justified to consider non-24-hour sleep-wake syndrome as a more developed stage of DSPS.

I could find only three cases of ASPS reported in the literature, and two were found in abstracts. They appeared after the original development of the ASDC Nosology in 1979, suggesting that unpublished syndromes seen in clinical practice may influence official classifications.

The first case was a 63-year-old woman who customarily slept from 2100 to 0600 hours and complained of insomnia (Kamei et al. 1979). She was placed in 20-day temporal isolation, during which she first showed a 23-hour circadian period length. After an unreported but brief interval of a few days, her period length lengthened to 24 hours and finally to 24.5 hours. She continued to complain of insomnia because of intervening wakefulness during sleep.

The second case was a 62-year-old man who slept between 1830 and 0300 hours (Moldofsky et al. 1986). He remained refreshed mornings but often napped 1–2 hours in the afternoon. Oral temperature peak was at 1400. Polysomnography beginning at 2330 hour revealed 4.5 hours of sleep with mild apnea (AI = 17, minimum O_2 saturation = 82%). A four-nap MSLT beginning at 0900 showed a 2.3-minute sleep latency with one sleep-onset rapid eye movement (REM) period 16 minutes into the second nap. Past history included treatment for depression. After phase advance chronotherapy, the patient slept from 2300 to 0600 hours, and his oral temperature peak occurred at 1300.

A third patient was a 38-year-old woman who could not depart from mean bedtimes of 2122 and arising times of 0334 (Singer and Lewy 1989). When she did remain up past midnight, she would sleep until 0400 or 0500. It is unclear in the abstract, but she may have taken daytime naps.

Presumably because the endogenous period length shortens with increased age (Matsumoto and Morita 1987; Morin 1988), the major sleep period shifts somewhat earlier with age (Tune 1969). Because the two of the three reported patients with ASPS were both in their seventh decade, they may represent the tail of a normal distribution, especially the first case.

Irregular Sleep-Wake Schedule

Moore-Ede and colleagues (1982) published a 3-week sleep chart of a patient they described as having a "disrupted sleep-wake cycle." This chart shows some elements of a progressive delay in bedtimes superimposed on a basically haphazard pattern.

Hauri (1982) described a patient who, to win a lawsuit, stayed out of work, spending 2 years alone in his apartment, obtaining food from a 24-hour store. Twenty-four hour recordings revealed frequent short naps throughout the day and night. A lengthening major sleep period beginning around 0100 occurred through a 7-day recording period. All insomnia vanished after the patient settled the lawsuit and became self-employed.

The ICSD referred to severely brain-damaged patients in whom irregular sleep pattern is allegedly most common. It referenced Okawa and colleagues (1986), who reported indefinite sleep times in 7 of 12 unresponsive bedridden children fed by gastrostomy. However, in the two examples of such "dispersed" sleep shown, one patient had 76% of his sleep during the dark period, with naps every 3–4 hours beginning about 12 hours after the beginning of the major sleep period. The second patient slept about 64% of the time in what appeared to be 2- to 4-hour disrupted sleep periods that were set off by 1- to 2-hour periods where wake predominated. Severe alterations of non–rapid eye movement sleep with "monostage" sleep was observed. Body temperature and cortisol circadian rhythms were preserved. In a double-plotted figure of the sleep-wake rhythm meant to exemplify dispersed sleep, a major sleep period that occurred between 0 and 6 hours was evident, with naps occurring in rough periodicity at around 0800, 1300, and 0400. This raises questions about the alleged irregularity of the sleep wake rhythm.

Two studies of sleep patterns in demented adults found preservation of circadian sleep-wake patterns. In the first study, 30 demented and 14 age-matched control inpatients were observed by 72-hour polygraphic monitoring, with behavioral observations for wakefulness every half hour (Allen et al. 1989). The 24-hour profiles of sleep-wake behavior as well as the results of the polygraph were generally similar in the two groups, with sleep at night and in the early afternoon. Three of the demented patients, however, slept somewhat more days than nights, and the demented group showed more daytime slow-wave sleep. The overall circadian sleep-wake rhythm remained intact.

In another study, 16 female nursing home residents with a severe and fairly homogenous degree of dementia were observed hourly for sleep-wake behavior for 2 weeks. A 24-hour rhythm in the percentage of residents asleep peaked from about 2100 to 0400, with a tendency to awaken around 0100–0200, regardless of the individual's total daily sleep times (Regestein and Morris 1987). Both long-sleeping and short-sleeping residents manifested circadian sleep-wake rhythms.

Night-Shift Sleep Disorder

The situation of frequently time-zone shifting aircrews would seem analogous to that of shift workers. Czeisler and Allan (1987) stated that both jet lag and shift work require shifting of the circadian phase. Wever (1980) stated that the problems of rhythmological readjustment after schedule displacement may apply to shift work as well as to jet lag. Aircrews can probably remain on their home circadian rhythm only temporarily at their destination (C. A. Czeisler, G. S. Richardson, personal communications, 1990); the lengths of stay at their destination and the flight configurations vary, as do work shifts. Jet lag and shift work, therefore, may be generic terms applied to individuals who are least physically fit at the beginning of the morning shift (Ostberg 1973). Quoting primary sources such as in-house publications and doctoral dissertations, Rutenfranz and colleagues (1977) stated that about 20% of 9,000 shift workers surveyed had difficulty adapting to night work. A major complaint focused on noise during daytime sleep hours from children, traffic, aircraft, and telephones.

Dumont and colleagues (1988) canvassed 426 nurses with questionnaire items pertaining to the quality of sleep and vigilance. From a principal components analysis, they extracted questions that loaded on a quality of sleep factor. An index was figured for each respondent by multiplying the magnitude of her scale response to each item by its factor loading from the analysis. This index increased stepwise with number of years on the night shift, except for those with the most night work (mean = 13.4 years) who had the smallest score (i.e., the best sleep and vigilance).

Transmeridian aircrews have been much studied during shift work. Hauty and Adams (1966) found an increase of fatigue after multiple time-zone shifts that did not last as long as the resynchronization period for calcium or steroid excretions. Kurosaki and colleagues (1989) reported more sleepiness and diminished mood after polar flights from Tokyo to London. A questionnaire study done of 312 Air France flight personnel found that a variety of adjustments were made after long flights (e.g., remaining on local time, going to bed early in local time after a westward flight) (LaVernhe 1970). After accommodating to American time, poor sleep was reported by 75% of personnel reaccommodating to Paris time. However, most slept well by the second night, even though steroid and calcium excretions took 4 or 5 days to resynchronize with local time.

Summarizing questionnaire studies, it would seem that the different shift schedules induce different alterations in sleep pattern; that such alterations induce insufficient sleep in some, especially during an adjustment period after shift rotation; that night shift is associated with the subjectively worst sleep; but that some workers sleep subjectively better while on continued night shift. Thus shift work induces heterogenous responses.

Objective measurements. An early polygraphic study found that day sleep after night work was shortened a mean of 104 minutes compared with night sleep after day work in nurses (Ehrenstein et al. 1970). In contrast, Kripke and colleagues (1971) found little sleep disturbance in 10 night-working Air Force corpsmen, although abnormal polygraphic patterns such as frequent transitions between sleep stages were observed. The dim-light conditions of the antarctic winter gradually diminish slow-wave sleep in all workers (Paterson 1975). In this setting, the night shift induces diminished sleep with early rising for weeks after return to day shift, which coincides with an advance in the timing of the daily melatonin rhythm (Broadway and Arendt 1986). Among 16 train drivers with irregular work hours, day sleep after night sleep was about 3.3 hours shorter than night sleep, with shorter latency and less stage 1, 2, and REM (Torsvall et al. 1981). Day sleep will be longer after longer periods of night sleep deprivation, but nevertheless truncated (e.g., 2.9 hours after 50% deprivation versus 4.5 hours after 100% deprivation) (Akerstedt et al. 1983). An unusual shift work pattern in Japan consists of 24 hours work shift, during which 3.5 hours sleep is allowed alternating with 24 hours off. Day sleep beginning at 1100 hour on days off had more awakenings and more stage shifts (Matsumoto and Morita 1987). Among 19 males rotating work shifts, sleep duration was increasingly shortened the later in the night sleep began (Foret and Benoit 1974). Slow-wave sleep increased with lengthened duration of the prior wake period, in contrast to REM sleep, which was present in greater amounts at the end of the night regardless of bedtimes or prior wakefulness.

Sleepiness. However workers sleep while on the night shift, many of them feel sleepy when awake. When asked "Out of a week of day shifts, how many times do you usually nod off or fall asleep while at work?" 23% slept sometimes, whereas on analogous questions, 20% and 53% fell asleep on evening and night shifts, respectively (Coleman and Dement 1986). Of 1,000 train drivers on day trips, 8% admitted "dozing off on most trips" and 23% dozing off at least once, whereas 11%

and 59% respectively so responded for night trips (Akerstedt 1988). Monitored night train drivers manifested stigmata of sleepiness such as increased alpha activity and slow eye movements in 60% of cases; 20% manifested frank sleep while driving. On the basis of these and other polygraphic studies, Akerstedt estimated that 75% of night-shift workers were sleepy every night. Thus the sleepiness complaints of night workers are statistically normal phenomena.

Summary. The cause of night-shift sleep pattern is widely attributed to the inertia of a temporarily fixed propensity to sleep onset (Strogatz et al. 1987) with respect to rapid schedule shifts. Experimenters observe that the length and organization of sleep depend on which phase, ascending or descending, of the circadian temperature cycle it begins (Czeisler et al. 1980; Gillberg and Akerstedt 1982). The temperature cycle itself shows delayed peaks and flattened amplitudes in night workers (Smith 1979), implying distortion of bodily timing mechanisms. In practical terms, the weaker internal circadian synchronization of older persons (Wever 1975), plus their tendency to advance daily temperature peaks earlier into the daytime sleep period of the night worker (Matsumoto and Morita 1987), may account for why night work is less tolerated with advancing age. This may also account for the relative paucity of sleep abnormalities found in young subjects whose sleep had been shifted either by night work (Kripke et al. 1971) or experimentally (Webb et al. 1971), whereas older shift workers had polygraphically lower quality sleep after night work compared with younger ones (Matsumoto and Morita 1987; Torsvall et al. 1981). Thus inability to tolerate the night shift may be likened to the gradually decreasing tolerance for physically demanding work of all kinds that affects greater numbers of the population with advancing age. In any case, as-yet-undefined intolerance to temporal relocation of work hours (e.g., lessened sensitivities to external pacemakers or slowness of reentrainment) as well as age all predispose to sleep disturbances.

There may be other explanations, however, since circadian dislocation and age relate to all shift workers, but only 20% of them tolerate it poorly, not necessarily the oldest 20% (Rutenfranz et al. 1977; Thiis-Evensen 1958). In a masterful overview of shift work, Rutenfranz (1973) pointed out that many of the nonspecific complaints of night workers (e.g., malaise, fatigue, difficulty concentrating, irritability) could be attributed to sleep loss. However, there seemed to be a specific problem with gastrointestinal disturbances. This impression is consistent with observations by LaVernhe (1970) in flight personnel and Koller and colleagues (1978) in night-shift oil refinery workers. Gordon and colleagues (1986) found much heavier use of caffeine in shift workers as well as significantly increased use of alcohol (16% of men on variable shifts drank more than four drinks daily). On their repeated telephone interviews with more than 2,500 workers, they also found more job stress, severe emotional problems, and, not surprisingly, indigestion. Reviewers have explained some distress of shift work by means of social factors (e.g., frequent absences from the family, insufficient recreation, and disruption of family organization) (Monk 1989; Schaffler and Renemann 1976). It is not entirely clear, however, how distressing shift work actually is to the family. One study found a lower rate of divorces, a higher rate of marriage, and more children among shift workers, although they had more health-related complaints (Koller et al. 1978). The prevalence of health problems among shift workers when health status rather than questionnaire responses is considered may be the same as others. Epidemiological surveys of 8,603 men working shifts for 10 or more years showed no excess death nor any other apparent health effect of shift work (Taylor and Pocock 1972). Studies of 6,385 day workers and 7,963 shift workers revealed consistently less absenteeism among shift workers, despite the fact that 60% of them complained of sleep problems and 35% had gastric complaints. Those with peptic ulcers transferred to day work, however, had the same incidence of ulcers as day workers (Thiis-Evensen 1958). Thus subjective complaints of sleep disorders do not apparently translate into actual illness.

Although the sleep problems reported by shift workers are tolerated by most of them, as indicated by the majority who remain on shifts, it may nevertheless induce some impairment. Redesigning the work schedule to progress to later rather than earlier shifts at 8-day rather than 21-day intervals increased production at one plant (Czeisler et al. 1982). The mechanism of this improvement (e.g., less sleep disruption, less disruption of off-job activities, or less use of stimulants) was not investigated.

Summarizing much literature on shift work sleep disorder, there seems not much written in proportion to the vast numbers of shift workers. Any disturbance is heterogenous in the sense that work schedules vary widely in design, and in the sense that reactions to shift work vary from intolerance to preference. The night shift would seem most associated with both health complaints and sleepiness, of which the worker may not complain. Circadian rhythm dislocation, augmented daytime noise, and heavy use of stimulants may all lessen sleep quality.

Jet-Lag Sleep Disorder

Sleep quality diminishes after lengthy meridian flight, more so after eastward flights. Sleep after time change may be worse a few days after the change compared with immediately after the change. After both westward and eastward flights, sleep was generally more affected on night 5 than on night 1 (Nicholson et al. 1986), although sleep had recovered considerably by night 3 compared with night 1 among another eastward flying group (Sasaki et al. 1986). There is some evidence that sleep recovers in a zigzag, relapsing manner, rather than with constant improvement. Twelve placebo-treated travelers returning to San Francisco from Japan had about 1 hour less sleep than normal on nights 2 and 4. Of interest, hypnotic-treated travelers had less sleep on night 5. In any case, sleep did not steadily improve (Seidel et al. 1987). In a laboratory analogue, 6-hour phase-advanced subjects also recovered their total sleep times in a similar, zigzag manner (Monk 1989). Thus a complexity of interacting control mechanisms regulates the readapting sleep-wake cycle.

Inertia in the physiological control of the sleep-wake cycle will necessitate a readaptation period after sudden dislocation of the sleep schedule. Details of each individual readjustment after time-zone changes will vary widely, according to the host of constitutional, behavioral, and social factors that impinge on sleep.

It may be that the sleep distortions imposed by jet lag are insufficient to cause much functional impairment. For instance, among 11 pilots flying from San Francisco to London, Dement and colleagues (1986) found no differences in MSLT-measured sleepiness. Furthermore, compared with baseline, among 8 pilots who flew from San Francisco to Tokyo, these investigators found less rather than more sleepiness. Such findings are consistent with the faster recovery of task performance compared with circadian synchrony after eastward or westward 8- to 10-hour flights (Buck 1976; Hauty and Adams 1966). Performance rhythms have also been reported that shift in parallel with recovering circadian rhythms (Klein et al. 1972).

Circadian phenomena may not account for all the adjustments required after long jet flights. After a 12-hour flight westward to their home time, travelers had more subjective fatigue by scale ratings then they had on an eastward flight (Petrie et al. 1989). The above diversity of unexpected data suggests that the physiological effects on sleep after transmeridian flights are either poorly predictable or heterogenous or have yet to be adequately assessed.

Discussion and Recommendations

The major diagnostic criterion for DSPS would be the tendency for the major sleep period to drift progressively later.

With a virtually nonexistent data base, the question arises whether ASPS deserves a separate heading in a sleep classification. If it does, the diagnostic features of the syndrome would be difficult to base on published data. In only one of the two published cases were the actual sleep hours a presenting complaint. This would force the committee to compose a diagnostic entity based on a single case. Since the syndrome first appeared in the ASDC classification of 10 years ago, the dearth of literature would suggest that it is exquisitely rare. Some feel, however, that ASPS is fairly common among the elderly. Thus authors may be disinclined to write about the problem.

Faced with producing criteria for shift work sleep disorder, the ICSD simply defined it as any complaint of insomnia or excessive sleepiness associated with work during the habitual sleep phase, usually night work. In the text, it stated that "the disorder is usually able to be diagnosed by history," and its essential feature was that it was transient, according to work schedules. Where diagnosis was in doubt, it suggested a variety of investigations, but proposed that any sleep abnormality, rather than specific criteria, would be consistent with the disorder.

At this point it would seem that the mechanisms by which some are intolerably afflicted, some complain but work, and some prefer night work remain unclear. Biological clock phenomena associated with age, morningness-eveningness, and perhaps total sleep requirement may relate to such mechanisms. For the moment, any complaint of diminished sleep quality that disappears when work shifts are optimized would seem to stand as the major criterion. Whether this common reaction is a "disorder" or a "problem" (Webb 1989) may continue to be a matter of definition rather than of data.

Subjective worsening of sleep after transmeridian flight is widely acknowledged and is greater after night flights east and less after day flights west (Suvanto and Ilmaren 1987). Large variations in frequency, scheduling, and routes of flying, however, render *jet lag* a generic term. Thus reported observations will have rather general rather than specific meanings for the individual.

The irregular sleep-wake pattern or sleep-wake scheduling disorder, disorganized type, has little descriptive literature. Hauri's (1982) single case is the only one. The acerbate patient's irregular sleep-wake pattern (Okawa et al. 1986) rests on little information and is questionable. Even if it were more firmly established, however, it would hardly seem like an insomnia problem, since the essentials of a complaint, inadequate daytime functioning because of sleep problems, or even the presence of conventional EEG sleep patterns, are all lacking. Among demented adults, furthermore, the data indicate an intact circadian rhythm.

The Sleep Disorder Work Group elected to combine various disorders under a single rubric "Circadian Rhythm Sleep Disorder (Sleep-Wake Schedule Disorder)" as stated in the *DSM-IV Options Book* (American Psychiatric Association 1991). Specific subtypes were optionally included for delayed sleep phase type, and either "desynchronized type" to cover jet-lag and night-shift sleep disorders or delayed sleep phase type plus these two additional disorders listed separately. Advanced sleep phase type and disorganized type were deleted because they were considered too rare to include.

Another option might be to list criteria for these subtypes (Table 40–1).

Table 40–1. Proposed DSM-IV diagnostic criteria for Sleep Disorder subtypes

Delayed Sleep Phase Syndrome

A. A persistent drift of bedtimes increasingly later until an equilibrium is established between sleep phase and scheduled obligations. Cycles of sudden shifts to earlier bedtimes with subsequent drifts later may be seen.

B. A complaint of initial insomnia.

C. A 2-week sleep log demonstrating progressively later shifts in bedtime.

Options:
1. Persistent unsuccessful attempts to sleep and wake at earlier times.
2. Excessive sleepiness for abnormally long periods at the desirable rising time.
3. Disrupted work or social functioning due to sleep patterns.

Advanced Sleep Phase Syndrome

A. Persistent drift of bedtimes earlier, until an equilibrium is established between sleep phase and scheduled obligations.

B. A complaint of early morning awakening.

C. A 2-week sleep log demonstrating undesirable early bedtimes.

Non-24-Hour Sleep Phase Syndrome

A. Persistent drift of major sleep period scheduling through the 24-hour day.

B. Primary complaint of insomnia or excessive sleepiness.

C. Absence of other apparent causes of insomnia.

Options:
1. Have all three conditions in DSM-IV as independent conditions, despite the minuscule data base for the last two.
2. Combine these disorders, to make "Sleep-Wake Scheduling Disorder" or "Circadian Rhythm Sleep Disorder."
3. Admit only Delayed Sleep Phase Syndrome as a disorder and describe the other two as variants in the text.
4. Continue as in DSM-III-R.

Night-Shift Sleep Disorder

A. Primary complaint of insomnia or excessive daytime sleepiness associated with periods of night work.

B. Absence of sleep-related complaint during periods of day or afternoon work.

Option:
1. Consider it a Z code (analogous to V codes of DSM-III-R), rather than a disorder.

Disorganized Type (Irregular Sleep-Wake Pattern)

A. Primary complaint of insomnia or excessive sleepiness.

B. Haphazard, irregular, temporarily disorganized sleep-wake pattern with poorly discernible sleep-wake rhythm.

(continued)

Table 40–1. Proposed DSM-IV diagnostic criteria for Sleep Disorder subtypes *(continued)*

Options:
1. Omit irregular sleep-wake schedule disorder, disorganized type from DSM-IV.
2. Include a category that refers to irregular in-bed times rather than to irregular sleep-wake patterns.
3. Use the above modification of DSM-III-R criteria, which requires "poorly discernible" rather than "absent" daily major sleep period.
4. Leave this category as it was, a subtype of the major classification "Sleep-Wake Schedule Disorder."

Jet-Lag Sleep Disorder

A. Primary complaint of dyssomnia or of excessive daytime sleepiness.

B. Occurs after more than one rapid time-zone change.

C. Lasts longer than 3 days.

Option:
1. Lasts longer in days than half the number of time-zone changes flown.

References

Akerstedt T: Sleepiness as a consequence of shift work. Sleep 11:17–34, 1988

Akerstedt T, Torsvall L, Gillberg M: Sleep/wake disturbances in shift work: implications of sleep loss and circadian rhythms. Sleep Research 12:359, 1983

Allen R, Rosenthal N, Joseph-Vanderpool Jr, et al: Delayed sleep phase syndrome: polysomnographic characteristics. Sleep Research 18:133, 1989

American Psychiatric Association: Diagnostic and Statistical Manual of Mental Disorders, 3rd Edition, Revised. Washington, DC, American Psychiatric Association, 1987

American Psychiatric Association: DSM-IV Options Book: Work in Progress 9/9/91. Washington, DC, American Psychiatric Association, 1991

American Sleep Disorders Association, Diagnostic Classification Steering Committee: International Classification of Sleep Disorders: Diagnostic and Coding Manual. Rochester, MN, American Sleep Disorders Association, 1990

Broadway J, Arendt J: Delayed recovery of sleep and melatonin rhythms after nightshift in antarctic winter. Lancet 2:813–814, 1986

Buck L: Psychomotor test performance and sleep patterns of aircrew flying transmeridian routes. Aviat Space Environ Med 47:979–985, 1976

Coleman RM, Dement WC: Falling asleep at work: a problem for continuous operations. Sleep Research 15:265, 1986

Czeisler CA, Allan JS: Acute circadian phase reversal in man via bright light exposure: application to jet lag. Sleep Research 16:605, 1987

Czeisler CA, Weitzman ED, Moore-Ede MC, et al: Human sleep: its duration and organization depend on its circadian phase. Science 210:1264–1267, 1980

Czeisler CA, Moore-Ede MC, Coleman RM: Rotating shift work schedules that disrupt sleep are improved by applying circadian principles. Science 217:460–463, 1982

Dement WC, Seidel WF, Cohen SA, et al: Sleep and wakefulness in aircrew before and after transatlantic flights. Aviat Space Environ Med 57 (suppl):1314–1328, 1986

Dumont M, Montplaisir J, Infante-Rivard C: Insomnia index among nursing personnel with past experience of night work: results of a survey. Sleep Research 17:371, 1988

Eastman CL, Anagnopoulos CA, Cartwright RD: Can bright light entrain a free-runner? Sleep Research 17:372, 1988

Ehrenstein W, Mueller-Limmroth W, Schaffler K: Polygraphic sleep investigations comparing day-sleep after night work to night-sleep after day work in 8 nurses. Pflugers Arch 319:R121, 1970

Eliott AL, Mills NJ, Waterhouse JM: A man with too long a day. J Physiol (Lond) 211:30P–31P, 1971

Ferber R, Boyle MD: Delayed sleep phase syndrome versus motivated sleep phase delay in adolescents. Sleep Research 12:239, 1983

Foret J, Benoit O: Structure of sleep in shift workers. Electroencephalogr Clin Neurophysiol 37:337–344, 1974

Gillberg M, Akerstedt T: Body temperature and sleep at different times of day. Sleep 5:378–388, 1982

Gordon NP, Cleary PD, Parlan CE, et al: The prevalence and health impact of shiftwork. Am J Public Health 76:1225–1228, 1986

Hathaway SR, McKinley JC: Minnesota Multiphasic Personality Inventory, Revised. Minneapolis, MN, University of Minnesota, 1970

Hauri P: The Sleep Disorders, 2nd Edition. Kalamazoo, MI, Upjohn, 1982

Hauty GT, Adams T: Phase shifts of the human circadian system and performance deficit during the periods of transition, II: West-East flight. Aerospace Medicine 10:1027–1033, 1966

Joseph-Vanderpool JR, Kelly KG, Schulz PM, et al: Delayed sleep phase syndrome revisited: preliminary effects of light and triazolam. Sleep Research 17:381, 1988

Kamei R, Hughes L, Miles L, et al: Advanced-sleep phase syndrome studied in a time isolation facility. Chronobiologia 6:115, 1979

Kamgar-Parsi B, Wehr TA, Gillin JC: Successful treatment of human non-24-hour sleep-wake syndrome. Sleep 6:257–264, 1983

Klein KE, Wegmann HM, Hunt BI: Desynchronization of body temperature and performance circadian rhythm as a result of outgoing and homegoing transmeridian flights. Aerospace Medicine 43:119–132, 1972

Kokkoris CP, Weitzman D, Pollak CP, et al: Long-term ambulatory temperature monitoring in a subject with a hypernychthemeral sleep-wake cycle disturbance. Sleep 1:177–190, 1978

Koller M, Jundi M, Cervinka R: Field studies of shift work at an Austrian oil refinery, I: health and psychosocial well being of workers who drop out of shift work. Ergonomics 10:835–847, 1978

Kripke DF, Cook B, Lewis OF: Sleep of night workers. Psychophysiology 7:377–384, 1971

Kurosaki Y, Sasaki M, Tanura M, et al: Mood changes of flight crew during multiple layover polar plight. Sleep Research 18:426, 1989

LaVernhe J: Effects of time-shift of air flights on flight personnel. Muenchener Medijinliche Wochenschrift 112:1746–1752, 1970

Luce GG: Biological rhythms in psychiatry and medicine (PHS Publ No 2088). Washington, DC, U.S. Government Printing Office, 1970

Matsumoto K, Morita Y: Effects of nighttime nap and age on sleep patterns of shift workers. Sleep 10:580–589, 1987

Miles LEM, Raynal DM, Wilson MA: Blind man living in normal society has circadian rhythms of 24.9 hours. Science 198:421–423, 1977

Moldofsky H, Musisi S, Phillipson EA: Treatment of a case of advanced sleep phase syndrome by phase advance chronotherapy. Sleep 9:61–65, 1986

Monk TH: Shift work, in Principles and Practice of Sleep Medicine. Edited by Kryger MH, Roth T, Dement WC. Philadelphia, PA, WB Saunders, 1989, pp 163–172

Moore-Ede MC, Sulzman FM, Fuller CA: The Clocks That Time Us. Cambridge, MA, Harvard University Press, 1982

Morgan R, Minors DS, Waterhouse JM: Does light rather than social factors synchronize the temperature rhythm of psychiatric patients? Chronobiologia 7:331–335, 1980

Morin LP: Age-related changes in hamster circadian period, entrainment and rhythm splitting. Journal of Biological Rhythms 3:237–248, 1988

Nicholson AN, Pascoe PA, Spencer MB, et al: Nocturnal sleep and daytime alertness of aircrew after transatlantic flights. Aviat Space Environ Med 57 (12 suppl):1342–1352, 1986

Okawa M, Takahashi K, Sasaki H: Disturbance of circadian rhythms in severely brain-damaged patients correlated with CT findings. J Neurol 233:274–282, 1986

Ostberg O: Interindividual differences in circadian fatigue patterns of shift workers. Br J Ind Med 30:341–351, 1973

Paterson RAH: Seasonal reduction of slow-wave sleep at an antarctic coastal station. Lancet 1:468–469, 1975

Pelayo RP, Thorpy MJ, Glovinsky P: Prevalence of delayed sleep phase syndrome among adolescents. Sleep Research 17:391, 1988

Petrie K, Conaglen JV, Thompson L, et al: Effect of melatonin on jet lag after long haul flight. BMJ 298:705–707, 1989

Regestein QR, Morris J: Daily sleep patterns observed among institutionalized elderly patients. J Am Geriatr Soc 35:767–772, 1987

Rutenfranz J: Pathogenic effects of exogenous rhythm disturbances. Verh Dtsch Ges Inn Med 79:31–37, 1973

Rutenfranz J, Colquhoun WP, Krauth P, et al: Biomedical and psychosocial aspects of shift work. Scand J Work Environ Health 3:165–182, 1977

Sasaki M, Kurosaki Y, Mori A, et al: Patterns of sleep-wakefulness before and after transmeridian flight in commercial airline pilots. Aviat Space Environ Med 57 (12, suppl):1329–1342, 1986

Schaffler K, Renemann HH: Sleep disturbance in cabin personnel after transmeridian long distance flights. Med Klin 71:1985–1995, 1976

Seidel WF, Cohen SA, Blinise NG, et al: Jet lag after eastward and westward flights. Sleep Research 16:639, 1987

Sherman B, Whysham C, Pfahl B: Age-related changes in the circadian rhythm of plasma cortisol in man. J Clin Endocrinol Metab 61:439–443, 1985

Singer CM, Lewy AJ: Case report: use of the dim light melatonin onset in the treatment of ASPS with bright light. Sleep Research 18:445, 1989

Smith D: A study of weekly and rapidly rotating shift workers. Int Arch Occup Environ Health 43:211–220, 1979

Strogatz SH, Kronauer RE, Czeisler CA: Circadian pacemaker interferes with sleep onset at specific times each day: role in insomnia. Am J Physiol 253:R172–R178, 1987

Suvanto S, Ilmaren J: Disturbances in sleep-wakefulness cycle of flight attendants after transmeridian flights. Sleep Research 16:645, 1987

Taylor PJ, Pocock SJ: Mortality of shift and day workers. 1956–68. Br J Ind Med 29:201–207, 1972

Thiis-Evensen E: Shiftwork and health. Industrial Medicine and Surgery 27:493–497, 1958

Thorpy MJ, Korman E, Spielman AJ, et al: Delayed sleep phase syndrome in adolescents. J Adolesc Health Care 9:22–27, 1988

Torsvall L, Akerstedt T, Gillberg M: Age, sleep and irregular work hours. Scand J Work Environ Health 7:196–203, 1981

Tune GS: Sleep and wakefulness in a group of shift workers. Br J Ind Med 26:54–58, 1969

Webb WB: What is a sleep disorder? APSS Newsletter 4:25, 1989

Webb WB, Agnew HW, Williams RL: Effect of sleep of a sleep period time displacement. Aerospace Medicine 42:152–155, 1971

Weber AL, Cary MS, Connor N, et al: Human non-24-hour sleep/wake cycles in an everyday environment. Sleep 2:347–354, 1980

Weitzman D, Czeisler C, Coleman R, et al: Delayed sleep phase syndrome: a biological rhythm disorder. Sleep Research 8:221, 1979

Weitzman ED, Czeisler CA, Coleman RM, et al: Delayed sleep phase syndrome, a chronobiological disorder with sleep-onset insomnia. Arch Gen Psychiatry 38:737–746, 1981

Wever R: The meaning of circadian periodicity for older people. Verh Dtsch Ges Pathol 59:100–180, 1975

Wever RA: Phase shifts of human circadian rhythms due to shifts of artificial zeitgebers. Chronobiologia 7:303–327, 1980

Wollman M, Lavie P: Hypernychthemeral sleep-wake cycle: some hidden regularities. Sleep 9:324–334, 1986

Chapter 41

REM-Related Parasomnias and Other Parasomnias

Michael J. Sateia, M.D.

Statement of the Issues

Two subcategories of the "Parasomnias" section of the International Classification of Sleep Disorders (ICSD) (American Sleep Disorders Association 1990) nosology are addressed here. ICSD has chosen to identify a distinct grouping for rapid eye movement (REM)–related parasomnias—those disorders that arise as a result of the unique physiology and mentation that is associated with REM sleep. All of these disorders would be classified under the "Parasomnias" section of DSM-III-R (American Psychiatric Association 1987). "Nightmares" (dream anxiety attacks) is the only diagnosis of this group that is specifically coded, the remainder being classified as "Parasomnia Not Otherwise Specified." There are several issues to be addressed. Does current scientific information justify a separate designation of "REM-related parasomnias" and is such a designation of relevance for psychiatry? To what extent does available evidence support a consistent set of diagnostic findings that occur with sufficient predictability as to constitute a meaningful clinical profile and are these findings of utility with respect to differential diagnosis with other sleep-related disorders? In light of these findings, what is the relevance of these disorders to clinical psychiatry?

The questions that must be addressed for the purpose of classification are relatively straightforward. Is a separate category for "REM-related parasomnias" warranted? If so, what disorders should be specifically coded within this category? Should any of the disorders listed under "other parasomnias" in ICSD be given specific coding in DSM-IV, or should they simply be grouped under "Parasomnia Not Otherwise Specified"?

Significance of the Issues

The overriding significance of the issues related to classification of these disorders lies in the extent to which DSM-IV will adhere to the ICSD template, as opposed to maintaining the more conservative DSM-III-R approach. Other issues that are specific to given diagnoses are discussed under the relevant diagnosis.

Methods

References cited in the ICSD bibliography for each diagnosis were reviewed. References from these articles were consulted for additional relevant material. A Medline search (BRS Colleague) was conducted for all primary diagnoses listed in the ICSD classification for REM-related and other parasomnias. The general search frame was from 1965 to 1990, English language, and human subjects only. Search terms and resulting numbers of references were as follows: nightmares, 291; sleep paralysis, 57; REM behavior disorder, 14; REM sleep-related sinus arrest, 1; sinus arrest with sleep, 4; sleep-related painful erections, 2; snoring, 336; sleep/bruxism, 50; sleep/tooth grinding, 5; tooth clenching/sleep, 18; bruxism/nocturnal, 30; bruxism/psych, 19; bruxism/stress, 7; bruxism/anxiety, 1; sudden unexplained death, 5; primary enuresis, 33; enuresis/day/nocturnal, 64; dystonia/nocturnal, 5; and hypnogenic paroxysmal dystonia, 7. Studies were then selected according to criteria and issues described under each diagnostic heading. For the diagnoses REM behavior disorder, REM sinus arrest, sleep-related painful erections, nocturnal paroxysmal dystonia, and sudden unexplained nocturnal death, all available literature was reviewed. A literature review of impaired sleep-related penile tumescence was not conducted for reasons noted in that section of the text.

Results

Nightmares (Dream Anxiety Attacks)

This diagnosis is included under the "Parasomnias" in DSM-III-R. It is listed as a "REM-related Parasomnia" in the ICSD system. The criteria set forth in the two systems do not differ significantly from one another in most respects. They are based to a great extent on the descriptions of Fisher and colleagues (1970a, 1970b) and Mack (1970). More recent studies do not call the current criteria into question—with the possible exception of investigations pertaining to posttraumatic "nightmares."

In a letter to the editor of *Sleep*, Ross and colleagues (1989) discussed the failure of DSM-III-R to acknowledge "Post-traumatic Stress Disorder" as part of the differential diagnosis for Dream Anxiety Disorder. Although Ross and colleagues did not argue for inclusion of a separate diagnosis of "Dream Anxiety Episodes Related to Another Mental Disorder" at that time, they suggested that future evidence may favor inclusion of such a diagnosis. Both DSM-III-R and ICSD acknowledged an increased incidence of psychopathology in adults with frequent nightmares. This has been documented in multiple studies (Fisher et al. 1970a; Hartmann et al. 1981, 1987b; Kales et al. 1980) by means of psychological testing or clinical interview. Where explicit diagnostic criteria have been applied (Hartmann et al. 1981), psychiatric diagnoses (primarily borderline and schizotypal personality disorder and schizophrenia) have been documented in as many as 50% of these patients. However, no systematic analysis of differences (with respect to phenomenology, physiology, treatment response, or otherwise) between the nightmares of individuals with well-documented psychopathology and those of other long-term nightmare sufferers were identified. Thus there seems little basis at this time for drawing a distinction between these groups. However, the literature does suggest the possibility that posttraumatic nightmares may differ in certain respects from classical dream anxiety attacks. These differences are briefly delineated in the following section.

Multiple reports described the frequency of nightmares following traumatic events and, specifically, in individuals with posttraumatic stress disorder, although explicit criteria for the diagnosis of posttraumatic stress disorder are not clearly applied in most cases (Astrøm et al. 1989; DeFazio et al. 1975; Goldstein et al. 1987; Kinzie et al. 1984). Only a few of these reports contain any detail regarding characteristics of the "nightmare" episodes that are relevant to diagnostic criteria for Dream Anxiety Disorder (Greenberg et al. 1972; Hefez et al. 1987; Kramer et al. 1982, 1987; Schlosberg and Benjamin 1978; van der Kolk et al. 1984). These studies vary with respect to the types of trauma, duration from traumatic event(s) to time of study, application of diagnostic criteria for associated psychopathology (especially posttraumatic stress disorder), frequency of reported nightmares, and reported detail of associated sleep and nightmare features. Research design included experimental REM awakenings in some studies, whereas reports from non–rapid eye movement (NREM) sleep were obtained only after spontaneous awakening.

The profile of posttraumatic nightmares that emerges is inconclusive. Of 17 patients in these studies who experienced nightmares during polysomnography (PSG), 5 had NREM (stage 2) episodes only, 6 had both REM and NREM episodes, and 6 had only REM-related occurrences. Reports of associated features emphasize the repetitive nature of content, reiteration of real events, increased body movement, and increased vocalization. Although timing of nightmare events is not consistently reported, these studies suggest a higher rate of occurrence during the first half of the night.

Should posttraumatic nightmares be classified as dream anxiety attacks? The DSM-III-R system and the proposed ICSD nosology would classify them as such. ICSD noted that "nightmares that follow trauma can sometimes occur from NREM sleep especially from stage 2 sleep." Three major possibilities exist: 1) posttraumatic nightmares are essentially dream anxiety attacks, with some degree of "spillover" into NREM; 2) these episodes represent, as Schlosberg and Benjamin (1978) seemed to suggest, a variation of partial arousal disorder; or 3) they are entities unto themselves, distinguishable from Dream Anxiety Disorder and partial arousal.

At this time, there are insufficient data to resolve this issue. It should be emphasized that posttraumatic nightmares do, in fact, conform in most major respects to the descriptive criteria of DSM and ICSD, even though significant underlying psychological and physiological differences may exist. This issue requires further investigation inasmuch as significant differences between nightmares of the posttraumatic variety and classical Dream Anxiety Disorder may be reflected in dissimilarity of course, prognosis, or treatment response.

REM Behavior Disorder

REM behavior disorder has been described only fairly recently. Schenck and colleagues (1986, 1987) reported a total of nine cases. Two additional cases have been reported by Salva and Guilleminault (1986). Ishigooka and colleagues (1985) provided a single case report of probable REM behavior disorder. A similar syndrome has been described in relation to alcohol and sedative-hypnotic withdrawal (Hishikawa et al. 1981). No controlled studies pertaining to any aspect of REM behavior disorder have been published as of this writing.

Although the total number of reported cases is small, a reasonably well-defined and clinically recognizable syndrome emerges. The differential diagnosis of this disorder would include partial arousal disorders, posttraumatic nightmares, complex partial seizures, dream anxiety attacks (nightmares), and other sleep-related confusional states associated with obstructive sleep apnea or organic mental disorders. As of this writing, there has been no systematic investigation regarding the distinction of REM behavior disorder from any of these disorders.

Case studies suggest a relationship to organic disorder (neurological and withdrawal syndromes) in at least 40% of cases. The REM behavior disorder of patients with the "symptomatic" variety was not distinguishable from that of patients with "idiopathic" REM behavior disorder on clinical or polysomnographic grounds. Thus there is no basis at the present time for attempting to distinguish these "subtypes," although this issue may eventually prove relevant to matters of pathophysiology, course, or treatment.

Although detailed psychiatric evaluation has not been conducted for the majority of these patients, no consistent psychopathology has been identified.

REM behavior disorder is relevant to psychiatry on several grounds: 1) it is a behavioral disturbance; 2) its differential includes a number of other sleep disorders that are relevant to psychiatry and that will be coded in DSM-IV; and 3) it occurs as a function of dream activity. Despite the limited data yet available, REM behavior disorder should be considered for inclusion as a distinct diagnostic entity in DSM-IV. However, it may prove difficult to construct non-PSG dependent criteria that will reliably distinguish the disorder from night terrors/sleepwalking. The ICSD system utilizes PSG findings in both major and minimal criteria. Without laboratory-dependent findings, criteria for the diagnosis are essentially reduced to 1) agitated, semi-purposeful, violent, or harmful behaviors during sleep; and 2) movement associated with dream mentation. Clinical reports would suggest that the "dream mentation" associated with REM behavior disorder can be distinguished from the fragmentary or single image reports more often associated with partial arousal events. Unfortunately, this impression has not been subjected to scientific scrutiny. It is tempting to suggest that a "dream recall"-related criterion would aid in making the distinction, but the accuracy of this as a critical diagnostic distinction is open to question. Field trials may be useful in establishing the reliability of a distinction between partial arousal and REM behavior disorder without the help of PSG.

Sleep Paralysis

Sleep paralysis has been described primarily as an ancillary symptom of narcolepsy. In its "isolated" or "familial" forms, it has received relatively little attention. Although its manifestations in narcoleptic and isolated or familial forms are descriptively similar, if not identical, the mechanistic relationships have never been clearly elaborated. Polygraphic recording of sleep paralysis in a nonnarcoleptic subject has not been accomplished.

The literature devoted to the isolated variety consists largely of incidence surveys. Studies of primarily Caucasian populations have found incidence statistics of 5%–16% (Everett 1963; Goode 1962; Penn et al. 1981), with the exception of Ness' (1978) study of the so-called old hag phenomenon in Newfoundlanders, in whom he reported a 60% incidence of one or more lifetime episodes. In non-Caucasian groups, much higher incidences have been reported, including a 40%–50% rate in blacks (Bell et al. 1984, 1986) and a 40% incidence in Japanese ("Kanashibari") (Fukuda et al. 1987). In the latter study, the investigators suggest that the apparent differences in incidence among races are not real, but rather a function of cultural familiarity with the phenomenon, yielding higher recognition and response rates. They further asserted that isolated sleep paralysis, being a common occurrence, is a physiological variant, not a pathological entity. Soft evidence suggests that individuals may be predisposed to episodes as a result of psychological stress or disruption of the sleep-wake cycle (Folkard et al. 1984; Fukuda et al. 1987; Snyder 1983). Although it is inviting to conclude that a qualitative, as well as quantitative, difference exists between individuals with rare episodes of isolated sleep paralysis and those with frequent occurrence, there is no sound basis in the literature for this contention.

The case of familial sleep paralysis is somewhat different. Roth and colleagues (1968) described a familial form of the disorder and posited an X-linked dominant mode of transmission by the mother. It is significant to note episodes in the familial form are more likely to occur at sleep onset than those seen in the isolated variety, raising the possibility that the familial form may have more in common with the narcoleptic presentation of sleep paralysis than it does with the isolated type.

The preliminary impression, based on very limited data, is that familial sleep paralysis is a distinct pathological condition that may account for the majority of cases in which the episodes occur frequently, whereas isolated sleep paralysis is a physiological variant.

Although sleep paralysis is of some potential relevance to psychiatry with respect to differential diagnosis (e.g., "psychogenic stupor"), this relevance is rather limited. The small body of literature devoted to psychodynamic explanations of the disorder antedates modern sleep disorders medicine and is entirely subjective.

REM Sinus Arrest

This ICSD diagnosis rests largely on a description of four patients with sinus arrest of up to 9 seconds in phasic REM (Guilleminault et al. 1984). Symptoms of the disorder consist, at most, of vague chest discomfort and syncopal episodes. Establishment of the diagnosis rests entirely on PSG recording. The disorder is of no direct relevance to psychiatry.

Sleep-Related Painful Erections

There are only two well-described cases of sleep-related painful erections in the literature (Karacan 1971; Matthews and Crutchfield 1987). The disorder is of uncertain etiology and is apparently rare.

Impaired Sleep-Related Penile Erections

Nocturnal penile tumescence is a well-described phenomenon. Its evaluation has proven to be of considerable value as a diagnostic tool in the assessment of erection dysfunction, and there is no question about the need for psychiatrists to be well informed on this issue. Inclusion of this "diagnosis" in ICSD seems proper inasmuch as this is the diagnostic finding most relevant to the primary users of this nomenclature. However, the elevation of this "biological marker" of dysfunction to diagnostic status in DSM-IV may be ill advised. The disorder or diagnosis that is being addressed is erection dysfunction (as it pertains to waking sexual function)—*not* impaired sleep-related erection. Discussion of symptoms, etiology, course, associated features, prognosis, and treatment pertain to impotence—not impaired sleep-related erection.

Snoring

Most of the literature related to snoring is concerned primarily with obstructive sleep apnea syndrome. Inasmuch as this diagnosis is reviewed by Thorpy (Chapter 39, this volume), studies related primarily to obstructive sleep apnea syndrome were excluded. Research pertaining to upper airway physiology in snoring was also excluded on the grounds that it does not contribute information directly relevant to nosological issues. The remaining body of work is comparatively small and consists largely of epidemiologic studies of snoring as a risk factor for disease. This specific area is the subject of the following review.

Six major epidemiologic studies of snoring as a risk factor for disease were reviewed. These studies pertain to systemic hypertension, ischemic heart disease, and cerebrovascular disease. Studies of the prevalence of hypertension among habitual snorers have demonstrated an increased risk for hypertension in this group (Gislason et al. 1987; Hoffstein et al. 1988a; Koskenvuo et al. 1985; Norton and Dunn 1985). However, when corrections for body mass index are applied, the correlation is substantially weakened or negated. In addition, the one investigation (Hoffstein et al. 1988a) that pursued polysomnographic studies demonstrated that diastolic blood pressure was correlated with body mass index, respiratory disturbance index (RDI), and mean SaO_2 (arterial oxygen saturation), not with snoring index. Likewise, snoring was correlated with body mass index, RDI, and mean SaO_2, suggesting that weight and obstructive apneas are the critical intermediate variables between snoring and hypertension. Investigations of snoring and ischemic heart disease or cardiovascular disease have yielded similar results. In a prospective study (3-year follow), Koskenvuo and colleagues (1987) demonstrated an increased risk for ischemic heart disease and/or cardiovascular disease in habitual snorers. Risk was decreased but still significantly higher with correction for age, body mass index, and history of hypertension. Partinen and Palomaki (1985) found a significant association between snoring and cerebral infarct. Although no direct adjustments for body mass index were made, the authors did point out that the history suggested a diagnosis of obstructive apnea in a number of habitual snorers and suggested that obstructive sleep apnea may explain a substantial amount of the risk for cardiovascular disease in this population.

These studies suffer from potential unreliability of reports, uncertain definitions of *habitual* and *occasional* snoring, and, in many cases, a failure to account for intermediate variables such as weight or the presence of underlying sleep-disordered breathing that may, in fact, be the critical determinants of vascular disease. In a meta-analysis of these epidemiologic studies, Waller and Bhopal (1989) concluded that, at the very least, "it is premature to describe snoring as a risk factor for cardiovascular disease" (p. 146). They suggested, as described above, that confounding variables may well account for much of the apparent risk associated with snoring.

Polysomnographic studies of pure snorers have been infrequent. In addition to the one study noted above (Hoffstein et al. 1988a), which is by far the largest ($N = 372$), four PSG investigations of snoring were identified. These studies have revealed increased blood pressure during sleep in heavy snorers, who showed "some" obstructive apnea (Lugaresi 1975); significant correlations between severity of snoring and nasal airway resistance in a population of 109 heavy snorers (50% of whom had an RDI > 5); and an association between severity of snoring and weight, RDI, and pharyngeal area (Hoffstein et al. 1988b). In a population of asymptomatic light snorers, Perez-Padilla and colleagues (1987) found that snoring was highest in slow-wave sleep and lowest in REM, whereas the converse held true for apnea and hypopnea. They also reported that continuous snoring can occur without decline in SaO_2. They suggested a continuum from light snoring to habitual snoring to obstructive sleep apnea syndrome. Berry and colleagues (1986) studied a subclinical population of heavy snorers and found that 39% had no apnea or hypopnea, 47% showed an RDI of 0–5, and 13% had an RDI greater than 5.

In conclusion, it has not been clearly demonstrated that snoring per se represents a significant risk factor for vascular disease. There is clearly a strong correlation between snoring and obstructive sleep apnea, but the precise natural history of heavy snoring and its relationship to obstructive sleep apnea syndrome have not been defined and will require long-term prospective study. The immediate relevance of snoring to psychiatry lies primarily in the extent to which it is associated with neuropsychiatric complications of obstructive sleep apnea syndrome. The social consequences of snoring are also germane, but, as of this writing, there have been no systematic studies of this issue.

Enuresis

This selective review of enuresis derives its focus from the fact that "functional enuresis" is currently classified in DSM-III-R under elimination disorders in the disorders usually first evident in infancy, childhood, or adolescence section. It is the intention of the Work Group for that section to retain this diagnosis. In an effort to define a specific association between sleep physiology or pathology and enuresis, a number of investigators have conducted PSG studies. Early studies by Gastaut and Broughton (1965) and Evans (1971) suggested that enuresis was associated with slow-wave sleep. Others found this to be true in enuretic children, whereas older groups (those in late adolescence or early adulthood) tended to wet the bed during lighter sleep or even in wakefulness (Ditman and Blinn 1955; Finley 1971). Ritvo and colleagues (1969) described three groups: enuresis during awake time and enuresis associated with or without arousal from sleep. The arousal group included four of the seven subjects. The authors postulated that this group was associated with a psychogenic etiology, whereas the "nonarousal" enuresis may occur as a result of deficient signals of bladder fullness. Other investigators formed theories, based on sleep studies, that enuresis occurred as a REM equivalent (Schiff 1965) or dream equivalent (Pierce et al. 1961).

Most studies have largely discredited this earlier work. Reporting on only four subjects, Kales and colleagues (1977) found that, although enuretic events tended to cluster in the first one-third of the night, the episodes were associated with different sleep stages in approximate proportion to the percentage of that sleep stage. In the most definitive study as of this writing, Mikkelsen and colleagues (1980) reached a similar conclusion regarding distribution in sleep stages from PSG analysis of 40 enuretic males, provided that the 5-minute period of stage 2 preceding slow-wave sleep was scored as stage 3/4. In contradistinction to the findings by Kales and colleagues, the enuretic events were spread more or less evenly throughout the night. No studies have identified any specific sleep pathology consistently associated with enuresis, although an association between increased upper airway resistance, obstructive apnea, and nocturnal enuresis has been reported in a limited number of cases (Grundfast and Wittich 1982; Guilleminault et al. 1976; Weider and Hauri 1985).

In summary, there is limited evidence of an association between any specific sleep physiology or pathology and enuresis.

Nocturnal Paroxysmal Dystonia

Nocturnal paroxysmal dystonia was initially described by Lugaresi and Cirignotta (1981, 1982). These initial reports on eight patients described short attacks (< 1 minute) of agitated movement consisting of twisting of trunk and coarse movement of limbs occurring up to 20 times per night. The case series has now been expanded to 12. All ages are affected (7–74 years), and there is no apparent sex bias. Episodes occur in NREM sleep and are preceded by signs of electroencephalographic (EEG) arousal. EEGs are normal in waking and sleep (including the period during attacks), although a grand mal seizure was recorded in one subject during a night of monitoring, and a history of daytime "spells," strongly suggestive of seizure activity, was elicited in several subjects. No familial predisposition was identified, and all subjects demonstrated a good response to carbamazepine, although other anticonvulsants were not effective. The investigators believe that these attacks are epileptic in nature. Lee and colleagues (1985) subsequently described a strikingly similar disorder affecting five members of a family. Phenomenology and associated physiological characteristics were virtually identical to those described by Lugaresi and Cirignotta, although the familial occurrence (postulated autosomal dominant inheritance) was, of course, at variance. Lee and colleagues argued against an epileptic origin on the basis of normal EEGs and nonspecificity of carbamazepine responsivity.

Similar attacks of longer duration were described in two patients (Lugaresi and Cirignotta 1984; Lugaresi et al. 1986). Motor disturbance was similar but episodes lasted up to about 1 hour, occurring in NREM sleep. There was no epileptic history in either individual, but one subject developed Huntington's chorea. No effective treatment has been found. The authors suggested that this variety is not epileptic but more likely related to underlying neurochemical disturbance. Lugaresi and Cirignotta (1984) stressed the similarity of these two entities (nocturnal paroxysmal dystonia with short and long attacks) to paroxysmal kinesigenic choreoathetosis and paroxysmal dystonic choreoathetosis, respectively.

ICSD classified this disorder under "other parasomnias" as opposed to grouping it with "Neurological Conditions." Although the etiology (or etiologies) is still somewhat uncertain, there seems to be relatively little doubt that the mechanisms are neurological in nature—probably epileptic in the short form and, possibly, degenerative in the long variety.

Bruxism

Bruxism is a common condition, conservatively estimated to be of clinical significance in approximately 5%–10% of the population (Reding et al. 1966). Sexes appear to be equally affected, as are adults and children. The study of bruxism must take into account the potential differences between diurnal and nocturnal bruxism. Unfortunately, this distinction has not often been clearly drawn in the past, although many investigations have been concerned only with individuals who grind at night. A number of arguments have been advanced as to why the nocturnal and diurnal presentations are different disorders, including the facts that diurnal bruxism is silent, that the mechanics of nocturnal bruxism cannot be duplicated by waking subjects, and that those with nocturnal bruxism do not report daytime grinding (Reding et al. 1968a, 1968b). The literature on bruxism consists largely of 1) studies related to dental aspects of teeth grinding, 2) analysis of personality and stress-related factors in bruxism, 3) physiological characteristics of bruxism and its relationship to sleep physiology, and 4) evaluation of treatment. In this review we focus on studies pertaining to psychological aspects of nocturnal bruxism and the relationship of grinding to sleep physiology.

Early reports concerning the psychological characteristics of those with bruxism were largely subjective and emphasized oral-aggressive tendencies. This literature will not be reviewed in detail. Vernallis (1955) produced one of the earliest efforts at objective assessment and found that bruxism (no distinction of diurnal versus nocturnal) correlated with elevated anxiety scores and "hyperactivity," as assessed by the Minnesota Multiphasic Personality Inventory (MMPI) (Hathaway and McKinley 1970) hypomanic scale. Other investigators also reported an association between anxiety and bruxism on psychological or medical inventories (Molin and Levi 1966; Thaller 1960). However, when nocturnal bruxism alone was examined, Reding and colleagues (1968b) found no significant differences from control subjects on the MMPI or the Cornell Medical Index (Brodman et al. 1949). More recent studies have examined the role of "stress" or situational anxiety on teeth grinding. Data have been presented suggesting that heightened stress on a given day results in increased bruxism that night (Hartmann et al. 1987a; Rugh and Harlan 1988; Rugh and Solberg 1975). Funch and Gale (1980) found no such relationship in a single case report, but did postulate a role for anticipatory stress (i.e., increased bruxism prior to stressful events).

A specific association between bruxism and DSM diagnoses has not been examined in any detail, although Hartmann and colleagues (1987a) found that none of 16 persons with bruxism met criteria for any DSM-III (American Psychiatric Association 1980) diagnosis. They did report a tendency among many patients toward fulfilling criteria for obsessive compulsive personality disorder. This finding is perhaps complemented by those of Hicks and Chancellor (1987), who described an increase in nocturnal bruxism among "Type A" college students.

These studies of the relationship between emotional disturbance, personality style or stress, and bruxism are difficult to interpret. As previously noted, early studies failed to distinguish between diurnal and nocturnal bruxism, a distinction that most investigators in the field believe to be significant. Methods of determining presence or degree of grinding vary considerably (subjective report, home electromyographic recording, laboratory electromyographic or acoustic recording). Analysis of "stress" factors are frequently based on subjective report in case study formats. Finally, as Glaros and Rao (1977) pointed out, many of these studies are correlational in nature and "[do] not allow for inference of causality" (p. 770). Thus one is left with the impression that, although it is likely that emotional disturbance, personality trait, and stress are likely to play a role in at least some cases of bruxism, the precise nature of this relationship is not clear.

Polysomnographic studies of bruxism suggest that grinding can occur in all sleep stages, although there is near complete agreement that it is least evident during deep sleep (Reding et al. 1964; Satoh and Harada 1973; Ware and Rugh 1988). A number of investigators have reported frequency of grinding to be highest during stage 2 sleep (Reding et al. 1968a; Tani et al. 1966; Weiselman et al. 1986); others have reported maximal frequencies in REM (Powell 1965; Reding et al. 1964). Bruxism has also been reported to occur commonly in waking and stage 1 (Gastaut and Broughton 1965; Ware and Rugh 1988).

Particular emphasis has been placed on bruxism as an arousal response. It has been noted that grinding is often preceded or accompanied by evidence of arousal in the form of K-complexes and increased cardiac and respiratory rates (Reding et al. 1968a; Satoh and Harada 1973; Tani et al. 1966). Satoh and Harada were able to elicit bruxism in response to experimentally induced arousal.

Ware and Rugh (1988) noted a particularly important distinction in their analyses of "destructive" versus "non-destructive" bruxism. Those in the former group, referred because of orofacial pain complaints, showed much higher levels of grinding in REM than those in the latter group, whose bruxism came to the attention of investigators as a result of referral for sleep complaints. They suggested that the orofacial pain and dysfunction may occur primarily as a result of loss of protective mechanisms during REM sleep. This finding is significant not only with respect to elaborating mechanisms of injury in bruxism, but also in underscoring the influence of referral source on the outcome of physiological studies. The group of patients with bruxism referred by dental or pain clinics ("destructive bruxers") may, in fact, differ significantly from those patients identified from other sources on a number of variables.

In summary, nocturnal bruxism appears to be a multidetermined disorder with psychological factors and sleep physiology as important contributors. Genetic predisposition, dental abnormalities, brain damage, and other factors may also contribute to development of bruxism in selected cases. Future research may provide greater discrimination among subgroups of nocturnal bruxism. Although psychological factors do appear to play a contributory role, the consequences of the disorder are primarily physical; as a result, these patients seldom present to psychiatry for diagnostic purposes.

Sudden Unexplained Nocturnal Death Syndrome

From 1981 to 1988, at least 117 cases of sudden unexplained nocturnal death were reported in the United States among Southeast Asian refugees (*Journal of the American Medical Association* 1988). The victims were predominantly young male immigrants from Laos, Kampuchea, and Vietnam. The Hmong tribe, predominantly of northern Laotian extraction, were particularly affected. Of the episodes witnessed from onset, all seem to have begun during sleep (Baron et al. 1983). Victims are described as exhibiting "choking, gasping, gurgling or labored respirations, without wheezing or stridor." They did not appear conscious and could not be aroused. Several were noted to exhibit signs of pulmonary edema or seizures.

Kirschner and colleagues (1986) reported on detailed postmortem evaluations of 18 hearts from victims of sudden unexplained nocturnal death syndrome. They found slight to significant cardiomegaly in 14 and anomalies of the conduction system in all but one. Otto and colleagues (1984) described three cases of "near-miss" sudden unexplained nocturnal death and offered convincing evidence that ventricular fibrillation was the primary mechanism underlying the event. The phenomenon is well known in Southeast Asian culture—referred to as "bangungut" in the Philippines, "pokkuri" in Japan, or "non-laitia" in Laos.

Since early recognition in this country, Munger (1987) identified 16 cases of apparent sudden unexplained nocturnal death in a Thai refugee camp, predominantly among members of the Green-Hmong group. Case control study indicated that risk was also associated with previous nonfatal sleep disturbance and a family history of sudden death.

Analysis of associated or predisposing nonorganic factors is limited largely to a case control study by Baron and colleagues (1983). They identified acute, stress-provoking situations within the 24 hours preceding death in only 4 of 41 cases whose families were interviewed. The case control study of 26 cases provided indirect evidence of possible stress-related factors, including a shorter period of time in the United States, greater financial instability, and poorer acculturation (language skills and job training) than found in control subjects.

Although the investigation clearly links these events to sleep, no further detail regarding the nature of the relationship to sleep is available as of this writing. The time from sleep onset to the event has varied from minutes to 8.5 hours (mean, 3.5 hours). None of the victims had any clear history of prior sleep disturbance or daytime sleepiness. Specifically, there was no history indicative of obstructive apnea or other sleep-disordered breathing. No related events have been recorded polygraphically. Folk wisdom in Southeast Asian cultures has associated these episodes with "nightmares," but the descriptions cited to support this view sound as compatible with agonal behavior as they do with nightmares or night terrors. Mellis and Katz (1988) reported that patients who were successfully aroused in the middle of an event have related terrifying dreams, but this information is anecdotal in nature. These authors hypothesized that a night terror and accompanying autonomic arousal is the precipitating event of ventricular fibrillation in cardiac-vulnerable individuals. The evidence for this association is weak.

In summary, current evidence suggests that these deaths are cardiac in nature, probably related to congenital abnormality of the conduction system. Although sleep physiology appears to be a significant component of the pathophysiology, the precise nature of this is altogether unclear. Thus the relationship of this dramatic syndrome to specific aspects of sleep physiology or to emotional disturbance has not been well established.

Discussion

The major overriding issue is whether or not to include a separate category for "REM-related parasomnias." There is merit to the argument for inclusion of such a category in that REM sleep physiology and mentation undoubtedly give rise to certain distinct clinical entities not observed in other sleep stages. The only "REM-related parasomnia" currently listed in DSM-III-R is nightmares. The literature on posttraumatic nightmares slightly weakens the "REM relatedness" of this diagnosis. This review suggests that none of the other ICSD REM-related parasomnias merit separate DSM-IV coding, with the possible exception of REM behavior disorder.

Thus to create a separate classification for REM-related parasomnias would be to create a class that, for DSM-IV purposes, has only one member (nightmares)—a member that itself contains exceptions to the definition of the class. The "other parasomnias" do not warrant separate diagnoses in DSM-IV, primarily because they are not of sufficient relevance to psychiatry, or, in the cases of enuresis and impaired sleep-related erections, because they belong elsewhere in the nosology.

Recommendations

The options for classifying "REM-related Parasomnias" are 1) establishment of a separate category within the parasomnia section for REM-related parasomnias, with coding for nightmares and, possibly, REM behavior disorder within this category (the ICSD approach); or 2) classification of nightmares under the general heading of parasomnias, lumping the remaining diagnoses (with the exception of partial arousal disorders, which are reviewed elsewhere) under the same general heading.

The alternatives for "other parasomnias" are similar: 1) establishment of a distinct category of "other parasomnias," with separate coding for one or more of the diagnoses contained in this section; or 2) lumping these diagnoses in the "Parasomnia Not Otherwise Specified" category. Although specific diagnoses were not included in the *DSM-IV Options Book* (American Psychiatric Association 1991), this remains an option.

For the reasons presented above, it seems most judicious to adhere largely to the DSM-III-R approach of including nightmares in the general "Parasomnia" section, without specification of "REM-related Parasomnias." Furthermore, the diagnoses listed in the "other parasomnias" section of ICSD should be included under the "Parasomnia Not otherwise Specified" heading in DSM-IV. The text that is included in the parasomnia section should be utilized 1) to establish linkages between the sleep disorders section and other DSM-IV sections for enuresis and nocturnal penile tumescence and 2) to identify relevant diagnoses, such as sleep paralysis or bruxism, that are not separately coded. (With respect to enuresis, it is important to bear in mind that this is currently listed in the disorders of childhood and adolescence. If enuresis remains in that section, as proposed, this would still require secondary sleep enuresis that occurs during adulthood to be classified in the sleep disorders section, under other parasomnias.)

References

American Psychiatric Association: Diagnostic and Statistical Manual of Mental Disorders, 3rd Edition. Washington, DC, American Psychiatric Association, 1980

American Psychiatric Association: Diagnostic and Statistical Manual of Mental Disorders, 3rd Edition, Revised. Washington, DC, American Psychiatric Association, 1987

American Psychiatric Association: DSM-IV Options Book: Work in Progress 9/9/91. Washington, DC, American Psychiatric Association, 1991

American Sleep Disorders Association, Diagnostic Classification Steering Committee: International Classification of Sleep Disorders: Diagnostic and Coding Manual. Rochester, MN, American Sleep Disorders, 1990

Astrøm C, Lunde I, Ortmann J, et al: Sleep disturbances in torture survivors. Acta Neurol Scand 79:150–154, 1989

Baron RC, Thacker SB, Gorelkin L, et al: Sudden death among Southeast Asian refugees. JAMA 250:2947–2951, 1983

Bell CC, Shakoor B, Thompson B, et al: Prevalence of isolated sleep paralysis in black subjects. J Natl Med Assoc 76:501–508, 1984

Bell CC, Dixie-Bell DD, Thompson B: Further studies on the prevalence of isolated sleep paralysis in black subjects. J Natl Med Assoc 78:649–659, 1986

Berry DT, Webb WB, Block AJ, et al: Sleep-disordered breathing and its concomitants in a subclinical population. Sleep 9:478–483, 1986

Brodman K, Erdmann AJ, Lorge I, et al: The Cornell Medical Index. JAMA 140:530, 1949

DeFazio VJ, Rustin S, Diamond A: Symptom development in Vietnam era veterans. Am J Orthopsychiatry 45:158–163, 1975

Ditman KS, Blinn KA: Sleep levels in enuresis. Am J Psychiatry 111:913–920, 1955

Evans JI: Sleep of enuretics (letter). BMJ 3:110, 1971

Everett HC: Sleep paralysis in medical students. J Nerv Ment Dis 136:283–287, 1963

Finley WW: An EEG study of the sleep of enuretics at three age levels. Clin Electroencephalogr 2:35–39, 1971

Fisher C, Byrne JV, Edwards A, et al: A psychophysiological study of nightmares. J Am Psychoanal Assoc 18:747–782, 1970a

Fisher C, Byrne JV, Edwards A, et al: REM and REM nightmares. International Psychiatry Clinics 7:183–187, 1970b

Folkard S, Concon R, Herbert M: Night shift paralysis. Experientia 40:510–512, 1984

Fukuda K, Miyasita A, Inugami M, et al: High prevalence of isolated sleep paralysis: Kanashibari phenomenon in Japan. Sleep 10:279–286, 1987

Funch DP, Gale EN: Factors associated with nocturnal bruxism and its treatment. J Behav Med 3:385–397, 1980

Gastaut H, Broughton R: A clinical and polygraphic study of episodic phenomena during sleep. Recent Advances in Biological Psychiatry 8:197–223, 1965

Gislason T, Aberg H, Taube A: Snoring and systemic hypertension: an epidemiological study. Acta Medica Scandinavica 222:415–421, 1987

Glaros AG, Rao SM: Bruxism: a critical review. Psychol Bull 84:767–781, 1977

Goldstein G, van Kammen W, Shelly C, et al: Survivors of imprisonment in the Pacific theater during World War II. Am J Psychiatry 144:1210–1213, 1987

Goode GB: Sleep paralysis. Arch Neurol 6:228–234, 1962

Greenberg R, Pearlman CA, Gampel D: War neuroses and adaptive functions of REM sleep. Br J Med Psychol 45:27–33, 1972

Grundfast KM, Wittich DJ: Adenotonsillar hypertrophy and upper airway obstruction in evolutionary perspective. Laryngoscope 92 (1 part 6):650–656, 1982

Guilleminault C, Eldridge FL, Simmons F, et al: Sleep apnea in eight children. Pediatrics 58:23–30, 1976

Guilleminault C, Pool P, Motta J, et al: Sinus arrest during REM sleep in young adults. N Engl J Med 311:1006–1010, 1984

Hartmann E, Russ D, van der Kolk B, et al: A preliminary study of the personality of the nightmare sufferer: relationship to schizophrenia and creativity? Am J Psychiatry 138:794–797, 1981

Hartmann E, Mehta N, Forgione A, et al: Bruxism: personality traits and other characteristics. Sleep Research 16:350, 1987a

Hartmann E, Russ D, Oldfield M, et al: Who has nightmares? the personality of the lifelong nightmare sufferer. Arch Gen Psychiatry 44:49–56, 1987b

Hathaway SR, McKinley JC: Minnesota Multiphasic Personality Inventory, Revised. Minneapolis, MN, University of Minnesota, 1970

Hefez A, Metz L, Lavie P: Long-term effects of extreme situational stress on sleep and dreaming. Am J Psychiatry 144:344–347, 1987

Hicks RA, Chancellor C: Nocturnal bruxism and type A-B behavior in college students. Psychol Rep 60:1211–1214, 1987

Hishikawa Y, Sugita Y, Teshima Y, et al: Sleep disorders in alcoholic patients with delirium tremens and transient withdrawal hallucinations—re-evaluation of the REM rebound and intrusion theory, in Psychophysiological Aspects of Sleep. Edited by Karacan I. Park Ridge, NJ, Noyes Medical Publications, 1981, pp 109–122

Hoffstein V, Rubinstein I, Mateika S, et al: Determinants of blood pressure in snorers. Lancet 2:992–994, 1988a

Hoffstein V, Chaban R, Cole P, et al: Snoring and upper airway properties. Chest 94:87–89, 1988b

Ishigooka J, Westendorp F, Oguchi T, et al: Somnambulistic behavior associated with abnormal REM sleep in an elderly woman. Biol Psychiatry 20:1003–1008, 1985

Journal of the American Medical Association: Leads from the MMWR: update: sudden unexplained death syndrome among Southeast Asian refugees—United States. JAMA 260:2033, 1988

Kales A, Kales J, Jacobson A, et al: Effects of imipramine on enuretic frequency and sleep stages. Pediatrics 60:431, 1977

Kales A, Soldatos CR, Caldwell AB, et al: Nightmares: clinical characteristics and personality patterns. Am J Psychiatry 137:1197–1201, 1980

Karacan I: Painful nocturnal erections. JAMA 215:1831, 1971

Kinzie JD, Fredrickson RH, Ben R, et al: Post-traumatic stress disorder among survivors of Cambodian concentration camps. Am J Psychiatry 141:645–650, 1984

Kirschner RH, Eckner FAD, Baron RC: The cardiac pathology of sudden unexplained nocturnal death in Southeast Asian refugees. JAMA 256:2700–2705, 1986

Koskenvuo M, Kaprio J, Partinen M, et al: Snoring as a risk factor for hypertension and angina pectoris. Lancet 1:893–896, 1985

Koskenvuo M, Kaprio J, Telakivi T, et al: Snoring as risk factor for ischaemic heart disease and stroke in men. BMJ 294:16–19, 1987

Kramer M, Kinney L, Scharf M: Sleep in delayed stress victims (abstract). Sleep Research 11:113, 1982

Kramer M, Schoen LS, Kinney L: Nightmares in Vietnam veterans. J Am Acad Psychoanal 15:67–81, 1987

Lee BI, Lesser RP, Pippenger CE, et al: Familial paroxysmal hypnogenic dystonia. Neurology 35:1357–1360, 1985

Lugaresi E: Snoring. Electroencephalogr Clin Neurophysiol 39:59–64, 1975

Lugaresi E, Cirignotta F: Hypnogenic paroxysmal dystonia: epileptic seizure or a new syndrome? Sleep 4:129–138, 1981

Lugaresi E, Cirignotta F: Nocturnal paroxysmal dystonia, in Sleep and Epilepsy. Edited by Sterman MB, Shouse MN, Passouant P. New York, Academic, 1982, pp 507–510

Lugaresi E, Cirignotta F: Two variants of nocturnal paroxysmal dystonia with attacks of short and long duration, in Epilepsy, Sleep and Sleep Deprivation. Edited by Degen R, Niedermeyer E. New York, Elsevier Science, 1984, pp 169–173

Lugaresi E, Cirignotta F, Montagna P: Nocturnal paroxysmal dystonia. J Neurol Neurosurg Psychiatry 49:375–380, 1986

Mack JE: Nightmares and Human Conflict. Boston, MA, Little, Brown, 1970

Matthews BJ, Crutchfield MB: Painful nocturnal penile erections associated with rapid eye movement sleep. Sleep 10:184–187, 1987

Mellis RB, Katz B: Night terrors and sudden unexplained nocturnal death. Med Hypotheses 26:149–154, 1988

Mikkelsen EJ, Rapoport JL, Nee L, et al: Childhood enuresis, I: sleep patterns and psychopathology. Arch Gen Psychiatry 37:1139–1144, 1980

Molin C, Levi L: A psycho-odontologic investigation of patients with bruxism. Acta Odontol Scand 24:373–391, 1966

Munger RG: Sudden death in sleep of Laotian-Hmong refugees in Thailand: a case control study. Am J Public Health 77:1187–1190, 1987

Ness RC: The old hag phenomenon as sleep paralysis: a biocultural interpretation. Cult Med Psychiatry 2:15–39, 1978

Norton PG, Dunn EV: Snoring as a risk factor for disease: an epidemiological survey. BMJ 291:630–632, 1985

Otto CM, Tauxe RV, Cobb LA, et al: Ventricular fibrillation causes sudden death in Southeast Asian immigrants. Ann Intern Med 100:45–47, 1984

Partinen M, Palomaki H: Snoring and cerebral infarction. Lancet 2:1325–1326, 1985

Penn NE, Kripke DF, Scharff J: Sleep paralysis among medical students. J Psychol 107:247–252, 1981

Perez-Padilla JR, West P, Kryger M: Snoring in normal young adults: prevalence in sleep stages and associated changes in oxygen saturation, heart rate, and breathing pattern. Sleep 10:249–253, 1987

Pierce CM, Whitman RM, Maas JW, et al: Enuresis and dreaming: experimental studies. Arch Gen Psychiatry 4:166–170, 1961

Powell RN: Tooth contact during sleep: association with other events. J Dent Res 44:959–967, 1965

Reding GR, Rubright WC, Rechtschaffen A, et al: Sleep pattern of tooth-grinding: its relationship to dreaming. Science 145:725–726, 1964

Reding GR, Rubright WC, Zimmerman SO: Incidence of bruxism. J Dent Res 45:1198–1204, 1966

Reding GR, Zepelin H, Robinson JE, et al: Nocturnal teeth-grinding: all-night psychophysiologic studies. J Dent Res 47:786–797, 1968a

Reding GR, Zepelin H, Monroe LJ: Personality study of nocturnal teeth-grinders. Percept Mot Skills 26:523–531, 1968b

Ritvo ER, Ornitz EM, Gottlieb F, et al: Arousal and nonarousal enuretic events. Am J Psychiatry 126:77–84, 1969

Ross RR, Ball WA, Morrison AR: Revising the differential diagnosis of the parasomnias in DSM III-R (letter). Sleep 12:287–289, 1989

Roth B, Buuhova S, Berkova L: Familial sleep paralysis. Schweizer Archiv fur Neurologie, Neurochirurgie und Psychiatrie 102:321–330,1968

Rugh JD, Harlan J: Nocturnal bruxism and temporomandibular disorders. Adv Neurol 49:329–341, 1988

Rugh JD, Solberg WK: Electromyographic studies of bruxist behavior before and during treatment. California Dental Association Journal 3:57, 1975

Salva MA, Guilleminault C: Olivopontocerebellar degeneration, abnormal sleep, and REM sleep without atonia. Neurology 36:576–577, 1986

Satoh T, Harada Y: Electrophysiological study on tooth-grinding during sleep. Electroencephalogr Clin Neurophysiol 35:267–275, 1973

Schenck CH, Bundlie SR, Ettinger MG, et al: Chronic behavioral disorders of human REM sleep: a new category of parasomnia. Sleep 9:293–308, 1986

Schenck CH, Bundlie SR, Patterson AL, et al: Rapid eye movement sleep behavior disorder: a treatable parasomnia affecting older adults. JAMA 257:1786–1789, 1987

Schiff SS: The EEG, eye movements and dreaming in adult enuresis. J Nerv Ment Dis 140:397–404, 1965

Schlosberg A, Benjamin M: Sleep patterns in three acute combat fatigue cases. J Clin Psychiatry 39:546–549, 1978

Snyder S: Isolated sleep paralysis after rapid time-zone change ("jet lag") syndrome. Chronobiologia 10:377–379, 1983

Tani K, Yoshii N, Yoshino I, et al: Electroencephalographic study of parasomnia: sleep-talking, enuresis and bruxism. Physiol Behav 1:241–243, 1966

Thaller JL: The use of the Cornell Medical Index to determine the correlation between bruxism and the anxiety state. J Periodontol 31:138–140, 1960

van der Kolk B, Blitz R, Burr W, et al: Nightmares and trauma: a comparison of nightmares after combat with lifelong nightmares in veterans. Am J Psychiatry 141:187–190, 1984

Vernallis FF: Teeth-grinding: some relationships to anxiety, hostility and hyperactivity. J Clin Psychol 11:389–391, 1955

Waller PC, Bhopal RS: Is snoring a cause of vascular disease? an epidemiological review. Lancet 1:143–146, 1989

Ware JC, Rugh JD: Destructive bruxism: sleep stage relationship. Sleep 11:172–181, 1988

Weider DJ, Hauri PJ: Nocturnal enuresis in children with upper airway obstruction. Int J Pediatr Otorhinolaryngol 9:173–182, 1985

Weiselman G, Permann R, Korner E, et al: Distribution of muscle activity during sleep bruxism. Eur Neurol 25 (suppl 2):111–116, 1986

Chapter 42

Sleep Disorders Related to Another Mental Disorder

Eric A. Nofzinger, M.D.

Statement of the Issues

In this literature review, I focus on whether the classification system as outlined in DSM-III-R (American Psychiatric Association 1987) for sleep disorders and mental disorders should be altered for DSM-IV. I first clarify the DSM-III-R categories, then cite subsequent developments in the field of sleep disorders medicine and psychiatric sleep research that are germane to a conceptualization of a classification system for sleep disorders and mental disorders.

In DSM-III-R there were no specific guidelines about diagnosing a separate sleep disorder when a mental disorder was concurrently present. Since sleep abnormalities are common accompanying symptoms of a variety of mental disorders, specific guidelines are necessary to help the clinician distinguish between sleep symptoms of another mental disorder versus a sleep disorder warranting clinical attention independent from the mental disorder. I highlight research defining the sleep abnormalities associated with mental disorders 1) to verify that abnormalities in sleep accompany individual mental disorders and 2) to determine whether the abnormality in sleep warrants independent clinical attention so that separate diagnostic classification of the sleep disorder is indicated.

This chapter is adapted from Nofzinger EA: "Sleep Disorders Related to Another Mental Disorder (Non-Substance/Primary): A DSM-IV Literature Review." *The Journal of Clinical Psychiatry* 54:244–255, 1993.

Significance of the Issues

Two major developments in sleep medicine have occurred since the development of DSM-III-R. First, the multidisciplinary field of sleep medicine has altered its own classification system for sleep disorders. The previous system, the 1979 Association of Sleep Disorders Centers' (ASDC) Diagnostic Classification of Sleep and Arousal Disorders, was revised to form the International Classification of Sleep Disorders (ICSD) (American Sleep Disorders Association 1990). Second, based on a literature search described below, roughly 40% of all articles published on sleep disorders and mental disorders in the past 25 years have appeared since the development of DSM-III-R in the mid-1980s (Figure 42–1).

The ICSD was developed by the American Sleep Disorders Association in association with the European Sleep Research Society, the Japanese Society of Sleep Research, and the Latin American Sleep Society. Completed in 1990, it represented the combined efforts of a multidisciplinary Diagnostic Classification Steering Committee, who surveyed sleep disorders specialists around the world for comments on the validity and clinical utility of the preceding classification system, the ASDC. The major shift in focus of the new system (which also represents a

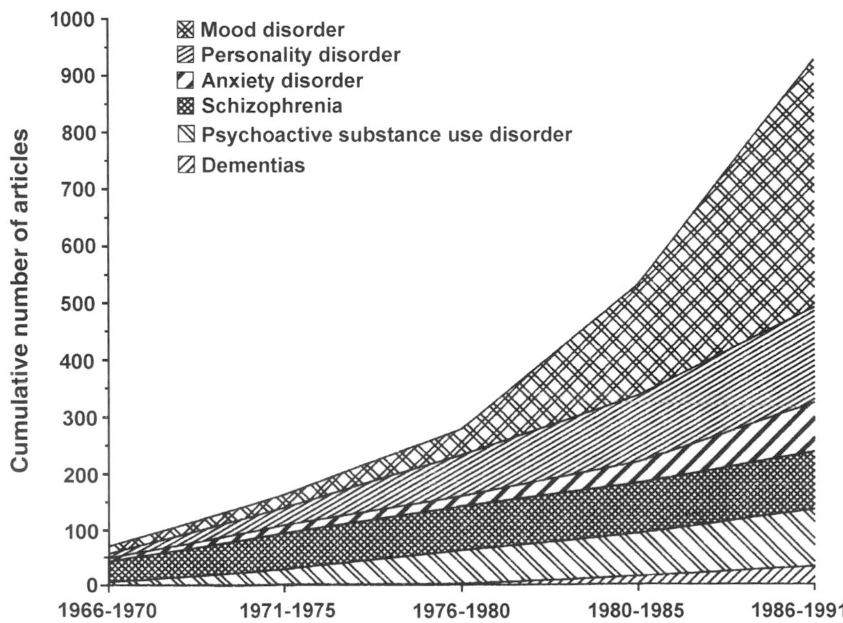

Figure 42–1. Number of articles published on sleep and mental disorders 1966–1991 according to type of mental disorder.

departure from the current DSM-III-R system) is the emphasis on the *pathophysiologic basis* of the sleep disorder in contrast to emphasis on the *presenting clinical complaint.* In the ICSD, sleep disorders associated with mental disorders are classified separately from other sleep disorders, recognizing that the pathophysiologic basis of the sleep disruption is the mental disorder itself. It further subclassifies the mental disorders as Psychosis, Mood Disorders, Anxiety Disorders, Panic Disorder, and Alcoholism, suggesting characteristic disturbances of sleep for each. The DSM-III-R system follows the previous ASDC in its broad symptom-based categories, either insomnia or hypersomnia, and subclassifications of sleep disorders related to another mental disorder, to a known organic factor or as primary.

The literature over the past three decades has revealed several important observations concerning the relationship between sleep and mental disorders. The first observation is that mental disorders are often accompanied by changes in sleep. Several questions have emerged from this observation. What is the relationship between the clinical complaint and objective findings? Are there electroencephalographic (EEG) or polysomnographic correlates of the complaint? Are the changes in sleep central to the pathophysiology of the disorder? Can sleep studies be useful diagnostic tools for mental disorders?

Sleep disorders specialists have recognized a frequent association between disrupted sleep and mental disorders. Of all patients presenting to sleep disorders centers with a complaint of insomnia, the most frequent diagnosis is insomnia related to a primary psychiatric condition (35%) (Coleman et al. 1982). The next most frequent cause of insomnia is a closely related condition, psychophysiological insomnia (15%) (Coleman et al. 1982). It is clear that a nosology of sleep disorders for psychiatrists should reflect the high incidence of sleep disorders associated with mental disorders recognized by sleep disorders specialists.

A study by Ford and Kamerow (1989) highlights an additional relationship between sleep and mental disorders: that is, disrupted sleep is often present prior to the onset of a psychiatric disturbance, suggesting that in some instances the mental disorder may be caused by the sleep disruption itself. As part of the National Institute of Mental Health Epidemiologic Catchment Area study (Regier et al. 1984), respondents with persistent insomnia or hypersomnia over a 1-year period had significantly higher rates of new cases of both Major Depression and Anxiety Disorders compared with those whose initial sleep disturbance resolved. The resolution of sleep disturbances was associated with a decreased incidence of new psychiatric disorders, suggesting that early recognition and treatment of sleep disorders provides an opportunity to prevent psychiatric disorders.

The relationships between sleep and mental disorders can be summarized as follows: 1) sleep disruptions oftentimes are associated with primary mental disorders; 2) mental disorders are often implicated as etiologic factors in patients whose chief complaint is a disturbance of sleep; and 3) disturbances of sleep may precede mental disorders and be etiologic factors in the mental disorder itself. Due to the varied and complex relationships between sleep and mental disorders, it is important that a psychiatric nosology accurately reflect these relationships.

Methods

All primary source references listed in the ICSD for sleep disorders associated with the following mental disorders were reviewed: Psychoses, Mood Disorders, Anxiety Disorders, Panic Disorders, and Alcoholism. The references from each of these sources were also reviewed. A Medline search (BRS Colleague) was conducted for each of the above-listed disorders and sleep. A Medline search was also conducted for sleep and each of the following disorders generally following the DSM-III-R classification of mental disorders: Schizophrenia, Psychotic Disorders, Delusional Disorder, Mood Disorders, Bipolar Disorder, Seasonal Affective Disorder, Anxiety Disorder, Somatoform Disorder, Generalized Anxiety Disorder, Social Phobia, Simple Phobia, Obsessive-Compulsive Disorder, Adjustment Disorder, Posttraumatic Stress Disorder, Panic Disorder, Dissociative Disorder, Personality Disorder, and Borderline Personality Disorder. The general search frame was from 1966 to 1992, English language, and human subjects only, in which the mental disorder and sleep were the major focus. To explore longitudinal trends in psychiatric sleep research, the number of articles published in 4-year increments from 1966 to 1992 for sleep and major psychiatric disorders as well as for the disorder alone were tabulated. Selected review articles (Buysse and Kupfer 1990; Gierz et al. 1987; Soldatos et al. 1987) and book chapters (Vogel et al. 1989; Walsh and Sugerman 1989) relevant to each of the above disorders and sleep were also reviewed for additional references. Emphasis for inclusion of an article in the review was given to articles that 1) were published in peer-reviewed journals; 2) had adequate sample sizes; 3) included adequate control groups; 4) listed both subjective and objective polysomnographic measures; and 5) had well-defined patient populations based on established criteria, who were reliably diagnosed and were distinct from comparison groups.

Results

Sleep disorders associated with mental disorders in the ICSD (Psychoses, Mood Disorders, Anxiety Disorders, Panic Disorders, and Alcoholism) are reviewed first. Other mental disorders that are not covered in the ICSD review, but for which either specific sleep disorders are known to exist or for which there has been considerable research interest, are then reviewed. In general, in the review I highlight the ICSD descriptions of these disorders, then review the relevant literature that either supports or refutes the reported findings as outlined in the ICSD. For each sleep profile of a specific mental disorder, distinctions are made between the research relevance, pathophysiology, and clinical relevance. Each of these is important to consider in determining whether to modify, or add to, existing sleep disorders as outlined in DSM-III-R.

Psychoses

The ICSD lists the essential features of Psychoses as psychiatric disorders characterized by the occurrence of delusions, hallucinations, incoherence, catatonic behavior, or inappropriate affect that causes impaired social or work functioning. Included in this category are Schizophrenia, Schizophreniform Disorder, Drug Psychoses, Organic Psychoses, Delusional Disorder, Other Psychotic Disorders, Childhood Psychoses, Psychotic Decompensation, and Unspecified Functional Psychoses. The primary disturbances of sleep can be either insomnia or excessive sleepiness. In the description of sleep in psychoses, the ICSD describes marked sleep continuity disturbances in acute psychotic decompensation and suggests that there may be persistent disturbances in sleep in chronic or remitted psychotic disorders. Polysomnographic features include individual variability, increased sleep latency, decreased total sleep time, increased waking after sleep onset, sleep fragmentation, decreased slow-wave sleep, shortened rapid eye movement (REM) latency, variability in REM time, and an increase in REM density. The bibliography cites only sleep studies in Schizophrenia.

Although supporting some of the assertions in the ICSD description, the literature in sleep in Schizophrenia is mixed with enough controversial findings to make identifying specific sleep or polysomnographic findings in Schizophrenia difficult. Early studies on sleep in Schizophrenia were driven by the "REM intrusion" hypothesis: since there appears to be a similarity between mental products during dreaming and those during a psychotic exacerbation, Schizophrenia may involve weakening of the usual physiological boundaries between dreaming and waking (e.g., Vogel 1974; Wyatt et al. 1971). Several experiments were designed to test this notion (e.g., Benson and Zarcone 1985; Vogel 1968). A variety of physiological and mental products that were thought to be specific to either the waking or dreaming state were monitored during waking and sleeping. The distributions of the events between waking and REM sleep were compared among patients with Schizophrenia and control subjects. A number of variables were studied. Although the initial hypothesis regarding the intrusion of a dreamlike state into wakefulness in individuals with Schizophrenia was not confirmed, there does appear to be some support for the notion that individuals with Schizophrenia show abnormally reduced rebound of REM sleep following REM sleep deprivation. The clinical relevance of this finding remains to be seen.

In contrast to the literature on REM sleep abnormalities in Schizophrenia, studies on non–rapid eye movement (NREM) sleep have been more consistent in finding reduced slow-wave or delta sleep in individuals with Schizophrenia when compared with control subjects (e.g., Ganguli et al. 1987; Hiatt et al. 1985). The clinical significance of this finding is uncertain since reduced slow-wave sleep is found in a variety of conditions, including other psychiatric disorders, aging, and chronic medical illnesses, and is not always related to a sleep complaint by the patient. Whether reduced slow-wave sleep is related to a specific subset of individuals with Schizophrenia, identifies a pathophysiologic process, or is related to treatment outcome is unclear, although work is being conducted in this area—for example, relationship between slow-wave sleep and 5-hydroxyindoleacetic acid (5-HIAA) or ventricular enlargement (Van Kammen et al. 1988). Longitudinal studies of patients with Schizophrenia suggest that there is considerable variability over the course of an exacerbation of Psychosis (Kupfer et al. 1990). Severe disruptions in sleep, including reduced total sleep time, REM time, and percentage, with prolonged REM latencies are noted in the acute psychotic state. With recovery, NREM and REM sleep return to normal, although REM recovery may lag behind NREM recovery.

Aside from the Mood Disorders, which are reviewed below, little work has been done in identifying sleep disturbances in other nonschizophrenic psychoses.

Mood Disorders

The ICSD lists as the essential features of Mood Disorders one or more episodes of depression, or partial or full manic or hypomanic episodes. Included within this description are Major Depression, Dysthymia, Bipolar Disorder, Cyclothymia, and Seasonal Affective Disorder. The essential disturbances of sleep are reported to be typically insomnia and, less commonly, excessive sleepiness. The insomnia of depression is described as difficulty in falling asleep, sleep continuity disturbances, and "early morning awakening"—waking earlier in the morning than usual and being unable to fall back asleep. Distinctions are made between the sleep of depression and that of acute mania in which shorter sleep durations are due to reductions in the need for sleep. Also sleeping more, or hypersomnia, is reported to be seen in bipolar depression and some in dysthymic patients.

The ICSD lists several polysomnographic features of Mood Disorders. The most characteristic feature is short REM latency. Other REM sleep abnormalities include increased REM sleep and increased density of REMs, particularly in the first REM period. Sleep continuity disruptions include prolonged sleep latency and frequent awakenings throughout the night. Changes in sleep architecture include reduced delta sleep, with a shifting of delta sleep to the second NREM period. Bipolar depression is associated with higher sleep efficiency and complaints of daytime sleepiness, in contrast to unipolar depression. The sleep of patients in a hypomanic or manic episode is characterized by profound inability to fall asleep, with short REM latencies, short sleep durations, and reduced delta sleep. Patients with secondary depression following a medical illness are reported to show disruptions and reduced REM sleep. The characteristic findings of sleep changes in depression are reported to be present in at least 90% of cases, helping to clarify the diagnosis and aid in planning treatment recommendations.

There is a large body of literature to support the presence of characteristic sleep changes in depression. Over the years 1965–1990, 529 articles focused on sleep and depression. In the literature from 1984 to 1990, which shows 603 references to sleep and mental disorders, 266 (44%) of these are related to depression. In this time, 122 (46%) of the studies on sleep and depression focused on the REM sleep changes in depression. This accumulated body of literature supports the following sleep characteristics of depression: 1) sleep continuity disturbances such as prolonged sleep latency, increased nocturnal awakenings, and early morning awakenings; 2) diminished slow-wave sleep (stages 3 and 4), with shifting of slow-wave sleep and activity from the first to the second NREM period; and 3) changes in REM sleep including the earlier occurrence of REM sleep in the night (i.e., "shortened REM latency"), a shift of REM sleep earlier in the night, and increased frequency of eye movements during REM sleep (increased "REM density") (e.g., Akiskal et al. 1982; Gillin and Borbély 1985; Reynolds and Kupfer 1987).

Although the literature is clear regarding the characteristic sleep changes observed in depression, there are several other questions currently being addressed by psychiatric sleep researchers in the area of depression (Buysse and Kupfer 1990). One area of questioning surrounds the notion of the specificity of the sleep changes in depression. Can depression be distinguished from other psychiatric disorders on the basis of EEG sleep findings? Can subtypes of depression be separated from one another by EEG sleep profiles? Other areas of questioning address the neurobiology of depression. Are the sleep changes specific to the acute state of depression or are they indicative of trait markers? Are they present before or after an episode of depression? Are they present in family members? How are they changed by treatment? Do they predict treatment response, either with medications or with psychotherapy? How do the changes evolve into remission from depression?

Although the literature addressing these questions is still developing, some trends have begun to emerge. Although the overall pattern of sleep described above does appear to be sensitive to depression, individual aspects of the pattern, such as reduced REM latency, have been noted in other conditions and are not in themselves specific indicators of depression (Zarcone et al. 1987). Aging, severity of depression, and certain subtypes of depression appear to be associated with distinct sleep profiles (e.g., Akiskal et al. 1984; Nofzinger et al. 1991; Reynolds et al. 1985; Thase et al. 1986). The sleep changes appear to be more of a trait than state marker, present throughout the course of depression (e.g., Hauri et al. 1974; Rush et al. 1986) and noted in family members of depressed individuals (e.g., Giles et al. 1987). Currently there is insufficient evidence to suggest that there are specific aspects of sleep that predict medication or psychotherapy response. Reduced REM latency and reduced delta wave ratio (the average delta counts in first NREM period/the average delta counts in second NREM period) seem to be associated with increased recurrence of depression (Kupfer et al. 1990). Pharmacologic and chronobiologic probes such as cholinergic REM sleep induction (e.g., Sitaram et al. 1984) and sleep deprivation (e.g., Reynolds et al. 1990) are being used to explore the neurobiology of depression. There is evidence to suggest that sleep abnormalities are important in the pathophysiology of depression (e.g., Vogel 1975). Alterations in the sleep-wake cycle result from at least two forms of treatment for depression: pharmacotherapy and sleep deprivation. "Arousal-type REM sleep deprivation" has been suggested as a common mechanism of action for these treatments. However, other treatments for depression, such as electroconvulsive therapy and antidepressants, which do not affect REM sleep, do not appear to have this as their mechanism of action.

Anxiety Disorders (Excluding Panic)

Disorders included in this category are Generalized Anxiety Disorder, Anxiety State Unspecified, Social Phobia, Simple Phobia, Obsessive-Compulsive Disorder, Adjustment Disorder (with anxious features?), and Posttraumatic Stress Disorder. The essential features of sleep associated with Anxiety Disorders are a sleep-onset or maintenance insomnia due to excessive anxiety and apprehensive expectation about one or more life circumstances. It is distinguished from psychophysiological insomnia by the generalized nature of the anxiety seen in Anxiety Disorders in contrast to the focus of anxiety around the sleep complaint in the case of psychophysiological insomnia. The polysomnographic features of Anxiety Disorders are reported to be mostly nonspecific changes of increased sleep latency, decreased sleep efficiency, increased amounts of stage 1 and 2 sleep, and decreased slow-wave sleep. Sleep in the Anxiety Disorders is reported to be distinct from the sleep of depression in that the Anxiety Disorders do not show the characteristic REM sleep changes such as reduced REM latency that are associated with depression.

There has been little research on sleep in Generalized Anxiety Disorder as a separate diagnostic entity from other Anxiety Disorders. Most studies have been done with heterogeneous populations of subjects with Generalized Anxiety Disorder in combination with Panic Disorder, Obsessive-Compulsive Disorder, Schizotypal Personality Features, and concurrent or past history diagnoses of Dysthymia or Major Depression (e.g., Papadimitriou et al. 1988; Reynolds et al. 1983). The trends noted in the literature, which require further validation, include prolonged sleep latencies, decreased sleep efficiency, and reduced total sleep time. REM sleep–related abnormalities characteristic of depression have not been demonstrated.

The literature on sleep disorders in Posttraumatic Stress Disorder is conflicting (e.g., Kramer and Kinney 1988; Ross et al. 1989), with variable explanations for the clinically observed insomnia and repetitive traumatic dreams characteristic of the disorder. Aside from generalized alterations in the sleep-wake cycle, such as reduced sleep efficiency and reductions in delta sleep, which are not clearly distinct from those of other Anxiety Disorders, there is no consistent view about the pathophysiologic nature of the repetitive traumatic dream or the stage of sleep from which it arises.

The literature on sleep in Obsessive-Compulsive Disorder is scarce and does not yield a clear picture of how to categorize the disorder biologically in relation to other major categories of mental disorders (Insel et al. 1982). Profiles include several features to suggest a biological relationship with the other Anxiety Disorders, such as reduced sleep time and a shift of sleep staging from delta sleep to the lighter stages of sleep; however, the occurrence of reduced REM latencies suggests a possible link with affective disorders. Studies of sleep deprivation in Obsessive-Compulsive Disorder (Joffe and Swinson 1988) yielded responses that were more compatible with Panic Disorder as opposed to affective disorders. Based on the paucity of sleep studies in this disorder, comments about a specific sleep profile in Obsessive-Compulsive Disorder should be considered tentative.

Panic Disorder

Included in this category are Panic Disorder with and without Agoraphobia. Panic episodes can be associated with sudden awakenings from sleep, which may be the primary sleep complaint. The polysomnographic features listed in the ICSD for Panic Disorder are marginally increased sleep latency and decreased sleep efficiency, with panic episodes occurring in NREM sleep, often in the transition from stage 2 sleep to slow-wave sleep.

A review of the current literature does not support a diagnostic categorization of sleep abnormalities associated with Panic Disorder as distinct from those of other Anxiety Disorders (e.g., Grunhaus et al. 1986; Mellman and Uhde 1989). The major sleep abnormalities include prolonged sleep latencies, reduced sleep efficiency, and reductions in total sleep time in the absence of distinct changes in REM sleep. These are the same findings noted in other Anxiety Disorders. Recent efforts have focused on characterization of "panic" episodes, which occur during sleep primarily due to the heuristic value of clarifying the biological foundations of panic episodes (Mellman and Uhde 1989). Panic episodes during sleep are assumed to be devoid of a psychological etiology of the panic attack. Examination of these episodes is proposed to provide a window to the understanding of daytime "spontaneous" panic episodes. It is not clear if there is a separate population of patients who present with only sleep panic attacks. Most studied have occurred in patients with concurrent Panic Disorder. There is no information that describes the incidence of these episodes in nonpanic Anxiety Disorders or other psychiatric conditions, which would be necessary prior to concluding that these episodes are distinct entities. The polysomnographic profile suggests that the "sleep panic" episodes represent arousals from NREM sleep. It is not clear if they are distinct from either night terrors or from the disturbing arousals that have been described in Posttraumatic Stress Disorder, each of which has similarities in both clinical profile and occurrence in EEG sleep stage.

At this time it remains unclear whether the similarities in polysomnographic sleep profiles for the Anxiety Disorders suggest common biological foundations or whether the sleep-wake regulators are reacting in a similar but limited fashion to biologically heterogeneous conditions.

Alcoholism

The ICSD describes Alcoholism as excessive alcohol intake applying to both Alcohol Abuse and Dependency. Included in this category are Chronic Alcoholism, Acute Alcoholism, Alcohol Abuse, Alcoholic Psychoses, Korsakoff's Psychosis, and Delirium Tremens. The essential feature of the sleep disturbances can be either insomnia or excessive sleepiness. The effects of alcohol on sleep are described over three periods: acute alcohol use, chronic excessive use, and abstinence. Acute use is described to induce sleepiness and reduce wakefulness for the first 3–4 hours of sleep, with subsequent increases in wakefulness occasionally associated with anxiety dreams in the latter half of the night. With chronic excessive alcohol use, sleep is reported to be fragmented, with short periods of deep sleep interrupted by brief arousals or periods of restlessness. With abstinence, sleep is initially characterized by profound disruption, including insomnia, and nightmares. Although sleep improves over time, light sleep and increased vulnerability to other sleep-disrupting factors are reported to persist even after short-term (2-week) abstinence.

The polysomnographic features listed in the ICSD describe the objective sleep abnormalities over the three periods of alcohol use: acute, chronic, and abstinence. Acutely, alcohol is reported to reduce wakefulness and REM sleep and increase delta sleep over the first 3–4 hours of sleep, with subsequent increases (rebound) in REM sleep and wakefulness over the latter half of the night. With chronic use, sleep becomes fragmented, with frequent arousals, increased slow eye movements during stage 2 sleep, and increased alpha activity in the EEG during slow-wave sleep. In short-term abstinence, sleep is reported to show profound sleep disruption, short sleep times, and increased REM sleep with profound reductions in slow-wave sleep. Sleep times and REM sleep tend to normalize after acute abstinence. However, slow-wave sleep is reported to continue to be reduced for several years and may never return to baseline values. Review of the literature supports each of these well-defined sleep changes in acute and chronic use as well as in abstinence (e.g., Gross and Hastey 1976; Porkny 1978; Zarcone 1979).

Discussion

Recommendations for the DSM-IV classification of sleep disorders associated with mental disorders should be grounded on existing classification systems with reference to the literature either in support of new systems of classification or suggesting maintenance of current categories. The existing classification systems described above include the DSM-III-R, the ASDC, and the ICSD.

Any translation of the literature in sleep and mental disorders, in which the goal is the clarification of a nosologic system, should be made with an understanding of the forces that shape the overall climate in which the research is being conducted (Grob 1991). In the 1960s, when psychoanalysis was a predominant force in psychiatry, interest in sleep followed closely the psychodynamic importance of the dream. The discovery of a psychophysiological marker for a recurrent dreaming period, the REM during sleep, offered a window to further observation of dreams and their psychological and physiological significance (Aserinsky and Kleitman 1953; Dement and Kleitman 1957). The similarity between dream mentation and psychotic states provided the foundation for a hypothesis of psychotic states as some manifestation of dreamlike mentation intruding into wakefulness. This notion fueled much of the research in sleep and Schizophrenia in the 1960s and early 1970s. This is reflected by the finding that close to 50% of all research in sleep and mental disorders in the latter half of the 1960s was in Schizophrenia (Figure 42–1).

Research over the past two decades in sleep and mental disorders shifted to an emphasis on understanding the neurobiology of mental disorders as reflected in alterations in the sleep-wake cycle produced by individual disorders. Objectively, this can be seen by the shift in the literature in recent years to a focus on sleep abnormalities in depression, accounting for roughly 60% of all research on sleep and mental disorders over this time (Figure 42–1). Taking into account the proliferation of both psychiatric research and the shift in psychiatric sleep research to

Affective Disorders, the literature on sleep and Affective Disorders in recent years accounts for roughly a quarter of all research conducted on sleep and mental disorders since 1966. The major emphasis of this literature focuses on REM sleep changes as putative biological markers of the disorder or on sleep deprivation as a treatment of the disorder. It is apparent in viewing this trend that the research emphasis in sleep disorders and mental disorders has followed overall trends in psychiatric research shaped by a variety of social, political, and economic forces in which nosologic strategies based on neurobiologic and empirically based guides to treatment decisions have become predominant (Sabshin 1990).

Within this historical perspective it can be seen that the research on sleep and mental disorders has proliferated not entirely because of the presence of a specific complaint about sleep in patients, a sleep disorder per se, but rather as a technical tool used as a window to the neurobiology of psychiatric disorders. The majority of the literature addresses the importance of furthering our understanding of the neurobiology of the individual disorders in the hope of ultimately improving our therapeutic efforts. Clarifying a nosology of sleep disorders associated with mental disorders, although a natural consequence of the accumulated literature, has not been the primary focus.

The patient's subjective distress due to sleep disruption is variable between psychiatric disorders. In some instances, such as depression, the presenting clinical complaint is often related to a disruption in sleep, emphasizing the subjective distress noted by the patient. In other disorders, such as the manic phase of Bipolar Affective Disorder, the clinical concern revolves around the management of the acute psychotic phase, even though it is recognized that there may be an associated decreased need for sleep. Given the variability in the clinical subjective complaint between mental disorders, it is reasonable to continue the current DSM-III-R tradition of including the sleep complaint as a symptom in the diagnostic criteria for the mental disorder itself.

The identification by the ICSD that mental disorders are important factors in the pathophysiology of certain sleep disorders has been empirically verified in more than three decades of psychiatric sleep research. In comparison with control subjects, the literature review above clearly recognizes abnormalities in the objective polysomnographic profiles in patients diagnosed with Schizophrenia, Mood Disorders, Anxiety Disorders, Panic Disorders, and Alcoholism. The observation that the most frequent diagnosis of insomnia for patients presenting to a sleep disorders center is insomnia related to a mental disorder (Coleman et al. 1982) lends further epidemiologic support for the morbidity associated with the sleep disruption. Both from pathophysiologic and clinical perspectives then, it is clear that sleep disorders related to mental disorders warrant separate diagnostic classification from other sleep disorders. It is also clear that independent clinical attention to a sleep disorder as separate from the underlying mental disorder is sometimes warranted since the impaired daytime functioning or distress can be seen as secondary to the marked sleep disruption of some mental disorders.

Although the literature is clear that mental disorders are associated with subjective and objective disturbances in sleep, there remains considerable controversy in the field regarding the specificity of sleep profiles that distinguish one mental disorder from another, or for that matter, a mental disorder from a general medical sleep disorder. Certain polysomnographic abnormalities, such as sleep continuity disruptions, and loss of delta, or stages 3 and 4 sleep, can be found in a variety of mental disorders and general medical sleep disorders. A characteristic pattern of REM sleep described above under Mood Disorders appears to be more specific for depression. However, individual REM abnormalities, such as a reduced REM latency, have been found, although less reliably, in a variety of other conditions, such as drug withdrawal states, Schizophrenia, Narcolepsy, and the "normal" population. With regard to specificity of sleep findings reported in the ICSD, the literature review suggests that the reported profiles should be seen as general trends that await further clarification and validation before being recognized as specific to an individual disorder.

Despite the lack of specific sleep profiles for individual psychiatric disorders, the ICSD system of categorizing sleep disorders related to individual mental disorders appears to be conceptually sound (although the disorders listed are limiting in scope). For DSM-IV, classifying sleep disorders as related to an unspecified mental disorder when the mental disorder is known would not accurately reflect the specificity of the clinical assessment, thereby eliminating therapeutically useful information. Allowing the clinician to diagnose the sleep disorder as related to a mental disorder with the option of specifying the individual disorder from a full complement of DSM-IV diagnoses would allow greater flexibility in diagnostic accuracy and provide a window for future research in sleep and mental disorders.

Recommendations

A review of the literature suggests that there is sufficient empirical support for the classification of sleep disorders related to mental disorders. Adoption of the ICSD system highlighting that the pathophysiologic nature of the disorder is related to the mental disorder is conceptually sound. It is clinically useful to continue to identify the specific mental disorder to which the sleep disorder is being attributed, recognizing the limitations of the objective assessment of sleep in defining specific sleep profiles for individual sleep disorders. In addition, the DSM-III-R criteria for insomnia or hypersomnia related to another mental disorder should be modified in DSM-IV by adding the specific guideline that the sleep disorder is "sufficiently severe to warrant independent clinical attention," especially since sleep disorders are so frequently encountered as a symptom of other mental disorders.

Future research efforts should focus on 1) further clarification of the specificity of sleep findings for individual disorders; 2) further definition of sleep disorders related to mental disorders versus associated sleep symptoms of mental disorders; 3) exploration of the clinical relevance of individual sleep findings with respect to clinical course and treatment response; 4) elucidation of the role of disrupted sleep as an etiologic factor, an associated feature, or as a lasting scar of a mental disorder; and 5) clarification of the morbidity of disrupted sleep on the functional capacity of the individual, in terms of both subjective and objective sleep abnormalities.

References

Akiskal HS, Lemmi H, Yerevanian B, et al: The usefulness of REM latency test in psychiatric diagnosis: a study of 81 depressed outpatients. Psychiatry Res 7:101–110, 1982

Akiskal HS, Lemmi H, Dickson H, et al: Chronic depressions, part 2: sleep EEG separation of primary dysthymic disorders from chronic depressions. J Affective Disord 6:287–295, 1984

American Psychiatric Association: Diagnostic and Statistical Manual of Mental Disorders, 3rd Edition, Revised. Washington, DC, American Psychiatric Association, 1987

American Sleep Disorders Association, Diagnostic Classification Steering Committee: International Classification of Sleep Disorders: Diagnostic and Coding Manual. Rochester, MN, American Sleep Disorders Association, 1990

Aserinsky E, Kleitman N: Regularly occurring periods of eye motility and concomitant phenomena during sleep. Science 118:273–274, 1953

Association of Sleep Disorders Centers: Diagnostic classification of sleep and arousal disorders. Sleep 2:1–137, 1979

Benson KL, Zarcone VP: Testing the REM sleep intrusion hypothesis of schizophrenia. Psychiatry Res 15:163–173, 1985

Buysse DJ, Kupfer DJ: Diagnostic and research applications of electroencephalographic sleep studies in depression: conceptual and methodological issues. J Nerv Ment Dis 178:405–413, 1990

Coleman RM, Roffwarg HP, Kennedy SJ, et al: Sleep-wake disorders based on a polysomnographic diagnosis: a national cooperative study. JAMA 247:997–1103, 1982

Dement W, Kleitman N: The relation of eye movements during sleep to dream activity: an objective method for the study of dreaming. J Exp Psychol 53:339–346, 1957

Ford DE, Kamerow DB: Epidemiologic study of sleep disturbances and psychiatric disorders: an opportunity for prevention? JAMA 262:1479–1484, 1989

Ganguli R, Reynolds CF III, Kupfer DJ: EEG sleep in young, never-medicated, schizophrenic patients: a comparison with delusional and nondelusional depressives and with healthy controls. Arch Gen Psychiatry 44:36–45, 1987

Gierz M, Campbell SS, Gillin JC: Sleep disturbances in various nonaffective psychiatric disorders. Psychiatr Clin North Am 10:565–581, 1987

Giles DE, Roffwerg HP, Rush AJ: REM latency concordance in depressed family members. Biol Psychiatry 22:910–924, 1987

Gillin JC, Borbély AA: Sleep: a neurobiological window on affective disorders. Trends Neurosci 8:537–542, 1985

Grob GN: Origins of DSM-I: a study in appearance and reality. Am J Psychiatry 148:421–431, 1991

Gross MM, Hastey JM: Sleep disturbances in alcoholism, in Alcoholism: Interdisciplinary Approaches to an Enduring Problem. Edited by Tarter RE, Suguman A. Reading, MA, Addison-Wesley, 1976, pp 257–309

Grunhaus L, Rabin D, Harel Y, et al: Simultaneous panic and depressive disorders: clinical and sleep EEG correlates. Psychiatry Res 17:251–259, 1986

Hauri P, Chernik D, Hawkins D, et al: Sleep of depressed patients in remission. Arch Gen Psychiatry 31:386–391, 1974

Hiatt JF, Floyd TC, Katz PH, et al: Further evidence of abnormal NREM sleep in schizophrenia. Arch Gen Psychiatry 42:797–802, 1985

Insel TR, Gillin JC, Moore A, et al: The sleep of patients with obsessive-compulsive disorder. Arch Gen Psychiatry 39:1370–1377, 1982

Joffe RT, Swinson RP: Total sleep deprivation in patients with obsessive-compulsive disorder. Acta Psychiatr Scand 77:483–487, 1988

Kramer M, Kinney L: Sleep patterns in trauma victims with disturbed dreaming. Psychiatr J Univ Ottawa 13:12–16, 1988

Kupfer DJ, Frank E, McEachran AB, et al: Delta sleep ratio: a biological correlate of early recurrence in unipolar affective disorder. Arch Gen Psychiatry 47:1100–1105, 1990

Mellman TA, Uhde TW: Electroencephalographic sleep in panic disorder. Arch Gen Psychiatry 46:178–184, 1989

Nofzinger EA, Thase ME, Reynolds CF III, et al: Hypersomnia in bipolar depression, part 1: a comparison with narcolepsy using the multiple sleep latency test. Am J Psychiatry 148:1177–1181, 1991

Papadimitriou GN, Kerkhofs M, Kempenaers C, et al: EEG sleep studies in patients with generalized anxiety disorder. Psychiatry Res 26:183–190, 1988

Porkny AD: Sleep disturbances, alcohol and alcoholism: a review, in Sleep Disorders: Diagnosis and Treatment. Edited by Williams RL, Karacan I. New York, Wiley, 1978, pp 389–402

Regier DA, Myers JK, Kramer M, et al: The NIMH Epidemiologic Catchment Area program: historical context, major objectives, and study populations characteristics. Arch Gen Psychiatry 41:934–941, 1984

Reynolds CF III, Kupfer DJ: Sleep research in affective illness: state of the art circa 1987. Sleep 10:199–215, 1987

Reynolds CF III, Shaw DM, Newton TF, et al: EEG sleep in outpatients with generalized anxiety: a preliminary comparison with depressed outpatients. Psychiatry Res 8:81–89, 1983

Reynolds CF III, Kupfer DJ, Taska LS, et al: EEG sleep in elderly depressed, demented, and healthy subjects. Biol Psychiatry 20:431–442, 1985

Reynolds CF, Buysse DJ, Kupfer DJ, et al: Rapid eye movement sleep deprivation as a probe in elderly subjects. Arch Gen Psychiatry 47:1128–1136, 1990

Ross RJ, Ball WA, Sullivan KA, et al: Sleep disturbance as the hallmark of post-traumatic stress disorder. Am J Psychiatry 146:697–707, 1989

Rush AJ, Erman MK, Giles DE, et al: Polysomnographic findings in recently drug free and clinically remitted depressed patients. Arch Gen Psychiatry 43:878–884, 1986

Sabshin M: Turning points in twentieth-century American psychiatry. Am J Psychiatry 147:1267–1274, 1990

Sitaram N, Gillin JC, Bunney WE Jr: Cholinergic and catecholaminergic receptor sensitivity in affective illness: strategy and theory, in Neurobiology of Mood Disorders. Edited by Post RM, Ballenger JC. Baltimore, MD, Williams & Wilkins, 1984, pp 629–651

Soldatos CR, Vela-Bueno A, Kales A: Sleep in psychiatric disorders. Psychiatr Med 4:119–132, 1987

Thase ME, Kupfer DJ, Ulrich RF: EEG sleep in psychotic depression: a valid subtype? Arch Gen Psychiatry 43:886–893, 1986

Van Kammen WB, Peters JL, Goetz KL, et al: Diminished slow wave sleep and ventricular enlargement in schizophrenia. Schizophr Res 1:164–165, 1988

Vogel GW: REM deprivation III dreaming and psychosis. Arch Gen Psychiatry 18:312–329, 1968

Vogel GW: Dreaming and schizophrenia. Psychiatric Annals 4:63–77, 1974

Vogel GW: A review of REM sleep deprivation. Arch Gen Psychiatry 32:749–761, 1975

Vogel GW, Reynolds CF III, Akiskal HS, et al: Psychiatric disorders, in Principles and Practice of Sleep Medicine. Edited by Kryger MG, Roth T, Dement WC. Philadelphia, PA, WB Saunders, 1989, pp 413–430

Walsh JK, Sugerman JL: Disorders of initiating and maintaining sleep in adult psychiatric disorders, in Principles and Practice of Sleep Medicine. Edited by Kryger MH, Roth T, Dement WC. Philadelphia, PA, WB Saunders, 1989, pp 448–455

Wyatt R, Termini BA, Davis J: A review of the literature 1960–1970, part II: sleep studies. Schizophr Bull 4:45–66, 1971

Zarcone VP: Alcoholism and sleep, in Pharmacology of the States of Alertness. Edited by Passonant P, Oswald I. Oxford, Pergamon, 1979, pp 9–38

Zarcone VP, Benson KL, Berger PA: Abnormal latencies in schizophrenia. Arch Gen Psychiatry 44:45–48, 1987

Chapter 43

Sleep Disorders Associated With Neurological Disorders

Michael J. Sateia, M.D.

Statement of the Issues

A subdivision of sleep disorders associated with neurological disorders is complicated by several factors. Sleep-related issues become relevant to the extent to which 1) there are consistent sleep-related abnormalities that are a significant component of the clinical profile; 2) there are sleep-related abnormalities that are useful in establishing the diagnosis of the primary (neurological) disorder; 3) there are aspects of the primary disorder that are substantially influenced by sleep physiology; and 4) sleep-related findings are of scientific value in understanding the pathophysiology of the primary disorder, or the physiology of sleep itself. The relative importance of each of these factors varies with the particular neurological diagnosis that one is addressing. Moreover, the types of sleep pathology that are observed in this group of disorders cover the full spectrum of sleep disorders.

Inasmuch as sleep disorders may complicate virtually any neurological condition, at least in an indirect manner, it is arbitrary to some extent to select a given subset for discussion. It would appear that the International Classification of Sleep Disorders (ICSD) (American Sleep Disorders Association 1990) has selected a particular subgroup based on the extent to which 1) the sleep pathology occurs as a direct result of the disorder and 2) the association of the neurological condition with sleep disorders has received adequate attention in the literature. The ICSD diagnoses can be further subdivided into three groups: degenerative diseases (Alzheimer's, Parkinson's, Fatal Familial Insomnia, and other degenerative disorders); seizure disorders (sleep-related epilepsy and status epilepticus of sleep); and sleep-related headaches. In this review I focus on the degenerative disorders, in that they are of greatest relevance to psychiatry. I address several questions. Is there a consistent set of sleep-related findings that occurs with sufficient predictability as to be considered an inherent component of the clinical profile? Are these findings of diagnostic utility with respect to differential diagnosis with other neuropsychiatric or sleep disorders? Are ancillary sleep disorders that may complicate the clinical profile observed at a higher than expected frequency in association with the condition? What is the relevance of these findings to clinical psychiatry? To the extent to which sleep-related findings associated with any given neurological disorder satisfy these criteria, then separate criteria for that disorder may be warranted. Otherwise, sleep disorders that are associated with neurological conditions should be combined under a general heading without specification of separate diagnoses within that heading. As is the case with sleep disorders secondary to medical disorders, a decision must be reached regarding whether that heading should be phenomenologically directed (e.g., insomnia due to organic [neurological] condition) or etiologically directed (e.g., sleep disorders secondary to neurological disorders).

Significance of the Issues

In that the ICSD has established a category of "Sleep disorders associated with neurological disorders," internosologic consistency suggests that such a category must be seriously considered for DSM-IV. Establishment of a separate category for neurological disorders may also have scientific and clinical value inasmuch as unique aspects of sleep disorders due to neurological conditions are highlighted by separate classification. However, this approach represents somewhat of a departure from DSM-III-R (American Psychiatric Association 1987) and must be justified on the basis of scientific merit and clinical relevance.

In addition, it should be noted that a separate classification for neurological disorders would, in effect, lump dyssomnias (e.g., insomnia associated with Alzheimer's disease) and parasomnias (e.g., nocturnal complex partial seizures) into a single category—a decision that tends to violate the distinction drawn between these broad categories both in DSM-III-R and elsewhere in the ICSD system. Such a decision is not in keeping with the DSM emphasis on grouping by phenomenology as opposed to etiology.

Methods

Articles and book chapters noted in the bibliography section of the appropriate ICSD diagnoses were reviewed. References from these articles were consulted for additional relevant material. A Medline search (BRS Colleague) was conducted for all primary neurological diagnoses and appropriate synonyms referenced "with sleep." This search yielded the following numbers of references for each category: Dementia with sleep, 36; Alzheimer's disease with sleep, 24; Parkinson's disease with sleep, 54; Hereditary progressive dystonia with sleep, 3; Olivopontocerebellar degeneration with sleep, 4; and Huntington's disease with sleep, 2. Studies were then selected from the search results based on criteria described above. Selection was further guided by the following considerations: 1) use of matched control groups and/or other diagnostic comparison groups, 2) employment of objective criteria for subject selection, 3) use of objective measures for determination of sleep-related findings, and 4) adequate distinction of diagnostic subtypes and severity rating. Studies that were designed primarily to investigate treatment effects were not included unless they contained data considered directly relevant to diagnostic issues. Similarly, investigations that pertained primarily to etiologic considerations were not included.

Results

Dementia

The majority of controlled studies of sleep in dementia patients utilize polysomnographic (PSG) analysis of sleep as the primary investigative tool. These studies consist largely of comparisons between dementia patients and age-matched control subjects on a variety of PSG measures. Although most of these studies have attempted to distinguish senile dementia of the Alzheimer's type (SDAT) from multi-infarct dementia, mixed dementia, and other forms of dementia, this is not always the case. Comparisons of data are complicated further by variation in types of control groups, severity rating, medication status of subjects, definition of sleep variables analyzed, degree of screening for complicating sleep disorders, adequacy of assessment for other neuropsychiatric variables (e.g., depression), and control of environmental variables (e.g., daily routine and sleep-wake schedule).

With respect to PSG data derived largely from studies of patients with SDAT, there is general agreement regarding disruption of sleep continuity as evidenced by decreased sleep efficiency, increased number of awakenings, and increased wake after sleep onset (Bliwise et al. 1989; Feinberg et al. 1967; Prinz et al. 1982a, 1982b; Reynolds et al. 1985a). A loss of stage 2 transients (spindles/K-complexes) and its corollary, an increase in "indeterminate" non–rapid eye movement (NREM) has also been well documented (Allen et al. 1983, 1987; Reynolds et al. 1985a), as have significant declines in slow-wave sleep (Allen et al. 1983; Bliwise et al. 1986, 1989; Martin et al. 1986; Prinz et al. 1982a). The data are somewhat less clear with respect to parameters related to rapid eye movement (REM). Decreased REM percentage and absolute REM time have been described in several studies (Allen et al. 1983, 1987; Feinberg et al. 1967; Prinz et al. 1982a, 1982b); others have failed to find a significant difference from control subjects (Bliwise et al. 1986; Loewenstein et al.

1982). REM latencies are reportedly increased, but, in most cases, only if intervening wake time is included in the definition (Bliwise et al. 1986, 1989; Prinz et al. 1982a, 1982b; Vitiello et al. 1984). This suggests that increased REM latency may be a reflection of the sleep continuity disturbance in dementia, as much as it is an abnormality in inherent timing of the NREM/REM cycle.

Discriminant function analyses utilizing sleep variables have been employed to distinguish demented patients from control subjects. Prinz and colleagues (1982b) reported 90% correct classification using percentage of waking of time in bed, percentage of stage 3/4 time in bed, and percentage of REM time in bed. Vitiello and colleagues (1984) obtained 89% correct classification of moderately to severely demented patients using total REM time, although no measures were reliable in distinguishing mildly demented patients from control subjects in their population. Bliwise and colleagues (1989) found only 65% correct identification employing the most discriminating REM latency definition.

Correlations of sleep parameters with cognitive function have produced variable results. Prinz and colleagues (1982a) described a positive correlation between percentage of REM and Wechsler Adult Intelligence Scale (WAIS) (Wechsler 1981) and Clinical Dementia Rating Scale (Hughes et al. 1982) scores. Feinberg and colleagues (1967) reported that WAIS (verbal and performance) was significantly correlated with number of awakenings and percentage of wake time in bed. Reynolds and colleagues (1985a) found an association between stage number (indeterminate NREM) and scores on the Mini-Mental State (Folstein et al. 1975).

Findings regarding the intactness of circadian rhythm in dementia patients have likewise produced varying conclusions. Based on the extent of percentage of wake time in bed, number of nighttime arousals and awakenings, and increase in daytime napping, several investigators have concluded that the normal circadian rhythm of sleep-wake is replaced by an arrhythmic distribution of sleep-wake across the 24 hours (Prinz et al. 1982a; Reynolds et al. 1988). Others have suggested that the basic sleep-wake cycle remains intact (Allen et al. 1983, 1987; Bliwise et al. 1988). Prinz and colleagues (1984) found that the circadian regulation of temperature cycle was intact in SDAT patients. It should be noted that these studies differ with respect to the methods employed in assessing day-night distribution of sleep, definitions of disrupted rhythm, severity of dementia, and control of environmental variables (especially daily routine of patients).

Comparisons of SDAT patients with other patient populations (non-SDAT dementia, other degenerative or psychiatric diagnoses) are few, with the exception of the work of Reynolds and others comparing dementia and depression (discussed later). Allen and colleagues (1987) found no significant difference in sleep variables between a group of SDAT patients and patients with multi-infarct or mixed dementia. Martin and colleagues (1986) reported a significant increase in intermediate wake time in patients with Korsakoff's psychosis as compared with a group of SDAT patients. The most extensive work in the area of interdiagnostic comparisons involving dementia is that of Reynolds and colleagues, who have attempted to discriminate dementia from depression on the basis of sleep-related variables. In a series of articles (Reynolds et al. 1983, 1985a, 1988), they demonstrated correct classification of patients at a 70%–80% rate of accuracy employing discriminant function analyses that included REM latency, REM percentage, sleep continuity measures, and determination of phasic activity (REM/stage 2). Similar rates were achieved with application of analyses to a new population. One measure (sleep continuity) was demonstrated to have significant predictive value regarding course and outcome at 2-year follow-up.

Several investigators have examined the frequency of sleep-disordered breathing in dementia. Most studies have demonstrated a significant increase in respiratory disturbance (apnea or hypopnea) in SDAT or multi-infarct dementia (Erkinjuntti et al. 1987; Hoch et al. 1986, 1989; Mant et al. 1988; Reynolds et al. 1985b), with 42%–72% of subjects demonstrating a respiratory disturbance index > 5. The frequency of apnea or hypopnea correlated with severity of dementia in two studies (Erkinjuntti et al. 1987; Reynolds et al. 1985b). Mant and colleagues found no difference in sleep-disordered breathing by type of dementia, whereas Erkinjuntti and colleagues noted a nonsignificant trend toward higher respiratory disturbance index in multi-infarct dementia as compared with SDAT. Hoch and colleagues (1989) reported that degree of respiratory disturbance was not predictive of overnight mental status changes or disruptive nocturnal behavior, although Bliwise and colleagues (1986) found an inverse correlation between lowest SaO_2 (arterial oxygen saturation) and overnight level of disorientation. Paradoxically, the control subjects in the report by Bliwise and colleagues showed a significantly greater number of desaturations than dementia patients. Smallwood and colleagues (1983) found no significant increase of sleep-disordered breathing in a medically healthy, nonobese, normotensive population of Alzheimer's patients.

No extensive studies of non-PSG sleep-related variables in dementia were identified. Evans (1987) reported that "sundowning" tended to distinguish elderly demented from nondemented patients, although the difference was not statistically significant. In a prospective clinicopathological study, Molsa and colleagues (1985) found that nocturnal confusion was one of three clinical variables that had significant value in discriminating SDAT from multi-infarct and combined dementias.

Parkinsonism

The literature on sleep-related variables in parkinsonism consists largely of studies of baseline PSG data and analysis of drug effects on PSG-determined sleep parameters, with a very limited number of other investigations related to respiratory disturbance during sleep, movement in sleep, endocrine factors, and non-PSG sleep-related symptoms. PSG studies are confounded by use of mixed groups (e.g., idiopathic, encephalitic), inadequate control of treatment variables (surgery, medication), absence of severity ratings, imprecise or confusing definitions of PSG variables, and, in almost all cases, complete inattention to the degree of dementia and depression among subjects.

In summary, PSG data reveal general agreement regarding an increase in sleep latency, stage 1, number of arousals, and waking time in bed (Apps et al. 1985; Bergonzi et al. 1974, 1975; Emser et al. 1988; Friedman 1980; Kales et al. 1971; Mouret 1975; Wein et al. 1979). Spindle activity has been reported to be decreased in several studies (Emser et al. 1988; Ferrari et al. 1964; Myslobodsky et al. 1982; Puca et al. 1973). Slow-wave sleep is typically decreased (Bergonzi et al. 1974; Emser et al. 1988; Friedman 1980; Kales et al. 1971; Wein et al. 1979), although some investigators have found no difference from control subjects or normative data (Apps et al. 1985; Bergonzi et al. 1975; Mouret 1975).

As is the case with SDAT and other dementias, data regarding REM variables are somewhat less clear. Most investigators report a significant decrease in total REM time or REM percentage (Apps et al. 1985; Bergonzi et al. 1975; Emser et al. 1988; Friedman 1980; Mouret 1975), but others have found no difference (Kales et al. 1971; Wein et al. 1979). Subjects in these latter two studies were not clearly drug free. REM latency, where reported, does not seem to differ significantly from control subjects (Apps et al. 1985; Kales et al. 1971; Wein et al. 1979). The same caveat regarding possible medication effects applies here.

Attempts at correlation of PSG variables with severity or diagnostic subgroups have been very limited. Friedman (1980) found a significant negative correlation between severity and average duration of REM periods and total REM time, as well as a positive correlation of severity with number of awakenings. Mouret (1975) identified two subgroups of patients with Parkinson's disease. The first, those with repetitive blinking before sleep onset, showed no significant differences from "controls" (drawn from other literature) on PSG variables, whereas the second group, those with a lack of atonia in REM, showed decreased REM duration and increased stages 1 and 2.

The etiology of the sleep disturbance seen in parkinsonian patients is quite unclear. Many investigators who have examined sleep in these patients have done so in the hope that, by studying individuals with functional dopaminergic and, to a lesser extent, other bioaminergic deficiencies, one might gain further information regarding basic aspects of sleep physiology. Unfortunately, these investigators have, for the most part, failed to consider that sleep disturbance in these patients may be as much a function of associated abnormalities (e.g., pain, movement disturbance, depression, respiratory disturbance) as they are reflective of the primary neurochemical-neurophysiologic disturbance.

Of what importance is this to DSM-IV? Although etiologic considerations are not, in their own right, of concern in a phenomenologically based system, the argument for parceling out a specific neurological disorder is, perhaps, strengthened by the demonstration that a primary component of the pathophysiology of the disorder is responsible for the sleep disturbance. Such a relationship has not been clearly demonstrated for parkinsonism.

For example, Goetz and colleagues (1987) reported on the relationship among pain, depression, and sleep alteration in 95 patients with idiopathic Parkinson's disease. They found that 43%–46% of these patients described pain that was believed to be related to their Parkinson's. Depression was significantly increased among the pain population. Sleep disturbance was positively correlated with both depression and pain in these patients. Greenberg and Pearlman (1970) reported that total REM time was inversely proportional to degree of depression in subjects, although objective criteria for depression were not utilized.

Few attempts have been made to analyze data according to type of parkinsonism. Efthimiou and colleagues (1987) found decreased total sleep time in postencephalitic patients compared with untreated idiopathic patients, but the parkinsonism was more severe in the former group.

Studies of treatment effects were reviewed. Comparisons are difficult because of varying drug regimens, dosages, and treatment duration before follow-up PSG. On the whole, these investigations do not contribute information that is very useful to diagnostic considerations.

Comparisons of parkinsonian groups with other disorders on sleep-related variables are rare. In fact, the only relevant study identified was that of Emser and colleagues (1988), who compared sleep changes in patients with Parkinson's disease and Huntington's disease with control subjects. Sleep changes in Parkinson's patients were much the same as described above, whereas Huntington's patients did not differ significantly from control subjects except for an increase in spindle activity.

Other Cerebral Degenerative Disorders

"Other cerebral degenerative disorders" includes a vast array of rather diverse disorders. Many disorders that might be included have not been investigated with respect to sleep-related findings and are, therefore, not included in this discussion. Those studies that have yielded PSG or other data that are pertinent to sleep have typically included small numbers of patients, and therefore the information presented should be considered preliminary in nature. Because many of these diagnoses involve movement disorders, many of the investigations have focused on analysis of movement in sleep.

Four studies of sleep in Huntington's disease are pertinent. Although there is consensus regarding the presence of sleep disturbance, at least in advanced stages of the illness, agreement seems limited to this. Hansotia and colleagues (1985) reported no clinical abnormalities in two patients with mild disease, although wake after sleep onset and REM latency were increased. Five moderately severe patients showed clinical insomnia; increased sleep latency, wake after sleep onset, and REM latency; and decreased sleep efficiency and total sleep time. Trends toward increased stage 1 and decreased stage 3/4 and REM were noted. Spindles and K-complexes were described as "normal" but not subjected to statistical analysis of frequency or amplitude. Emser and colleagues (1988) reported no differences in sleep-stage distribution between 10 Huntington's patients (severity unspecified) and control subjects, but did find a significant increase in spindle activity. Sishta and colleagues (1974) had previously reported an absence of sleep spindles or K-complexes in Huntington's patients during barbiturate-induced sleep.

Olivopontocerebellar degeneration has been studied to a limited extent with regard to PSG data, sleep-disordered breathing, and movement in sleep. Neil and colleagues (1980), reporting on PSG analysis of two patients, noted decreased REM and slow-wave sleep, with phasic components of REM being reduced out of proportion to tonic components. Mild-to-moderate sleep continuity disturbance was also described. REM latency was normal. Salva and Guilleminault (1986) reported two cases of olivopontocerebellar degeneration exhibiting REM sleep without atonia. They also found a tendency toward increased stage 1 and, possibly, decreased REM latency, at least in advanced stages of the disease. Several investigators have described the occurrence of sleep-disordered breathing in olivopontocerebellar degeneration (Chokroverty et al. 1984; Salazar-Grueso et al. 1988).

Reports of sleep in various dystonic conditions have focused primarily on movement abnormalities. In a series of investigations of patients with hereditary progressive dystonia with marked diurnal fluctuation, Segawa and colleagues (1976, 1983, 1988) found that tonic components of sleep were relatively normal, whereas phasic components (body movements and REMs) were not. Patients demonstrated a pattern of diminished movement in undisturbed sleep. Jankel and colleagues (1983) described poor sleep efficiency, increased sleep latency and number of awakenings, and a significant increase in high-voltage spindle activity in four patients with dystonia musculorum deformans. Wein and Golubev (1979) reported similar findings in patients with advanced torsion dystonia.

Fatal Familial Insomnia

E. Lugaresi and colleagues (1986), Medori and colleagues (1985), and A. Lugaresi and colleagues (1987) described a syndrome of progressive insomnia and dysautonomia resulting from degeneration of anterior and dorsomedial thalamic nuclei. Extensive physiologic data were obtained on only one patient, although the disorder had apparently affected 13 of his relatives. An autosomal dominant mode of transmission is posited. The course is rapidly downhill, progressing to stupor, coma, and death. In later stages of the disease, physiologic recordings showed no tracings that could be clearly identified as sleep, although apparent abortive attempts at REM (decreased electromyogram tone, REMs, desynchronized electroencephalographic, and dreamlike episodes) were noted. Circadian rhythm of temperature and endocrine function were absent. Pronounced dysregulation of the autonomic nervous system was also described.

The authors suggested that the disorder can be distinguished from other thalamic degenerative disorders by the specificity and localization of degeneration, the rapidity of course, the pronounced abnormality of sleep (not described in other syndromes), and the intactness of cognitive function.

Discussion

The disorders reviewed in this section represent only a small subset of neurological disorders. They are, however, among those that have been most thoroughly investigated. The findings presented do provide ample documentation that these neurological disorders are associated with various disturbances of sleep at a higher than expected frequency and that, in many cases, it is possible to distinguish afflicted patients from age-matched control subjects on the basis of objective criteria, largely PSG in nature. However, the nature of these findings is such that they do not provide a solid basis for the contention that the observed abnormalities are *specific* to the disorder—nor do they clearly support the notion that the sleep disturbances are *direct* products of the underlying neuropathophysiology of these disorders, in many cases.

To a great extent, the findings related to tonic aspects of sleep are those observed in a multitude of disorders—diminished total sleep, sleep continuity disturbances, and relative declines in slow-wave sleep and REM. The vast majority of the literature surveyed addresses the distinction between a given neurological disorder and control subjects. There is virtually no literature that addresses the issue of distinguishing among different neurological disorders on the basis of sleep-related variables. Thus any diagnostic classification system that attempts to establish sleep-related criteria specific to a particular neurological disorder must, in fact, rely heavily on nonsleep-related (i.e., clinical-neurological) criteria in its approach. Such is the case with the ICSD system. The end product of this approach is that the sleep-related "criteria" are not so much specific diagnostic markers as they are descriptions of the variety of sleep disturbances that may be observed in association with the neurological condition.

The "Cognitive Impairment Disorders" section of DSM-IV faces a somewhat similar dilemma in that it attempts to classify a general condition (i.e., cognitive impairment) that may be attributable to a variety of different medical or neurological conditions. The approach taken is to classify these disorders as "due to a General Medical Condition" with reference to an accompanying Axis III diagnosis. This is the most appropriate solution to the DSM classification of sleep disorders associated with neurological disorders. There is not sufficient justification for inclusion of specific neurological disorders on Axis I, and to do so would be incompatible with the approach taken in other sections.

The DSM-III-R system would parcel the sleep disorders associated with neurological conditions into various sections—specifically, insomnia or hypersomnia related to a known organic factor, or parasomnia not otherwise specified. This raises the difficult issue of whether the neurological (and medical) disorders should be classified according to phenomenology of sleep disorder (as in DSM-III-R or the "old" Association of Sleep Disorders Centers [1979] system) or according to etiologic considerations (which ICSD leans to, for the most part). To the extent that one wishes to adhere to the ICSD system as a "template" for DSM-IV, the choice would be to include, at minimum, a category of "Sleep Disorders due to a General Medical Condition." In doing so, however, one must be conscious of the fact that this potentially combines "dyssomnias" and "parasomnias" into a single category—a decision that, in some respects, violates the distinction that is drawn between these two broad categories elsewhere in ICSD. A compromise solution to this difficulty is suggested below.

A final conundrum arises with respect to how one classifies certain sleep disorders associated with neurological disease that appear as primary diagnoses elsewhere in ICSD. For example, sleep apnea has been reported in association with degenerative neurological disorders. Some studies indicate that they are seen at a higher-than-expected frequency, suggesting that the pathophysiology of the neurological illness is, at least in part, directly responsible for the occurrence of apnea. From the information available, it is not clear whether ICSD would classify this sleep apnea under "neurological conditions" or under "obstructive (or central) sleep apnea syndrome." This point requires further clarification.

Recommendations

The three major alternatives for classification of these disorders under DSM-IV are 1) retaining a division of dyssomnias and parasomnias by utilizing two categories—

"Dyssomnias associated with neurological disorders" and "Parasomnias associated with neurological disorders"; 2) maintaining the ICSD approach of lumping all medical or neurological-related sleep disorders—"Sleep Disorders due to a General Medical Condition"; or 3) returning the specific sleep disorder to a phenomenologic "home base," with designation as a "secondary" disorder—for example, "Secondary dyssomnia (insomnia)" or "Dyssomnia (insomnia) associated with known organic condition," with specification of the neurological disorder on Axis III. The results of this review suggest that much of the sleep pathology associated with neurological disorders is nonspecific and does not warrant separate coding for each neurological disorder on Axis I. It is recommended that the disorders be classified under the general heading of "Secondary Sleep Disorders due to a General Medical Condition" and that the symptom presentation (insomnia, hypersomnia, or unspecified) be identified. This approach, in effect, combines the most useful aspects of the options outlined above. As discussed in the review of medical disorders, this is most compatible with the former DSM system and the new ICSD system, while not overstepping the boundaries of current knowledge and information.

References

Allen SR, Stahelin MB, Seiler WO, et al: EEG and sleep in aged hospitalized patients with senile dementia: 24 hour recordings. Experientia 39:249–255, 1983

Allen SR, Seiler WO, Stahelin HB, et al: Seventy-two hour polygraphic and behavioral recordings of wakefulness and sleep in a hospital geriatric unit: comparison between demented and nondemented patients. Sleep 10:143–159, 1987

American Psychiatric Association: Diagnostic and Statistical Manual of Mental Disorders, 3rd Edition, Revised. Washington, DC, American Psychiatric Association, 1987

American Sleep Disorders Association, Diagnostic Classification Steering Committee: International Classification of Sleep Disorders Association: Diagnostic and Coding Manual. Rochester, MN, American Sleep Disorders Association, 1990

Apps MC, Sheaff PC, Ingram DA, et al: Respiration and sleep in Parkinson's disease. J Neurol Neurosurg Psychiatry 48:1240–1245, 1985

Association of Sleep Disorders Centers: Diagnostic classification of sleep and arousal disorders. Sleep 2:1–137, 1979

Bergonzi P, Chiurulla C, Cianchetti C, et al: Clinical pharmacology as an approach to the study of biochemical sleep mechanisms: the action of L-dopa. Confinia Neurologica 36:5–22, 1974

Bergonzi P, Chiurulla C, Gambi D, et al: L-dopa plus dopa decarboxylase inhibitor: sleep organization in Parkinson's syndrome before and after treatment. Acta Neurol Belg 75:5–10, 1975

Bliwise D, Tinklenberg J, Davies H, et al: Sleep patterns in Alzheimer's disease. Sleep Research 15:49, 1986

Bliwise DL, Pursley AM, Dement WC: Day/night relationships of observed sleep/wakefulness (S/W) in aged nursing home patients. Sleep Research 17:72, 1988

Bliwise DL, Tinklenberg J, Yesavage JA, et al: REM latency in Alzheimer's disease. Biol Psychiatry 25:320–328, 1989

Chokroverty S, Sachdeo R, Masdeu J: Autonomic dysfunction and sleep apnea in olivopontocerebellar degeneration. Arch Neurol 41:926–931, 1984

Efthimiou J, Ellis SJ, Hardie RJ, et al: Sleep apnea in idiopathic and postencephalitic parkinsonism. Adv Neurol 45:275–276, 1987

Emser W, Brenner M, Stober T, et al: Changes in sleep in Huntington's and Parkinson's disease. J Neurol 235:177–179, 1988

Erkinjuntti T, Partinen M, Sulkava R, et al: Sleep apnea in multi-infarct dementia and Alzheimer's disease. Sleep 10:419–425, 1987

Evans LK: Sundown Syndrome in institutionalized elderly. J Am Geriatr Soc 35:101–108, 1987

Feinberg I, Koresko RL, Heller N: EEG sleep patterns as a function of normal and pathological aging in man. J Psychiatr Res 5:107–144, 1967

Ferrari E, Puca FM, Margherita G: Le anomalie dei fusi da sonno nei parkinsoniani. Riv Neurol 34:48–55, 1964

Folstein MF, Folstein SE, McHugh PR: Mini-Mental State: a practical method for grading the cognitive state of patients for the clinician. J Psychiatr Res 12:189–198, 1975

Friedman A: Sleep pattern in Parkinson's disease. Acta Med Pol 21:193–199, 1980

Goetz CG, Wilson RS, Tanner CM, et al: Relationships among pain, depression, and sleep alterations in Parkinson's disease. Adv Neurol 45:345–347, 1987

Greenberg R, Pearlman CA: L-dopa, parkinsonism, and sleep. Psychophysiology 7:314, 1970

Hansotia P, Wall R, Berendes J: Sleep disturbances and severity of Huntington's disease. Neurology 35:1672–1674, 1985

Hoch CC, Reynolds CF, Kupfer DJ, et al: Sleep-disordered breathing in normal and pathological aging. J Clin Psychiatry 47:499–503, 1986

Hoch CC, Reynolds CF, Nebes RD, et al: Clinical significance of sleep-disordered breathing in Alzheimer's disease. J Am Geriatr Soc 37:138–144, 1989

Hughes CP, Berg L, Cohen LA, et al: A new clinical scale for the staging of dementia. Br J Psychiatry 140:566–572, 1982

Jankel WR, Allen RP, Niedermeyer E, et al: Polysomnographic findings in dystonia musculorum deformans. Sleep 6:281–285, 1983

Kales A, Ansel RD, Markham CH, et al: Sleep in patients with Parkinson's disease and normal subjects prior to and following levodopa administration. Clin Pharmacol Ther 12:397–406, 1971

Loewenstein RJ, Weingartner H, Gillin JC, et al: Disturbances of sleep and cognitive functioning in patients with dementia. Neurobiol Aging 3:371–377, 1982

Lugaresi E, Medori R, Montagna P, et al: Fatal familial insomnia and dysautonomia with selective degeneration of thalamic nuclei. N Engl J Med 315:997–1003, 1986

Lugaresi A, Baruzzi A, Cacciari E, et al: Lack of vegetative and endocrine circadian rhythms in fatal familial thalamic degeneration. Clin Endocrinol (Oxf) 26:573–580, 1987

Mant A, Saunders NA, Eyland AE, et al: Sleep-related respiratory disturbance and dementia in elderly females. J Gerontol 43:M140–144, 1988

Martin PR, Loewenstein RJ, Kaye WH, et al: Sleep EEG in Korsakoff's psychosis and Alzheimer's disease. Neurology 36:411–414, 1986

Medori R, Gambetti P, Montagna P, et al: Familial progressive insomnia, impairment of the autonomic functions, degeneration of thalamic nuclei: a new disease? Neurology 35 (suppl 1):145, 1985

Molsa PK, Paljarvi L, Rinne JO, et al: Validity of clinical diagnosis in dementia: a prospective clinicopathological study. J Neurol Neurosurg Psychiatry 48:1085–1090, 1985

Mouret J: Differences in sleep in patients with Parkinson's disease. Electroencephalogr Clin Neurophysiol 38:653–657, 1975

Myslobodsky M, Mintz M, Ben-Mayor V, et al: Unilateral dopamine deficit and lateral EEG asymmetry: sleep abnormalities in hemi-Parkinson's patients. Electroencephalogr Clin Neurophysiol 54:227–231, 1982

Neil JF, Holzer BC, Spiker DG, et al: EEG sleep alterations in olivopontocerebellar degeneration. Neurology 30:660–662, 1980

Prinz PN, Peskind ER, Raskind M, et al: Changes in the sleep and waking EEGs of nondemented and demented elderly subjects. J Am Geriatr Soc 30:86–93, 1982a

Prinz PN, Vitaliano PP, Vitiello MV, et al: Sleep, EEG and mental function changes in senile dementia of the Alzheimer's type. Neurobiol Aging 3:361–370, 1982b

Prinz PN, Christie C, Smallwood R, et al: Circadian temperature variation in healthy aged and in Alzheimer's disease. J Gerontol 39:30–35, 1984

Puca FM, Bricolo A, Turella G: Effect of L-dopa or amantadine therapy on sleep spindles in parkinsonism. Electroencephalogr Clin Neurophysiol 35:327–330, 1973

Reynolds CF, Spiker DG, Hanin I, et al: Electroencephalographic sleep, aging, and psychopathology: new data and state of the art. Biol Psychiatry 18:139–155, 1983

Reynolds CF, Kupfer DJ, Taska LS, et al: EEG sleep in elderly depressed, demented, and healthy subjects. Biol Psychiatry 20:431–442, 1985a

Reynolds CF, Kupfer DJ, Taska LS, et al: Sleep apnea in Alzheimer's dementia: correlation with mental deterioration. J Clin Psychiatry 46:257–261, 1985b

Reynolds CF, Kupfer DJ, Houck PR, et al: Reliable discrimination of elderly depressed and demented patients by electroencephalographic sleep data. Arch Gen Psychiatry 45:258–264, 1988

Salazar-Grueso EF, Rosenberg RS, Roos RP: Sleep apnea in olivopontocerebellar degeneration: treatment with trazodone. Ann Neurol 23:399–401, 1988

Salva MA, Guilleminault C: Olivopontocerebellar degeneration, abnormal sleep, and REM sleep without atonia. Neurology 36:576–577, 1986

Segawa M, Hosaka A, Miyagawa F, et al: Hereditary progressive dystonia with marked diurnal fluctuation. Adv Neurol 14:215–233, 1976

Segawa M, Igawa C, Ogiso M, et al: Polysomnographic examination of dystonia syndrome. Electroencephalogr Clin Neurophysiol 56:57–58P, 1983

Segawa M, Nomura Y, Tanaka S, et al: Hereditary progressive dystonia with marked diurnal fluctuation: consideration of its pathophysiology based on the characteristics of clinical and polysomnographical findings. Adv Neurol 50:367–376, 1988

Sishta SK, Troupe A, Marszalek KS, et al: Huntington's chorea: an electroencephalographic and psychometric study. Electroencephalogr Clin Neurophysiol 36:387–393, 1974

Smallwood RG, Vitiello MV, Giblin EC, et al: Sleep apnea: relationship to age, sex, and Alzheimer's dementia. Sleep 6:16–22, 1983

Vitiello MV, Bokan JA, Kukull WA, et al: Rapid eye movement sleep measures of Alzheimer's-type dementia patients and optimally healthy aged individuals. Biol Psychiatry 19:721–734, 1984

Wechsler D: Wechsler Adult Intelligence Scale—Revised. San Antonio, TX, Psychological Corporation, 1981

Wein A, Golubev V: Polygraphic analysis of sleep in dystonia musculorum deformans. Waking and Sleeping 3:41–50, 1979

Wein A, Golubev V, Yakhno N: Polygraphic analysis of sleep and wakefulness in patients with Parkinson's syndrome. Waking and Sleeping 3:31–40, 1979

Chapter 44

Sleep Disorders Associated With a General Medical Condition

Michael J. Sateia, M.D.

Statement of the Issues

The International Classification of Sleep Disorders (ICSD) (American Sleep Disorders Association 1990) has chosen to include a number of specific medical disorders in the category of sleep disorders associated with a general medical condition, although those chosen for inclusion clearly do not constitute an exhaustive listing. These disorders were presumably chosen on the basis of 1) the degree to which sleep physiology influences the medical condition, 2) the degree to which nocturnal manifestations of the medical condition may influence sleep physiology, and (perhaps) 3) the volume of available literature pertaining to the associations noted. The medical disorders included are quite disparate, both with respect to the types of disorder as well as to their possible effects on sleep or their manifestations during sleep—that is to say, they have little in common except that they are all presumably medical disorders (see fibromyalgia later) that may be manifest in sleep or are exacerbated by sleep physiology.

Hence, interdiagnostic comparisons have little relevance in this category. Moreover, the types of sleep disorders associated with these conditions are multiple, even within a single medical condition. For example, the 1979 Association of Sleep Disorders Centers (ASDC) nosology would classify gastroesophageal reflux as a parasomnia. Yet the current ICSD description also makes note of insomnia as a complication of gastroesophageal reflux. Likewise, the focus of a complaint pertaining to nocturnal asthma may be on the asthmatic episode itself (parasomnia) or on the sleep disturbance engendered by the respiratory condition (dyssomnia–insomnia). Depending on the nature of the primary complaint, DSM-III-R (American Psychiatric Association 1987) would classify these conditions under "insomnia [or, in some cases, hypersomnia] related to a known organic condition," or under "parasomnia not otherwise specified." Although there are certain advantages in emphasizing the medical aspects of these conditions in a nosology constructed for multidisciplinary use (ICSD), these advantages are not as clear in a system designed primarily for use by psychiatrists. Thus the primary issue is whether to retain a separate category for "medical disorders" (as in ICSD) or to employ a symptom-oriented approach (e.g., dyssomnia [insomnia] related to *X* medical condition). If the former approach is elected, should individual medical diagnoses be specified and criteria generated for each?

Significance of the Issues

Although a desire for internosologic consistency underscores the advisability of maintaining the ICSD designation of "Sleep Disorders Associated With Medical Conditions," this inclination must be tempered by the necessity of establishing a sound scientific basis for deviation from the DSM-III-R classification system. In light of this, the literature pertaining to these diagnoses must be reviewed with the following questions in mind. To what extent is there a consistent set of sleep-related findings that occurs with sufficient predictability as to be considered an inherent component of the clinical profile? Are these findings of diagnostic utility with respect to differential diagnosis with other medical, psychiatric, or sleep disorders? To what extent do unique aspects of sleep physiology contribute to the genesis, maintenance, or exacerbation of these conditions? What is the relevance of these findings to clinical psychiatry? To the extent that there are well-documented, consistent, and specific sleep-related findings associated with these medical conditions *that are relevant to clinical psychiatry*, they should be classified under the general heading of "medical disorders" with specification of individual diagnoses within this group, as warranted by above criteria. Otherwise, they should be classified as "Secondary Sleep Disorders" with specification of the medical condition on Axis III.

Methods

References in the ICSD bibliography were reviewed for all major headings. The references of these articles were reviewed for additional material, according to guidelines described in each subsection below. Medline search (BRS Colleague) was conducted for each topic. Specific search headings are provided below. The general frame of search was from 1965 to 1990, English language, and human subjects only.

Results of each search are indicated below. Articles were reviewed by title and abstract (where available). Criteria of selection for further review are included in the following subsections.

Fibromyalgia

A Medline search was conducted for the following (with their number of references): Fibromyalgia, 222; Fibrositis syndrome, 51; and Rheumatic pain modulation disorder, 6. Searches excluded previous search terms (e.g., fibrositis not fibromyalgia). The search results were then reviewed by title and abstract with the following criteria for inclusion: 1) analysis of psychological factors or sleep physiology, 2) original data, and 3) inclusion of controls. Selected review articles were also included, primarily for consultation of references pertaining to the stated issues. This process yielded 43 primary references, which form the basis of this review.

Chronic Obstructive Pulmonary Disease (COPD)

Medline search was conducted for the following (with their number of references): Chronic obstructive pulmonary disease with sleep, 51 titles; and Chronic obstructive lung disease with sleep, 17. Search results were reviewed by title and abstract with the following criteria for inclusion: 1) changes in ventilation or arterial blood gases (with clinical application) associated with sleep or specific sleep stages, 2) control of breathing in sleep (with clinical application), 3) arrhythmia in sleep with COPD, 4) distinction among different types of sleep-disordered breathing, 5) quality of sleep in COPD, and 6) effects of sleep loss or deprivation on ventilation in COPD. Selected reviews were also consulted. This process yielded 31 articles which formed the basis of the review. Articles addressing basic pulmonary physiology and treatment effects were not reviewed except as they provided data pertinent to the inclusion criteria described above.

Asthma

Medline search was conducted for Asthma with sleep. This search yielded 48 titles or abstracts that were then reviewed with the following criteria for inclusion: 1) breathing patterns during sleep in asthmatic patients, 2) association of asthmatic episodes with specific sleep stages, 3) effects of sleep physiology on nocturnal asthma, 4) the role of sleep versus other aspects of circadian rhythm or sleep deprivation studies, 5) psychological factors in sleep affecting nocturnal asthma, and 6) sleep patterns in asthmatic patients. Reviews, case reports, and studies of treatment effect or associated conditions were included only to the extent to which they provided data relevant to inclusion criteria. This process yielded 20 articles for further review.

Nocturnal Cardiac Ischemia

Medline search was conducted for Angina with sleep, Cardiac ischemia with sleep, Myocardial infarct with sleep, and Coronary with sleep. This search yielded 53 references that were then reviewed by title or abstract with the following criteria for inclusion: 1) sleep patterns in angina, 2) association of angina with sleep stages, and 3) association of other sleep disorders with nocturnal angina. Hemodynamic, biochemical, and treatment effect studies were reviewed only if they contributed data relevant to inclusion criteria noted above. This process yielded seven articles for further review.

Gastroesophageal Reflux

Medline search was conducted for Gastroesophageal reflux with sleep and Reflux with sleep, yielding 17 articles. These articles were concerned primarily with reflux in infancy, acid clearance during sleep, and esophageal pressures in sleep. None of these articles were pertinent to nosologic issues, and the review was limited to the ICSD bibliography.

Results

Fibromyalgia

Fibromyalgia (fibrositis syndrome) is a common disorder, accounting for a significant percentage of outpatient visits for rheumatic-related disease. Although it has been extensively researched in recent years, no well-defined organic substrates of the disorder have been identified. This fact, coupled with clinical observations and research on the psychological profiles of this population, has led some to speculate that primary fibromyalgia syndrome (PFS) may be a direct expression of psychological disturbance or, at least, that psychological factors are causally related to the disorder. It is this issue that is of greatest relevance to DSM-IV and that is reviewed herein. Additionally, investigations of sleep physiology in PFS are briefly discussed. Is there sufficient support for a cause-and-effect relationship between psychological disturbance psychiatric disorder and PFS to warrant inclusion of the syndrome as a distinct diagnostic entity in DSM-IV? If not, how should the disorder be classified?

The terms *fibromyalgia* and *fibrositis syndrome* should generally be considered synonymous. The term "fibrositis" is used here when the investigators in question have chosen to use this term. Elsewhere, the preferred term "fibromyalgia" is used.

Psychological assessment. Evaluation of psychological factors in fibromyalgia patients have addressed two major questions: 1) Is there an increased incidence of psychological disturbance among these patients? and 2) Is there evidence for a specific relationship between fibromyalgia and affective disorder? Most studies have employed rheumatoid arthritis patients as a control population and utilize specific diagnostic criteria for selection of fibromyalgia patients.

Payne and colleagues (1982) reported Minnesota Multiphasic Personality Inventory (MMPI) (Hathaway and McKinley 1970) data on 32 fibrositis patients. They found significant elevations on six scales (hysteria, hypochondriasis, psychopathic deviate, paranoia, schizophrenia, and hypomania) compared with rheumatoid arthritis control subjects and patients with other forms of arthritis. They noted greater variability on the MMPIs of fibrositis patients. The investigators concluded that fibrositis patients were more psychologically disturbed and that the disturbance may take a variety of different forms. Similar results were obtained by Wolfe and colleagues (1984), who found a significant increase in the percentage of "psychological disturbance" by MMPI in primary fibrositis patients, when compared with rheumatoid arthritis control subjects. Ahles and colleagues (1984) reported that 31% of PFS patients had MMPI profiles indicative of "psychological disturbance." However, in a reanalysis of their data using more contemporary MMPI norms, this number was reduced to 17.8% (Ahles et al. 1986). Although this percentage still represented a significantly higher incidence of psychological disturbance in PFS patients when compared with rheumatoid arthritis patients or control subjects, it is suggested that contemporary norms may provide a more accurate representation of the degree of psychopathology. More recent data (Ahles et al. 1991) confirm the lower incidence of psychologically disturbed MMPI profiles in PFS patients, using contemporary norms (17.1% by original norms versus 8.5% by contemporary norms). The latter percentage is not significantly different from the percentage of rheumatoid arthritis patients with psychological disturbance.

A more relevant issue in addressing the relationship between PFS and psychopathology may be analysis of the occurrence of psychiatric diagnoses in this population. Hudson and colleagues (1985), employing the National Institute of Mental Health Diagnostic Interview Schedule (Robins et al. 1981) and Hamilton Rating Scale for Depression (Hamilton 1960), reported a lifetime prevalence of major depressive disorder of 71% among PFS patients, with 26% meeting criteria for a current episode. The onset of mood disorder preceded symptoms of PFS in approximately two-thirds of patients. Tariot and colleagues (1986) contributed a brief report on seven PFS patients, six of whom met DSM-III (American Psychiatric Association 1980) criteria for major depression. Both of these studies described an increased incidence of major affective disorder, dysthymia, or substance abuse in the families of patients.

Findings such as this have fueled speculation that PFS may represent an expression or variant of depressive illness. However, subsequent reports have failed to confirm the finding of an increased incidence of depression or, for that matter, any other psychiatric diagnosis in these patients. Kirmayer and colleagues (1988) found no significant difference between PFS and rheumatoid arthritis patients with respect to lifetime prevalence of depressive disorder or likelihood to report depressive symptoms. Ahles and colleagues (1987) found no difference between PFS and rheumatoid arthritis patients on the Zung Depression Scale (Zung 1965), although they did note that a subgroup (about 30%) of each of the two populations had significant depressive symptomatology. Clark and colleagues (1985) found no differences between fibromyalgia patients and control subjects drawn from a general medical population on Beck Depression Inventory (Beck et al. 1961), State-Trait Anxiety Scale (Spielberger 1975), or Hopkins Symptom Checklist—90 (Derogatis 1983) scores. Efforts to identify biological markers indicative of affective disorder in this group have been unsuccessful. Only 1 of 23 fibrositis patients showed nonsuppression on dexamethasone suppression test, although 6 of the 23 met criteria for major depression by the Diagnostic Interview Schedule (Hudson et al. 1984). Gupta and Moldofsky (1986) compared sleep physiology and symptoms in small samples of dysthymic and fibrositis patients. Based on these measures, they concluded that the two disorders were not related.

Sleep physiology. In a series of investigations, Moldofsky and colleagues have studied sleep physiology in fibrositis (synonymously labeled "Rheumatic Pain Modulation Disorder"). They demonstrated an overnight increase in muscle tenderness and aching associated with a non–rapid eye movement (NREM) electroencephalographic disturbance, characterized particularly by intrusion of alpha activity (Moldofsky et al. 1975). Experimental induction of a similar syndrome of musculoskeletal pain and tenderness was achieved by stage 4 sleep deprivation (Moldofsky and Scarisbrick 1976). These investigators concluded that internal arousal mechanisms, possibly related to emotional distress, give rise to disturbance in sleep physiology, thereby disrupting restorative functions of deep sleep. This line of reasoning has been extended to include other potential sources of increased arousal in sleep that may give rise to a fibrositis-like syndrome of NREM sleep disturbance and musculoskeletal and psychological symptoms. Specifically, this constellation has been reported in association with periodic leg movement in sleep (Moldofsky et al. 1984), sleep apnea syndrome (Molony et al. 1986), rheumatoid arthritis (Moldofsky et al. 1983), and postaccident pain (Saskin et al. 1986). These studies are, in general, somewhat compromised by lack of control subjects and relatively small sample sizes, but offer at least preliminary evidence of a causal relationship between arousal-alpha NREM anomaly and fibromyalgia.

Discussion of fibromyalgia. The existing data regarding psychological factors and fibromyalgia do not allow firm conclusions to be drawn. The MMPI results suggest an increased incidence of psychological disturbance, but are subject to questions of validity in light of more recent information regarding reanalysis utilizing contemporary norms. In addition, questions have been raised regarding the validity of the MMPI in assessing psychological disturbance in pain-related conditions (Smythe 1984), although an analysis by Leavitt and Katz (1989) suggested that physical illness and pain do not account for the increased incidence of psychological disturbance in fibromyalgia.

Even if one does accept that these patients have a greater degree of psychological disturbance, the psychometric results certainly do not elaborate the exact nature of cause-and-effect relationships nor do they provide much information regarding the specific nature of any psychological disturbance. Rather, they suggest a high degree of variability in this area. Investigations that have attempted to establish criteria-based psychiatric diagnoses in fibromyalgia patients have, for the most part, failed to identify formal disorders. The impression derived from several studies is that these patients may have a greater likelihood to report somatic symptoms that are atypical or without medical explanation, although sufficient evidence of somatization disorder is lacking.

Thus fibromyalgia represents a complicated syndrome of uncertain etiology. Psychological factors may play a significant etiologic role, possibly via disturbance in sleep physiology, but this remains uncertain. Although the disorder is of considerable heuristic interest among sleep disorders specialists and, perhaps, rheumatologists, it has little direct relevance to psychiatry, and establishment of a causal linkage to psychopathology is tenuous.

COPD

Most sleep studies of COPD have focused on blood gas alterations and related findings. Although there are highly significant findings in these areas, the issues are of relatively little importance for most clinical psychiatrists. A limited number of studies have been conducted on sleep disturbance in COPD patients.

Sleep studies of COPD patients have revealed that many of these patients experience marked deterioration of respiratory status in sleep, especially during rapid eye movement (REM) sleep (Catterall et al. 1983; Coccagna and Lugaresi 1978; DeMarco et al. 1981; Hudgel et al. 1983; Littner et al. 1980; Manni et al. 1988). These investigations have suggested that oxyhemoglobin desaturations during sleep are not primarily a function of upper airway obstructive apneas (although acute declines in SaO_2 related to such apneas may coexist in these patients and are typically associated with increased negative intrathoracic pressure). Hypoxic episodes related to COPD itself are more sustained and are associated with decreased respiratory effort (Arand et al. 1981). There is reasonably strong evidence to suggest that individuals with lower waking baseline pO_2 and greater CO_2 retention ("blue bloaters") are significantly more predisposed to major oxygen desaturation than those with more normal waking blood gases ("pink puffers") (Catterall et al. 1983; DeMarco et al. 1981; Perez-Padilla et al. 1987).

Clinical experience suggests that sleep disturbance is common among patients with COPD. Subjective reports of poor sleep (derived from sleep questionnaire) were documented by Cormick and colleagues (1986), who described a significant increase in difficulty falling asleep and maintaining sleep, as well as an increase in daytime sleepiness, in 50 COPD patients compared with age-matched control subjects. These investigators studied 16 patients overnight and reported that degree of arousal in sleep was inversely correlated with SaO_2 level. A similar relationship between arousal and frequency of desaturation was previously described by Fleetham and colleagues (1982). Manni and colleagues (1988) reported increased sleep latency, stage 1, and arousal, and decreased total sleep time and sleep efficiency in 11 COPD patients, but found that sleep parameters were worse in those patients with milder ventilatory impairment. Thus, although it seems clear that COPD patients are comparatively poor sleepers, the exact nature of the cause-and-effect relationship between hypoxia and arousal remains uncertain. Cormick and colleagues suggested that degree of sleep disturbance may conform to a bell-shaped distribution when plotted against severity of COPD—that is, sleep in late-stage COPD patients may improve. This theory, however, has not been tested.

No objective measures of daytime sleepiness in COPD were identified.

Asthma

Studies of the relationship between sleep and asthma have focused on four basic questions. Does sleep physiology per se influence the nocturnal course of asthma and, if so, what specific physiological factors are at play? What is the distribution of asthmatic episodes across the night and how might this relate to issues of sleep physiology addressed in the first question? How is sleep affected by asthma? Do sleep-specific psychological factors play a role in the genesis of nocturnal asthma?

Early studies noted the temporal association between the nocturnal nadir of corticosteroid levels and diminished peak expiratory flow rates (PEFR), leading some investigators to suspect that nocturnal asthma may arise as a result of diminished endogenous steroid activity (Reinberg et al. 1963; Soutar et al. 1975). However, Soutar and colleagues also reported that cortisol infusion was not successful in preventing the decline in PEFR in five of six subjects, casting doubt on a direct causal relationship. Efforts to determine if sleep physiology per se (as opposed to other physiological aspects of circadian rhythm) are contributory to nocturnal asthma have produced mixed results. Catterall and colleagues (1986) measured morning PEFR in 12 asthmatic patients—once after a normal night of sleep and again after a night of sleep deprivation. They found that PEFR morning values were significantly higher after the sleep deprivation night compared with those after a night of sleep. The conclusion was that sleep itself is an important factor in determining overnight bronchoconstriction. In a somewhat similar design, Hetzel and Clark (1979) found that keeping patients awake until 3:00 A.M. did not prevent a decline in PEFR in 6 of 11, leading them to conclude that other aspects of circadian rhythm, and not sleep per se, were responsible for nocturnal bronchoconstriction.

Analysis of sleep-stage distribution of asthmatic episodes is likewise inconclusive. Isaa and Sullivan (1985) recorded six attacks from four patients—one in stage 1/2, three in stage 3/4, and two in REM. Kales and colleagues (1968, 1970) found that the frequency of episodes was decreased in the first one-third of the night, but reported no clear-cut relationship to any specific sleep stage, including REM. Montplaisir and colleagues (1982) noted that asthmatic subjects had less REM sleep in the first third of the night. Although no attacks occurred during stage 3/4 sleep, no difference was noted in frequency of episodes in NREM versus REM sleep. The authors speculated that stage 3/4 sleep may provide some degree of protection against occurrence of asthmatic episodes.

With respect to quality of sleep, most studies reported a relatively nonspecific disturbance of sleep. In a large survey of the general adult population, Klink and Quan (1987) found that asthma was associated with significant increases in the incidence of reported difficulty initiating and maintaining sleep, excessive daytime sleepiness, and nightmares, although the coexistence of chronic bronchitis resulted in dramatically higher rates. A follow-up study of 139 patients recently discharged from the hospital revealed "regular sleep disturbance" due to wheezing in 54 (39%) (Bucknall et al. 1988). Catterall and colleagues (1982) reported that although total sleep time and REM percentage did not differ between asthmatic patients and control subjects, the former slept less well, with increased awakening and stage 1 sleep. Kales and associates (1968, 1970) also described increased awakening, as well as decreased total sleep time and stage 4. As in the study of Catterall and colleagues, REM percentages were not different.

Finally, only one controlled study of the relationship between psychological factors in sleep and asthma was identified. Monday and colleagues (1987) reported that asthmatic patients 1) described more episodes of a "vivid impression" of dreaming without specific dream recollection following spontaneous awakening or experimental post-REM awakenings, 2) used shorter sentences in dream narration, and 3) had no dream recall when they were awakened during an episode of asthma. They suggested that conflictual material occurring during REM or other sleep stages may play a role in the genesis of nocturnal asthmatic episodes, but that the material is repressed on awakening.

Nocturnal Cardiac Ischemia

A relatively high frequency of nocturnal angina and myocardial infarction in sleep has been described for many years. This has led investigators to evaluate the possible contributions of circadian rhythm and sleep physiology to nocturnal ischemia. Specific studies of cardiovascular physiology during sleep are not relevant to the diagnostic issues addressed herein and were not reviewed. A brief review of the association of angina with sleep and specific sleep stages is presented.

Several studies have suggested that nocturnal cardiac ischemia is specifically associated with REM. Nowlin and colleagues (1965) described four patients in whom 32 of 39 episodes of nocturnal angina occurred during REM. Murao and colleagues (1972) studied 12 patients who had 58 episodes of cardiac ischemia, of which 24 were during REM and 21 in the awake state. Only one of the patients had any ischemia in NREM. King and colleagues (1973) contributed a case report of Prinzmetal's angina during REM, and Otsuka and colleagues (1988) reported on 47 episodes of nocturnal Prinzmetal's angina in 8 patients of which 55% occurred in REM and 45% followed an arousal or awakening. There were no NREM-related episodes. Although these data provide strong support for an association between nocturnal cardiac ischemia and REM sleep, others have failed to identify a clear relationship with REM (Broughton and Baron 1978; Cassano et al. 1981; Maggini et al. 1976).

A limited number of studies suggest that sleep may be disturbed in patients with angina. Karacan and colleagues (1969) found total sleep time to be approximately the same in angina patients and in control subjects, but noted greater variability among patients. Sleep efficiency and stage 3/4 were decreased, whereas sleep latency and percentage stage wake, 1, and 2 were increased. Maggini and colleagues (1976) likewise reported increased waking and stage 1 and felt that sleep disruption was especially related to nights with ischemic episodes.

A high incidence of sleep-disordered breathing in patients with coronary artery disease was described in a study by De Olazabal and colleagues (1982). They reported that 13 (76%) patients studied had breathing disturbance in sleep (11 with obstructive apnea and 2 with Cheyne-Stokes breathing). Mean respiratory disturbance index in apneic patients was 20.

Trypanosomiasis (Sleeping Sickness)

Trypanosomiasis is of extremely limited relevance to psychiatry and is largely limited to Africa; a detailed review was not conducted. Schwartz and Escande

(1970) provided a single case report in English of polysomnographic recording of an affected individual.

Gastroesophageal Reflux and Peptic Ulcer Disease

The literature on these topics, as related to sleep, consists almost entirely of investigations of nocturnal acid secretion and clearance, esophageal sphincter pressures, and peristalsis during sleep. Although very pertinent to the underlying physiology of these disorders, this literature contributes little to the nosologic issues at hand and was not reviewed. It has been documented that most episodes of gastroesophageal reflux actually occur during arousals, rather than in sleep (Dent et al. 1980). Gastroesophageal reflux must be considered in the differential diagnosis of obstructive sleep apnea, nocturnal choking, angina, or laryngospasm of other origin. It may also contribute to the occurrence of nocturnal asthma in children (Buts et al. 1986), although Hughes and colleagues (1983) found no such relationship.

No literature dealing specifically with differential diagnosis of these disorders, as they pertain to sleep, was found.

Discussion

These results provide clear documentation that 1) a variety of significant medical problems may be manifest during sleep; 2) sleep physiology can exacerbate underlying medical conditions; and 3) to a lesser extent, there are disturbances in the quality and quantity of sleep that can occur as a result of these medical conditions. However, it must be noted that much of the available data pertain to the pathophysiology and clinical significance of the medical condition, as manifest in sleep. Although this is certainly germane to an understanding of the medical problems and is of clear clinical significance to those nonpsychiatric specialists primarily responsible for the management of these disorders, it is of comparatively little relevance for most psychiatrists. Information regarding the effects of these medical conditions on sleep is scanty and, for the most part, suggests nonspecific sleep disturbance that does not distinguish among the different diagnoses.

As a result of this, any classification system that attempts to establish sleep-related criteria specific to these disorders must, in fact, rely heavily on nonsleep-related (i.e., clinical-medical) criteria in its approach, as reflected in the ICSD system. In addition, it should be noted that inclusion of these disorders under a single heading of "sleep disorders associated with medical conditions" will, in effect, result in a lumping of dyssomnias and parasomnias into a single category—a decision that seems to violate the distinction maintained between these two categories elsewhere in ICSD and in DSM-III-R.

Recommendations

The alternatives for categorization include the following: 1) A distinct category of "sleep disorders associated with medical disorders" with specification of diagnoses within this category (e.g., "sleep disorders associated with COPD"). This is the ICSD approach. 2) A distinct category of "Secondary Sleep Disorders" without specification of individual diagnoses. The relevant medical diagnosis may be specified on Axis III. Text may include discussion of the most significant medical conditions. 3) No separate category for medical disorders, with return of the primary complaint to its appropriate phenomenologic category (i.e., dyssomnia—insomnia or excessive sleepiness—secondary to organic condition [specified on Axis III] or parasomnia not otherwise specified). It seems unlikely that the parasomnia not otherwise specified component (e.g., to designate nocturnal asthmatic episodes or angina) would be used to any significant extent by psychiatrists.

The case of primary fibromyalgia (fibrositis syndrome) is somewhat different from the remainder of the diagnoses in this section because, unlike the other disorders, it *may* arise primarily as a result of sleep-related disturbance. It does not appear that current information warrants inclusion of a specific DSM-IV diagnosis for this disorder. However, the nature of the disorder creates some uncertainty as to how it should be classified. Our present understanding of the pathophysiology (limited as it may be) indicates that, for now, it should be classified with other medical disorders. However, future research may suggest that it should be classified as a primary dyssomnia or secondary to mental disorder.

What arises most clearly from the literature review is that there is not sufficient basis for singling out the sleep disorder(s) associated with any one of these medical conditions by establishment of separate criteria. For the most part, the sleep disorders observed are not specific to the medical condition in question, and diagnostic criteria would, of necessity, be more strongly oriented toward characteristics of the medical condition—a practice that would be inappropriate for DSM-IV.

However, there is heuristic value in establishing a distinct general heading for sleep disorders secondary to medical disorders. A compromise that would allow for this approach, while still specifying the relevant sleep-related symptom, would be to include separate designations for symptom type under the general heading (e.g., Secondary Sleep Disorder due to General Medical Condition—insomnia). Medical condition would be specified on Axis III. This position is most compatible with DSM-III-R and ICSD and is recommended for DSM-IV.

References

Ahles TA, Yunus MB, Riley SD, et al: Psychological factors associated with primary fibromyalgia syndrome. Arthritis Rheum 27:1101–1106, 1984

Ahles TA, Yunus MB, Gaulier B, et al: The use of contemporary MMPI norms in the study of chronic pain patients. Pain 24:159–163, 1986

Ahles TA, Yunus MB, Masi AT: Is chronic pain a variant of depressive disease? the case of primary fibromyalgia syndrome. Pain 29:105–111, 1987

Ahles TA, Khan SA, Yunus MB, et al: Psychiatric status of patients with primary fibromyalgia, patients with rheumatoid arthritis, and subjects without pain: a blind comparison of DSM-III diagnoses. Am J Psychiatry 148:1721–1726, 1991

American Psychiatric Association: Diagnostic and Statistical Manual of Mental Disorders, 3rd Edition. Washington, DC, American Psychiatric Association, 1980

American Psychiatric Association: Diagnostic and Statistical Manual of Mental Disorders, 3rd Edition, Revised. Washington, DC, American Psychiatric Association, 1987

American Sleep Disorders Association, Diagnostic Classification Steering Committee: International Classification of Sleep Disorders: Diagnostic and Coding Manual. Rochester, MN, American Sleep Disorders Association, 1990

Arand DL, McGinty DJ, Littner MR: Respiratory patterns associated with hemoglobin desaturation during sleep in chronic obstructive pulmonary disease. Chest 80:183–190, 1981

Beck A, Ward CH, Mendelson M, et al: An inventory for measuring depression. Arch Gen Psychiatry 4:561–571, 1961

Broughton R, Baron R: Sleep patterns in the intensive care unit and on the ward after acute myocardial infarction. Electroencephalogr Clin Neurophysiol 45:348–360, 1978

Bucknall CE, Robertson C, Moran F, et al: Management of asthma in hospital: a prospective audit. BMJ 296:1637–1639, 1988

Buts JP, Barudi C, Moulin D, et al: Prevalence and treatment of silent gastro-esophageal reflux in children with recurrent respiratory disorders. Eur J Pediatr 145:396–400, 1986

Cassano GB, Maggini C, Guazzelli M: Nocturnal angina and sleep. Progress in Neuro-Psychopharmacology 5:99–104, 1981

Catterall JR, Douglas NJ, Calverley PM, et al: Irregular breathing and hypoxaemia during sleep in chronic stable asthma. Lancet 1:301–304, 1982

Catterall JR, Douglas NJ, Calverley PM, et al: Transient hypoxemia during sleep in chronic obstructive pulmonary disease is not a sleep apnea syndrome. Am Rev Respir Dis 128:24–29, 1983

Catterall JR, Rhind GB, Steward IC, et al: Effect of sleep deprivation on overnight bronchoconstriction in nocturnal asthma. Thorax 41:676–680, 1986

Clark S, Campbell SM, Forehand ME, et al: Clinical characteristics of fibrositis II: a "blinded" controlled study using standard psychological tests. Arthritis Rheum 28:132–137, 1985

Coccagna G, Lugaresi E: Arterial blood gases and pulmonary and systemic arterial pressure during sleep in chronic obstructive pulmonary disease. Sleep 1:117–124, 1978

Cormick W, Olson LG, Hensley MJ, et al: Nocturnal hypoxaemia and quality of sleep in patients with chronic obstructive disease. Thorax 41:846–854, 1986

DeMarco FJ Jr, Wynne JW, Block AJ, et al: Oxygen desaturation during sleep as a determinant of the "blue and bloated" syndrome. Chest 79:621–625, 1981

Dent J, Dodds WJ, Friedman RH, et al: Mechanisms of gastroesophageal reflux in recumbent asymptomatic human subjects. J Clin Invest 65:256–257, 1980

De Olazabal JR, Miller MS, Cook WR, et al: Disordered breathing and hypoxia during sleep in coronary artery disease. Chest 82:548–552, 1982

Derogatis LR: SCL-90-R Manual II. Towson, MD, Clinical Psychometric Research, 1983

Fleetham J, West P, Mezon B, et al: Sleep, arousals, and oxygen desaturation in chronic obstructive pulmonary disease. Am Rev Respir Dis 126:208–210, 1982

Gupta MA, Moldofsky H: Dysthymic disorder and rheumatic pain modulation disorder (fibrositis syndrome): a comparison of symptoms and sleep physiology. Can J Psychiatry 31:608–616, 1986

Hamilton M: A rating scale for depression. J Neurol Neurosurg Psychiatry 23:56–62, 1960

Hathaway SR, McKinley JC: Minnesota Multiphasic Personality Inventory, Revised. Minneapolis, MN, University of Minnesota, 1970

Hetzel MR, Clark TJH: Does sleep cause nocturnal asthma? Thorax 34:749–754, 1979

Hudgel DW, Martin RJ, Capehart M, et al: Contribution of hypoventilation to sleep oxygen desaturation in chronic obstructive pulmonary disease. J Appl Physiol 55:669–677, 1983

Hudson JI, Pliner LF, Hudson MS, et al: The dexamethasone suppression test in fibrositis. Biol Psychiatry 19:1489–1493, 1984

Hudson JI, Hudson MS, Pliner LF, et al: Fibromyalgia and major affective disorder: a controlled phenomenology and family history study. Am J Psychiatry 142:441–446, 1985

Hughes DM, Spier S, Rivlin J, et al: Gastroesophageal reflux during sleep in asthmatic patients. J Pediatr 102:666–672, 1983

Isaa FG, Sullivan EC: Respiratory muscle activity and thoracoabdominal motion during acute episodes of asthma during sleep. Am Rev Respir Dis 132:999–1004, 1985

Kales A, Beall GN, Bajor GF, et al: Sleep studies in asthmatic adults: relationship of attacks to sleep stage and time of night. Journal of Allergy 41:164–173, 1968

Kales A, Kales JD, Sly RM, et al: Sleep patterns of asthmatic children: all-night electroencephalographic studies. Journal of Allergy 46:300–308, 1970

Karacan I, Williams RL, Taylor WJ: Sleep characteristics in patients with angina pectoris. Psychosomatics 10:280–284, 1969

King MJ, Lir LM, Kaltman AJ, et al: Variant angina associated with angiographically demonstrated coronary artery spasm and REM sleep. Am J Med Sci 265:419–422, 1973

Kirmayer LJ, Robbins JM, Kapusta MA: Somatization and depression in fibromyalgia syndrome. Am J Psychiatry 145:950–954, 1988

Klink M, Quan SF: Prevalence of reported sleep disturbances in a general adult population and their relationship to obstructive airways disease. Chest 91:540–546, 1987

Leavitt F, Katz RS: Is the MMPI invalid for assessing psychological disturbance in pain related to organic conditions? J Rheumatol 16:521–526, 1989

Littner MR, McGinty DJ, Arand DL: Determinants of oxygen desaturation in the course of ventilation during sleep in chronic obstructive pulmonary disease. Am Rev Respir Dis 122:849–857, 1980

Maggini C, Guazzelli M, Castrogiovanni P, et al: Psychological and physiopathological study on coronary patients. Psychother Psychosom 27:210–216, 1976

Manni R, Cerveri I, Bruschi C, et al: Sleep and oxyhemoglobin desaturation patterns in chronic obstructive pulmonary disease. Eur Neurol 28:275–278, 1988

Moldofsky H, Scarisbrick P: Induction of neurasthenic musculoskeletal pain syndrome by selective sleep stage deprivation. Psychosom Med 38:35–44, 1976

Moldofsky H, Scarisbrick P, England R, et al: Musculoskeletal symptoms and nonREM sleep disturbance in patients with "fibrositis syndrome" and healthy subjects. Psychosom Med 37:341–351, 1975

Moldofsky H, Lue FA, Smythe HA: Alpha EEG sleep and morning symptoms in rheumatoid arthritis, J Rheumatol 10:373–379, 1983

Moldofsky H, Tullis C, Lue FA, et al: Sleep-related myoclonus in rheumatic pain modulation disorder (fibrositis syndrome) and in excessive daytime somnolence. J Rheumatol 13:614–617, 1984

Molony RR, MacPeck DM, Schiffman PL, et al: Sleep, sleep apnea, and the fibromyalgia syndrome. J Rheumatol 13:797–800, 1986

Monday J, Montplaisir J, Malo J: Dream process in asthmatic subjects with nocturnal attacks. Am J Psychiatry 144:638–640, 1987

Montplaisir J, Walsh J, Malo J: Nocturnal asthma: features of attacks, sleep and breathing patterns. Am Rev Respir Dis 125:18–25, 1982

Murao S, Harumi K, Katayama S, et al: All-night polygraphic studies of nocturnal angina pectoris. Jpn Heart J 13:295–306, 1972

Nowlin JB, Troyer WG, Collins WS, et al: The association of nocturnal angina pectoris with dreaming. Ann Intern Med 63:1040–1046, 1965

Otsuka K, Yanaga T, Watanabe H: Variant angina and REM sleep. Am Heart J 115:1343–1346, 1988

Payne TC, Leavitt F, Garron DC, et al: Fibrositis and psychological disturbance. Arthritis Rheum 25:213–217, 1982

Perez-Padilla R, Conway W, Roth T, et al: Hypercapnea and sleep O_2 desaturation in chronic obstructive pulmonary disease. Sleep 10:216–223, 1987

Reinberg A, Ghata J, Sidi E: Nocturnal asthma attacks: Their relationship to the circadian adrenal cycle. J Allergy 34:323–330, 1963

Robins LN, Helzer JE, Croughan J, et al: National Institute of Mental Health Diagnostic Interview Schedule: its history, characteristics, and validity. Arch Gen Psychiatry 38:381–389, 1981

Saskin P, Moldofsky H, Lue FA: Sleep and post traumatic rheumatic pain modulation disorder (fibrositis syndrome). Psychosom Med 48:319–323, 1986

Schwartz BA, Escande C: Sleeping sickness: sleep study of a case. Electroencephalogr Clin Neurophysiol 29:83–87, 1970

Smythe HA: Problems with the MMPI (editorial). J Rheumatol 11:417–418, 1984

Soutar CA, Costello J, Ijaduola O, et al: Nocturnal and morning asthma. Thorax 30:436–440, 1975

Spielberger CD: The measurement of state and trait anxiety: conceptual and methodological issues, in Emotions: Their Parameters and Measurement. Edited by Levi L. New York, Raven, 1975, pp 713–725

Tariot PN, Yocum D, Kalin NH: Psychiatric disorders in primary fibromyalgia (letter). Am J Psychiatry 143:812–813, 1986

Wolfe F, Cathey MA, Kleinheksel SM, et al: Psychological status in primary fibrositis and fibrositis associated with rheumatoid arthritis. J Rheumatol 11:500–506, 1984

Zung WWK: A self-rating depression scale. Arch Gen Psychiatry 12:63–67, 1965

Chapter 45

Substance-Induced Sleep Disorder

Eric A. Nofzinger, M.D.

Statement of the Issues

The International Classification of Sleep Disorders (ICSD) (American Sleep Disorders Association 1990) has listed a variety of sleep disorders in which the pathophysiology is presumed to stem from "extrinsic" sources (i.e., factors outside of the body). In this review I summarize the literature relevant to the following disorders listed in the current ICSD classification system under the heading extrinsic sleep disorders that have not been covered under the review on insomnia. In the review I focus on the following questions: What are the essential descriptive features of the disorder? Is there empirical support for the diagnosis? What has been the overall research focus and clinical relevance of the proposed disorders? In light of the available literature, how can the disorders best be conceptualized for psychiatric clinicians? Are the disorders adequately described in the DSM-III-R (American Psychiatric Association 1987) diagnostic system? If not, what alternative classification schemes should be used?

Significance of the Issues

The DSM-IV nosology should 1) allow for classification of a sleep disorder secondary to a substance of abuse due to well-recognized substance-induced sleep disturbances, 2) include a multiaxial diagnostic system recognizing the importance of the substance abuse as a separate disorder, and 3) recognize the distinction between specific substance-induced sleep disorders and unspecified "organic" sleep disorders. In the following review I outline the empirical basis for these claims.

Methods

All primary source references listed in the ICSD for the following sleep disorders were reviewed: food allergy insomnia, nocturnal eating (drinking) syndrome, hypnotic-dependent sleep disorder, stimulant-dependent sleep disorder, alcohol-dependent sleep disorder, and toxin-induced sleep disorder. The references from each of these sources were also reviewed. A Medline search (BRS Colleague) was conducted on each of the above-listed sleep disorders for 1965 to 1992, selecting only English-language reports of human subjects. This yielded 127 articles for review. Selected review articles were also reviewed, as were the primary references listed in each of these review articles. Although all relevant research within the area was reviewed, priority for inclusion as a primary reference for the literature review was given to articles that 1) were published in peer-reviewed journals, 2) had adequate sample sizes, 3) included control groups, 4) listed both subjective and objective sleep measures, and 5) had well-defined patient populations based on established criteria and who were reliably diagnosed and distinct from comparison groups.

Results

The first two extrinsic sleep disorders according to the ICSD classification system that were not reviewed under the general topic of insomnia are food allergy insomnia and nocturnal eating (drinking) syndrome. These are primarily childhood sleep disorders and, although not sleep disorders that are secondary to substances of abuse, they are "substance-induced."

Food Allergy Insomnia

This disorder is characterized by frequent arousals that are temporally associated with a food or drink and accompanied by other allergic manifestations, such as psychomotor agitation, lethargy, respiratory disturbances, skin irritation, gastrointestinal upset, and elevated serum antibodies against the allergen. Only two references to papers citing cow's milk allergy in infants are cited in ICSD (Kahn et al. 1985, 1987). The authors cautioned that "only the most persistent and severe cases [of infant insomnia] should be considered potential candidates for the diagnosis of milk allergy" (Kahn et al. 1987), reflecting their sense that the disorder is infrequent even in children who present with a complaint of insomnia. No reports in adults are known, and no replications of this work have been reported aside from the group who presented the initial findings. The pathophysiology of the insomnia is unknown, but presumably involves physical discomfort associated with having the allergy. The polysomnographic profiles reported were nonspecific, with increased arousals and reduced sleep time.

Nocturnal Eating (Drinking) Syndrome

The essential features of this disorder are recurrent awakenings and inability to return to sleep without eating or drinking. It is thought to be primarily a disorder of infancy, but may occur in adults as well. The ingestion of large quantities of food or drink is presumed to be based on psychological and physiological conditioning factors. At this time there are no empirical studies documenting this condition. References cited in ICSD (Ferber 1987; Stunkard et al. 1955) described clinical experiences, but no peer-reviewed papers describing this condition are known. Although it is suggested to occur in the adult population, there are no empirical studies documenting this condition in adults.

Hypnotic-Dependent Sleep Disorder

The essential features of hypnotic-dependent sleep disorder include insomnia or excessive sleepiness that is associated with tolerance to or withdrawal from hypnotic medications. Within this framework, the specific type of disorder will depend on whether the patient presents during the initiation, maintenance, or withdrawal of the medication. The sleep disturbances are determined by the characteristic physiological responses caused by hypnotic medications and are attributed to this "extrinsic" factor rather than intrinsic characteristics of the individual using the medication. The patterns described in the ICSD are either 1) the subjective worsening of insomnia on abrupt withdrawal of a hypnotic, or "rebound" insomnia, or 2) development of tolerance and subsequent need to increase the dosage of the hypnotic to obtain the same hypnotic benefit, often resulting in impaired daytime performance from the elevated dosage. Well-defined polysomnographic changes are cited that accompany the changes in sleep tendency and subjective state. Changes associated with chronic use include decreased stages 1, 3, and 4 and rapid eye movement (REM) sleep, increased stage 2 sleep, fragmented sleep with frequent transitions between the different stages of sleep, decreased K-complexes and delta waves, and increased 14–18 Hz "pseudo-spindles." Phasic REMs can be reduced also. During hypnotic withdrawal, severe subjective and objective sleep disruptions can occur, before sleep stages return to baseline levels. Measures of daytime sleepiness such as the Multiple Sleep Latency Test indicate increased sleepiness with chronic use.

In general, there is an adequate empirical data base to support the above assertions (Adam et al. 1976; Gillin et al. 1989; Kales et al. 1969, 1974, 1978, 1983; Roehrs et al. 1986), although individual variability exists between hypnotics, depending on their specific pharmacokinetic profile. Hypnotics with short half-lives used in high dosages tend to be more problematic with respect to alterations in the sleep-wake cycle, referred to as rebound insomnia. Hypnotics with longer half-lives tend to be more problematic with respect to residual effects on daytime performance and daytime sleepiness. As with many of the sleep-wake disturbances, the subjective effects on daytime performance or hypersomnia may or may not coincide with objective measures of sleepiness determined polysomnographically. Although much research has focused on acute treatment and withdrawal of hypnotics, controversy remains with respect to chronic use of individual hypnotics and their effects on hypnotic efficacy and residual effects on daytime performance, both in terms of objective and subjective measures.

Stimulant-Dependent Sleep Disorder

The essential features of stimulant-dependent sleep disorder include a reduction of sleepiness or suppression of sleep by central stimulants, and resultant alterations in wakefulness following drug abstinence. Specific stimulant agents include phenylethylamines (ephedrine, amphetamines), cocaine, thyroid hormones, xanthine derivatives (caffeine, theophylline), and peripheral sympathomimetics (decongestants, bronchodilators, pressor agents). Two general patterns of sleep-wake disruption are seen. The first is insomnia secondary to initiation, increase in the dosage, or shifting the stimulant administration closer to bedtime. The second is a period of exhaustion and hypersomnia, which can occur secondary to sleep deprivation from stimulant use, or from withdrawal. Specific polysomnographic features of stimulant use include increased sleep latency, decreased total sleep time, increased spontaneous awakenings, prolonged REM latency, and decreased REM time. Features associated with stimulant withdrawal include reduced sleep latency, increased total sleep time, and REM rebound, characterized by reduced REM latency and increased REM time and percentage. Multiple sleep latency testing during withdrawal is reported to be suggestive of narcolepsy, with mean sleep latencies less than 10 minutes during daytime naps.

The literature supports the above-cited polysomnographic changes in the sleep-wake cycle, as well as similarities between different agents, such as amphetamines, caffeine, and cocaine (Connell 1958; Ellinwood 1969; Kalant 1966; Nausieda 1979; Oswald 1969; Watson et al. 1972). Most of the literature, however, is concerned not with the adverse consequences of these substances on sleep-wake cycles, but rather on their efficacy in improving waking performance during shift work and conditions with daytime sleepiness, such as narcolepsy (e.g., Mitler et al. 1986; Walsh et al. 1990). In the case of cocaine, the above sleep disturbances are generally reported as side effects, but the euphoric effects of the drug generally override treatment-seeking on the basis of a primary sleep disturbance. Thus the effects of stimulants on sleep-wake disruptions have been described primarily in performance of studies and not in studies aimed at specific sleep disorders secondary to the use of stimulants. Although it is reasonable to suspect that there may be a population of patients in whom disruption of sleep may be secondary to stimulant use, the sleep literature in general gives little description of this population.

Alcohol-Dependent Sleep Disorder

The essential feature of alcohol-dependent sleep disorder is the assisted initiation of sleep onset by the sustained ingestion of ethanol. The ICSD distinguishes this disorder from sleep-wake disruptions due to alcoholism by defining this as a rare disorder in which the primary purpose of alcohol is to aid sleep onset. Other descriptive features of this syndrome include the intake of alcohol 3–4 hours prior to sleep onset, initial hypnotic benefit with increased arousal from sleep later in the night as the alcohol blood level declines, eventual tolerance to the hypnotic effects after prolonged nightly use, and withdrawal, if reductions in alcohol intake are attempted. The polysomnographic features include increased stages 3 and 4 sleep, REM sleep fragmentation with increased REM activity, and marked sleep continuity disruptions in the latter half of the night as the ethanol blood level declines.

Review of the literature supports the above sleep and polysomnographic findings in the case of acute, brief use of alcohol in nonalcoholic subjects. However, the major focus of most of the research literature is in the effects of alcoholism on sleep, either acute or chronic (Gross et al. 1973; Johnson et al. 1970; Pokorny 1978; Rundell et al. 1977; Williams and Salamy 1972; Zarcone 1983). The major findings on sleep in acute use include an initial hypnotic effect early in the night with disruptions in sleep in the second half of the night; suppression of REM sleep early in the night with some rebound of REM sleep in the second half of the night; and increased stages 3 and 4 sleep in the early portions of the night. The major chronic effects of alcohol on sleep include marked sleep continuity disturbances, decreased stages 3 and 4 sleep, and increased transitions between different stages of sleep throughout the night. These long-term effects have been reported to be present for as long as 50 months into abstinence. There has been little emphasis in the literature on a separate syndrome of alcohol use solely as a hypnotic agent in the absence of concerns about a diagnosis of alcoholism itself.

Toxin-Induced Sleep Disorder

The essential feature of toxin-induced sleep disorder is insomnia or excessive sleepiness produced by poisoning with heavy metals or organic toxins. The specific toxins mentioned include mercury, lead, arsenic, and copper. In the description of the disorder, the ICSD describes that either central nervous system activation or depression would be expected to cause alterations in either the subjective or objective measures of sleeping and waking function. However, no information about polysomnographic measures is available. The ICSD also notes that complications secondary to the sleep syndrome are minor relative to the organ toxicity, including renal failure, coma, and death in severe cases.

Discussion

In the ICSD, each of the above disorders fell into the subcategory of extrinsic sleep disorders within the broader category of dyssomnias. In addressing the overall questions of how best to classify the above disorders that will be of most benefit and utility to the field of psychiatry, I focus in the following discussion on 1) the degree to which these disorders actually fit into an overall schematic theme of extrinsic disorders, 2) the degree to which the empirical literature actually supports the diagnoses as outlined in the ICSD, 3) potential ways of classifying the disorder according to DSM-III-R criteria, and 4) suggestions for classification that would best benefit the psychiatric practitioner.

Food allergy insomnia is a proposed sleep disorder that is most relevant to child psychiatry. Food allergy insomnia fits well into a classification system describing an extrinsic factor, the allergen, which disrupts the sleep-wake schedule. The literature review suggests that the resultant insomnia is nonspecific, may be related to illness alone, and is an infrequent sleep disorder to be considered only after other common sources of sleep disorders in children have been excluded. According to DSM-III-R criteria, this disorder would be classified as insomnia related to a known organic factor. Other possibilities for classification would include 1) the creation of a new category for this disorder in DSM-IV, 2) the creation of a general category of secondary sleep disorders in which case this disorder would be secondary to the allergy, or 3) the creation of a category for substance-induced sleep disorder in which case the substance would be the allergen. Other considerations would be for creation of a distance category of pediatric sleep disorders, highlighting that this is in general a consideration in infants. Aside from the fact that this is a diagnosis that should be considered in an infant who might present to a child psychiatrist when other sleep disorders have been excluded, the relevance to psychiatry for including such a diagnosis is unclear, given the infrequency and nonspecific nature of this disorder. Overall this disorder would best be classified within a general category such as secondary sleep disorders.

Nocturnal eating (drinking) syndrome also has been described primarily as a disorder of childhood. The degree to which this is an "extrinsic" disorder is uncertain, since learning or conditioning factors initiate the process, and physiological circadian changes may "intrinsically" perpetuate the pattern of voluminous nocturnal feedings. There is little empirical support for this diagnosis aside from clinical experience. According to DSM-III-R criteria, this disorder would likely be classified as a primary insomnia similar to the concept of learned or psychophysiological insomnia in an adult population. Alternatives for classification of nocturnal eating (drinking) include 1) the creation of a separate category for this disorder or 2) the creation of a separate diagnostic group related to parent-child problems associated with sleep disorders since the problem would appear to lie in the parent-child interaction. Although these concerns may stimulate future diagnostic classification systems, I suggest at the current time that this diagnosis requires further empirical validation prior to establishing this as a diagnostic entity.

Hypnotic-dependent sleep disorder, stimulant-dependent sleep disorder, alcohol-dependent sleep disorder, and toxin-induced sleep disorder can all be seen as related in some way to an extrinsic substance; however there are likely overlapping intrinsic factors for some that might predispose to use or abuse of a specific agent. For hypnotics, stimulants, and alcohol, there is empirical support for well-recognized effects on the sleep-wake cycle. It is less clear if there is a specific group of patients for whom a specific sleep disorder is present. For example, in alcohol-dependent sleep disorder, there is little empirical support for a subset of patients who use alcohol primarily as a hypnotic and who are not alcoholic. For stimulants, insomnia is a well-recognized side effect, but it is questionable whether there is a specific group of patients who present for evaluation of sleep disorders for this side effect alone. There appears to be no empirical support for specific sleep disorders secondary to toxins aside from clinical observations of alterations in central nervous system activation noted in the course of toxin ingestion.

According to DSM-III-R, these disorders would be classified as either insomnia or hypersomnia related to a known organic factor. Use of this classification would result in lumping of these disorders along with other medical disorders that may disrupt the sleep-wake cycle and present as a sleep disorder. Alternatively, if the substance abuse was felt to be primary, the appropriate DSM-III-R diagnosis would list the substance abuse or dependence as the primary disorder, using the sleep disturbance as an associated feature. Creation of a specific category of sleep disorder for each substance as has been done in the ICSD does not appear to be supported by the literature review. In a general way, a separate diagnostic heading for the substances in the sleep disorders section would highlight the fact that sleep-wake disruptions are significant comorbid conditions and recognize the importance of ruling out occult problems secondary to substance abuse in the patient with a disrupted sleep-wake schedule.

From the perspective of the psychiatric clinician, the overriding clinical concern when faced with a patient who is using substances with abuse potential and who also has a sleep complaint is the possibility of substance abuse itself, with its consequent impact on the overall functioning of the individual. For this reason it would appear wise at the current time to continue in the DSM-III-R tradition of classifying the substance abuse or dependence as the primary diagnosis when appropriate. In those instances in which a diagnosis of substance abuse can be excluded, and in which the predominant clinical picture is one of a sleep disorder that is temporally related to the use of a substance with well-known effects on the sleep cycle, then it would appear reasonable to have a separate diagnostic entity. This diagnostic category is supported by the literature review, which documents clear effects both subjectively and objectively secondary to these substances.

Recommendations

At this time the literature review suggests that the ICSD extrinsic sleep disorders, including food allergy insomnia, nocturnal eating (drinking) syndrome, hypnotic-dependent sleep disorder, stimulant-dependent sleep disorder, alcohol-dependent sleep disorder, and toxin-induced sleep disorder, require further validation as well as demonstration of their clinical utility in psychiatry before being adopted for use in DSM-IV. Review of the literature, however, does point to specific alterations in the sleep-wake cycle induced by certain medications, which may be separate from disorders of substance abuse or dependence, which would warrant a separate diagnostic category for substance-induced sleep disorder for inclusion in DSM-IV. Since the review also recognized specific abnormalities associated with a particular substance, it is appropriate to designate the specific substance that is implicated. Review of the literature also supports the notion that a specific type of sleep disorder (e.g., insomnia, hypersomnia) is associated with specific medications. It also depends on the stage of drug use—acute intoxication, withdrawal, or persistent use—so that both the type of sleep disorder and the stage of use should be specified in the diagnostic categorization of the substance-induced sleep disorder.

References

Adam K, Adamson L, Brezinova V, et al: Nitrazepam: lastingly effective but trouble on withdrawal. BMJ 1:1558–1560, 1976

American Psychiatric Association: Diagnostic and Statistical Manual of Mental Disorders, 3rd Edition, Revised. Washington, DC, American Psychiatric Association, 1987

American Sleep Disorders Association, Diagnostic Classification Steering Committee: International Classification of Sleep Disorders: Diagnostic and Coding Manual. Rochester, MN, American Sleep Disorders Association, 1990

Connell PH: Amphetamine Psychosis (Maudsley Monograph No 5). London, Chapman & Hall, 1958

Ellinwood E: Amphetamine psychosis: a multidimensional process. Seminars in Psychiatry 1:208–226, 1969

Ferber R: The sleepless child, in Sleep and Its Disorders in Children. Edited by Guilleminault C. New York, Raven, 1987, pp 141–163

Gillin JC, Spinwebber CL, Johnson LC: Rebound insomnia: a critical review. J Clin Psychopharmacol 9:161–172, 1989

Gross MM, Goodenough DR, Hasten J: Experimental study of sleep in chronic alcoholics before, during and after four days of heavy drinking, with a non-drinking comparison. Ann N Y Acad Sci 215:254–275, 1973

Johnson LC, Burdick A, Smith J: Sleep during alcohol intake and withdrawal in the chronic alcoholic. Arch Gen Psychiatry 22:406–418, 1970

Kahn A, Mozin MJ, Casimir G, et al: Insomnia and cow's milk allergy in infants. Pediatrics 76:880–884, 1985

Kahn A, Mozin MJ, Rebuffat E, et al: Difficulty in initiating and maintaining sleep associated with cow's milk allergy in infants. Sleep 10:116–121, 1987

Kalant O: Amphetamines: Toxicity and Addiction. Springfield, IL, Charles C Thomas, 1966

Kales A, Malinstrom EJ, Scharf MB, et al: Psychophysiological and biochemical changes following use and withdrawal of hypnotics, in Sleep, Physiology and Pathology. Edited by Kales A. Philadelphia, PA, JB Lippincott, 1969, pp 331–343

Kales A, Bixler E, Tan T, et al: Chronic hypnotic drug use: ineffectiveness, drug withdrawal insomnia and dependence. JAMA 227:511–517, 1974

Kales A, Scharf MB, Kales J: Rebound insomnia: a new chemical syndrome. Science 201:1039–1041, 1978

Kales A, Soldatos CR, Bixler EO, et al: Rebound insomnia and rebound anxiety: a review. Pharmacology 26:121–137, 1983

Mitler MM, Shafer R, Hajdukovich R, et al: Treatment of narcolepsy: objective studies on methylphenidate, pemoline, and protriptyline. Sleep 9:260–264, 1986

Nausieda PA: Central stimulant toxicity, in Handbook of Clinical Neurology. Edited by Vinken PJ, Bruyn G. Amsterdam, Elsevier-North Holland, 1979, pp 37:223–297

Oswald I: Sleep and dependence on amphetamine and other drugs, in Sleep: Physiology and Pathology. Edited by Kales A. Philadelphia, PA, JB Lippincott, 1969, pp 317–330

Pokorny AD: Sleep disturbances, alcohol, and alcoholism: a review, in Sleep Disorders: Diagnosis and Treatment. Edited by Williams RL, Karacan I. New York, Wiley, 1978, pp 233–260

Roehrs T, Kribbs N, Zorick F, et al: Hypnotic residual effects of benzodiazepines with repeated administration. Sleep 9:309–316, 1986

Rundell OH, Williams HL, Lester BK: Sleep in alcoholic patients: longitudinal findings, in Alcohol Intoxication and Withdrawal, Volume 3B. Edited by Gross MM. New York, Plenum, 1977, pp 389–402

Stunkard AJ, Grace WJ, Wolfe HG: The night eating syndrome. Am J Med 7:78–86, 1955

Walsh JK, Muehlbach MJ, Humm TM, et al: Effect of caffeine on physiological sleep tendency and ability to sustain wakefulness at night. Am J Psychiatry 101:271–273, 1990

Watson R, Hartmann E, Shildkraut J: Amphetamine withdrawal: affective state, sleep patterns and MHPG excretion. Am J Psychiatry 129:263–269, 1972

Williams HL, Salamy A: Alcohol and sleep, in The Biology of Alcoholism. Edited by Kissin B, Begleiter H. New York, Plenum, 1972, pp 435–483

Zarcone VP: Sleep and alcoholism, in Sleep Disorders: Basic and Clinical Research: Advances in Sleep Research, Vol 6. Edited by Chase M, Weitzman E. New York, Spectrum, 1983, pp 319–333

Index

Page numbers printed in **boldface** *type refer to tables.*

D

E

F

I

M

N

O

P

R

S

W

Y

Z